TEXTBOOK OF OBSTETRIC ANAESTHESIA

TEXTBOOK OF OBSTETRIC ANAESTHESIA

Edited by

Rachel E Collis FRCA
Consultant Anaesthetist
University Hospital of Wales
Cardiff

Felicity Plaat FRCA
Consultant Anaesthetist
Department of Anaesthesia
Queen Charlotte's Hospital
London

John Urquhart FRCA
Consultant Anaesthetist
West Suffolk Hospital
Bury St Edmunds

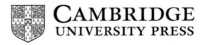

CAMBRIDGE
UNIVERSITY PRESS

CAMBRIDGE UNIVERSITY PRESS
Cambridge, New York, Melbourne, Madrid, Cape Town, Singapore,
São Paulo, Delhi, Dubai, Tokyo, Mexico City

Cambridge University Press
The Edinburgh Building, Cambridge CB2 8RU, UK

Published in the United States of America by Cambridge University Press, New York

www.cambridge.org
Information on this title: www.cambridge.org/9780521174183

First published 2002
Digitally reprinted by Cambridge University Press 2010

A catalogue record for this publication is available from the British Library

ISBN 978-0-521-17418-3 Paperback

Contents

Contributors

Jonathan Allsop
CONSULTANT
Department of Obstetrics and Gynaecology
Addenbrooke's Hospital
Cambridge

Rachel Collis
CONSULTANT ANAESTHETIST
University Hospital of Wales
Cardiff

Jason Cooper
CONSULTANT ANAESTHETIST
Department of Obstetrics and Gynaecology
North Staffordshire Hospital
Stoke-on-Trent

Girish Dhond
CONSULTANT ANAESTHETIST
Guildford Nuffield Hospital
Guildford

Toby Fay
CONSULTANT OBSTETRICIAN
Nottingham City Hospital
Nottingham

Roshan Fernando
CONSULTANT ANAESTHETIST
Royal Free Hospital
London

Paul Howell
CONSULTANT ANAESTHETIST
St Bartholomew's Hospital
London

Michael Hudspith
CONSULTANT ANAESTHETIST
Norfolk and Norwich Acute NHS Trust
Norwich

Sarah Hughes
CONSULTANT ANAESTHETIST
Southampton General Hospital
Southampton

Neena Navaneetham
CONSULTANT IN OBSTETRICS AND GYNAECOLOGY
George Eliot Hospital
Nuneaton

Nigel Penfold
CONSULTANT ANAESTHETIST
West Suffolk Hospital
Bury St Edmunds

Janet Pickett
CONSULTANT IN ANAESTHESIA
Addenbrooke's Hospital
Cambridge

Felicity Plaat
CONSULTANT ANAESTHETIST
Department of Anaesthesia
Queen Charlotte's Hospital
London

CM Price
CONSULTANT ANAESTHETIST
Southampton General Hospital
Southampton

Saxon Ridley
DIRECTOR OF CRITICAL CARE
Norfolk and Norwich Acute NHS Trust
Norwich

Andy Shennan
CONSULTANT OBSTETRICIAN
Fetal Health Research Group
St Thomas' Hospital
London

Bryony Strachen
CONSULTANT OBSTETRICIAN
St Michael's Hospital
Bristol

John Urquhart
CONSULTANT ANAESTHETIST
West Suffolk Hospital
Bury St Edmunds

Stephanie Watts
CONSULTANT ANAESTHETIST
Barnet Hospital
Hertfordshire

Mike Wee
CONSULTANT ANAESTHETIST
Poole Hospital NHS Trust
Poole

1

HISTORY OF OBSTETRIC ANALGESIA AND ANAESTHESIA

Janet A. Pickett

'Should you scratch deeply enough a man
of pioneering spirit, the chances are that
you will draw Scottish blood'

JM Horton

The 19th January 1847 marks the beginning of obstetric anaesthesia. On this day James Young Simpson (Fig. 1.1), Professor of Midwifery at the University of Edinburgh, administered ether to a mother with a contracted pelvis undergoing a difficult delivery.[1] Although the infant was stillborn the mother experienced no pain. Simpson wrote later, 'whilst this agent [ether] has been used extensively, and by numerous hands, in the practice of surgery, I am not aware that any one has hitherto ventured to test its applicability to the practice of midwifery. I am induced, therefore, to hope that the few following hurried and imperfect

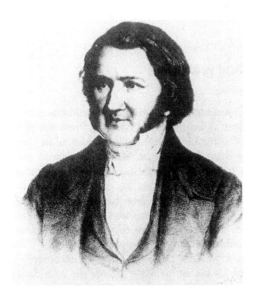

Figure 1.1   James Young Simpson (1811–1870).

notes, relative to its employment in obstetric cases, may not ... prove uninteresting to the profession' (Fig. 1.2).[2]

INHALATIONAL ANALGESIA AND ANAESTHESIA

ETHER

James Young Simpson was born in 1811 at Bathgate near Edinburgh to, 'respectable but by no means wealthy parents'.[3] Financially assisted by elder brothers, James attended the University of Edinburgh from where he graduated in 1830 with a degree in medicine. He subsequently obtained an MD for a thesis on 'Death from Inflammation' from the same university. Thereafter he progressed from assistant to the Professor in Pathology to a Lecturer's post in Midwifery. During 1839 the Chair of Midwifery at the University became vacant and the new professor was to be elected by 33 members of Edinburgh's Town Council. Simpson campaigned vigorously, accruing election expenses of £500.[4] In 1840 at the age of 29 years he was duly appointed to the Midwifery Chair.

Simpson was a success, 'He was a most impressive and instructive teacher ... there was no need to call the roll or take cards, as was the custom in Edinburgh, at Simpson's lecture. Every seat was occupied by no more persuasion than the attractiveness of the lecturer ... At home, his consulting rooms were crowded with patients who had heard of his fame, and who came from all quarters of the world to consult him. Medical men came from every country eager to see something of his practice, and to have the pleasure of an interview with so celebrated a man'.[3]

In 1846, 6 years after Simpson's appointment, news quickly spread of William Morton's successful demonstration of ether anaesthesia in Boston and of Robert

Addition to Part First:

ORIGINAL COMMUNICATION.

Notes on the Employment of the Inhalation of Sulphuric Ether in the Practice of Midwifery. By J. Y. SIMPSON, M.D., Professor of Midwifery in the University of Edinburgh.

Figure 1.2   Title page from James Simpson's first communication on the use of ether anaesthesia for obstetric practice.[1]

Liston's employment of the same for a leg amputation in London. Simpson realized the potential for his midwifery practice. He rapidly obtained apparatus for ether administration and on the 19th January 1847 Simpson gave the first ever obstetric anaesthetic. Other cases quickly followed, 'Within the last month I have had opportunities of using the inhalation of ether in the operation of turning, in cases of the employment of the long and of the short forceps, as well as in several instances in which the labour was of a natural type'.[2] Simpson was delighted to have found a means of reducing the agonies of labour and its consequences, 'in modifying and obliterating the state of conscious pain, the nervous shock otherwise liable to be produced by such pain, particularly whenever it is extreme, and intensely waited for and endured, is saved to the constitution'.[2] Protheroe Smith was the first to use ether anaesthesia for midwifery in England, 'To Professor Simpson justly belongs the merit of first employing ether by inhalation in midwifery practice ... I may perhaps, however, be allowed to observe, that I had the privilege of first exhibiting the ether in obstetric cases in England'.[5] Reports of ether anaesthesia during labour also came quickly from France and Germany. On the 7th April 1847 Nathan Cooley Keep was the first to administer ether for obstetric practice in the USA.[6] Walter Channing, Professor of Obstetrics at Harvard University, soon followed.

Simpson, meanwhile, had become obsessed with the alleviation of pain during childbirth. On receiving a letter of appointment as the Queen's Physician-Accoucher in Scotland, Simpson wrote to his brother, 'Flattery from the Queen is perhaps not common flattery but I am far less interested in it than in having delivered a woman this week without any pain, while inhaling sulphuric ether. I can think of naught else'.[7] There were however properties of ether that Simpson disliked – the unpleasant smell, the large quantities required and the tendency to produce bronchial irritation.

CHLOROFORM

Simpson began to investigate other volatile fluids. David Waldie, a Scottish chemist working in Liverpool, directed him towards an agent known as chloroform and suggested that it possessed anaesthetic properties. At his home in Queen Street in Edinburgh, Simpson and two of his assistants, Matthews Duncan and George Keith, self-experimented during the autumn and winter of 1847 with various agents. On the evening of the 4th of November they successfully demonstrated the anaesthetic properties of chloroform. 'In searching for another object among some loose paper after

coming home very late one night my hand chanced to fall upon it [chloroform] and I poured some of the fluid into tumblers before my assistants Dr Keith and Dr Duncan and myself. Before sitting down to supper we all inhaled the fluid and were all 'under the mahogany' in a trice to my wife's consternation and alarm'.[7] The energetic Simpson then wasted no time – he administered chloroform to an obstetric patient the very next day, reported its use to the Medico-Chirurgical Society of Edinburgh 5 days later and gave 'Notice of a New Anaesthetic Agent' on 12th November 1847.[8,9] By the 20th of November he had published in the Lancet, 'I have employed it [chloroform], with few and rare exceptions, in every case of labour that I have attended, and with the most delightful results ... I have now seen an immense amount of maternal pain and agony saved by its employment'.[10]

INITIAL REACTIONS

Medical profession

Supporters

The introduction of obstetric anaesthesia provoked a furious debate. Edward Murphy, Professor of Midwifery at the University College Hospital in London, was a staunch supporter. With reference to chloroform he wrote, 'It is *the most valuable assistant in the management of labours that has ever been discovered*. The patient goes through her labour quietly, without those distressing exclamations of agony, painful to her friends and embarrassing to the practitioner, and a favourable recovery is, I might say, insured'.[11] Walter Channing in the USA was similarly enthusiastic and published his influential '*Treatise on etherization in childbirth*' in 1848.[12]

Opposition

Other members of the medical profession vigorously objected to obstetric anaesthesia, particularly if it was given to ease an uncomplicated labour. Many believed that labour pains were an essential prerequisite to a successful outcome and they strongly attacked Simpson for his interference with this process. One of the most venomous critics was Robert Barnes, Lecturer in Midwifery from London, 'We may judge, by the character of the pains, and the expression the woman gives to her sufferings, not only of the stage of labour, but also of its duration, its difficulties, and its complications ... Does Dr Simpson imagine that any one rational man, accustomed to act upon calm reflection and logical deduction from facts, will thus be dragooned into adopting, in every case of natural labour, the use of a hazardous and doubtful agent?'.[13] Rankin, a surgeon from Carluke in Scotland expressed his opinion, 'Art has no portion in ordinary parturition, which, in all strictness, is a natural function ... no responsible person would readily administer to a female in labour, during five or six hours, through the medium of the delicate tissues of the lungs, diluted though it be by the atmosphere, an agent [chloroform] so powerful – so fatal!'[14] Opposition also came from abroad – most importantly from Charles Delucina Meigs an eminent obstetrician at Jefferson Medical College in Philadelphia. Meigs also firmly believed that labour pains were there for a purpose and that it was unsafe to intervene, 'Should I exhibit the remedy for pain to a thousand patients in labour, merely to prevent the physiological pain, and for no other motive – and if I should in consequence destroy only one of them, I should feel disposed to clothe me in sack cloth, and cast ashes on my head for the remainder of my days'.[15]

Church

'In *sorrow* thou shalt bring forth children'. Simpson was concerned that he would be accused of contravening the divine will. In 1847 he published his *Answer to the religious objections advanced against the employment of anaesthetical agents in midwifery and surgery*[16] arguing skilfully that the Hebrew word interpreted as 'sorrow' in fact meant 'labour, toil or physical exertion' i.e. women were to work during labour rather than to experience pain. Although much has been made of the religious objections to anaesthesia for childbirth, Farr argues that searches of contemporary medical, theological and lay literature gave little evidence for this and that Simpson's pamphlet was written to forestall religious objections which, in the event, did not arise.[17,18]

Lay public

The concept of anaesthesia for childbirth was initially regarded with reservation. Public opinion, however gradually changed, despite medical opposition. In 1847 James Moffat of Edinburgh commented, 'Medical men will, no doubt ... insist on mothers continuing to endure, in all their primitive intensity, all the agonies of childbirth, as a proper sacrifice to the conservatism of the doctrine of the desirability of pain ... But husbands will scarcely permit the sufferings of their wives to be perpetuated, merely in order that the tranquillity of this or that medical dogma be not rudely disturbed. Women themselves will betimes rebel against enduring the usual tortures and miseries of childbirth, merely to subserve the caprice of their medical attendants'.[19]

Royal family

Connor and Connor suggest that in 1848, Queen Victoria expressed interest in the use of chloroform for the delivery of her sixth child. The evidence comes from a report in the *Hereford Times*, 'ACCOUCHMENT OF HER MAJESTY – Professor Simpson, the discoverer of chloroform, has received intimation that his services, in conjunction with Dr Locock, her Majesty's physician accoucher, will be required at Buckingham Palace on an approaching interesting occasion. Professor Simpson leaves Edinburgh for London some time next month, in order to be on attendance on Her Majesty'.[20] Simpson's services were, in fact not used on this occasion, but 5 years later on 7th April 1853 there is no doubt that Dr John Snow, London's premier anaesthetist, administered chloroform to Queen Victoria for the birth of her eighth child. The Queen was 'much gratified with the effect of the chloroform'.[21]

It is often suggested that this 'royal example' greatly influenced the acceptability of obstetric anaesthesia. Again examination of contemporary evidence does not support this. The event was largely ignored by lay newspapers, and although reported by the medical press, subsequent correspondence suggests that Queen Victoria's use of chloroform did not influence those doctors already opposed to obstetric anaesthesia.[20]

As Simpson had predicted it was the lay public who ultimately played the most important role in the acceptance of obstetric anaesthesia, 'Obstetricians may oppose it, but I believe our patients themselves will force the use of it upon the profession'.[10]

METHODS OF ADMINISTRATION

In his original description of the use of chloroform Simpson detailed that, 'No special kind of inhaler or instrument is necessary for its exhibition. A little of the liquid diffused upon the interior of a hollow-shaped sponge, or pocket-handkerchief, or a piece of linen or paper, and held over the mouth and nostrils, so as to be fully inhaled, generally suffices in about a minute or two to produce the desired effect'.[10] Under Simpson's influence the administration of chloroform was conducted in this manner throughout Scotland, and in many parts of the continent. In England however the situation was different. John Snow regarded the Scottish method of administration as 'somewhat slovenly, and not very cleanly'.[22] He designed his own inhaler for the administration of chloroform for surgical use and commented, 'I nearly always employ, in obstetric cases, the inhaler that I use in surgical operations ... I find the inhaler much more convenient of application than a handkerchief, and it contains a supply of chloroform which lasts for some time, thereby saving the trouble of constantly pouring out more'.[23] Snow also questioned the depth of anaesthesia required for the parturient during labour, 'Dr. Simpson ... naturally adopted the plan which is usually followed in surgical operations, making the patient unconscious at once, and keeping her so to the end of labour ... Drs Murphy and Rigby were, I believe, amongst the first to state that relief from pain may often be afforded in obstetric cases, without removing the consciousness of the patient; and I soon observed the same circumstance'.[23]

DRAWBACKS OF CHLOROFORM

Within 3 months of the introduction of chloroform to anaesthetic practice an unexplained death had been reported. Others followed, although more commonly in relation to general surgical procedures. Simpson argued that parturients were less at risk, 'I am not aware of any death in Scotland or elsewhere from the use of chloroform in midwifery ... nor, indeed, does the obstetric patient run anything like the risk of the surgical patient; for, in midwifery, though the anaesthetic is required to be given for a far longer period, it does not require to be given so deeply as in surgery'.[24] Indeed Simpson was very trusting in his administration of chloroform, 'After once beginning its use at an obstetric case, I generally leave its exhibition to be continued by the nurse, or by any intelligent friend of the patient who may be in the room'.[24] In spite of the potential hazards, the use of chloroform for labour analgesia was to continue into the 20th century. In 1911 A. Goodman Levy demonstrated the cause of the unexpected deaths – ventricular fibrillation of the heart occurring under light anaesthesia.[25]

OTHER INHALATIONAL AGENTS

Nitrous oxide

Stanislav Klikovich was the first to describe the use of nitrous oxide analgesia for labour in 1880 (Fig. 1.3).[26,27] He prepared nitrous oxide in his own laboratory in St. Petersburg. Oxygen was then added so that the final preparation was 80% nitrous oxide and 20% oxygen. His instructions on how a woman should inhale this mixture were quite clear, 'She should breathe out as fully as possible and then inhale as deeply as possible from the mouthpiece. If the inspired mixture is kept for a short time in the lungs before being expelled, the effect is achieved quicker and the gas consumption is greatly reduced. The

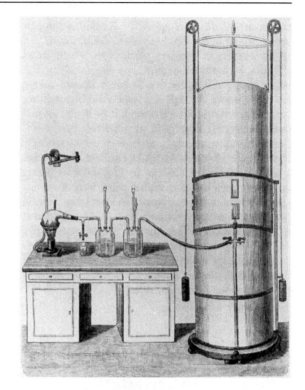

Figure 1.3   Stanislav Klikovich's method for preparing nitrous oxide. Ammonium nitrate was heated in the glass retort on the left and the evolved gas purified by passage through the Wolff bottles containing ferrous sulphate acidified with sulphuric acid and potassium hydroxide respectively. The nitrous oxide was then stored in the gasometer on the right. (Reproduced with permission from Ref. 27, Blackwell Science Ltd.)

woman must be warned that she may feel intoxicated for a short time ... Inhalation should begin a minute or half a minute before the expected pain ... If, however, the inhalations are started late, the commencing pain will often prevent the woman from taking deep breaths and the anaesthesia will not be completely successful'.[27] Sadly, Klikovich's technique was not widely copied.

In 1912 Arthur Guedel described an inhaler for the self-administration of nitrous oxide and air for use during 'small office surgery'.[28] This was followed in 1915 by two further descriptions of the use of nitrous oxide for labour analgesia: with 0–3% oxygen when given by J. Clarence Webster, 'Pure nitrous oxide gas or gas with oxygen (3 per cent) may be employed. The former is, perhaps, most universally applicable. It may be used in private houses as well as in hospitals, the necessary apparatus being small, compact and easily transported';[29] or with 0–10%

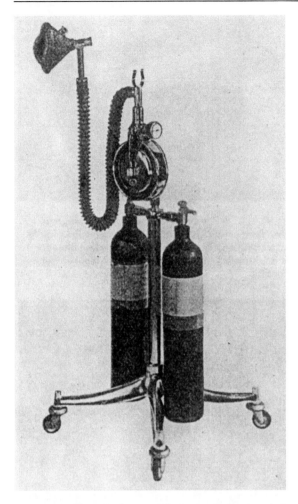

Figure 1.4 The Minnitt gas and air apparatus – hospital model. (Reproduced with permission from Ref. 32.)

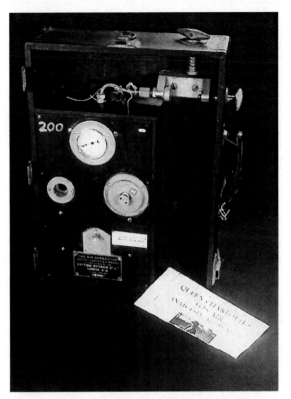

Figure 1.5 The Queen Charlotte's apparatus for the administration of gas and air. (Permission from The Mushin Anaesthetic Equipment Library, University Hospital of Wales, Cardiff.)

oxygen when administered by Frank Lynch, 'Gas [nitrous oxide] is the ideal drug for conducting labours. It is the most volatile of anesthetics, acts most quickly, and its effects pass away most rapidly. It is practically free from danger even when analgesia is continued for many hours'.[30] In 1934 Robert James Minnitt a general practitioner and honorary anaesthetist to the Liverpool Maternity Hospital designed, with the help of Charles King, his first 'gas (nitrous oxide)-and-air' machine. By 1936, 400 of the machines were in use and the apparatus was approved by the Central Midwives Board.[31] Minnitt described the soothing influence of gas-and-air, 'After the administration has commenced, an obvious change occurs in the labour ward. In a place previously filled with groans, comparative peace and quiet reign'.[32] The Minnitt gas-and-air apparatus

was widely used for the next 25 years (Figs 1.4 and 1.5). During 1961 Tunstall of Aberdeen gave his preliminary report of a 50% nitrous oxide and 50% oxygen mixture contained in one cylinder.[33] This coincided with reports of unreliability in the Minnitt apparatus and hypoxic gas mixtures (as little as 3–4% oxygen) being delivered to parturients.[34–36] Tunstall's mixture of 50% nitrous oxide and 50% oxygen (Entonox) was approved by the Central Midwives Board in 1965 and has retained an important role in inhalational obstetric analgesia up to the present day (Fig. 1.6).

Divinyl ether

This agent was first described for obstetric use in 1934 by Wesley Bourne.[37] Later Bourne suggested that divinyl ether was particularly useful for obstetric anaesthesia in general practice, 'Vinyl ether would seem to offer an opportunity for replacing the much more dangerous chloroform … almost any one can

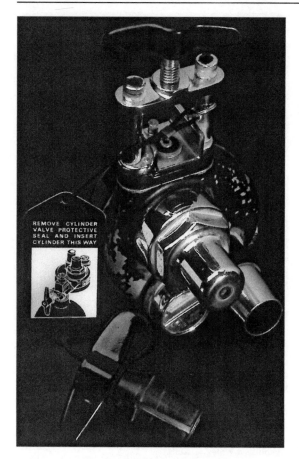

Figure 1.6   An early Entonox demand regulator valve. (Permission from The Mushin Anaesthetic Equipment Library, University Hospital of Wales, Cardiff.)

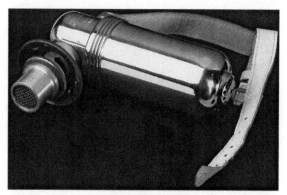

Figure 1.7   A hand-held Trilene vaporiser designed to give a low concentration of trilene. Suitable for midwife administration. (Permission from The Mushin Museum of Anaesthetic Equipment, University Hospital of Wales, Cardiff.)

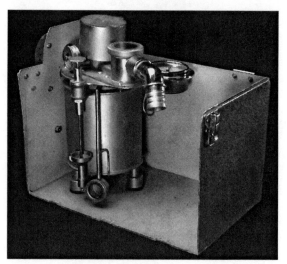

Figure 1.8   The Emotril Trilene vaporiser. Placed in a box for maximum up-right portability, with weak mixture control and thermometer for improved regulation of Trilene concentration. Widely used by midwives before 1970. (Permission from The Mushin Museum of Anaesthetic Equipment, University Hospital of Wales, Cardiff.)

give vinyl ether with much greater safety than when chloroform is given with special care'.[38]

Cyclopropane

The first report of cyclopropane for labour analgesia was again by Wesley Bourne in 1934.[39] Its use was further promoted by Harold Griffith in 1935, 'Cyclopropane gives such deep, quiet, safe anaesthesia … that it has replaced chloroform and ether in my private obstetrical practice'.[40] Bonica in 1967 considered cyclopropane to be one of the best agents for inhalational analgesia in obstetrics.[41]

Trichloroethylene

John Elam reported favourably on trichloroethylene (trilene) analgesia in 1942 (Fig. 1.7), 'I would especially call attention to its use in midwifery for it appears to have very little effect on the uterine muscle, and a weak mixture of trilene and air will give an analgesia similar to that obtained with gas and oxygen'.[42] Freedman described the use of an inhaler for trilene and air in 1943.[43] Accurate drawover inhalers were later approved for use under the supervision of midwives in 1955 – the Emotril and Tecota Mark 6 machines (Fig. 1.8).

Methoxyflurane

The first reports of the extensive use of methoxyflurane in obstetrics came from Fernando Hudon in

1961 and 1962, 'The outstanding features of the drug are the rapidity of induction, high level of analgesia under a light plane of anaesthesia, very low incidence of vomiting, minimal depression of uterine contractions, minimal respiratory depression of the fetus, quiet and rapid recovery'.[44,45] Major et al from Cardiff in 1967 reported that a fixed inhaled concentration of 0.35% methoxyflurane provided good obstetric analgesia without unacceptable side effects.[46] Midwives were allowed to administer 0.35% methoxyflurane from the Cardiff inhaler from 1970 onwards.

Isoflurane

Isoflurane was first reported for labour analgesia in 1975.[47] Tunstall, administering 0.75% isoflurane in oxygen with contractions for the first stage of labour, found lower pain scores than with Entonox but at the expense of increased drowsiness.[48] Wee et al compared isoflurane 0.2%/Entonox with Entonox alone and found that the former provided superior analgesia with higher but not clinically significant drowsiness scores.[49]

Enflurane

The analgesic efficacy of enflurane 1% in air was compared with Entonox by McGuinness and Rosen in 1984 – pain scores were significantly lower with enflurane, but drowsiness scores were higher.[50]

Desflurane

The use of desflurane 1.0–4.5% and oxygen for vaginal delivery was described by Abboud et al in 1995. Satisfactory analgesia was achieved but several mothers had amnesia for the delivery.[51]

THE HISTORY OF MENDELSON'S SYNDROME

In 1847 when inhalational anaesthesia was first introduced to obstetric practice, Caesarean deliveries were rarely performed. During the first half of the 20th century as the procedure became more common, one of the gravest dangers of deep inhalational anaesthesia was exposed – the acid aspiration syndrome described by Curtis Mendelson in 1946.[52] Mendelson reviewed 44 016 pregnancies at the Lying-In Hospital in New York and reported 66 cases of aspiration of stomach contents into the lungs – an incidence of 0.15%. All patients had been anaesthetized with gas/oxygen/ether. Aspiration was recorded as having definitely occurred in the delivery room in 68%. Of these cases the character of the aspirated material was solid in five and liquid in forty-five. Mendelson described the unpleasant consequences, 'Obstructive reactions occurred in

the five patients that aspirated solid material. Three of these cases had complete obstruction; two died of suffocation on the delivery table, whereas the third recovered after coughing up a large piece of meat. Two of the five patients had incomplete obstruction with massive atelectasis, and both recovered after coughing up the obstructing material … a very different type of reaction was observed in the 40 patients that aspirated liquid material. For lack of any existing description, this type of reaction may best be likened to an acute asthmatic attack. Apparently liquid gastric contents were aspirated into the lungs, while the laryngeal reflexes were abolished during general anesthesia. The actual aspiration often escaped recognition. Cyanosis, tachycardia, and dyspnoea developed … auscultation over the involved areas revealed numerous wheezes, rales, and rhonchi. High pulse and respiratory rates were common, often reaching values of 160 and 40 respectively. Evidence of cardiac failure frequently appeared, and occasionally culminated in pulmonary edema'. Mendelson subsequently performed a series of experiments using rabbit models to determine the pathology of these two distinct aspiration syndromes. 'After aspiration of solid undigested food the picture is invariably that of obstruction … following aspiration of liquid containing hydrochloric acid the animals develop a syndrome similar in many respects to that observed in the human following liquid aspiration'. Mendelson concluded that the incidence of aspiration could be reduced by withholding oral feeding in labour and by the wider use of regional anaesthesia. He also advocated alkanization of stomach contents prior to general anaesthesia to minimize the consequences of aspiration.

OPIOID ANALGESIA AND SEDATION

OPIOID ANALGESIA

Morphine

Morphine was isolated from crude opium by Friedrich Sertürner in 1805.[53] Its use in main stream obstetrics was delayed until after the invention of the hypodermic syringe and hollow needle. The German physician Kormann recommended hypodermic administration of morphine for labour analgesia, but problems with the use of narcotics for this purpose were soon recognized.[54]

Twilight-sleep

The administration of morphine and scopolamine in combination was introduced by von Steinbüchel of Graz in 1902.[55] Gauss of Freiburg developed the method further. He gave slightly larger doses of morphine and scopolamine, followed by repeated injections of scopolamine alone, in a regimen which became known as twilight-sleep (Dämmerschlaf): 'a period of amnesia results, during which time painful sensations, which may be felt, are not stored up in the memory to haunt the patient after the ordeal is over'.[56] Gauss claimed to have attained complete amnesia in 80% of his patients.[57] Many members of the medical profession recognized the potentially serious side effects of the isolated administration of scopolamine – neonatal respiratory depression and restless mothers. 'Occasionally there is an irregular movement of the hands and at times there is considerable motor restlessness, the patient moving about in bed and sometimes getting out of bed. The patient frequently talks to herself and will answer questions which have been self-given; and in about one and one-half per cent of the cases there is some mental excitation, generally of a mild degree; though occasionally this may be so marked as to require restraint'.[56] The women however had little recall of painful labours and therefore considered it to be an acceptable technique. In spite of the reluctance of many doctors to advocate twilight-sleep, women demanded access to it, particularly in the USA, where an organization named the National Twilight Sleep Association was formed. Two events subsequently took place which limited the success of this movement – firstly one of the associations' leaders, Mrs Francis X Carmody, died suddenly during childbirth and secondly the outbreak of world war one diminished enthusiasm for anything 'German'.[58,59] In spite of this loss of popular support twilight-sleep continued to be used quite extensively over the next 30 years.

Pethidine

Pethidine was synthesized in 1939 in Germany[60] and first used for labour analgesia in 1940. Compared to equipotent doses of morphine, pethidine is said to produce less neonatal respiratory depression – possibly due to morphine penetrating the fetal nervous system more easily.[61] None the less the pethidine concentration in fetal blood is still about 70% of the concentration in maternal blood[62] and neonatal respiratory depression is well documented.[63,64] Midwives have been allowed to prescribe and administer pethidine since 1950. This ease of availability has allowed it to develop as the most commonly used systemic opioid for labour analgesia in the UK – despite the limitations of pethidine as an effective analgesic. Holdcroft and Morgan, and Beazly et al found that 40–75% of women receiving intramuscular pethidine during labour had ineffective pain

relief.[65,66] In an effort to improve analgesia, pethidine has been administered intravenously by patient controlled analgesia (PCA) systems. Adverse effects may be less than following intramuscular injection and analgesia better although reports are variable.[67] Shorter acting opioids such as fentanyl, alfentanil and remifentanil have also been administered by PCA systems, usually when regional analgesia has been contraindicated.[68–70]

Naloxone, an opioid receptor antagonist, was introduced by Clarke in 1971[71] and has proved to be an invaluable tool in the treatment of opioid induced neonatal respiratory depression.

OTHER SEDATIVES IN LABOUR

Chloral hydrate, tincture of opium and bromide was a popular mixture during the latter half of the 19th century, used to produce sleep during labour. It was replaced by the barbiturates following the introduction of barbitone by Emil Fischer and von Mering in 1903. Rectal ether, ether and oil, and antihistamines have also been used for their sedative properties.[72] Bepko et al reported on the use of parenterally administered diazepam during labour in 1965, 'Parenteral administration of 20–40 mg of diazepam to 81 women during labour produced no untoward effects upon mother or baby. The drug markedly reduced apprehension, and pain associated with it, blurred the memory of labor ... the medication exerted no apparent influence upon Apgar scores in the neonates, or upon length of labor or anesthesia requirements'.[73]

REGIONAL ANALGESIA AND ANAESTHESIA

SPINAL ANAESTHESIA

Carl Koller of Vienna was the first to utilize local anaesthesia for surgery – he performed an eye operation using cocaine in 1884.[74] J. Leonard Corning, a neurologist from New York, accidentally produced spinal analgesia in 1885 whilst experimenting with cocaine on the spinal nerves of dogs.[75] During 1891 both Quincke and Wynter were responsible for making the performance of a lumbar puncture a straightforward clinical procedure.[76,77] August Bier in 1898 was the first to use planned spinal anaesthesia for surgery.[78] Tuffier, of Paris, later reported on the use of spinal anaesthesia for lower abdominal procedures.[79]

Oscar Kreis, an assistant obstetrician at the Women's Hospital in Basel, administered the first spinal for obstetric use in 1900 – analgesia for operative vaginal delivery.[80] During the same year Marx from New York described intrathecal cocaine for labour analgesia. Marx also discussed the importance of watching cerebrospinal fluid escape from the needle hub prior to injecting local anaesthetic solution, 'a *sina qua non* to an absolute analgesia is the escape of subarachnoid fluid before the cocaine solution is injected, and by its escape I am in positive position to state that the needle is in the canal. There is no other guide'.[81] The importance of the curves of the vertebral canal and the use of gravity in the control of the level of spinal analgesia was first realized by Arthur Barker of London in 1906, 'it has for a long time past appeared to me that if we are to aim at localizing our spinal analgesia to any particular region of the cord we ought to employ the force of *gravity* acting upon an injected compound of greater density than that of the liquor spinalis. This would sink to the most dependent part of the canal open to it independent of any displacement of the cerebro-spinal fluid. Here it would remain more or less undiluted in contact with the structures around'.[82,83]

In 1907 Henry Dean was the first to describe continuous spinal anaesthesia, 'In some cases the anaesthesia tends to disappear before the operation is completed ... It is necessary, therefore, to be prepared to give another injection during the operation, and with this in view I have so arranged the exploring needle that it can be left *in situ* during the operation, so that at any moment another dose can be injected without moving the patient beyond a slight degree'.[84]

George Pitkin popularized spinal anaesthesia for obstetric use in the USA and described 'controllable spinal anaesthesia' in 1928, 'The results were so satisfactory in 89 cases of instrumental deliveries, versions, breech cases, and prolonged labors ... the technique of controlling the anaesthetic solution and limiting its contact to those strands of the cauda equina that pierce the tip of the dural sac, forming the sacral nerves is relatively simple with the use of gliadin (the mucilaginous content of wheat starch) which prevents dissemination or mixing of the anaesthetic solution with the spinal fluid until the anaesthetic agent has been absorbed' (Fig. 1.9).[85] Continuous spinal anaesthesia using a 'ureteral catheter' was described by Major Edward Tuohy in 1945.[86]

Complications of spinal anaesthesia

Aorto-caval compression

Spinal analgesia and anaesthesia in obstetric practice has waxed and waned in popularity. There were early fatalities from circulatory collapse when pregnant mothers were given spinal anaesthetics for Caesarean section. Holmes in 1958 suggested that, 'the mechanism

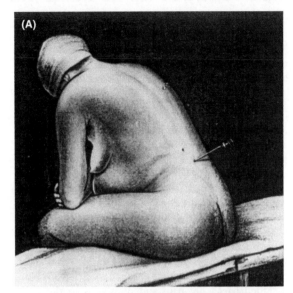

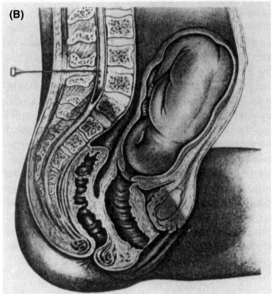

Figure 1.9   (A) The sitting posture as described by George Pitkin for controllable spinal anaesthesia – 'the elbows rest on the knees, the head is bent forward, and the back is bowed out'. (B) The result of George Pitkin's controllable spinal anaesthesia – anaesthesia of the tissues as illustrated by the shaded area. (Reproduced with permission from Ref. 86, American College of Surgeons.)

in sudden circulatory collapse during Caesarean section under spinal analgesia is a combination of the effects of occlusion of the inferior vena cava and reduction of peripheral vascular resistance on cardiac output'. He felt that, 'vigilant supervision will focus attention on an early decline of cardiac output, in which case venous return and cardiac filling can be restored by turning the patient on to one side and raising her legs'.[87] Ephedrine was first used to counteract hypotension in spinal anaesthesia in 1926.[88,89] Wollman and Marx described volume preloading in 1968.[90]

Neurological

Another concern with spinal anaesthesia was the possibility of permanent neurological deficit – this anxiety reached a peak following the infamous Woolley and Roe case in 1947[91,92] and Foster Kennedy's 1950 publication entitled 'The grave spinal cord paralyses caused by spinal anesthesia'.[93] In 1954 Robert Dripps and Leroy Vandam published the results of their long-term follow-up of 8460 patients who received 10 098 spinal anaesthetics. They reported, 'minor neurological sequelae of sufficient frequency and severity to suggest strongly a causal relationship to spinal anaesthesia. These included backache; pain and numbness in the buttocks, thighs, legs, and feet; and occasional instances of weakness in the leg muscles. The majority of these complaints were transient and disappeared completely with the passage of time … a good many of these findings could be related to the trauma of lumbar puncture and can be prevented or minimized by improvement in technique. The remainder suggest a relation to the injection of the anaesthetic solution into the subarachnoid space. The factors that lead to neurological disease insofar as the injection of the anaesthetic solution is concerned have never been elucidated despite extensive animal experimentation and case analysis in human beings. We are convinced, however, on the basis of this study, that major neurological damage need not follow spinal anaesthesia; we found none'.[94] The technique of continuous spinal anaesthesia still remains relatively unpopular – the cauda equina syndrome was reported following several cases in the USA in 1991.[95]

Post-spinal headaches

Post-spinal headaches, however, remained a problem for the obstetric population, Selwyn Crawford, using 23 or 25 gauge Quincke needles, reported an incidence of headache amongst women of 16.3%.[96] The development of spinal needles with new bevel designs such as the Whitacre and Sprotte needles has reduced the incidence of post-spinal headache dramatically[97,98] and allowed spinal anaesthesia to become almost routine for elective and many emergency Caesarean sections (Fig. 1.10).

CAUDAL ANAESTHESIA

Sicard and Cathelin working independently in Paris both described the sacral approach to the epidural

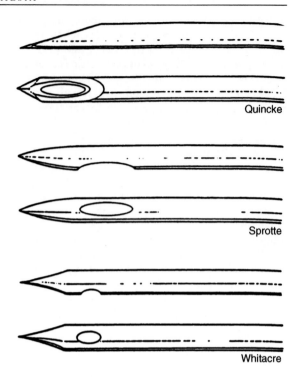

Figure 1.10   Quincke, Sprotte and Whitacre spinal needle tips. (Reproduced with permission from Morgan P. Spinal anaesthesia in obstetrics. *Can J Anaesth* 1995; 42: 1145–1163.)

space in 1901.[99–101] Eight years later Walter Stoeckel performed 141 caudal blocks in parturients but due to the local anaesthetic agents available at the time was only able to produce short-lived analgesia (the average duration was 1–1½ h).[102,103] Bonar and Meeker in 1923 carried out further caudal blocks in the obstetric population but again the duration of analgesia was of less than 2 h, 'The field of usefulness of this means of anaesthesia in normal delivery will greatly increase, when a means has been devised to prolong the anaesthetic action of an epidural injection for at least six or seven hours. Such an anaesthesia should find widespread use, and might become the anaesthetic of choice in normal delivery'.[104] Such anaesthesia was described on 12th January 1931 when Eugen Aburel presented a paper entitled 'L'anestésie locale continue (prolongée) en obstetrique' at a meeting of the Obstetric and Gynaecological Society of Paris. He described continuous caudal and lumbo-aortic plexus block for the relief of pain in childbirth.[105] In later years Aburel also studied the afferent innervation of the uterus – he concluded that the uterus had a double sensory innervation, sympathetic and cerebrospinal fibres.[106] Unfortunately since his work was published in only french and rumanian medical journals, Aburel's pioneering

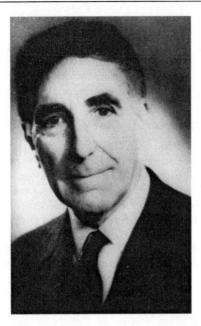

Figure 1.11   Eugen Bogdan Aburel (1899–1975). (Reproduced with permission from Ref. 107, Blackwell Science Ltd.)

contributions to obstetric analgesia remained largely unknown (Fig. 1.11).[107]

In 1933 John Cleland produced his classic work on the nerve supply of the uterus and identified the pathways of uterine pain, unaware of Aburel's previous investigations.[108] The year 1942 saw the publication of two landmark papers by Edwards and Hingson. The first was '*Continuous caudal anesthesia in obstetrics*' – 'We consider this form of anesthesia to be an improvement over the conventional type of peridural anesthetic administered by a single injection. In this latter procedure, the time limit of satisfactory anesthesia is from forty-five minutes to two and a half hours, while with continuous caudal administration, the anesthesia can be safely prolonged indefinitely. The maximum time of effective anesthesia during labor, in our experience, has been thirteen hours'.[109] This was followed by a second report entitled '*Continuous caudal analgesia*' (Fig. 1.12) – 'We are convinced that continuous caudal analgesia will give complete relief of pain to the parturient with absolute safety to her and her baby, provided the procedure is supervised by a specially trained person. We have found that the ideal person for this responsibility is an obstetrician who has been fundamentally trained in the specialized form of

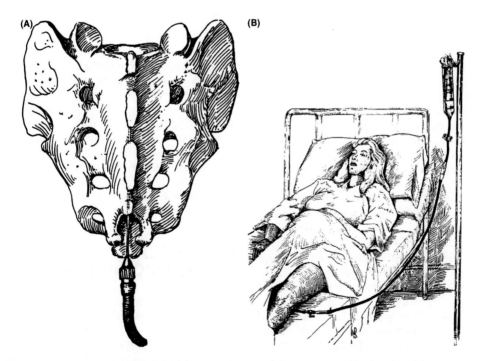

Figure 1.12   Continuous caudal anaesthesia: (A) 17 gauge needle inserted into the sacral canal. (B) Graduated cylinder containing procaine solution, clamp, rubber tubing and glass adapter. (Reproduced with permission from Block N, Rochberg S. Continuous caudal anesthesia in obstetrics. *Am J Obstet Gynecol* 1943; **45**: 645–650.)

anesthesiology. We have also observed that in some instances the specially trained obstetrician's nurse is able to make some of the subsequent injections and to determine the progress of the parturient with absolute safety'.[110] Hingson, in particular, popularized continuous caudal analgesia for labour throughout the USA. In 1949 he wrote, 'After a personal experience with this technique in 12 000 cases, and after training 2,000 physicians, who have reported its use in 260 scientific papers in eight languages for 600 000 deliveries, I am convinced that it offers effective and humane relief, without suggestion or hypnotism, to normal and handicapped mothers, for the delivery of normal and premature babies. This opinion is shared by the 80 American obstetricians who have each managed more than a thousand deliveries under continuous caudal analgesia'.[111]

LUMBAR EPIDURAL

Fidel Pagés, a Spanish surgeon working in Madrid, described a lumbar epidural block in 1920, 'Last November, whilst giving a spinal anaesthetic, it occurred to me to block the nerves between the intervertebral spaces and the meninges rather than pierce the dura ... I used a Type A Novocaine–epinephrine preparation containing 375 mg of Novocaine and 25 ml of normal saline in a galley pot, injecting it through the needle which was lying between the 2nd and 3rd lumbar vertebrae ... Analgesia gradually increased until, 20 min after the injection, it was sufficient to permit the repair of a right inguinal hernia without the patient experiencing any discomfort. This result encouraged us to study the method further and we called it Segmental Anaesthesia'.[112,113] Lumbar epidural anaesthesia was further developed 10 years later by Achile Dogliotti of Milan.[114] During 1936 Charles Odom, a surgeon at the Charity Hospital of Louisiana, reported the use of lumbar epidural anaesthesia for Caesarean section and both normal and abnormal obstetric deliveries.[115] Curbelo of Cuba was the first to describe the use of a catheter technique in the lumbar epidural space in 1949.[116] Continuous lumbar epidural analgesia for parturients using a Tuohy needle and plastic tubing was described by Flowers et al in 1949[117] and later advocated by Philip Bromage in 1961, 'The technique appears to offer many theoretical and practical advantages for the prolonged relief of pain in difficult labour. Over 500 women in labour have been treated by this method of continuous epidural analgesia, the majority in the last two years. This number is due to the increasing popularity of the method with obstetricians and patients alike'. However Bromage warned, 'Continuous epidural analgesia is not a technique for the occasional anaesthetist, and its use should be confined to institutions with proper staffing facilities. Although epidural puncture in itself is relatively easy, given care and a good pair of hands, the management of the continuous technique in labour does require a degree of skill and judgement which is unlikely to be attained without special training and experience'.[118]

The development of the epidural service

In Britain, epidural analgesia for childbirth developed during the late 1960s, enhanced by the appearance of bupivacaine in 1963. The first 24 h 'on demand' epidural service to a delivery unit was established at the Queen Mother's Hospital in Glasgow in 1964. Donald Moir reported on a large series of continuous lumbar epidural blocks in 1968.[119] Approval was given in 1970 by the Central Midwives Board for midwives to administer epidural top-ups. Epidural anaesthesia also became increasingly used for Caesarean section. In 1980 Thorburn and Moir described a technique of epidural anaesthesia for Caesarean section with a 98% success rate and an acceptably low incidence of intra-operative pain.[120]

Opioids were first injected into the epidural space in 1979.[121] Cooper et al demonstrated in 1991 that the addition of opioids to epidural solutions for labour analgesia reduced the dose of local anaesthetic agent required.[122]

'Walking epidurals' were first described by Collis and Morgan from Queen Charlotte's Hospital in London in 1993, utilizing the technique of combined spinal–epidural analgesia.[123] The intrathecal component provides analgesia of rapid onset whilst the epidural catheter allows further doses of low dose local anaesthetic and opioid to be administered as the spinal block diminishes. The minimal motor block allows mothers to mobilize during labour. The choice of epidural analgesia for labour is now widely available – in 1997 a survey in the UK showed that 90% of maternity units offered a 24 h epidural service. Many units additionally offered 'walking' epidurals.[124]

HISTORY OF PSYCHOPROPHYLAXIS

'Natural Childbirth' was advocated by Grantly Dick Read, a London obstetrician, in 1933.[125] Read believed that the presence of fear activated the sympathetic nervous system and this in turn produced the pain of labour – abolition of fear by developing the appropriate mental attitude would result in a pain free labour. Women therefore needed to be re-educated about the anticipation of pain. Fernand Lamaze, in the 1950s,

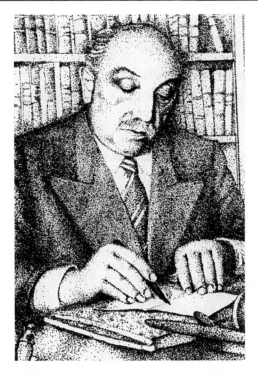

Figure 1.13   Dr Fernand Lamaze. (Reproduced with permission from Ref. 58.)

supported the idea that instruction in the physiology of pregnancy and labour, breathing exercises and relaxation techniques would help to reduce pain from delivery (Fig. 1.13).[126] Leboyer in 1975 suggested manoeuvres to minimize the neonate's first separation experience. He advocated birth in a quiet and darkened room, the newly delivered baby being placed on his mother's abdomen and delayed clamping of the cord.[127] A randomized clinical trial of the Leboyer approach was however shown to offer no advantage over a gentle, conventional approach in terms of infant and maternal outcomes.[128]

IMPACT OF OBSTETRIC ANAESTHESIA ON THE NEW-BORN

A careful collection of cautious and accurate observations will no doubt be required, before the inhalation of sulphuric ether is adopted to any great extent in the practice of midwifery. It will be necessary to ascertain its precise effects, both upon the action of the uterus, and of the assistant abdominal muscles: its influence if any, upon the child.

James Young Simpson[2]

James Simpson commented on the importance of understanding the effects of anaesthetic agents on both the 'child' and on uterine action. Walter Channing in his '*Treatise on etherization in childbirth*' remarked on the fact that he had been unable to detect the odour of ether at the cut ends of the umbilical cord and therefore implied that ether did not cross the placenta.[12] Channing's opinion gave early acceptability to the use of anaesthesia for midwifery.[129]

In 1853 John Snow remarked upon the placental transfer of chloroform and ether, 'It is quite certain that the fetus must receive a portion of the chloroform into its circulation, as it does of any other medicine which is absorbed into the blood of the mother: and when sulphuric ether was the agent employed, its odour could be perceived in the child's breath after birth. The fetus must therefore, be influenced by the chloroform, though generally to a less extent than its mother, as it receives its dose only at second-hand. It has seemed in some cases that the child was less acutely sensible to the cold air than usual at the time of its birth: and when the mother is unconscious from chloroform, I have not seen it kick and scream in the violent way, and grasp the bed clothes with the force, during the first minute after its birth, that is often observed under other circumstances'.[23] The observations of John Snow, and others, made little impact on the popularity of inhalational anaesthesia for obstetric pain relief for at least another 25 years.

Paul Zweifel in 1877 published the definitive experiments which confirmed that chloroform crossed the placenta – he provided evidence of chloroform in umbilical blood and in urine of new-born infants.[130] Zweifel also established the placental transfer of oxygen, using a light absorption technique to demonstrate a difference in oxygen content between umbilical arterial and venous blood.[131] Although Zweifel's work demonstrated beyond doubt that drugs did cross the placenta, it still did not immediately alter obstetric practice or increase concerns for the safety of the fetus. The implications of Zweifel's findings were only finally accepted with the introduction of 'twilight-sleep'. Problems with neonatal respiratory depression soon became apparent and the risks of the placental transfer of drugs from mother to fetus could no longer be ignored. It is now accepted that all drugs that enter the maternal circulation will cross the placenta to some extent, unless they are broken down or altered during the transfer.

Apgar scores

In the mid 19th century, when obstetric anaesthesia commenced, maternal mortality was very high and scant attention was given to the condition of the neonate. As maternal mortality improved it was gradually recognized that the condition of the neonate was also an important indicator of obstetric care. Virginia Apgar, an anaesthetist working in New York, was the first, in 1953, to describe a simple, reliable system for evaluating new-born infants. She suggested a score of 0, 1 or 2 given for each of five variables – heart rate, respiratory effort, muscle tone, colour and reflex irritability, allowing assessment of the neonate one or more minutes after birth.[132] The scoring system enabled the effects of differing treatments and methods of analgesia given to the mother to be compared in regards to their effects on the condition of the neonate.

EFFECTS OF ANAESTHESIA ON LABOUR

The fact, that chloroform can and does induce inertia of muscular fibre, both voluntary and involuntary, when given in sufficient dose, is now well-established ... chloroform may produce alarming results in midwifery practice, and that, if given at all, it should be in small quantities only.
Charles Delucina Meigs[15]

The possible detrimental effects of chloroform and ether on uterine activity were recognized at a relatively early stage. John Snow realized the depressant action of chloroform on uterine activity, but felt that this could be controlled by the amount of the agent given: 'It was said that, in some of the early cases in which chloroform was employed, the uterine contractions were so much enfeebled by it, that delivery had ultimately to be accomplished by the use of forceps. It is not improbable that the over free use of this agent might lead to such a result; but I believe it would not arise from its judicious use. It has happened that, in all the cases of manual and instrumental delivery in which I have given chloroform, it was exhibited only in consequence of the operation: for the other cases in which I have administered it have all terminated without artificial assistance'.[23] Snow also acknowledged that on some occasions a reduction in uterine activity could be useful to the obstetrician. 'Dr. Snow, in opening the subject, said that ... Some objections had arisen from the supposed necessity of inducing a deep state of insensibility, and he was of the opinion that if it were requisite to cause the same amount of insensibility in midwifery, as is required in operations in which the knife is used, that would be a valid objection ... But this amount of insensibility was not required in obstetric practice unless to arrest or diminish strong uterine action for a few minutes to facilitate turning the child'.[133] Gradually it became standard practice to minimize the amount of anaesthetic agent given unless anaesthesia was required for operative delivery.

Regional anaesthesia

Clelland's description of the nerve pathways mediating labour pain allowed for greater thoughts on the effects of analgesic drugs on uterine function. The introduction of continuous caudal analgesia by Hingson and Edwards meant that analgesia was commenced at a comparatively early stage in labour. Problems with prolonged labour soon became apparent. Controversy still exists today about the effects of epidural analgesia on the progress of labour and on the incidence of Caesarean section.[134]

HISTORY OF AUDIT AND THE OBSTETRIC SOCIETIES

The confidential enquiries into maternal deaths in England and Wales

The enquiry began in 1952. Since 1985 the report for England and Wales has been combined with those from Scotland and Northern Ireland, and published as a UK report (Fig. 1.14). This report has been described as the 'most influential clinical self-audit in the world'[135] and includes discussion of maternal deaths attributed solely to obstetric anaesthesia.

Obstetric Anaesthetists' Association

Tom Bryson had the original idea of an association for anaesthetists working within the UK with a particular interest in obstetric anaesthesia. The inaugural meeting of the Obstetric Anaesthetists' Association (OAA) was held in 1969. Selwyn Crawford was elected as the first president. The OAA now has a membership in excess of 1500. Annual meetings are organized and research grants awarded. The OAA also publishes recommended minimum standards for obstetric anaesthesia services,[136] and the *International Journal of Obstetric Anesthesia* is the official journal.

Society for Obstetric Anesthetia and Perinatology (SOAP)

Robert Hustead hosted the first meeting of the newly formed Society for Obstetric Anesthesia and Perinatology in Kansas City, Missouri in 1969. Today, SOAP has a membership of about 1200 and is the official sub-specialty component of the American Society of Anesthesiologists. An annual meeting is held every Spring. *Anesthesiology* is the official journal.

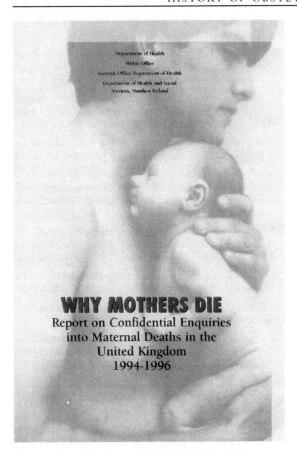

Figure 1.14   Front cover – Report on Confidential Enquiries into Maternal Deaths in the UK 1994–1996. Department of Health, Welsh Office, Scottish Office Department of Health, Department of Health and Social services, Northern Ireland. Crown copyright is reproduced with the permission of the Controller of Her Majesty's Stationery Office.

REFERENCES

Note: Epigraph has been taken from Horton JM. Norman Dott 1897–1973. *Proc Hist Anaesth Soc* 1995; **17**: 58.

1. *Mon J Med Sci* 1847; **1**: 639–640.

2. Simpson JY. Notes on the employment of the inhalation of sulphuric ether in the practice of midwifery. *Mon J Med Sci* 1847; **1**: 721–728.

3. Obituary, Sir James Young Simpson. *Med Times Gaz* 1870; **1**: 530–532.

4. Hale-White W. Sir James Young Simpson. In: Hale-White W (ed) *Great doctors of the nineteenth century*. London: Edward Arnold and Co., 1935, p 146.

5. Smith P. On the use of chloroform in midwifery practice. *Lancet* 1847; **2**: 572–574.

6. Keep NC. The Letheon administered in a case of labor. *Boston Med Surg J* 1847; **36**: 226.

7. Shepherd JA. The introduction of general anaesthesia. In: Shepherd JA (ed) *Simpson and Syme of Edinburgh*. Edinburgh and London: E and S Livingstone Ltd, 1969, pp 77–102.

8. Thomas KB. The early use of chloroform with some notes on certain apparatus designed for its delivery. *Anaesthesia* 1971; **26**: 348–362.

9. Gaskell E. Three letters by Sir James Young Simpson. *Br Med J* 1970; **2**: 414–416.

10. Simpson JY. On a new anaesthetic agent more efficient than sulphuric ether. *Lancet* 1847; **2**: 549–550.

11. Murphy EW. Chloroform in midwifery. *Assoc Med J* 1856; **1**: 86–88.

12. Channing W. *A treatise on etherization in childbirth*. Boston: William D Ticknor and Co., 1848.

13. Barnes R. Observations on Dr. Simpson's anaesthetic statistics. *Lancet* 1847; **2**: 677–678.

14. Rankin DR. On the employment of chloroform in medical practice. *Lancet* 1848; **2**: 181–182.

15. Meigs CD. Letter to Prof. J.Y. Simpson, dated 18th February 1848. In: Meigs CD (ed) *Obstetrics: the science and the art*, 4th edn. Philadelphia: Blanchard and Lea, 1863, p 358.

16. Simpson JY. *Answer to the religious objections advanced against the employment of anaesthetic agents in midwifery and surgery*. Edinburgh: Sutherland and Knox, 1847.

17. Farr AD. Early opposition to obstetric anaesthesia. *Anaesthesia* 1980; **35**: 896–907.

18. Farr AD. Early opposition to obstetric anaesthesia. *Anaesthesia* 1981; **36**: 541–542.

19. Moffat J. Observations on anaesthesia in midwifery in answer to Dr Barnes. *Lancet* 1848; **1**: 97–98.

20. Connor H, Connor T. Did the use of chloroform by Queen Victoria influence its acceptance in obstetric practice? *Anaesthesia* 1996; **51**: 955–957.

21. Dunn PM. Dr John Snow (1813-58) of London: pioneer of obstetric anaesthesia. *Arch Dis Child* 1996; **75**: F141–F142.

22. Snow J. *On chloroform and other anaesthetics*. London: 1858, p 79.

23. Snow J. On the administration of chloroform during parturition. *Assoc Med J* 1853; **1**: 500–502.

24. Simpson JY. Chloroform in Scotland. *Med Times Gaz* 1852; **4**: 627–628.

25. Levy AG. Sudden death under light chloroform anaesthesia. *J Physiol* 1911; **42**: iii–vii.

26. Marx GF, Katsnelson T. The introduction of nitrous oxide analgesia into obstetrics. *Obstet Gynecol* 1992; **80**: 715–718.

27. Richards W, Parbrook GD, Wilson J. Stanislav Klikovich. *Anaesthesia* 1976; **31**: 933–940.

28. Guedel AE. The office anesthetic for small surgery, nitrous oxide and air, self-administered. *NY Med J* 1912; **95**: 387–388.

29. Webster JC. Nitrous oxide gas analgesia in obstetrics. *JAMA* 1915; **64**: 812–813.

30. Lynch FW. Nitrous oxide gas analgesia in obstetrics. *JAMA* 1915; **64**: 813.

31. Sced A. The Minnitt gas–air apparatus. *Proc Hist Anaesth Soc* 1995; **18**: 38–39.

32. Minnitt RJ. Self-administered analgesia for the midwifery of general practice. *Proc Roy Soc Med* 1934; **27**: 1313–1318.

33. Tunstall ME. Obstetric analgesia – the use of a fixed nitrous oxide and oxygen mixture from one cylinder. *Lancet* 1961; **2**: 964.

34. Cole PV, Nainby-Luxmoore RC. The hazards of gas and air in obstetrics. *Anaesthesia* 1962; **17**: 505–518.

35. Nainby-Luxmoore RC. Further hazards of gas and air in obstetrics. *Anaesthesia* 1964; **19**: 421–423.

36. Moir DD, Bisset WIK. An assessment of nitrous oxide apparatus used for obstetric analgesia. *J Obstet Gynaecol Br Comm* 1965; **72**: 264–268.

37. Bourne W. Divinyl oxide anaesthesia in obstetrics. *Lancet* 1934; **1**: 566–567.

38. Bourne W. Vinyl ether obstetric anesthesia for general practice. *JAMA* 1935; **105**: 2047–2051.

39. Bourne W. Cyclopropane anaesthesia in obstetrics. *Lancet* 1934; **2**: 20–21.

40. Griffith HR. Cyclopropane anesthesia. *Curr Res Anesth Analg* 1935; **14**: 253–256.

41. Bonica JJ. *Principles and practice of obstetric analgesia and anesthesia*, vol 1. Oxford: Blackwell Scientific Publications, 1967, p 381.

42. Elam J. Trichlorethylene anaesthesia. *Lancet* 1942; **2**: 309.

43. Freedman A. Trichlorethylene–air analgesia in childbirth. *Lancet* 1943; **2**: 696–697.

44. Hudon F. Methoxyflurane. *Can Anaesth Soc J* 1961; **8**: 544–550.

45. Boisvert M, Hudon F. Clinical evaluation of methoxyflurane in obstetrical anaesthesia: a report on 500 cases. *Can Anaesth Soc J* 1962; **9**: 325–330.

46. Major V, Rosen M, Mushin WW. Concentration of methoxyflurane for obstetric analgesia by self-administered intermittent inhalation. *Br Med J* 1967; **4**: 767–770.

47. Hicks JS, Shnider SM, Cohen H. *Abst Sci Paper ASA Ann Meet* 1975, Chicago, pp 99–100.

48. McLeod DD, Ramayya GP, Tunstall ME. Self-administered isoflurane in labour. A comparative study with Entonox. *Anaesthesia* 1985; **40**: 424–426.

49. Wee MYK, Hasan MA, Thomas TA. Isoflurane in labour. *Anaesthesia* 1993; **48**: 369–372.

50. McGuinness C, Rosen M. Enflurane as an analgesic in labour. *Anaesthesia* 1984; **39**: 24–26.

51. Abboud TK, Swart F, Zhu J, Donovan MM, Peres da Silva E, Yakal K. Desflurane analgesia for vaginal delivery. *Acta Anaesthesiol Scand* 1995; **39**: 259–261.

52. Mendelson CL. The aspiration of stomach contents into the lungs during obstetric anesthesia. *Am J Obstet Gynecol* 1946; **52**: 191–204.

53. Macht DI. The history of opium and some of its preparations and alkaloids. *JAMA* 1915; **64**: 477–481.

54. Schaer HM. History of pain relief in obstetrics. In: Marx GF, Bassell GM (eds) *Obstetric analgesia and anesthesia*. Amsterdam: Elsevier/North Holland Biomedical Press 1980, p 10.

55. Von Steinbüchel R. Vorläufige mittheilung uber die anwendung von skopolamin-morphium injektionen in der geburtshilfe. *Zentralbl Gynakol* 1902; **30**: 1304–1306.

56. Knipe WHW. The Freiburg method of dämmerschlaf or twilight sleep. *Am J Obstet Gynecol* 1914; **70**: 884–909.

57. Gauss CJ. Geburten in künstlichem dämmerschlaf. *Archiv für Gynäkologie* 1906; **78**: 579–631.

58. Pitcock CDH, Clark RB. From Fanny to Fernand: the development of consumerism in pain control during the birth process. *Am J Obstet Gynecol* 1992; **167**: 581–587.

59. Caton D. The influence of feminists on the early development of obstetric anesthesia. *Bull Anesth Hist* 1998; **16**(4): 4–7, 23.

60. Eisleb O, Schaumann O. Dolantin, ein neuartiges spasmolytikum und analgetikum (chemisches und pharmakologisches). *Dtsch Med Wochenschr* 1939; **65**: 967–968.

61. Way WL, Costley EC, Way EL. Respiratory sensitivity of the newborn infant to meperidine and morphine. *Clin Pharmacol Ther* 1965; **6**: 454–461.

62. Crawford JS, Rudofsky S. The placental transmission of pethidine. *Br J Anaesth* 1965; **37**: 929–933.

63. Shnider S, Moya F. Effects of meperidine on the newborn infant. *Am J Obstet Gynecol* 1964; **89**: 1009–1015.

64. Koch G, Wendel H. The effect of pethidine on the postnatal adjustment of respiration and acid-base balance. *Acta Obstet Gynecol Scand* 1968; **47**: 27–37.

65. Holdcroft A, Morgan M. An assessment of the analgesic effect in labour of pethidine and 50 per cent nitrous oxide in oxygen (Entonox). *J Obstet Gynaecol Br Comm* 1974; **81**: 603–607.

66. Beazly JM, Leaver EP, Morewood JHM, Bircumshaw J. Relief of pain in labour. *Lancet* 1967; **1**: 1033–1035.

67. Scrutton M. Systemic opioid analgesia. In: Reynolds F (ed) *Pain relief in labour*. London: BMJ publishing group, 1997, pp 102–103.

68. Kleiman SJ, Wiesel S, Tessler MJ. Patient-controlled analgesia (PCA) using fentanyl in a parturient with a platelet function abnormality. *Can J Anaesth* 1991; **38**: 489–491.

69. Dar AQ, Wilson R, Lyons G. Use of patient-controlled intravenous alfentanil analgesia during labour. *Int J Obstet Anesth* 1997; **6**: 209.

70. Jones R, Pegrum A, Stacey RGW. Patient-controlled analgesia using remifentanil in the parturient with thrombocytopenia. *Anaesthesia* 1999; **54**: 461–465.

71. Clark RB. Transplacental reversal of meperidine depression in the fetus by naloxone. *J Ark Med Soc* 1971; **68**: 128–130.

72. Rushman GB, Davies NJH, Atkinson RS. Obstetric anaesthesia. In: Rushman GB, Davies NJH, Atkinson RS (eds) *A short history of anaesthesia*. Oxford: Butterworth-Heinemann, 1996, pp 131–136.

73. Bepko F, Lowe E, Waxman B. Relief of the emotional factor in labor with parenterally administered diazepam. *Obstet Gynecol* 1965; **26**: 852–857.

74. Koller C. On the use of cocaine for producing anaesthesia on the eye. *Lancet* 1884; **2**: 990–992.

75. Corning JL. Spinal anaesthesia and local medication of the cord. *NY Med J* 1885; **42**: 483–485 (reprinted in 'Classical File'. *Sur Anesthesiol* 1960; **4**: 331–335).

76. Quincke H. Die lumbalpunction des hydrocephalus. *Berliner Klinische Wochenschrift* 1891; **28**: 929–933, 965–968.

77. Wynter WE. Four cases of tubercular meningitis in which paracentesis of the theca vertebralis was performed for the relief of fluid pressure. *Lancet* 1891; **1**: 981–982.

78. Bier A. Versucheüber cocainisirung des rückenmarkes. *Deutsche Zeitschrift für Chirurgie* 1899; **51**: 361–369 (translated and reprinted in 'Classical File'. *Sur Anesthesiol* 1962; **6**: 352–358).

79. Tuffier T. Anesthésie médullaire chirurgicale par injection sous-arachnoïdienne lombaire de cocaïne; technique et résultats. *La Semaine Médicale* 1900; **43**: 167–169.

80. Kreis O. Uber Medullarnarkosen bei gebärenden. *Zentralbl Gynakol* 1900; **28**: 724–729.

81. Marx S. Analgesia in obstetrics produced by medullary injections of cocaine. *Philadel Med J* 1900; **6**: 857–859.

82. Barker AE. A report on clinical experiences with spinal analgesia in 100 cases. *Br Med J* 1907; **1**: 665–674.

83. Lee JA. Arthur Edward James Barker 1850–1916, British pioneer of regional analgesia. *Anaesthesia* 1979; **34**: 885–891.

84. Akhtar M. Henry Percy Dean – an early British pioneer of spinal analgesia. *Anaesthesia* 1972; **27**: 330–333.

85. Pitkin GP, McCormack FC. Controllable spinal anaesthesia in obstetrics. *Surg Gynecol Obstet* 1928; **47**: 713–726.

86. Tuohy EB. The use of continuous spinal anesthesia utilizing the ureteral catheter technic. *JAMA* 1945; **128**: 262–264.

87. Holmes F. Spinal analgesia and caesarean section – maternal mortality. *J Obstet Gynaecol Br Emp* 1957; **64**: 229–232.

88. Ockerblad NF, Dillon TG. The use of ephedrine in spinal anesthesia. *JAMA* 1927; **88**: 1135–1136.

89. Rudolf RD, Graham JD. Notes on sulphate of ephedrin. *Am J Med Sci* 1927; **173**: 399–408.

90. Wollman SB, Marx GF. Acute hydration for prevention of hypotension of spinal anesthesia in parturients. *Anesthesiology* 1968; **29**: 374–380.

91. Cope RW. The Woolley and Roe case – Woolley and Roe versus Ministry of Health and others. *Anaesthesia* 1954; **9**: 249–270.

92. Hutter CDD. The Woolley and Roe case: a reassessment. *Anaesthesia* 1990; **45**: 859–864.

93. Kennedy F, Effron AS, Perry G. The grave spinal cord paralyses caused by spinal anesthesia. *Surg Gynecol Obstet* 1950; **91**: 385–398.

94. Dripps RD, Vandam LD. Long-term follow-up of patients who received 10,098 spinal anesthetics – failure to discover major neurological sequelae. *JAMA* 1954; **156**: 1486–1491.

95. Rigler ML, Drasner K, Krejcie TC et al. Cauda equina syndrome after continuous spinal anesthesia. *Anesth Analg* 1991; **72**: 275–281.

96. Crawford JS. Experience with spinal analgesia in a British obstetric unit. *Br J Anaesth* 1979; **51**: 531–535.

97. Shutt LE, Valentine SJ, Wee MYK, Page RJ, Prosser A, Thomas TA. Spinal anaesthesia for caesarean section: comparison of 22-gauge and 25-gauge whitacre needles with 26-gauge quincke needles. *Br J Anaesth* 1992; **69**: 589–594.

98. Cesarini M, Torrielli R, Lahaye F, Mene JM, Cabiro C. Sprotte needle for intrathecal anaesthesia for caesarean section: incidence of postdural puncture headache. *Anaesthesia* 1990; **45**: 656–658.

99. Sicard JA. Les injections medicamenteuses extra-durales par voie sacro-coccygienne. *Comptes Rendus Hebdomadaires des Séances et Mémoires de la Société de Biologie (Paris)* 1901; **53**: 396–398.

100. Cathelin F. Une nouvelle voie d'injection rachidienne. Méthode des injections épidurales par le procédé du canal sacré. Applications à l'homme. *Comptes Rendus Hebdomadaires des Séances et Mémoires de la Société de Biologie (Paris)* 1901; **53**: 452–453.

101. Meehan FP. Historical review of caudal epidural analgesia in obstetrics. *Midwifery* 1987; **3**: 39–45.

102. Stoeckel W. Über sakrale Anästhesie. *Zentralbl Gynakol* 1909; **33**: 1–15.

103. Doughty A. Walter Stoeckel (1871–1961) – a pioneer of regional analgesia in obstetrics. *Anaesthesia* 1990; **45**: 468–471.

104. Bonar BE, Meeker WR. The value of sacral nerve block anesthesia in obstetrics. *JAMA* 1923; **81**: 1079–1083.

105. Aburel E. L'anesthésie locale continue (prolongée) en obstétrique. *Bulletin de la Société d'Obstétrique et Gynécologie de Paris* 1931; **20**(12 January): 35–37.

106. Aburel E. La topographie et le mécanisme des doulerus de l'accouchement avant la période d'expulsion. *Comptes Rendus Hebdomadaires des Séances et Mémoires de la Société de Biologie (Paris)* 1930; **103**: 902–904.

107. Curelaru I, Sandu L. Eugen Bogdan Aburel (1899–1975) – the pioneer of regional analgesia for pain relief in childbirth. *Anaesthesia* 1982; **37**: 663–669.

108. Cleland JGP. Paravertebral anaesthesia in obstetrics. *Surg Gynecol Obstet* 1933; **57**: 51–62.

109. Edwards WB, Hingson RA. Continuous caudal anesthesia in obstetrics. *Am J Surg* 1942; **57**: 459–464 (reprinted in 'Classical File'. *Sur Anesthesiol* 1980; **24**: 272–280).

110. Hingson RA, Edwards WB. Continuous caudal analgesia – an analysis of the first ten thousand confinements thus managed with the report of the authors' first thousand cases. *JAMA* 1943; **123**: 538–546.

111. Hingson RA. Continuous caudal analgesia in obstetrics, surgery and therapeutics. *Br Med J* 1949; **2**: 777–781.

112. Pagés F. Anestesia metamérica. *Revista de Sanidad Militar,* Madrid, 1921; **11**: 351–365, 385–396 (translated in 'Classical File'. *Sur Anesthesiol* 1961; **5**: 326–338).

113. De Lange JJ, Cuesta MA, Cuesta De Pedro A. Fidel Pagés Miravé (1886–1923) – the pioneer of lumbar epidural anaesthesia. *Anaesthesia* 1994; **49**: 429–431.

114. Dogliotti AM. Eine neue methode der regionären anästhesie: die peridurale segmentäre anästhesie. *Zentralblatt für Chirurgie* 1931; **58**: 3141–3145.

115. Odom CB. Epidural anesthesia. *Am J Surg* 1936; **34**: 547–558.

116. Curbelo MM. Continuous peridural segmental anesthesia by means of a ureteral catheter. *Curr Res Anesth Analg* 1949; **28**: 13–23.

117. Flowers CE, Hellman LM, Hingson RA. Continuous peridural anesthesia and analgesia for labor, delivery and cesarean section. *Curr Res Anesth Analg* 1949; **28**: 181–189.

118. Bromage PR. Continuous lumbar epidural analgesia for obstetrics. *Can Med Assoc J* 1961; **85**: 1136–1140.

119. Moir DD, Willocks J. Epidural analgesia in British obstetrics. *Br J Anaesth* 1968; **40**: 129–138.

120. Thorburn J, Moir DD. Epidural analgesia for elective caesarean section. *Anaesthesia* 1980; **35**: 3–6.

121. Behar M, Olshwang D, Magora F, Davidson JT. Epidural morphine in treatment of pain. *Lancet* 1979; **1**: 527–529.

122. Murphy JD, Henderson K, Bowden MI, Lewis M, Cooper GM. Bupivacaine versus bupivacaine plus fentanyl for epidural analgesia: effect on maternal satisfaction. *Br Med J* 1991; **302**: 564–567.

123. Collis RE, Baxandall ML, Srikantharajah ID, Edge G, Kadim MY, Morgan BM. Combined spinal epidural analgesia with the ability to walk throughout labour. *Lancet* 1993; **341**: 767–768.

124. Burnstein R, Buckland R, Pickett JA. A survey of epidural analgesia for labour in the United Kingdom. *Anaesthesia* 1999; **54**: 634–640.

125. Read GD. *Natural childbirth.* London: Heinemann, 1933.

126. Lamaze F. *Painless childbirth.* London: Burke Publishing Company, 1958.

127. Leboyer F. *Birth without violence.* New York: Alfred A Knopf, 1975.

128. Nelson NM, Enkin MW, Saigal S, Bennett KJ, Milner R, Sackett DL. A randomized clinical trial of the Leboyer approach to childbirth. *N Engl J Med* 1980; **302**: 655–660.

129. Caton D. Obstetric anesthesia and concepts of placental transport – a historical review of the nineteenth century. *Anesthesiology* 1977; **46**: 132–137.

130. Zweifel P. Der Uebergang von chloroform und salicylsaüre in die placenta, nebst bemerkungen über den icterus neonatorum. *Archiv für Gynäkologie* 1877; **12**: 235–257.

131. Zweifel P. Die respiration des fötus. *Archiv für Gynäkologie* 1876; **9**: 291–305.

132. Apgar V. A proposal for a new method of evaluation of the newborn infant. *Curr Res Anesth Analg* 1953; **32**: 260–267.

133. Chloroform in midwifery. *Lancet* 1849; **1**: 99.

134. Miller AC. The effects of epidural analgesia on uterine activity and labor. *Int J Obstet Anesth* 1997; **6**: 2–18.

135. Willats SM. Confidential enquiries into maternal deaths in the United Kingdom 1991–1993. *Int J Obstet Anesth* 1997; **6**: 73–75.

136. Obstetric Anaesthetists Association. *Recommended minimum standards for Obstetric Anaesthesia Services.* Obstetric Anaesthetists Association, 1995.

2

MATERNAL PHYSIOLOGY

Jonathan Allsop, Neena Navaneetham & Jason Cooper

INTRODUCTION

As pregnancy progresses, changes in maternal physiology support the growing fetus, prepare for birth and allow the newborn child to thrive. These changes begin early in pregnancy, before fetal demand is great and are driven by placental hormones. The changes more than compensate for increasing fetal demands as the pregnancy progresses. Most systems have returned to normal by 6 weeks after the pregnancy has ended.

A thorough knowledge of the physiological changes in pregnant women is required to avoid misinterpretation of symptoms, signs and results of investigations. This is essential for the management of both normal and abnormal pregnancy.

HAEMATOLOGY

BLOOD VOLUME

One of the earliest and most fundamental changes in pregnancy is an increase in blood volume. This is detectable by the sixth week,[1] is greatest during the second trimester and reaches a plateau at 34–36 weeks. At term the blood volume is around 48% greater than non-pregnant values.[2] This represents an additional 2l of fluid accommodated in the maternal circulation. Greater increases may be seen in multiparous women and multiple pregnancies. The trigger to the increased blood volume is thought to be hormonal. Oestrogen stimulates uterine growth and the low resistance circuit created contributes to a fall in mean arterial pressure. This leads to activation of the renin–angiotensin axis and ultimately to renal retention of water and sodium by aldosterone. Oestrogen may directly increase plasma renin activity. Progesterone is a vasodilator and contributes to this process: It enhances aldosterone production but inhibits the effects of aldosterone on the renal tubules. Potassium secretion by the renal tubule is reduced[3] and the secretion of atrial natriuretic peptide in pregnancy is increased.[4]

Part of the increase in blood volume occurs through an increase in plasma volume. This can be measured using Evans blue dye that binds to plasma proteins, or by injecting radio-labelled albumin and measuring its dilution. By 34 weeks the plasma volume is 1250 ml greater than before conception.[5] Plasma volume then remains stable for the rest of the pregnancy. There is also an increase in total red cell mass.[1] The increase in the number of red cells appears to start slightly later than the changes in plasma volume, towards the end of the first trimester and shows a steady rise until

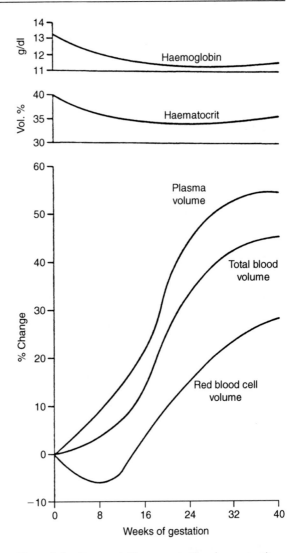

Figure 2.1   Haemoglobin concentration, haematocrit, blood volume, plasma volume and red blood cell volume during pregnancy.

term. The increment of plasma volume with each week of gestation exceeds the rise in red cell mass throughout pregnancy, the point of greatest difference being at 28–30 weeks of gestation.[2] By term the red cell mass is increased by around 15–20% over non-pregnant levels (Fig. 2.1). Such a rise is dependent on maternal stores of iron. In those who begin pregnancy with borderline iron stores, even without clinical evidence of anaemia, a much smaller increase in red cell mass is seen unless the diet is supplemented with iron.

Because plasma volume and red cell mass change at different rates and to differing degrees, haemoglobin concentration and haematocrit also change with gestation. In iron replete individuals, the haemoglobin concentration and haematocrit fall progressively throughout the first and second trimesters to a nadir of 15–20% below pre-pregnancy values. Both values rise slightly in the third trimester but still remain below non-pregnant levels. This dilutional effect is sometimes referred to as the physiological anaemia of pregnancy. In general a haemoglobin concentration of at least 11.5 g/dl is regarded as normal in pregnancy. Values less than this cannot be assumed to be due to physiological change. Pathology should be sought and treated.

The increased blood volume of pregnancy enhances circulation to the uterus, meets the excretory demands of the kidneys and compensates for blood loss at delivery. The latter is in the range of 500 ml for a spontaneous vaginal delivery[6] though instrumental vaginal delivery is associated with higher blood loss. The typical blood loss at Caesarean section is around 1000 ml.[6,7]

In normal pregnancy the red cell indices remain unchanged apart from red cell volume, which shows a small increase.

WHITE BLOOD CELLS

There is a relative leukocytosis in pregnancy with the white cell count rising to 12×10^9/l at term.[8] During labour, counts as high as $25–30 \times 10^9$/l have been noted. Most of the increase are granulocytes, with lymphocytes and monocytes remaining unchanged. Granulocyte increase is driven by cortisol and oestrogen.

COAGULATION

Pregnancy is associated with enhanced blood coagulability and platelet turnover. Greater platelet production matches the increase in platelet activation and consumption.[9] Factors VII, VIII, IX, X and XII are all present in higher concentration.[10,11] Fibrinogen concentration may double from 3 to 6 g/l. It should be noted that the rise in fibrinogen will cause a marked increase in erythrocyte sedimentation rate, making this marker unhelpful for following inflammatory conditions in pregnancy.[12] C-reactive protein is also increased in pregnancy, particularly in labour.[13] The prothrombin and partial thromboplastin times are slightly decreased as would be expected with the higher concentrations of clotting factors.[14]

Plasminogen concentration is markedly raised in pregnancy as are fibrin degradation products suggesting increased fibrinolysis.[15] This is offset by plasminogen

Table 2.1 Coagulation at term

Parameter	Change*
Factor I (fibrinogen)	+100%
Factor II (prothrombin)	No change
Factor V (proaccelerin)	No change
Factor VII (proconvertin)	+100%
Factor VIII (antihemophilic factor)	+150%
Factor IX (Christmas factor)	+100%
Factor X (Stuart–Power factor)	+30%
Factor XI (thromboplastin antecedent)	+40%
Factor XII (Hageman factor)	+30%
Factor XIII (fibrin-stabilizing factor)	−50%
Platelet count	−5%
Prothrombin time	Shortened (20%)
Partial thromboplastin time	Shortened (20%)
Bleeding time	Shortened (10%)
Fibrin degradation products	+100%

*Changes relative to values for non-pregnant individuals.

activator inhibitors, produced by the placenta. Antithrombin III concentration decreases.[11]

Overall in pregnancy there appears to be a state of accelerated but compensated fibrinolysis.[15]

The platelet count is slightly reduced in pregnancy with 8% of women becoming mildly thrombocytopenic by term (Table 2.1).[16,17]

PLASMA PROTEINS

The total plasma protein concentration in pregnancy falls from 70 to 60 g/l largely because of a reduced plasma albumin concentration, (this falls from 35 to 25 g/l by term). The production of albumin remains constant but as plasma volume rises, plasma albumin concentration falls. The globulin concentration increases slightly. Overall the effect is to reduce colloid osmotic pressure (from 288 to 277 mOsm/kg) and to increase the risk of oedema formation. This is particularly important in those mother's with cardio-respiratory compromise, who may develop pulmonary oedema.[18] Plasma cholinesterase activity decreases by 30% during pregnancy,[19] although this is not clinically significant (Table 2.2).

Table 2.2 Plasma proteins and colloid osmotic pressure

	Non-pregnant	Term
Albumin↓ (g%)	4.4	3.4
Globulin↑ (g%)	2.9	3.1
A/G ratio*	1.5	1.1
Total protein (g%)	7.3	6.5
COP** (mmHg)	26	22

*Albumin to globulin ratio.
**Colloid osmotic pressure.

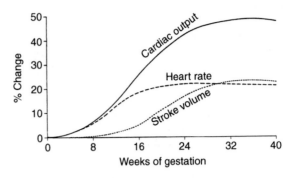

Figure 2.2 Haemodynamic parameters during pregnancy.

THE PUERPERIUM

Immediately after delivery, if blood loss has not been excessive, there is a further rise in blood volume. As extravascular fluid returns to the intravascular space, the haematocrit and haemoglobin concentration fall. Renal excretion of water occurs within the first week of the puerperium and a rise in the haematocrit follows. At the end of the puerperium the blood volume falls to 10% above pre-pregnancy levels.[20] In iron replete individuals the haemoglobin concentration and haematocrit rise to non-pregnant levels by 6 weeks after delivery.

Colloid osmotic pressure is uniformly lowered in the early postpartum period, in some cases to levels which increase the risk of pulmonary oedema in susceptible individuals.[21]

Plasma albumin concentration and colloid osmotic pressure usually return to normal within 6 weeks of delivery. Plasma cholinesterase levels may be slightly lower after delivery.[19]

Clotting factors initially increase in the puerperium. Increased levels of antithrombin III and plasminogen activators, which slightly offset the tendency to thrombosis at this time, accompany this. The coagulation and fibrinolytic systems revert to normal over the ensuing 6 weeks after delivery.[22] Plasma fibrinolysis returns to normal within hours of delivery.[23]

THE CARDIOVASCULAR SYSTEM

INTRODUCTION

The cardiovascular system undergoes remarkable change in pregnancy. These changes enhance the blood supply to the uterus, maintain fetal growth, and support changes in the breast in preparation for lactation. Increased circulation to the maternal kidneys enhance excretion and to the skin enhance heat loss through radiation.

Most of the cardiovascular changes are well underway by the first 8 weeks of pregnancy.[24] Longitudinal studies have shown that significant changes take place long before they are functionally necessary[25]. Fetal requirements are exceeded for the duration of the pregnancy (Fig. 2.2).

The stimulus behind cardiovascular adaptation is probably endocrine. There is a marked decrease in systemic vascular tone, perhaps induced by prostaglandins.[26] This triggers a compensatory increase in heart rate and stroke volume and activation of volume restoring mechanisms. A high flow, low resistance circulation is thus established in early pregnancy.[27] Oestrogen infusions has been shown to mimic the changes of reduced systemic vascular resistance and increased cardiac output.[28] Non-pregnant women receiving oestrogen demonstrate enhanced myocardial contractility.[29]

CLINICAL FINDINGS

The apex beat is palpated in the fourth intercostal space and lateral to the left mid-clavicular line. On auscultation the first heart sound is usually loud and may be split. There is reduced variation of the second sound with respiration. A third heart sound is commonly heard. A systolic murmur, loudest along the left sternal edge, is heard in most pregnant women.[30] This, may be due to regurgitation across a dilated tricuspid valve.[31] Diastolic murmurs are uncommon and a pathological cause should be sought. A continuous murmur is occasionally heard and usually is attributable to blood flow through the internal mammary vessels.[32]

The arterial pulse rate is increased by up to 16 beats/min[33] and the pulse is collapsing in nature.

CHEST X-RAY AND ECHOCARDIOGRAPH

Radiological investigation reveals the heart to be displaced upwards and rotated with a slight increase in the cardiothoracic ratio. There is straightening of the upper left cardiac border with increased prominence of the pulmonary conus.

Echocardiography shows a small increase in heart size due to increased venous filling.[29] Left ventricular hypertrophy is seen and begins in the first trimester.[34]

THE ELECTROCARDIOGRAM

The electrocardiogram (ECG) reflects the altered heart position with left axis deviation of 15° or more. There may be an S wave in lead 1 and a Q or inverted T wave in lead 3. No Q wave should be seen in lead AVF. The QRS complex tends to be of lower voltage in pregnancy, with depressed ST segments and low voltage T waves in the left chest leads. Atrial and ventricular extrasystoles are common.

CARDIAC OUTPUT

One of the most profound changes in pregnancy is the increase in cardiac output. When measured at 36–38 weeks of pregnancy, cardiac output is increased by 43% compared with measurements made at 11–13 weeks postpartum.[35] The increase in cardiac output is progressive during the first and second trimesters and is detectable as early as 8 weeks gestation.[24] Cardiac output does not change further in the third trimester. The increase in cardiac output is due to increases in both heart rate and stroke volume.

Heart rate increases first and rises by up to 16 beats/min by term.[33] Stroke volume increased from 65 ml before pregnancy to 83 ml in the second trimester.[24] Combined Doppler and cross-sectional echocardiography have been used to assess cardiac function in pregnancy.[36] There is great variation between and within individuals. Primarily, increased maternal vascular volume drives the haemodynamic changes (Table 2.3). Because the maternal heart responds to an increased pre-load by increasing stroke volume, pathology that limits diastolic flow through the ventricles is poorly tolerated.

AORTO-CAVAL COMPRESSION

The greatest rise in cardiac output is seen in the first and second trimesters. The amount and direction of change in the third trimester has been the subject of great controversy as values vary depending on the position of the subject when the measurement

Table 2.3 Haemodynamic changes at term	
Parameter	Change*
Cardiac output	+50%
Stroke volume	+25%
Heart rate	+20%
Left ventricular end-diastolic volume	Increased
Left ventricular end-systolic volume	No change
Ejection fraction	Increased
Left ventricular stroke work index	No change
Pulmonary capillary wedge pressure	No change
Central venous pressure	No change
Systemic vascular resistance	−20%

*Changes relative to values for non-pregnant individuals.
From Conklin KA. *Semin Anesth* 1991; **10**: 221–234.

is made. Maternal hypotension associated with the supine position in late pregnancy was first recognized in 1942.[37] That this was due to inferior vena caval compression, rather than displacement of the heart and diaphragm was not initially appreciated. Eleven per cent of term pregnant women made to lie on their backs developed hypotension within 3–7 min.[38] In 1965 Kerr injected radio-opaque dye and showed that the term uterus impeded venous return by obstructing the inferior vena cava.[39] There was some collateral return via the paravertebral and azygous systems and through the ovarian veins. Such collateral flow was often not sufficient to prevent a drop in right atrial pressure and cardiac output. An additional factor was compression of the aorta by the uterus, increasing after-load and again reducing cardiac output. Angiography in women in the third trimester has shown that in the supine position the aorta is both compressed and displaced[40] reducing placental perfusion in the supine position.[41] As would be expected, there is evidence to suggest reduced fetal cerebral oxygenation if the mother adopts the supine position at term.[42]

Cardiac output studies in primiparous women who consented to pulmonary artery catheterization between 36 and 38 weeks gestation have been carried out. Cardiac output, which was 6.6 l/min in the left lateral position, fell to 6.0 l/min in the supine position and 5.4 l/min in the standing position.[43] The importance of avoiding aorto-caval compression in late pregnancy cannot be overstated. The supine position must always be avoided though in a few women aorto-caval compression may still occur in the semi-recumbent position, or even whilst standing. It may be in these cases that the collateral venous system is poorly developed or that increased parasympathetic tone increases the likelihood of bradycardia.[45] Aorto-caval compression is also more likely to develop in multiple-pregnancy, polyhydramnios, and maternal obesity, and can occur from as early as the beginning of the second trimester.

If aorto-caval compression is allowed to persist, symptoms of the supine hypotensive syndrome occur. The mother begins to feel anxious, sweaty, nauseated and eventually becomes profoundly hypotensive. Abnormal fetal heart rate patterns may develop, signifying fetal compromise through hypoxia and acidosis.[44] Treatment consists of turning the patient from the supine to the lateral position with the administration of oxygen to the mother.[46]

If compensatory reflexes are obtunded or abolished by regional or general anaesthesia, then marked maternal hypotension and fetal distress may develop in the supine position. If the full lateral position is impractical, for example, during a Caesarean section, then 15° of lateral tilt must be achieved. During cardiac arrest it is necessary to undertake Caesarean delivery of a fetus in order to increase the chances of maternal survival if cardiopulmonary resuscitation remains ineffective after 5 minutes, to alleviate the effects of aorto-caval compression.[47]

BLOOD PRESSURE

There is a gradual fall in blood pressure during pregnancy.[48] Systolic blood pressure falls on average by 5–10 mmHg, whilst the fall in diastolic blood pressure is of the order of 10–15 mmHg.[49] This difference results in an increase in pulse pressure. Systolic and diastolic blood pressure reaches their lowest values in the second trimester and then increase to reach pre-pregnancy levels again at term. It must be remembered that the first blood pressure measurement recorded in the patient's maternity record is usually taken during the first trimester when the normal decrease in blood pressure has already begun.

VASCULAR RESISTANCE

Systemic and pulmonary vascular resistance both decrease significantly in pregnancy.[35] The former is in part related to the development of a low resistance utero-placental circulation and is in part due to progesterone driven vasodilatation. The blood vessels of pregnant women show increased refractoriness to angiotensin II.[50] This may be mediated by endothelial and platelet derived prostaglandins. Reliable measurements of prostaglandins are difficult to obtain because of their low plasma concentrations, but metabolites of the vasodilator prostacyclin are markedly increased in pregnancy.[51] Less information is available about the vasoconstrictor thromboxane, but one of its breakdown products has been found in decreased concentrations in pregnancy.[52] Progesterone may modulate prostaglandin mediated vascular responsiveness to angiotensin II.[53] Nitric oxide is also likely to be an important regulator of maternal blood pressure.[54] Calcitonin gene related peptide has been found to be increased in pregnancy and may have a role in promoting vasodilatation and increased cardiac output.[55]

Although vascular resistance is lowered, the increased blood flow is not uniformly distributed. By term the blood flow to the uterus has increased from a pre-pregnancy level of 50–190 to 700–800 ml/min. The uterus receives approximately 10% of the cardiac output. Blood flow to the breasts doubles, to make up 2% of the cardiac output. These increases are largely at the expense of blood flow to the splanchnic bed and skeletal muscle. The proportion of blood flow to the kidney, skin, brain and coronary circulations remains unaltered although the absolute flow is increased. Enhanced blood flow to the skin allows dissipation of heat from the uterine circulation, as the fetus is 1°C warmer than the mother.

CENTRAL VENOUS PRESSURE

No significant changes in central venous pressure or pulmonary capillary wedge pressure have been found in normal pregnancy when compared with values measured at 11–13 weeks post-partum.[35] This reflects the marked reduction in systemic and pulmonary vascular resistance which accommodates the increased intravascular volume at normal vascular pressures. As colloid osmotic pressure falls in pregnancy,[56] the normal pulmonary capillary wedge pressure implies a greater risk of pulmonary oedema if, for example, large volumes of crystalloid are administered.[57]

ARTERIO-VENOUS OXYGEN DIFFERENCE

Oxygen consumption increases by approximately 16% in pregnancy. Because there is a proportionally greater rise in cardiac output, the arterio-venous oxygen difference decreases by 26%.[58] The reduced arterio-venous oxygen difference in pregnancy indicates that oxygen delivery exceeds oxygen consumption. More oxygen is therefore returned to the heart in pregnancy, supporting the notion that the slightly reduced haemoglobin concentration is of no consequence.

LABOUR

Cardiac output increases further in labour. Basal cardiac output between uterine contractions increases by 13% in the first stage of labour, compared with pre-labour values, as a result of an increase in stroke volume. During contractions there is a further increase in cardiac output, as a result of increases in both stroke volume and heart rate. Late in the first stage of labour, cardiac output increases by 34% with each contraction. Within 24 h of delivery, all haemodynamic variables return to pre-labour values.[59] Each uterine contraction pushes a further 300 ml of blood back into the central circulation.[60] Some of the increased cardiac output occurs because of the pain and apprehension of labour and can be partly attenuated by effective pain relief.[61]

ECG studies have shown that all patients develop a sinus tachycardia in labour (mean maximum heart rate 138/min) and that premature ventricular contractions are common.[62]

PUERPERIUM

Cardiac output remains elevated for the first 24 h after delivery and then falls progressively.[63] Cardiac output measured by Doppler and cross-sectional echocardiography showed a fall from a mean of 7.42 l/min at 38 weeks to 4.96 l/min at 24 weeks after delivery (a decrease of 33%). Most of this decrease (28%) had occurred by 2 weeks after delivery. This was associated with a 20% reduction in heart rate and an 18% reduction in stroke volume. No differences were found between lactating and non-lactating mothers.[64] The persistent elevation in the early puerperium is due to autotransfusion of blood from the uterus re-entering the central circulation. Relief of aorto-caval obstruction and rapid mobilization of extracellular fluid also contributes. This is obviously influenced by the amount of blood lost at delivery.

Maternal blood pressure is initially reduced but tends to increase toward the end of the first postnatal week.

THE RESPIRATORY SYSTEM

INTRODUCTION

The marked changes in the respiratory system in pregnancy occur in tandem with changes in the cardiovascular system, resulting in increased oxygen uptake and carbon dioxide elimination.

ANATOMY

Generalized vasodilatation occurs in the skin and mucous membranes in pregnancy.[65] This effect is due to progesterone mediated relaxation of vascular smooth muscle. Capillary engorgement of the mucosal lining of the nose, oropharynx and larynx may lead the pregnant woman to report voice changes, difficulty with nasal breathing and occasionally episodes of epistaxis.[66] Oedema due to pre-eclampsia or upper respiratory tract infection is likely to exacerbate this.

Profound changes also occur in the lower respiratory tract in pregnancy. Although the diaphragm is elevated (up to 4 cm), this is not entirely due to uterine enlargement, but also the result of an increase in chest wall circumference because of splaying of the ribs. The sub-costal angle increases from 68° to 103°[67] and the circumference of the thoracic cage increases by 5–7 cm. Many women are aware of these changes in their rib cage during pregnancy, especially as they begin in the first trimester, long before the uterus impinges on the diaphragm. Elevation does not appear to hinder diaphragmatic movement. Indeed: fluoroscopy studies have shown that excursion increases by 1–2 cm. The diaphragmatic contribution to ventilation becomes proportionately greater as the abdominal muscles are less active in pregnancy.[68] By term, inspiration is largely accomplished by diaphragmatic movement.[69]

RADIOGRAPHY

The lung markings on chest X-ray are essentially normal, though occasionally they may be accentuated as a result of increased filling of the pulmonary vascular tree and a reduction in lung volume in expiration.

LUNG VOLUMES

During pregnancy, the tidal volume increases gradually with gestation. By term it is almost 40% greater than in non-pregnant women.[70] Functional residual capacity falls progressively starting in the second trimester. Upward displacement of the relaxed diaphragm causes a reduction in functional residual capacity by as much as 25%.[71] Similar reductions occur in the residual volume and expiratory reserve volume.[72] Functional residual capacity falls further when supine.[73] The increase in tidal volume and inspiratory reserve volume is roughly equivalent to the decrease in residual volume and expiratory reserve volume. The total lung capacity is slightly reduced but the vital capacity is unchanged (Fig. 2.3).[74]

Minute ventilation is increased by 40% in pregnancy.[70] This change is detectable by 6 weeks. The increase is

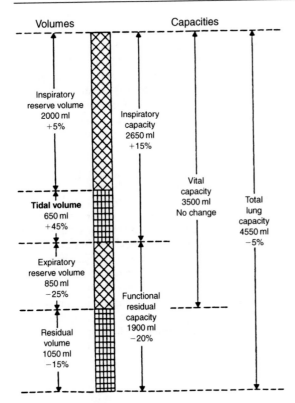

Volumes   Capacities

Inspiratory
reserve volume
2000 ml
+5%

Inspiratory
capacity
2650 ml
+15%

Tidal volume
650 ml
+45%

Vital
capacity
3500 ml
No change

Total
lung
capacity
4550 ml
−5%

Expiratory
reserve volume
850 ml
−25%

Functional
residual
capacity
1900 ml
−20%

Residual
volume
1050 ml
−15%

Figure 2.3   Lung volumes and capacities at term gestation in absolute volumes and as the percentage change from non-pregnant values.

largely due to an increased tidal volume as respiratory rate changes little. Alveolar ventilation rises by a similar degree; thus the ratio of dead space to tidal volume remains unchanged in pregnancy.[75] Physiological dead space may increase due to dilatation of the smaller bronchioles.[76]

The increased minute ventilation, which occurs early in pregnancy, is probably due to progesterone which lowers the carbon dioxide response threshold of the respiratory centre,[77] and may act as a primary stimulant.[78] Increased minute ventilation has been found in the second half of the menstrual cycle when circulating progesterone levels are increased.[79] (Indeed progesterone has been used as a therapeutic respiratory stimulant in patients with Pickwickian syndrome.[80]) The production of carbon dioxide is increased as the pregnancy advances,[81] but the changes of increased ventilation and reduced P_aCO_2 precede this.

Normal oxygen consumption in non-pregnant women at rest is 250 ml/min. In pregnancy this is increased by up to 16% by the demands of the uterus and its contents and also the increased maternal cardiac, renal

and respiratory activity.[82] The respiratory quotient increases from a pre-pregnancy value of 0.76–0.83 in late pregnancy.[83]

AIRWAY RESISTANCE

Airway resistance depends on large airway calibre and is unchanged in pregnancy.[84] The potential bronchial dilatatory effects of progesterone and PGE_2 are matched by the reduced resting lung volume and PGF_2. Small airway volume, (estimated by measurement of closing volume), may increase slightly, but does not encroach on normal tidal volumes.[85]

BLOOD GASES

Increased minute ventilation reduces the alveolar and therefore the arterial partial pressure of carbon dioxide. In late pregnancy the P_aCO_2 is typically 3.6–4.3 kPa compared with 5.3 kPa in the non-pregnant state.[86] The fall in P_aCO_2 is even greater at high altitudes where pregnant women hyperventilate to a greater degree.[87] The low maternal P_aCO_2 facilitates the excretion of fetal carbon dioxide across the placenta. It is generally agreed that the process begins early in pregnancy and precedes the increase in oxygen demand. The consequent respiratory alkalosis is compensated by a reduced plasma bicarbonate (18 mEq/l). Plasma pH tends to be at the upper end of the normal range.[88]

The partial pressure of oxygen in maternal arterial blood is usually slightly increased.[89] Although oxygen consumption rises by 16%,[82] the cardiac output increases to a greater extent; thus the arterio-venous oxygen difference is reduced and venous admixture has less effect on P_aO_2.

P_aO_2 may drop when supine

Dependent airway closure is liable to occur during tidal breathing[73] in the supine position.

Aorto-caval compression reduces cardiac output oxygen, and extraction must therefore increase to compensate. Turning the mother to the lateral position will improve her oxygen saturation.[90]

GAS TRANSFER

Gas transfer falls by 15% in pregnancy because of the reduced haemoglobin concentration. There may also be an oestrogen related effect on the alveolar–capillary wall.[91]

DYSPNOEA

Many women notice dyspnoea in pregnancy, with almost half becoming symptomatic by 19 weeks gestation.[92] It is reported as a feeling of laboured or unnaturally difficult breathing. After 31 weeks, few mothers report an increase in their symptoms.

LABOUR

During labour there is a further increase in both respiratory rate and tidal volume, the magnitude of which largely correlates with the degree of pain experienced. Without analgesia, the labouring woman shows the greatest hyperventilatory response, with marked hypocapnia, (P_aCO_2 as low as 2 kPa).[93] Minute ventilation and oxygen consumption increases markedly as labour progresses.[94]

In the presence of effective neuraxial analgesia, the rises in minute ventilation and oxygen consumption that occur with uterine contractions are significantly attenuated.[95] During the active phase of the second stage, minute ventilation and oxygen consumption are increased despite provision of effective analgesia, because of the series of extreme valsalva manoeuvres required to deliver the fetus.

PUERPERIUM

Expiratory muscle strength is reduced for up to 4 h after normal delivery in healthy women. This is especially relevant after general anaesthesia as there is a reduced ability to cough after general anaesthesia.[96]

The return to pre-pregnancy respiratory physiology occurs within a fortnight of birth.

THE GASTROINTESTINAL TRACT

THE MOUTH

Hyperplastic gingivitis has been associated with pregnancy[97] and there is an increase in dental caries, possibly due to an increase in acidophilic bacteria, calcium deficiency and increased sex hormones.

THE UPPER GASTROINTESTINAL TRACT

Pregnancy is associated with a generalized relaxation and decreased motility of the gastrointestinal tract.[98] There are several theories to explain this which encompass the smooth muscle relaxing properties of progesterone,[99,100] decreased motilin levels[101] and mechanical factors.[102]

In 1941 Williams[102] published a treatise on heartburn in pregnancy. He noted that although not a threat to life, heartburn is certainly a contributor to a marked diminution in quality of life. He felt that it was related to temperament, being more common in the 'highly-strung'. He discounted the common theory at that time that it was related to gastric hyperacidity, and indeed, gastric acidity has since been shown to decease with gestation.[103] His data indicated that any fluid, of whatever acidity, could cause symptoms.

X-ray and fluoroscopic imaging has clarified the anatomic changes of the stomach during pregnancy. The long axis of the stomach is approximately parallel with the spinal column, with the lesser curve to the right and the cardia opposite the tenth dorsal vertebra. By term the uterus pushes the fundus upwards and into the left diaphragmatic cup. Simultaneously the axis of the stomach is rotated to the right by approximately 45° and the greater curvature approaches the cardia. This relatively horizontal position may hinder gastric emptying. The majority of pregnant women with heartburn investigated with barium screening, revealed no pathological anatomical alterations, although in three cases dilatation of the lower third of the oesophagus was noted.[102]

Heartburn is extremely common in women and is often believed to be part-and-parcel of normal pregnancy. Bassey[104] found that whilst 78.8% of Caucasians admitted to the symptom, only 9.8% of Nigerians did so. Both groups were UK residents. Nigerian women tend to have a diet high in carbohydrate and residue and are less likely to become constipated. Straining tends to displace the lower oesophageal sphincter into the thorax where reflux is more likely due to the negative resting pressure in the chest. Bassey, using oesophageal manometry, found that the lower oesophageal sphincter pressure in normal pregnancy was lower than in non-pregnant controls, and found that in two pregnant women with heartburn, the low resting sphincter pressures were present with the sphincters displaced into the thorax. He concluded that if upward displacement of the lower oesophageal sphincter causes heartburn in pregnancy, patients with a sphincter, which is partly displaced before pregnancy begins, must be more liable to develop pregnancy heartburn. He offered this as the explanation for the racial differences in the prevalence of this symptom.

GASTRIC EMPTYING

It is widely believed that gastric emptying is delayed in pregnancy. At present the evidence for this is poor, with several conflicting results. Early studies relied on radiological investigations, which would be considered unethical today. The results of such studies are themselves conflicting, suggested an increase in gastric emptying;[105] little difference[106] and delay in emptying.[102] Later studies using a water test meal and double sampling technique in non-pregnant, pregnant and labouring women revealed that mean gastric emptying time was significantly increased in pregnant women. However the mean volume of fluid remaining in the stomach 30 minutes after eating was not significantly increased in this group. In those experiencing heartburn and all those in labour, there was clear evidence of impaired emptying. In the latter, the physiological effects of the pain and emotional disturbance associated with labour,[107] were assumed to be the cause. However, recent work indicates that delay in gastric emptying may in fact be due to administration of narcotics in labour.[108,109]

The rate of paracetamol absorption has been used to study gastric emptying. As paracetamol is not absorbed from the stomach but from the upper small bowel, the rate of absorption depends on the rate of gastric emptying, hence the value of this type of investigation. Simpson and colleagues[110] found that absorption of paracetamol was delayed in women who were 12–14 weeks gestation compared with non-pregnant controls. This study was followed by that of Macfie and colleagues[111] also using paracetamol absorption, which failed to demonstrate any significant delay in gastric emptying during the three trimesters of pregnancy. The authors suggested that the delay found in the earlier study could have been due to the study group adopting the supine position, which may exaggerate the tendency to delay. Stanley and colleagues[112] studied paracetamol absorption immediately after a meal and found a slight, but not significant, delay in gastric emptying present by 14–16 weeks gestation when compared with non-pregnant values.

Motilin is a possible mediator of changes in gastric emptying in pregnancy. Motilin is required for the initiation of antro-duodenal migration, therefore low levels might cause hypomobility. It has been shown that plasma motilin and somatostatin (an inhibitor of motilin release) are both significantly increased in the third trimester of pregnancy and postpartum compared with non-pregnant controls. This finding does not support the concept of motilin playing a role in the gastrointestinal hypomobility of pregnancy, rather it may be postulated that raised levels may be a compensatory mechanism to restore any postulated diminution of gastrointestinal mobility.[113] Christofides and colleagues[101] found the opposite and reported decreased motilin levels between 16–36 weeks gestation.

THE SMALL BOWEL

Small bowel transit time has been shown to be significantly increased in pregnancy.[114] The transit of a mercury-loaded bag was followed by screening with an image intensifier in 30 volunteers. This delay could explain the common complaint of constipation in pregnant women. Absorption itself is more efficient in the small bowel in pregnancy, further adding to the problems of constipation.[115]

THYROID FUNCTION IN PREGNANCY

The thyroid gland, usually impalpable, and weighing approximately 10–20 g in the non-pregnant woman, enlarges in pregnancy. This is due to relative hyperstimulation of the gland in early pregnancy, which is exaggerated by associated iodine deficiency. Pre-existing goitres and nodules may also enlarge.[116]

Levels of the thyroid hormones T3 and T4 fluctuate in pregnancy. Hepatic synthesis of thyroxine-binding globulin (TBG), is stimulated by high levels of oestrogen. Both total and free T3 and T4 are raised in early pregnancy and suppress thyroxine-stimulating-hormone (TSH) occasionally resulting in levels usually associated with hyperthyroidism.[117]

Human chorionic gonadotrophin, secreted by the placenta, has been demonstrated to have a thyroid stimulating effect, both in vitro and in vivo. It is structurally similar to TSH, with which it shares an alpha subunit. An inverse correlation between serum hCG and TSH levels is clearly demonstrated in women with hyperemesis gravidarum, twin pregnancies, and hydatidiform mole, in whom the levels of serum hCG are higher than normal.[118] Women with trophoblastic tumours may develop overt hyperthyroidism, which resolves with the treatment of the tumour. Antithyroid drugs are occasionally required, especially if the patient becomes symptomatic, or develops extremely raised levels of T3 and T4.[119]

In the third trimester the levels of free T3 and T4 decrease with a corresponding increase in TSH. This may be due to an increased demand for thyroxine by the fetus. The levels of serum TBG and total T3 and T4 however, continue to rise, although hCG levels plateau. Several studies have suggested that the thyroid stimulating activity in late pregnancy is thought to be due to another, as yet undiscovered hormone or growth factor.[120] Thyroid disease is the fifth most common disorder in the general obstetric medicine clinic.[121] If thyroid dysfunction is missed there is an increased risk of fetal loss. Autoimmune hyperthyroidism has been shown to increase the risk of meiotic non-dysfunction and Down's syndrome, as well as other chromosomal anomalies.[122] The risk of spontaneous abortion, intrauterine growth retardation, fetal and neo-natal death are all increased in women with pre-existing hyperthyroidism.[123] Hypothyroidism is associated with anovulatory menstrual cycles and is therefore rare in pregnancy. When it does occur it is also associated with a high risk of fetal loss. Thyroxine is required for development of the fetal central nervous system. The fetal thyroid gland cannot meet the demand, and maternal thyroid hormones cross the placenta. Autoimmune antibodies that stimulate or block the effect of TSH also cross the placenta and can cause transitory hyper- or hypothyroidism in the neonate.[124] The relative risk of postnatal depression is thought to be 1.7 in patients with autoimmune thyroid dysfunction.[125]

THE MUSCULOSKELETAL SYSTEM

CALCIUM HOMEOSTASIS

Maternal calcium levels are affected by the demands of the growing fetus. The fetus is hypercalcaemic compared to its mother and approximately 30 g of calcium is transferred across the placenta under the influence of parathyroid hormone related peptide, secreted by the fetal parathyroid glands. Pregnancy and lactation result in bone de-mineralization, which starts early in the first trimester. These changes occur mainly in trabecular bone, and the overall effect is a deficit on average of 3.6% in bone density.[126]

Heparin prophylaxis for 7 weeks has been shown to produce symptomatic vertebral fractures in 2.2% of pregnant women, with a loss in bone density of 5.2% in trabecular bone.[127] Lactation not only reduces oestrogen levels but leads to a loss of 4–6 mg/kg of calcium per day. The resulting loss of bone density has been estimated at 6% over a 6-month period.[128] However women who breast-feed for 6 months or more or who become pregnant again within 18 months, were not found to be more at risk.[129,130]

Back pain during pregnancy occurs frequently, sometimes as early as the first trimester. It is suggested that back pain starting in pregnancy may have a completely different aetiology to that pre-dating pregnancy.[131] Peri-partum pelvic pain is associated with primaparity, especially at a later age, large babies, twin pregnancies, operative vaginal delivery and flexion of the spine during childbirth. It does not appear to be causally associated with delivery by Caesarean section,

or neuraxial block for anaesthesia or analgesia. It is thought to be due to a strain on the ligaments of the pelvis and spine from hormonal effects, muscle weakness and fetal weight, as well as pre-pregnancy ligamentous injury.[132]

RELAXIN

Relaxin is a hormone or hormone complex produced by the ovaries in pregnancy. In animal studies it has been found to relax pelvic joints, inhibit the uterine myometrium, and soften and increase the distensibility of the cervix and lower uterine segment.[133] Its effect may increase the mothers susceptibility to back strain and injury.

THE SPINE

The pregnant uterus presses the aorta and inferior vena cava against the bodies of the lumbar vertebrae, causing engorgement of the extradural venous plexuses. At 32 weeks gestation, complete occlusion of the inferior vena cava may occur in the supine position. The engorged vertebral veins push the dura posteriorly, away from the wall of the vertebral canal, resulting in a reduction in the volume of cerebrospinal fluid at that level. The reduction in the capacity of the extradural and subarachnoid space may contribute to pregnancy-induced enhancement of regional anaesthesia.[134] The pH of cerebrospinal fluid is raised and P_aCO_2 lowered very early in pregnancy, but the relevance of this is not known.[135]

THE KIDNEYS AND LOWER URINARY TRACT

RENAL FUNCTION

Effective renal plasma flow (ERPF) is increased by up to 80% in early pregnancy, but falls to 60% in the third trimester. This increase is due to the relative hypervolaemia of pregnancy, an increased cardiac output, and the increased secretion of hormones such as aldosterone, cortisol, prolactin and human placental lactogen.[136]

The glomerular filtration rate (GFR) is elevated by 50% above the non-pregnant level throughout pregnancy. The filtration fraction (GFR/ERPF) is significantly reduced in early pregnancy but rises until almost that of the non-pregnant patient during the third trimester.[137]

Serum uric acid levels fall below non-pregnant levels by 8 weeks gestation. However, after 24 weeks, the concentration increases steadily to above non-pregnant values at term and remains elevated for up to 12 weeks postpartum. This is thought to be due to alterations in the renal handling of uric acid, which is re-absorbed in increasing amounts as pregnancy progresses, causing an increase in maternal serum concentrations.[138]

URETERIC AND BLADDER CHANGES

The size of the kidneys within 1 week of delivery has been found to be increased by up to 2 cm, with a mean shrinkage of 1 cm occurring over the following 6 months. Non-obstructive dilatation of the lumbar segment of the right ureter is almost always present, and the left ureter is often also dilated.[139] The ureters are compressed by the gravid uterus or engorged ovarian veins, the left ureter being relatively spared by the interposition of the sigmoid colon.

Raised levels of gonadotrophins and progesterone cause tissue oedema and hypertrophy of ureteric muscle, causing the ureters to become hypotonic and dilated. The epithelium of the bladder and urethra are relatively hyperaemic and high oestrogen levels cause squamous metaplasia in the urethral epithelium.[140]

Pregnancy and vaginal delivery are a major contributory factors for stress incontinence, due to damage of the pelvic floor fascia, musculature and their innovation.[141] Pelvic floor exercises during pregnancy may be helpful in reducing stress incontinence in the later years.

Asymptomatic bacteriuria occurs in 2–10% of pregnancies. The hypotonicity of the ureters increases the likelihood of reflux of urine; 25% of women will develop symptomatic upper urinary tract infection, which may result in premature labour. Scaring of the kidneys is a possible long-term effect.[142]

Urinary retention may occur post-delivery. Painless over-distention, if allowed to occur, may give rise to long-term voiding dysfunction.[143]

THE PANCREAS AND CARBOHYDRATE METABOLISM

Increased levels of progesterone and oestrogen in pregnancy are thought to cause hypertrophy of the beta islet cells of the pancreas.[144] These cells show an increased sensitivity to glucose and secrete more insulin, for a given serum concentration, compared to the non-pregnant state.[145] This is possibly in response to the rise in levels of hormones with anti-insulin activity such as cortisol, human placental lactogen, progesterone, prolactin and oestrogen, levels of which show a progressive rise from approximately

10 weeks onwards.[146] Gestational diabetes is a common problem.

Pregnancy has little or no effect on the alpha cells, and consequently there is little or no change in glucagon levels.[147]

Glucose crosses the placental barrier by facilitated diffusion. This appears to protect the fetus from excessively high maternal levels, and the fetal pancreas is protected from over stimulation by postprandial rises in maternal serum glucose levels.[148]

A small number of women intermittently excrete large amounts of glucose via the kidneys (as much as 1 g in 24 h). This is thought to be due to increased GFR and a diminished ability of the proximal and distal renal tubules to re-absorb a glucose load.[149] Glucosuria has to be distinguished from gestational diabetes by serial blood glucose measurements.

The insulin response returns to normal almost immediately after delivery[150] but the recovery of normal glucose homeostasis, takes 5–6 weeks.

REFERENCES

1. Hytten FE, Leitch I. Cardiovascular dynamics in the volume and composition of the blood. *The physiology of human pregnancy*, 2nd edn. Oxford: Blackwell Scientific Publications, 1971, p 1.

2. Pritchard JA. Changes in the blood volume during pregnancy and delivery. *Anesthesiology* 1965; **26**: 393–399.

3. Landau RL, Lugibihl K. Inhibition of the sodium-retaining influence of aldosterone by progesterone. *J Clin Endocrinol Metab* 1958; **18**: 1237–1245.

4. Cusson JR, Gutowska J, Rey E, Michon N, Boucher M, Larochelle P. Plasma concentration of atrial natriuretic factor in normal pregnancy. *New Engl J Med* 1985; **313**: 1230–1231.

5. Pirani BBK, Campbell DM, MacGillivray I. Plasma volume in normal first pregnancy. *J Obstet Gynaecol Br Comm* 1973; **80**: 884–887.

6. Pritchard JA, Baldwin RM, Dickey JC, Wiggins KM. Blood volume changes in pregnancy and the puerperium. II. Red blood cell loss and changes in apparent blood volume during and following vaginal delivery, cesarean section, and cesarean section plus total hysterectomy. *Am J Obstet Gynecol* 1962; **84**: 1271–1282.

7. Hood DD, Holubec DM. Elective repeat cesarean section. Effect of anesthesia type on blood loss. *J Reprod Med* 1990; **35**: 368–372.

8. Pitkin RM, Witte DL. Platelet and leukocyte counts in pregnancy. *JAMA* 1979; **242**: 2696–2698.

9. Tygart SG, McRoyan DK, Spinnato JA, McRoyan CJ, Kitay DZ. Longitudinal study of platelet indices

during normal pregnancy. *Am J Obstet Gynecol* 1986; **154**: 883–887.

10. Forbes CD, Greer IA. Physiology of haemostasis and the effect of pregnancy. In: Greer IA, Turpie AGG, Forbes CD (eds) *Haemostasis and thrombosis in obstetrics and gynaecology.* London: Chapman and Hall Medical, pp 1–25.

11. Van Royen EA, Ten-Cate JW. Antigen biological activity ratio for Factor VIII in late pregnancy. *Lancet* 1973; **ii**: 449–450.

12. Ozanne P, Linderkamp O, Miller FC, Meiselman HJ. Erythrocyte aggregation during normal pregnancy. *Am J Obstet Gynecol* 1983; **147**: 576–583.

13. Watts DH, Krohn MA, Wener M, Eschenbach DA. C-reactive protein in normal pregnancy. *Obstet Gynecol* 1991; **77**: 176–180.

14. Talbert LM, Langdell RD. Normal values of certain factors in the blood clotting mechanism in pregnancy. *Am J Obstet Gynecol* 1964; **90**: 44–50.

15. Gerbasi FR, Bottoms S, Farag A, Mammen E. Increased intravascular coagulation associated with pregnancy. *Obstet Gynecol* 1990; **75**: 385–389.

16. Sill PR, Lind T, Walker W. Platelet values during normal pregnancy. *Br J Obstet Gynaecol* 1985; **92**: 480–483.

17. Burrows RF, Kelton JG. Incidentally detected thrombocytopenia in healthy mothers and their infants. *New Engl J Med* 1988; **319**: 142–145.

18. Wu PY, Udani V, Chan L, Miller FC, Henneman CE. Colloid osmotic pressure: variations in normal pregnancy. *J Perinat Med* 1983; **11**: 193–199.

19. Leighton BL, Cheek TG, Gross JB, Apfelbaum JL, Shantz BB, Gutsche BB, Rosenberg H. Succinylcholine pharmacodynamics in peripartum patients. *Anesthesiology* 1986; **64**: 202–205.

20. Lund CJ, Donovan JC. Blood volume during pregnancy: significance of plasma and red cell volumes. *Am J Obstet Gynecol* 1967; **98**: 393–403.

21. Cotton DB, Gonik B, Spillman T, Dorman KF. Intrapartum to postpartum changes in colloid osmotic pressure. *Am J Obstet Gynecol* 1984; **149**: 174–177.

22. Bonnar J, McNicol GP, Douglas AS. Fibrinolytic enzyme system and pregnancy. *Br Med J* 1969; **3**: 387–389.

23. Bonnar J, McNicol GP, Douglas AS. Coagulation and fibrinolytic mechanisms during and after normal childbirth. *Br Med J* 1970; **2**: 200–203.

24. Capeless EL, Clapp JF. Cardiovascular changes in early phase of pregnancy. *Am J Obstet Gynecol* 1989; **161**: 1449–1453.

25. Clapp JF, Seaward BL, Sleamaker RH, Hiser J. Maternal physiologic adaptations to early human pregnancy. *Am J Obstet Gynecol* 1988; **159**: 1456–1460.

26. Broughton Pipkin F, Morrison R, O'Brien PMS. The effect of prostaglandin E$_1$ upon the pressor and hormonal response to exogenous angiotensin II in human pregnancy. *Clin Sci* 1987; **72**: 351–357.

27. Duvekot JJ, Cheriex EC, Pieters FA, Menheere PP, Peeters LL. Early pregnancy changes in hemodynamics and volume homeostasis are consecutive adjustments triggered by a primary fall in systemic vascular tone. *Am J Obstet Gynecol* 1993; **169**: 1382–1392.

28. Ueland K, Parer JT. Effects of estrogens on the cardiovascular system of the ewe. *Am J Obstet Gynecol* 1966; **96**: 400–406.

29. Rubler S, Damani PM, Pinto ER. Cardiac size and performance during pregnancy estimated with echocardiography. *Am J Cardiol* 1977; **40**: 534–540.

30. Cutforth R, MacDonald CB. Heart sounds and murmurs in pregnancy. *Am Heart J* 1966; **71**: 741–747.

31. Limacher MC, Ware JA, O'Meara ME, Fernandez GC, Young JB. Tricuspid regurgitation during pregnancy; two dimensional and pulsed Doppler echocardiographic observations. *Am J Cardiol* 1985; **55**: 1059–1062.

32. Tabatznik B, Randall TW, Hersch C. The mammary souffle of pregnancy and lactation. *Circulation* 1960; **22**: 1069–1073.

33. Clapp JF. Maternal heart rate in pregnancy. *Am J Obstet Gynecol* 1985; **152**: 659–660.

34. Robson SC, Hunter S, Boys RJ, Dunlop W. Serial study of factors influencing changes in cardiac output during human pregnancy. *Am J Physiol* 1989; **256**: H1060–H1065.

35. Clark SL, Cotton DB, Lee W, Bishop C, Hill T, Southwick J et al. Central hemodynamic assessment of normal term pregnancy. *Am J Obstet Gynaecol* 1987; **161**: 1439–1442.

36. Robson SC, Dunlop W, Moore W, Hunter S. Combined Doppler and echocardiographic measurement of cardiac output: theory and application in pregnancy. *Br J Obstet Gynaecol* 1987; **94**: 1014–1027.

37. Hansen R. Oshnmacht und schwangerschaft. *Klin Wochenschr* 1942; **21**: 241–245.

38. Howard BK, Goodson JH, Mengert WF. Supine hypotensive syndrome in late pregnancy. *Obstet Gynecol* 1953; **1**: 371–377.

39. Kerr MG. The mechanical effects of the gravid uterus in late pregnancy. *J Obstet Gynaecol Br Comm* 1965; **72**: 513–529.

40. Bieniairz J, Crottogini JJ, Curuchet E, Romero-Salinas G, Yoshida T, Poseiro J, Caldeyro-Barcia R. Aortocaval compression by the uterus in late human pregnancy. *Am J Obstet Gynecol* 1968; **100**: 203–217.

41. Abitbol MM. Aortic compression and uterine blood flow during pregnancy. *Obstet Gynecol* 1977; **50**: 562–570.

42. Aldrich CJ, D'Antona D, Spencer JAD, Wyatt JS, Peebles DM, Delpy DT, Reynolds EOR. The effect of maternal posture on fetal cerebral oxygenation during labour. *Br J Obstet Gynaecol* 1995; **102**: 14–19.

43. Clark SL, Cotton DB, Pivarnik JM, Lee W, Hankins GDV, Benedetti TJ, Phelan JP. Position

change and central hemodynamic profile during normal third-trimester pregnancy and postpartum. *Am J Obstet Gynecol* 1991; **164**: 883–887.

44. Huch A, Huch R, Schneider H, Rooth G. Continuous transcutaneous monitoring of fetal oxygen tension during labour. *Br J Obstet Gynaecol* 1977; **84**(suppl): 1–39.

45. Kauppila A, Koskinen M, Puolakka J, Tuimala R, Kuikka J. Decreased intervillous and unchanged myometrial blood flow in supine recumbency. *Obstet Gynecol* 1980; **55**: 203–205.

46. Buley RJR, Downing JW, Brock-Utne JG, Cuerden C. Right versus left lateral tilt for caesarean section. *Br J Anaesth* 1977; **49**: 1009–1015.

47. Walkamir MS (ed). *Advanced life support in obstetrics course syllabus. Maternal resuscitation* (UK suppl), 3rd edn. Kansas, Missouri: American Academy of Family Physicians, 1996.

48. Katz R, Karliner JS, Resnik R. Effects of a natural volume overload state (pregnancy) on left ventricular performance in normal human subjects. *Circulation* 1978; **58**: 434–441.

49. MacGillivray I, Rose GA, Rowe B. Blood pressure survey in pregnancy. *Clin Sci* 1969; **37**: 395–407.

50. Gant NF, Daley GL, Chand S, Whalley PJ, MacDonald PC. A study of angiotensin II pressor response throughout primigravid pregnancy. *J Clin Invest* 1973; **52**: 2682–2689.

51. Fitzgerald DJ, Entman SS, Mulloy K, FitzGerald GA. Decreased prostacyclin biosynthesis preceding the clinical manifestation of pregnancy-induced hypertension. Pathophysiology and natural history. *Circulation* 1987; **75**: 956–963.

52. Greer IA, Walker JJ, McLaren M, Bonduelle M, Cameron AD, Calder AA, Forbes CD. Immunoreactive prostacyclin and thromboxane metabolites in normal pregnancy and the puerperium. *Br J Obstet Gynaecol* 1985; **92**: 581–585.

53. Everett RB, Worley RJ, MacDonald PC, Gant NF. Modification of vascular responsiveness to angiotensin II in pregnant women by intravenously infused 5∝ dihydroprogesterone. *Am J Obstet Gynecol* 1978; **131**: 352–357.

54. Molnár M, Hertelendy F. N-nitro L-arginine, an inhibitor of nitric oxide synthesis, increases blood pressure in rats and reverses the pregnancy-induced refractoriness to vasopressor agents. *Am J Obstet Gynecol* 1992; **166**: 1560–1567.

55. Stevenson JC, MacDonald DWR, Warren RC, Booker MW, Whitehead M. Increased concentration of circulating calcitonin gene related peptide during normal human pregnancy. *Br Med J* 1986; **293**: 1329–1330.

56. Oian P, Malthau JM, Noddeland H, Fadnes HO. Oedema preventing mechanisms in subcutaneous tissue of normal pregnant women. *Br J Obstet Gynaecol* 1985; **92**: 1113–1119.

57. Gonik B, Cotton D, Spillman T, Abouleish E, Zavisca F. Peripartum colloid osmotic pressure changes: effects of controlled fluid management. *Am J Obstet Gynaecol* 1985; **151**: 812–815.

58. Palmer AJ, Walker AHC. The maternal circulation in normal pregnancy. *J Obstet Gynaecol Br Emp* 1949; **56**: 537–547.

59. Robson SC, Dunlop W, Boys RJ, Hunter S. Cardiac output during labour. *Br Med J* 1987; **295**: 1169–1172.

60. Hendricks CH. The hemodynamics of a uterine contraction. *Am J Obstet Gynecol* 1958; **76**: 969–982.

61. Hendricks CH, Quilligan EJ. Cardiac output during labor. *Am J Obstet Gynecol* 1956; **71**: 953–972.

62. Palmer CM. Maternal electrocardiographic changes in the peripartum period. *Int J Obstet Anesth* 1994; **3**: 63–66.

63. Robson SC, Boys RJ, Hunter S, Dunlop W. Maternal hemodynamics after normal delivery and delivery complicated by postpartum haemorrhage. *Obstet Gynecol* 1989; **74**: 234–239.

64. Robson SC, Hunter S, Moore M, Dunlop W. Haemodynamic changes during the puerperium; a Doppler and M-mode echocardiographic study. *Br J Obstet Gynaecol* 1987; **94**: 1028–1039.

65. Wong RC, Ellis CN. Physiologic skin changes in pregnancy. *Semin Dermatol* 1989; **8**: 7–11.

66. Leontic EA. Respiratory disease in pregnancy. *Med Clin N Am* 1977; **61**: 111–128.

67. Thompson KJ, Cohen ME. Studies on the circulation in pregnancy: II vital capacity observations in normal pregnant women. *Surg Gynecol Obstet* 1938; **66**: 591–603.

68. Gilroy RJ, Mangura BT, Lavietes MH. Rib cage and abdominal volume displacements during breathing in pregnancy. *Am Rev Respir Dis* 1988; **137**: 668–672.

69. Grenville-Mathers R, Trenchard HJ. The diaphragm in the puerperium. *J Obstet Gynaecol Br Emp* 1953; **60**: 825–833.

70. Lehmann V, Fabel H. Lungen funktionsuntersuchungen an schwangeren teil II: ventilation atemmechanik und diffisionkapazität. *Z Geburtsh Perinatolo* 1973; **177**: 397–410.

71. Novy MJ, Edwards MJ. Respiratory problems in pregnancy. *Am J Obstet Gynecol* 1967; **99**: 1024–1045.

72. Eng M, Butler J, Bonica JJ. Respiratory function in pregnant obese women. *Am J Obstet Gynecol* 1975; **123**: 241–245.

73. Russell IF, Chambers WA. Closing volume in normal pregnancy. *Br J Anaesth* 1981; **53**: 1043–1047.

74. Sims CD, Chamberlain GVP, de Swiet M. Lung function test in bronchial asthma during and after pregnancy. *Br J Obstet Gynaecol* 1976; **83**: 434–437.

75. Templeton A, Kelman GR. Maternal blood gases $(PAO_2–P_aO_2)$, physiological shunt and V_D/V_T in normal pregnancy. *Br J Anaesth* 1976; **48**: 1001–1004.

76. Pernoll ML, Metcalf J, Kovach PA, Wachtel R, Dunham MJ. Ventilation during rest and exercise in pregnancy and postpartum. *Resp Physiol* 1975; **25**: 295–310.

77. Lyons HA, Antonio R. The sensitivity of the respiratory centre in pregnancy and after the administration of progesterone. *Trans Assoc Am Physic* 1959; **72**: 173–180.

78. Skatrud JB, Dempsey JA, Kaiser DG. Ventilatory response to medroxyprogesterone acetate in normal subjects: time course and mechanism. *J Appl Physiol* 1978; **44**: 939–944.

79. White DP, Douglas NJ, Pickett CK, Weil JV, Zwillich CW. Sexual influence on the control of breathing. *J Appl Physiol* 1983; **54**: 874–879.

80. Sutton FD, Zwillich CD, Creagh CE, Pierson DJ, Weil JV. Progesterone for outpatient treatment of Pickwickian Syndrome. *Ann Intern Med* 1975; **83**: 476–479.

81. Spätling L, Fallenstein F, Huch A. The variability of cardiopulmonary adaptation to pregnancy at rest and during exercise. *Br J Obstet Gynaecol* 1992; **99**(suppl 8): 1–40.

82. Pernoll ML, Metcalfe J, Schlenker TL, Welch JE, Matsumoto JA. Oxygen consumption at rest and during exercise in pregnancy. *Resp Physiol* 1975; **25**: 285–294.

83. Knuttgen HG, Emerson K. Physiological response to pregnancy at rest and during exercise. *J Appl Physiol* 1974; **36**: 549–553.

84. Gazioglu K, Kaltreider NL, Rosen M, Yu PN. Pulmonary function during pregnancy in normal women and in patients with cardiopulmonary disease. *Thorax* 1970; **25**: 445–450.

85. Garrard GS, Littler WA, Redman CWG. Closing volume during normal pregnancy. *Thorax* 1978; **33**: 488–492.

86. Blechner JN, Cotter JR, Stenger VG, Hinkley CM, Prystowksy H. Oxygen, carbon dioxide and hydrogen ion concentrations in arterial blood during pregnancy. *Am J Obstet Gynecol* 1968; **100**: 1–6.

87. Sobrevilla LA, Cassinelli MT, Carcelen A, Malaga JM. Human fetal and maternal oxygen tension and acid base status during delivery at high altitude. *Am J Obstet Gynecol* 1971; **111**: 1111–1118.

88. Dayal P, Murata Y, Takamura H. Antepartum and postpartum acid–base changes in maternal blood in normal and complicated pregnancies. *J Obstet Gynaecol Br Comm* 1972; **79**: 612–624.

89. Andersen GJ, James GB, Mathers NP, Smith EL, Walker J. The maternal oxygen tension and acid–base status during pregnancy. *J Obstet Gynaecol Br Comm* 1969; **76**: 16–19.

90. Calvin S, Jones OW, Knieriem K, Weinstein L. Oxygen saturation in the supine hypotensive syndrome. *Obstet Gynecol* 1988; **71**: 872–877.

91. de Swiet M. Maternal pulmonary disorders. In: Creasy RK, Resnik R (eds) *Maternal–fetal medicine: principles and practice.* Philadelphia: W.B. Saunders, 1984, pp 781–794.

92. Milne JA, Howie AD, Pack AI. Dyspnoea during normal pregnancy. *Br J Obstet Gynaecol* 1978; **85**: 260–263.

93. Bonica JJ. Obstetric analgesia and anesthesia: recent trends and advances. *NY State J Med* 1970; **70**: 2079–2084.

94. Sangoul F, Fox GS, Houle GL. Effect of regional analgesia on maternal oxygen consumption during the first stage of labor. *Am J Obstet Gynecol* 1975; **121**: 1080–1083.

95. Hägerdal M, Morgan CW, Sumner AE, Gutsche BB. Minute ventilation and oxygen consumption during labor with epidural analgesia. *Anesthesiology* 1983; **59**: 425–427.

96. Gupta A, Johnson A, Johansson A, Berg G, Lennmarken C. Maternal respiratory function following normal vaginal delivery. *Int J Obstet Anesth* 1993; **2**: 129–133.

97. Loe H, Silness J. Periodontal disease in pregnancy. *Acta Odont Scand* 1963; **21**: 533–551.

98. Hytten FE. The alimentary system. In: Hytten FE, Chamberlain G (eds) *Clinical physiology in obstetrics.* Oxford: Blackwell Scientific Publications, 1991, pp 137–149.

99. Bruce LA, Behsudi FM. Progesterone effects on three gastrointestinal tissues. *Life Sci* 1979; **25**: 729–734.

100. Schaffer EA, Taylor PJ, Logan K, Gadomski S, Corenblum B. The effect of progestin on gallbladder function in young women. *Am J Obstet Gynecol* 1984; **148**: 504–507.

101. Christofides ND, Ghatei MA, Bloom SR, Borberg C, Gillmer MDG. Decreased plasma motilin levels in pregnancy. *Br Med J* 1982; **285**: 1453–1454.

102. Williams NH. Variable significance of heartburn. *Am J Obstet Gynecol* 1941; **42**: 814–819.

103. Campbell AM. Variable significance of heartburn (letter). *Am J Obstet Gynecol* 1941; **42**: 819.

104. Bassey OO. Pregnancy heartburn in Nigerians and caucasians with theories about aetiology based on manometric recordings from the oesophagus and stomach. *Br J Obstet Gynaecol* 1977; **84**: 439–443.

105. Hansen R. Zur physiologie des amgens in der schwangerschaft. *ZBL Gynakol* 1937; **61**: 2306–2309.

106. Boyden EA, Rigler LG. Initial emptying time of stomach in primigravidae as related to evacuation of biliary tract. *Proc Soc Experim Biol Med* 1944; **56**: 200–201.

107. Davison JS, Davison MV, Hay DM. Gastric emptying time in late pregnancy and labour. *J Obstet Gynaecol Br Comm* 1970; **77**: 37–41.

108. Geddes SM, Thorburn J, Logan RW. Gastric emptying following caesarean section and the effect of epidural fentanyl. *Anaesthesia* 1991; **46**: 1016–1018.

109. Holdsworth JD. Relationship between stomach contents and analgesia in labour. *Br J Anaesth* 1978; **50**: 1145–1148.

110. Simpson KH, Stakes AF, Miller M. Pregnancy delays paracetamol absorption and gastric emptying in patients undergoing surgery. *Br J Anaesth* 1988; **60**: 24–27.

111. Macfie AG, Magides AD, Richmond MN, Reilly CS. Gastric emptying in pregnancy. *Br J Anaesth* 1991; **67**: 54–57.

112. Stanley K, Magides A, Arnot M, Bruce C, Reilly C, McFee A, Fraser R. Delayed gastric emptying as a factor in delayed postprandial glycaemic response in pregnancy. *Br J Obstet Gynaecol* 1995; **102**: 288–291.

113. Holst N, Jenssen TG, Burhol PG. Plasma concentrations of motilin and somatostatin are increased in late pregnancy and postpartum. *Br J Obstet Gynaecol* 1992; **99**: 338–341.

114. Parry E, Shields R, Turnbull AC. Transit time in the small intestine in pregnancy. *J Obstet Gynaecol Br Comm* 1970; **77**: 900–901.

115. Montgomery TL, Pincus IJ. A nutritional problem in pregnancy resulting from extensive resection of the small bowel. *Am J Obstet Gynecol* 1955; **69**: 865–868.

116. Kennedy RL, Darné FJ. Disorders of the thyroid gland during pregnancy and the post-partum period. *Prog Obstet Gynaecol*, Studd J (ed) 1994; **11**: 125–140.

117. Glinoer D, De Nayer P, Bourdoux P. Regulation of the maternal thyroid during pregnancy. *J Clin Endocrin Metab* 1990; **71**: 276–287.

118. Kennedy RL, Darne F. The role of hCG in regulation of the thyroid gland in normal and abnormal pregnancy. *Obstet Gynecol* 1991; **78**: 298–307.

119. Desai RK, Norman RJ, Jialal I, Joubert SM. Spectrum of thyroid function abnormalities in gestational trophoblastic neoplasia. *Clin Endocrin* 1988; **29**: 583–592.

120. Kennedy RL, Darne J, Cohn M, Price A, Davies R, Blumsohn A, Griffiths H. Human chorionic gonadotrophin may not be responsible for thyroid stimulating activity in normal pregnancy serum. *J Clin Endocrin Metab* 1992; **74**: 260–265.

121. Girling JC. Thyroid disease and pregnancy. *Br J Hosp Med* 1996; **56**(7): 316–320.

122. Kennedy RL, Jones TH, Cuckle HS. Down's syndrome and the thyroid. *Clin Endocrin* 1992; **37**: 471–476.

123. Glinoer D, Soto MF, Bourdoux P, Lejeune B, Delange F, Lemore M, Kinthaert J, Robijn C, Grun J, De Nayer P. Pregnancy in patients with mild thyroid abnormalities: maternal and neonatal repurcussions. *J Clin Endocrin Metab* 1991; **73**: 421–427.

124. Montoro M, Collea JV, Frasier D. Successful outcome of pregnancy in women with hypothyroidism. *Ann Intern Med* 1981; **94**: 31–36.

125. Harris B, Othman S, Davies JA, Weppner GJ, Richards CJ, Newcombe RG, Lazarus JH, Parkes AB, Hall R, Phillips D. Association between postpartum thyroid dysfunction and thyroid antibodies. *Br Med J* 1992; **305**: 152–156.

126. Black AJ, Topping J, Durham B et al. Assessment of biochemical markers of bone turnover in pregnant women. *J Bone Miner Res* 1996; **11**: 5440–5442.

127. Shefras J, Farquharson RG. Bone density studies in pregnant women receiving heparin. *Eur J Obstet Gynaecol* 1996; **65**: 171–174.

128. Kalkwarf H, Specker B. Bone mineral loss during lactation. *Obstet Gynecol* 1995; **86**: 26–32.

129. Sowers M, Randolph J, Shapiro B, Jannausch M. A prospective study of bone density and pregnancy after an extended period of lactation with bone loss. *Obstet Gynecol* 1995; **85**(2): 285–289.

130. Bererhi H, Kolhoff N, Constable A, Nielsen SP. Multiparity and bone mass. *Br J Obstet Gynaecol* 1996; **103**(8): 818–821.

131. Kriastiansson P, Svardsudd K, von Schoultz B. Back pain during pregnancy: a prospective study. *Spine* 1996; **21**(6): 702–709.

132. Mens JM, Vleeming A, Stoeckart R, Stam HJ, Snijders CJ. Understanding peripartum pelvic pain. Implications of a patient survey. *Spine* 1996; **21**(11): 1363–1369.

133. Hall K. Relaxin. *J Reprod Fertil* 1960; **1**: 368–384.

134. Hirabayashi Y, Shimuzu R, Fukuda H, Saitoh K, Igarashi T. Soft tissue anatomy within the vertebral canal in pregnant women. *Br J Anaesth* 1996; **77**: 153–156.

135. Hirabayashi Y, Shimuzu R, Saitoh K, Fukuda H, Igarashi T. Acid base state of cerebrospinal fluid during pregnancy and its effect on spread of spinal anaesthesia. *Br J Anaesth* 1996; **77**: 352–355.

136. Dunlop W. Serial changes in renal haemodynamics during normal human pregnancy. *Br J Obstet Gynaecol* 1988; **88**: 1–9.

137. Davison JM, Hytten FE. Glomerular filtration during and after pregnancy. *J Obstet Gynaecol Br Comm* 1974; **81**: 588–595.

138. Lind T, Godfrey KA, Otun H. Changes in uric acid concentration during normal pregnancy. *Br J Obstet Gynaecol* 1984; **91**: 128–132.

139. Bailey RR, Rolleston GL. Kidney length and ureteric dilatation in the puerperium. *J Obstet Gynaecol Br Comm* 1971; **78**: 55–61.

140. Fainstat T. Ureteral dilatation in pregnancy: a review. *Obstet Gynaecol Surv* 1963; **18**: 845–849.

141. Ryhammer AM, Bek KM, Laurberg S. Multiple vaginal deliveries increase the risk of permanent incontinence of flatus and urine in normal premenopausal women. *Dis Colon Rectum* 1995; **38**: 1206–1209.

142. Williams JD. Bacteruria in pregnancy. In: Asscher AW, Brumfitt W (eds) *Microbial disease in nephrology.* Chichester: Wiley, 1986, pp 159–181.

143. Tapp AJS, Meire H et al. The effect of epidural analgesia in post partum voiding. *Neurol Urodyn* 1987; **6**(3): 235–237.

144. Baird JD. Some aspects of metabolism and hormonal adaptation to pregnancy. *Acta Endocrin Sup* 1986; **277**: 11–18.

145. Green IC, Taylor KW. Effects of pregnancy in the rat on the size and insulin secretory response of the Islets of Langerhans. *J Endocrin* 1972; **54**: 317–325.

146. Brudenell M, Doddridge MC. Diabetic pregnancy. *Current reviews in obstetrics and gynaecology.* Edinburgh: Churchill Livingstone, 1989.

147. Kuhl C. Glucose metabolism during and after pregnancy in normal and gestational diabetic women. *Acta Endocrin* 1975; **75**: 709–719.

148. Beard RW, Turner RC, Oakley N. Fetal response to glucose loading. Fetal blood glucose and insulin responses to hyperglycaemia in normal and diabetic pregnancies. *Postgrad Med J* 1971; **47**: 68–70.

149. Davison JM. Changes in renal function and other aspects of homeostasis in early pregnancy. *J Obstet Gynaecol Br Comm* 1974; **81**: 1003–1006.

150. Hytten F. Nutrition. *The clinical physiology of the puerperium.* London: Farrand Press, 1995, pp 77–117.

3

AUDIT IN OBSTETRIC ANAESTHESIA

John Urquhart

'Knowledge is itself power'
Francis Bacon

THE NEED FOR AUDIT

Participation in audit is a requirement for all in anaesthesia. Although audit was until recently an unfamiliar concept, there is now an imperative to be involved in the audit process, and it has become part of continuing professional development.[1] In the future this will become a legal responsibility with the enactment of the Government white paper on the Health Service, *The New NHS: Modern, Dependable.* Whether failure to do so might constitute a disciplinary issue, and whether the responsibility resides at the individual, department or trust level has yet to be resolved.

AUDIT VERSUS RESEARCH

There is a clear distinction between the processes of audit and research. Audit is a process of quality control; in medicine it is taken as the systematic peer review of clinical practice with the object of maintaining and improving the quality of that practice. Research, by contrast, is the discipline of improving medical care by expanding the known areas of medical science.

It is accepted that if the results of research are to be meaningful, they should be subjected to inferential statistical analysis. The standard for research is the randomized controlled trial, which is prospective, has a control group to which patients are allocated randomly, and where the treatment is concealed from both patient and researcher. Audit is frequently a retrospective process; randomization cannot take place, and statistical analysis is not usually valid.

Although publications may be obtained both through audit and research, audit rarely involves a departure from accepted clinical practice and does not have a control group. Hence ethics committee approval may not be needed for audit projects. They are easier to set up, quicker to perform and may lead to conclusions, and can be accomplished within the time a trainee will spend in any department of anaesthesia during his or her training.

The purpose of audit is to improve clinical practice. Collection of data and its subsequent analysis serves no purpose unless a conclusion can be drawn, which is then applied to the practice of an individual or a department. The expression 'closing the audit loop'

refers to the concept of a cycle as shown:

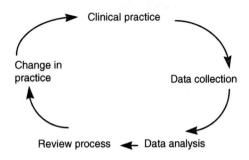

SUBJECTS FOR AUDIT

Audit may be performed in a number of different areas in obstetric anaesthesia with different purposes in mind as in Table 3.1.

DENOMINATOR DATA

Useful information can be obtained from the Department of Obstetrics and Gynaecology within a trust. Obstetricians are required by their royal college; the Royal College of Obstetricians and Gynaecologists, (RCOG), to collect quantitative data on the activity of their department (Box 3.1). These are raw numerical data and no qualitative conclusions may be drawn from them; however, they provide an excellent denominator for the activity and performance of the obstetric anaesthetic service.

Table 3.1	
QUANTITATIVE	**QUALITATIVE**
Department audit, NCEPOD, CEMD	Post delivery visiting, formal delivery unit ward rounds, maternal satisfaction
MORTALITY	**MORBIDITY**
NCEPOD, CEMD	Department M&M meetings, risk management groups
LOCAL	**NATIONAL**
Department audit	NCEPOD, CEMD
NCEPOD: National Confidential Enquiry into Perioperative Death; CEMD: Confidential Enquiries into Maternal Death; M&M meetings: Morbidity and Mortality meetings.	

1. Total number of women delivered (not the same as babies born, and does not include babies born out of hospital)
2. Total live births (includes twin births)
3. Total number of stillbirths, babies born inside and outside trust premises
4. Number of spontaneous vaginal deliveries
5. Number of assisted vaginal deliveries (forceps and ventouse)
6. Number of breech deliveries
7. Number of inductions of labour
8. Number of Caesarean sections performed, divided into elective and emergency indications

Box 3.1   RCOG data.

1. Patient name and unit number
2. Age, gravida, parity
3. Time of request and time of attendance, with free field to fill in for delay if greater than 30 min
4. Attending anaesthetist and grade
5. Indication, from a pick list including maternal request, multiple gestation, hypertensive disease and trial of scar
6. Procedure performed, from a tick list including spinal, epidural and combined spinal epidural
7. Complications, from a pick list including asymmetrical analgesia, failed analgesia and inadvertent dural puncture

Box 3.2   Suggested labour ward data.

NUMERATOR DATA

The collection of data describing the activity of an obstetric anaesthetic service is simply obtained. Broadly speaking, it is appropriate to generate one form for labour ward activity and one for theatre activity. From time to time, it may become necessary to redesign the forms when particular information is required for an audit project. Examples might include unilateral epidural block, inadvertent dural puncture, seniority of anaesthetist, or interval between decision and commencement of non-elective Caesarean section.

It is important to create data collection fields for all grades of staff to fill so that they are as simple as possible, in order to encourage compliance. In designing the fields, thought needs to be given to the way in which the data will be stored. Most departments will use a database such as Microsoft Access™, although for simple data a spreadsheet application such as Microsoft Excel™ is suitable. Suggested data for routine collection are shown in Box 3.2. Hand held computers can be very useful for data collection.[2] Data recorded by individual anaesthetists can be downloaded into a central computer database and then analysed in the usual way.

Annotation of different procedures for different situations – for example, whether epidural anaesthesia for Caesarean section was an extension of an existing epidural for labour, or sited *de novo* – can cause confusion and Gilbert and Cameron[2] have proposed the following nomenclature:

CS EP NEW	epidural inserted for Caesarean section (CS)
CS EP SIT	epidural *in situ*, extended for CS
CS GA	general anaesthetic for CS
CS GA SIT	general anaesthetic for CS, epidural *in situ*
CS SP	spinal anaesthesia for CS
CS SP SIT	spinal anaesthesia for CS, epidural *in situ*
FOR EP NEW	epidural inserted for forceps
FOR EP SIT	epidural *in situ*, extended for forceps
FOR SP	spinal anaesthetic for forceps
LAB EP CON	epidural infusion for analgesia for labour
LAB EP INT	epidural top-ups for analgesia in labour

It then becomes possible to describe quantitative performance of a department by employing data compiled from the accumulated data forms, in conjunction with data collected by midwives and obstetricians. Typical data are shown in Table 3.2.

QUALITATIVE AUDIT

Data derived by completion of audit forms with a numerator and a denominator provides local information which, when compared to national standards, provides quantitative audit of performance. The proportion of Caesarean sections performed under regional, rather than general anaesthesia indicates compliance with the recommendations of successive reports of CEMD; the proportion of procedures undertaken by consultant anaesthetists reflects adequacy of staffing. Numbers of instrumental delivery and Caesarean sections reflect obstetric practice and case mix and are largely outside the control of the anaesthetic service.

Postal questionnaires are popular and national surveys of obstetric anaesthetic practice can be backed by the

Table 3.2

Indicator	Number or %	Source
Pregnancies	971 533	per annum, UK, derived from CEMD[3]
Births	742 866	as above
Elective LSCS	7%	CEMD
Emergency LSCS	9%	CEMD
Total LSCS	16%	CEMD
Spontaneous vertex delivery	67.2%	Local data
Forceps delivery	6.8%	Local data
Ventouse delivery	3.1%	Local data
Regional analgesia in labour	36.5%	Local data
LSCS under GA	9%	Local data
LSCS under regional anaesthesia	91%	Local data

Obstetric Anaesthetists' Association (OAA). However postal surveys are unsatisfactory in a number of respects. Response rates are frequently poor, and one might speculate that it is the responses from the defaulters that might be the most informative. Studies with response rates of >70% are regarded by many as being capable of generating meaningful conclusions but this level of incomplete data would certainly not be accepted in the field of research.

Post-partum follow-up: Quality may be ascertained by interview with the mother in the puerperium. The anaesthetist conducting a postnatal ward round should be doing so in exactly the same way as he or she would after performing anaesthesia for any procedure. The opportunities offered in the postnatal setting are unlike those in the general surgical situation, as the patient – in this case the mother – may not have been ill in the first place, and the discussion is more likely to concentrate on overall satisfaction. Maternal expectations will be influenced by what she has read, what she has been told by friends and family and what she has been told at antenatal classes. Maternal satisfaction does not equate to complete anaesthesia but rather to the overall experience of childbirth of which pain relief is just a part, albeit a very important part and one which is high on the list of most mothers-to-be. Indeed this was emphasized by Shapiro et al,[4] who showed that maternal satisfaction was multifactorial. Robinson, Salmon and Yentis found that such factors included staffing, unit policies, quality of care, outcome, access, facilities, and maternal factors. These authors also discussed the difficulty of assessing maternal satisfaction.

The postnatal visit is essential, firstly so that complications can be excluded and secondly to assess the quality of the service offered.

At the author's hospital, the visits are made by consultant anaesthetists using a diary in which patient names are recorded when an anaesthetic procedure has been performed. This qualitative audit is in addition to the requirement for completion of audit forms and their inclusion in a database. In addition to assessing the service and dealing with the few complications arising, this provides opportunities to deal with anxieties and questions not disclosed at the time of delivery such as backache, posture and future analgesia. Finally, a record is made of who saw the mother before discharge.

NATIONAL AUDIT

The Confidential Enquiries into Maternal Deaths (CEMD) is the single longest-running medical audit project in the world.[3] It is envied by the profession and referred to in any discussion of maternal mortality. It is a rare example of an audit project which has had a profound effect on the conduct of obstetrics and on obstetric anaesthesia.

Confusion arises in some specialities and among the laity between CEMD and the National Confidential Enquiry into Perioperative Death, NCEPOD. These are different but complimentary projects and a comparison between the two is instructive (see Table 3.3).

DENOMINATORS IN CEMD

Three different denominators are in use, reflecting the different requirements for data (Box 3.3).

Definition	Reason
Deaths from obstetric causes per million women aged 15–44	Allows comparison with all other causes of death in this age group
Deaths from obstetric causes per 100 000 maternities	This examines the group representing the majority of women at risk
Deaths from obstetric causes per 100 000 estimated pregnancies	The least accurate, and only used when considering death in early pregnancy

Box 3.3

Table 3.3

	CEMD	NCEPOD
Started by	Beecher and Todd, 1952.	The Association of Anaesthetists of Great Britain and Ireland, 1956, who sampled 1000 cases.
Reporting	Every 3 years – the triennium.	Currently reports every year.
Sampling	Every death of a woman who is pregnant, or within 42 days of termination of pregnancy, from any cause related to or aggravated by pregnancy or its management, but not from accidental or incidental causes. Thus direct, indirect and fortuitous deaths. All are discussed in each report. Late deaths are those occurring between 42 days and 1 year.	All patients who die within 30 days of a surgical procedure, a sample of which are reviewed in detail. For example, the 1996/1997 report addressed gynaecological, head and neck, urological, oesophageal and spinal surgery; 1997/1998 examined deaths in the under 16 and the over 90 age groups, and 1998/1999 examined a 1:10 sample of all deaths.
Denominator	See below.	Unknown. The number and type of surgical procedures carried out in the UK is not recorded, and this is a perceived weakness in the audit.
Catchment	The whole of the UK has been included since 1984.	England, Wales and Northern Ireland, Channel Islands and Isle of Man. Scotland is not currently involved.
Responsibility	Consultant, midwife or general practitioner has a duty to inform the regional Director of Public Health of any death occurring while pregnant or within the subsequent year.	At present, data are supplied on a voluntary basis but co-operation will become a legal requirement. Deaths are reported by a nominated consultant in a Trust, usually a pathologist.

Since the Registrars General have precise knowledge of live births and stillbirths of 24 weeks or later, and there is a statutory requirement for the reporting of a maternal death to the Director of Public Health, these denominators are mostly sound. The exception is in the use of 'estimated pregnancies', as a number of pregnancies are spontaneously aborted by mothers who remain unaware of the fact they were pregnant in the first place. The figure for deaths per 100 000 maternities is flawed in that a completed death certificate may fail to identify the presence of pregnancy. This is emphasized by the disparity between deaths known to the Registrars General in 1994/1996 (producing a rate of 7.4 deaths per 100 000 maternities) as against the number known to the Enquiry for the same period, producing a rate of 12.2 deaths per 100 000 maternities.

TRENDS IN MATERNAL MORTALITY

As recently as just before the Second World War, maternal mortality was of the order of 5 per 1000

deliveries: this equates to 1:200, or, using the modern denominator, 500 per 100 000 maternities. A recent paper from Zimbabwe[5] identified a maternal mortality of 344 per 100 000 maternities. This illustrates the gulf that exists between the developed and developing world and the considerable advances which have been made in the UK since the setting up of the Health Service.

Although the figures from Great Britain 50 years ago are of the same magnitude as in Africa today, the major cause of death in the former was from puerperal sepsis. By contrast, McKenzie established that 77% of the deaths he saw were avoidable, and due to haemorrhage, thrombosis and hypertensive disease.

These conditions are exactly the same as have appeared in successive triennial reports in the UK. The causes are listed below in Table 3.4.

Haemorrhage has declined in importance as a cause of maternal mortality and this is attributed to the emphasis placed upon it in previous reports that advocated the multidisciplinary involvement in its

Table 3.4	
Cause of death	Number of cases (1997–1999)
Thrombosis and thromboembolism	35
Hypertensive diseases	15
Amniotic fluid embolism	8
Early pregnancy deaths (ectopic, etc.)	17
Sepsis	14
Haemorrhage	7
Other direct causes – genital tract trauma, etc.	7
Anaesthesia	3

Table 3.5	
Triennium	Number of deaths directly associated with anaesthesia
1985–1987	6
1988–1990	4
1991–1993	8
1994–1996	1
1997–1999	3

management and the institution of local protocols. These include the immediate availability and administration of blood and blood products along with the recognition of Caesarean hysterectomy as a life-saving procedure.

Thrombosis and thromboembolism remain important causes and there needs to be an awareness that this condition can occur in the first trimester. Thromboembolism after Caesarean section has been addressed by the prophylactic use of heparin in the post-delivery period.

Hypertensive disease continues to kill mothers despite the fact that its detection remains at the centre of antenatal care.

THE CONTRIBUTION OF ANAESTHESIA

Anaesthesia emerges with credit when reviewing the reports over the last decade. The number of deaths directly attributable to anaesthesia are shown in Table 3.5.

It is often stated that the reduction in the numbers of deaths attributable to anaesthesia has arisen from the increased use of regional anaesthesia both for Caesarean section and in labour, when emergency Caesarean section is envisaged. This may partially be so, but other factors are involved. Notable among them is the increased use of capnography at induction of general anaesthesia. This allows for early identification of correct placement of the tracheal tube at rapid sequence induction of anaesthesia. In a previous report, 1991–1993, there were eight deaths attributable to anaesthesia, in seven of which mismanagement of the airway was implicated. The routine use of

pulse oximetry, failed intubation policies and the trained, dedicated anaesthetic assistant, are also important. Two out of the three deaths in this triennium were associated with problems after the patient had been transfered to the ICU.

ANAESTHESIA AND LATE DEATHS: NO ROOM FOR COMPLACENCY

Descriptions of late deaths in which anaesthesia is involved are typically multifactorial events where substandard care is unusual. Pulmonary hypertension, congenital cardiac disease, cerebral haemorrhage and cystic fibrosis all appear in cases where there was anaesthetic involvement. Frequently the anaesthetic involvement included intensive care. This points to anaesthetists being increasingly involved in the management of the sick obstetric patient, whether on the delivery suite or the intensive care unit. This observation carries clear implications for staffing and consultant anaesthetic sessions.

NATIONAL QUALITATIVE AUDIT: OAA REGISTRIES

The emphasis, in national terms, has been on the confidential enquiries. Interest has recently increased in the development of registries of high-risk patients, through the auspices of the Obstetric Anaesthetists' Association (OAA).

CONCLUSIONS

Participation in audit is a contractual requirement for anaesthetists. Qualitative and quantitative data should be presented at local clinical governance meetings where the practice of closing the audit loop should be applied. The discussion of case reports can enhance the process. National audit has had profound effects on anaesthetic practice with maternal mortality declining. The anaesthetic contribution to the reduction in maternal mortality is considerable but as the role of the obstetric anaesthetist has expanded to cover management of the sick mother, more indirect anaesthetic deaths have been cited. Increasing consultant cover may improve the management of such patients with time.

REFERENCES

1. Implementation of proposals for continuing medical education. The Royal College of Anaesthetists, 1995.

2. Gilbert SS, Cameron AE. A system for audit of obstetric anaesthesia. *Int J Obstet Anesth* 1994; **3**: 146–148.

3. Lewis G, Drife JO. *Why mothers die: report on confidential enquiries into maternal deaths in the United Kingdom 1994–1996.* London: HMSO, 1998.

4. Shapiro A, Fredman B, Zohar E, Olsfanger D, Jedeikin R. Delivery room analgesia: an analysis of maternal satisfaction. *Int J Obstet Anesth* 1998; **7**: 226–230.

5. McKenzie AG. Operative obstetric mortality at Harare Central Hospital 1992–94: an anaesthetic view. *Int J Obstet Anesth* 1998; **7**: 237–241.

4

NON-REGIONAL ANALGESIA I: NON-PHARMACOLOGICAL METHODS

Mike Wee

THE NATURE OF LABOUR PAIN

Giving birth is a painful process. Labour pain measured using the McGill Pain Questionnaire[1] showed that it ranked high on the pain rating index superseded only by amputation of a digit and causalgia when compared with the acute and chronic pain syndromes (Fig. 4.1). Although prepared childbirth training did reduce the pain rating index score, the scores remained high.[2] The National Birthday Trust (NBT) survey of over 10 300 women in the United Kingdom reported that 93.5% of women experienced severe or unbearable pain sometime during their labour when asked shortly after delivery.[3] The percentage who admitted that they experienced severe or unbearable pain dropped to 65% when asked 6 weeks after delivery. This amnesia of severe pain was highlighted by Morgan et al[4] who reported that of the women who experienced severe pain in labour, 90% viewed the experience with satisfaction 3 months later. However, the fact that the pain is later forgotten does not make it any more bearable at the time. Although labour pain has been demonstrated to be more intense than most acute and chronic pain syndromes, there is an essential difference. In the majority of cases, there is a very positive outcome at the end of labour. This may explain the apparent amnesia of labour pain with time. However, if the outcome is a damaged fetus, the memory of a painful labour is less likely to fade. In a prospective study,[5] women expecting their first babies were found not so much to underestimate the pain of labour as to overestimate their ability to cope with it. An European multicentre study[6] of 611 nulliparous women from six large maternity units representing five European countries investigated maternal expectations and experiences with labour pain, pain relief and maternal satisfaction. Standardized interviews were undertaken during the last month of pregnancy and 24 h after delivery. Maternal expectations of labour pain and responses to the pre-delivery interview varied significantly between the centres, as did maternal knowledge and choice of analgesic techniques. The study found that the most satisfied women were those who expected more pain, those who were satisfied with the analgesia received and also those who had good pain relief. However, Morgan et al[7] found that epidural analgesia, which provided the best pain relief, did not necessarily equate with increased uptake of this method of pain relief nor improved maternal satisfaction with the birthing process. An explanation put forward was that parturients control the amount of pain they wish to tolerate and even though pain scores were high, the parturients were experiencing the level of pain they had expected.

CHARACTERISTICS OF LABOUR PAIN

- It is an individual experience
- The majority of parturients experience severe or unbearable pain
- Prepared childbirth may help to a limited extent
- Recollection of labour pain fades with time.

Clearly quality of analgesia is but one facet of a parturient's satisfaction with the birth experience. Pain relief in labour is a complex and controversial subject among the parturients themselves as well as those caring for them. Cultural factors, peer group pressures and personal aspirations all influence attitudes towards pain relief in labour. Some women may request epidural analgesia as their first choice, while others would prefer to choose almost any other method of analgesia before requesting an epidural. What is clearly important is the provision of information, support and choice of pain relief that can be tailored to the individual parturient. These will provide a measure of control for the parturient, which is an important factor. Participation in the decision-making process and information were deemed to be important for parturients' satisfaction[8] and associated with positive psychological outcomes.[9] The only person who can truly judge how much pain the parturient is experiencing and whether it is acceptable or not is the

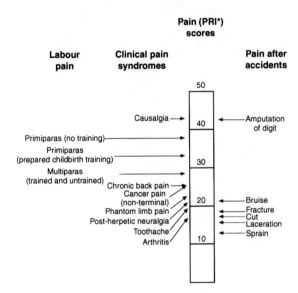

Figure 4.1 Comparison of pain scores using McGill Pain Questionnaire obtained from women in labour, patients from a pain clinic and emergency department (from Ref. 1, reproduced with permission from the author and publishers).

parturient herself. This may sound obvious but there are individuals, groups and organizations all purporting to be acting in the best interests of the parturient and yet not really taking into consideration the individual parturient's views.

FACTORS ASSOCIATED WITH MATERNAL SATISFACTION AND PAIN RELIEF

- Good analgesia
- The ability to choose type of analgesia
- Local information about methods of analgesia available
- Participation in the decision-making process
- Absence of pain does not necessarily equate to satisfaction
- Loss of sensation may equate to dissatisfaction.

CHILDBIRTH PREPARATION

The goals of childbirth preparation include giving information on the pregnancy, labour and delivery, training in relaxation exercises including breathing techniques, involvement of the spouse or partner in the preparation for childbirth and allaying anxieties due to ignorance.

INFORMATION

Women get their information from a variety of sources including friends and relatives, the media, books and magazines, healthcare personnel and increasingly the internet. The NBT survey of 1990[3] found that among the women attending antenatal classes, 54% attended a health centre, 38% a hospital and 8% National Childbirth Trust (NCT) classes. Midwives were considered important sources of information both antenatally and during the birthing process in 284 units (97.2%), the obstetrician in 166 units (56.8%) and the anaesthetist in 117 units (40%). The key role of the midwife is important. It is therefore imperative that anaesthetists should be more involved, not only in imparting information at antenatal classes, but are also involved in the continuing education of the obstetric

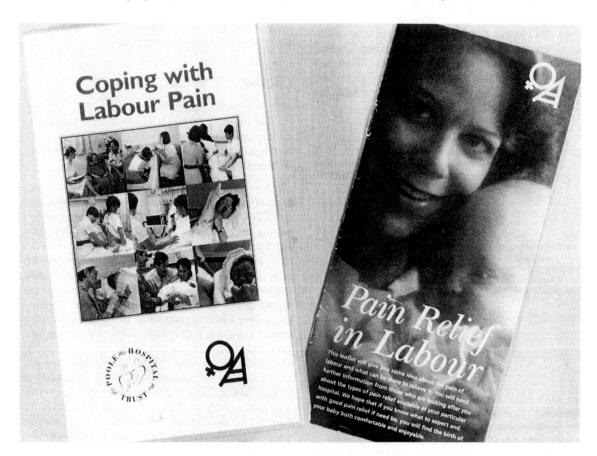

Figure 4.2   Pain relief booklet and video produced by the Obstetric Anaesthetists' Association.

team so that recent advances in obstetric anaesthesia and analgesia can be taught and the information passed on to women. Likewise, it is incumbent on anaesthetists to keep up to date with methods of analgesia that are less familiar to them. Consistency of information can be partly achieved by using common information media. Examples include the 'Pain Relief in Labour' booklet and the 'Coping with Labour Pain' video produced and distributed by the Obstetric Anaesthetists' Association (Fig. 4.2) where options of analgesia are discussed in a patient friendly format. It is also important that women are informed of the choices of analgesia available locally. One way of achieving this is the local use of a pain relief in labour algorithm[10] as shown in Fig. 4.3. It was shown in the NBT survey of 1990 that a great source of dissatisfaction among women in labour was to be deprived a form of analgesia because it was not available locally. Moreover, with the increasing tendency towards independent midwife-led units and birthing centres, where low-risk women are offered a nonmedical approach to childbirth, it is important that these women are fully informed of the limitations of analgesia choices available to them in order to avoid disappointment and dissatisfaction.

NON-PHARMACOLOGICAL STRATEGIES FOR PAIN RELIEF

(i)   Psychological techniques
(ii) Physical techniques
(iii) Other complementary techniques.

PSYCHOLOGICAL TECHNIQUES

- Environment
- Emotional support
- Natural childbirth
- Psychoprophylaxis
- Biofeedback
- Hypnosis.

Environment

The environment of the place of delivery may have an effect on the choice, provision and uptake of

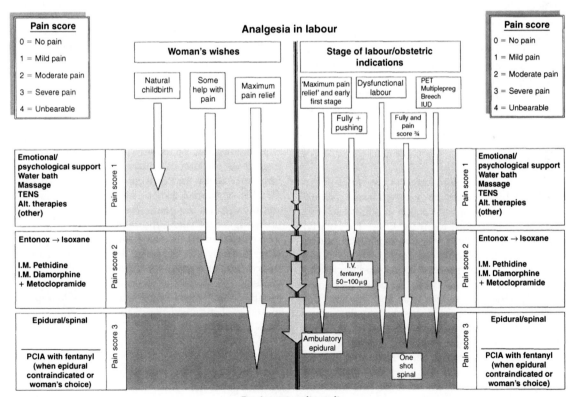

Poole maternity unit

Figure 4.3   Pain relief algorithm for use in the delivery suite (from Ref. 10, with permission).

analgesia. In a prospective non-randomized comparative study of uncomplicated labour and delivery in an alternative birthing centre in Denmark, and a conventional delivery suite within the same hospital, the usage of pethidine was four times greater in the conventional delivery suite.[11] A larger randomized Swedish study[12] comparing 1230 low-risk women in a birth centre and a conventional delivery suite demonstrated that the use of pethidine and Entonox was much lower in the birth centre. It was postulated that the environment of the birthing centre where the women were encouraged to mobilize, the 'relaxed attitude' and support of the staff as well as the ability to make choices might have contributed to this.

Emotional support

Emotional support is associated with a satisfying birth experience. Morgan et al[13] found that 61% of mothers felt that having a sympathetic midwife during labour was more beneficial than pain relief and the NBT survey of 1990 reinforced the view that the presence of a supportive partner, friend or relative was very helpful. The continuous presence of a supportive companion or 'doula' during labour may have beneficial effects.[14] A Cochrane database review[15] of 11 randomized controlled studies compared the effects of continuous support during labour with conventional care. Despite the large cultural differences, obstetric practices and conditions, the outcome was remarkably similar. The presence of a trained support person improved the physiological and psychological aspects of labour, delivery and the post-partum period for women.

Natural childbirth

Grantly Dick-Read is recognized as the father of the natural childbirth movement. His two books, *Natural childbirth* and *Childbirth without fear*, published in 1933 and 1944 led to interest in his work.[16,17] He asserted his belief that childbirth was not inherently painful and that the pain experienced during childbirth was largely a product of modern living leading to the fear-tension-pain vicious circle. He advocated antenatal preparation to reduce fear and tension and thereby relieving pain. Contrary to popular belief, Dick-Read did not condemn the use of analgesia where appropriate, but cautioned against routine use. Leboyer[18] described a modification of natural childbirth. He advocated childbirth in a dark quiet room, gentle massage of the newborn without routine suctioning and a warm bath soon after birth to limit the stresses of the birth process and limiting psychological trauma to the newborn.

Psychoprophylaxis

Ferdinand Lamaze[19] introduced the use of psychoprophylaxis or positive conditioning of the parturient, linked with education on the process of childbirth. The technique utilizes distraction and relaxation to focus on processes other than pain, thereby helping the parturient to cope with labour pain. Antenatal preparation is usually required a number of weeks before labour. Proponents of psychoprophylaxis point out that the technique is reliant on the parturient's conscious and co-operative efforts unlike hypnosis.

Biofeedback

Biofeedback is a technique utilizing two feedback methods to aid relaxation. The first involves voluntary muscle relaxation. Signals from the electromyography is fed back to the parturient in the form of audible clicks through an earpiece. A decrease in frequency of the audible clicks indicates relaxation. The second method utilizes skin conductance. When stressed, sympathetic activity causes sweating and increased skin conductance and this is reversed when the parturient is relaxed. St. James-Roberts et al[20] demonstrated that electromyographic as opposed to skin conductance biofeedback techniques could be taught effectively to aid relaxation in parturients. However, a review of studies by the Cochrane database by Simkin[21] was inconclusive in terms of its efficacy as a pain relieving method in labour.

Hypnosis

The use of hypnosis for childbirth is not new. There is a requirement of hypnotic suggestibility and the instruction of the technique is time consuming[22] both antenatally and during labour. Approximately 10–20% of women are not susceptible to hypnosis[23] and the eye-roll test grades the ability to roll the eyes upwards, which indicates hypnotic susceptibility.[24] The parturient is in a trance and receptive to positive suggestions by the hypnotist. In a randomized controlled trial of hypnosis in labour[25] no difference in epidural use could be demonstrated between the groups. Wahl[26] reported complications of hypnosis in obstetrics that ranged from acute states of anxiety to frank psychosis.

DISADVANTAGES OF PSYCHOLOGICAL SUPPORT

- Time consuming
- May generate unrealistic expectations

- Minimal evidence of efficacy of pain relief
- May generate feelings of guilt when other methods of pain relief are utilized.

The benefits of psychological methods for pain relief may be over-emphasized by certain groups and individuals. This may lead to over reliance on these methods by women. In reality, most women who plan not to use medication for pain relief do.[2,3] This may lead to feelings of disappointment, guilt and failure that are wholly unjustified. It is essential when using psychological techniques that a realistic approach to pain relief, including the option to use other methods, should be part and parcel of antenatal preparation. This will also be compatible to allowing greater maternal choice.[27] Failure to adopt this balanced approach could lead to emotional and psychological damage to both the parturients and their partners.[28]

PHYSICAL TECHNIQUES

- Immersion
- Transcutaneous electrical nerve stimulation (TENS)
- Massage
- Reflexology
- Acupuncture
- Water blocks.

Immersion (Hydrotherapy)

The use of warm water during labour to soothe the pain of labour has been used for centuries and came back in vogue recently for pain relief and birth. The House of Commons Health Committee's report[29] on maternal services recommended that all hospitals should provide women with the option of a birthing pool where possible. The sensation of warmth and pressure of the surrounding water may alleviate pain by inhibiting the transmission of pain and supporting the load of the gravid uterus. A Cochrane review of three trials involving 988 women showed no statistically significant differences between immersion and no immersion for pain relief, augmentation and duration of the first stage of labour, meconium stained liquor and perineal trauma.[30]

Transcutaneous electrical nerve stimulation

The use of TENS for pain relief in childbirth was introduced in the early 1980s. The NBT survey of 1990 showed that TENS was available in approximately 65% of units in the United Kingdom but used by fewer than 6% of women.[31] It appears to work best for low level pain and is therefore most effective earlier on in labour. It is also most efficacious for back

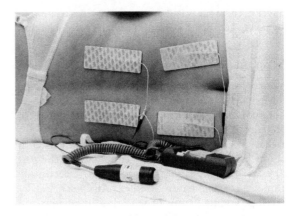

Figure 4.4   Transcutaneous electrical nerve stimulator (TENS) showing the position of the electrodes.

pain with two pairs of electrodes placed at the T_{10}–L_1 level and the S_2–S_4 level (Fig. 4.4). The modern TENS machine allows individual adjustment of the frequency and amplitude of electrical stimulation with some models allowing patient-controlled burst stimulation to coincide with peak contraction. The mechanism of action is based on the modification of pain via the 'gate theory' of pain transmission.[32] It has also been suggested that low frequency stimulation at 2 Hz acts through neuronal release of endorphins into the CSF.[33] A systematic review of eight randomized controlled trials investigating analgesic and adverse outcomes failed to demonstrate the pain relieving effect of TENS.[34]

Massage

The use of massage to release tension and aid relaxation is one of the oldest and simplest methods for soothing the pain of labour used by carers of the parturient. Massage techniques are used by about 20% of parturients in labour.[31] It has an effect similar to TENS in blocking the transmission of pain impulses as well as a form of support and distraction. Approximately 90% of women in the NBT survey who used massage rated it as either good or very good.

Reflexology

Reflexology has been practised for thousands of years in China and Egypt and introduced into the West by William Fitzgerald about 90 years ago. Reflexologists apply gentle pressure or massage to feet and hands to stimulate energy flow. Pressure on specific areas on the body are supposed to have a corresponding effect on a related area. Pressure around the ankle and radial aspect of the wrist is said to stimulate points relating to the pelvis, uterus and sacrum to ease the pain of labour.

Acupuncture

Acupuncture has a long history in Chinese medicine but its use for pain relief in labour and for Caesarean sections is limited. It has been used to treat a range of ailments of pregnancy including nausea, hyperemesis, backache and constipation.[35] Its use for pain relief in labour have been advanced by enthusiasts in the past 20 years in the West, with increasing use of electrically stimulated acupuncture needles. Analgesia usually develops within 30 min of starting acupuncture and studies in the West have demonstrated that acupuncture raises the pain threshold.[36] The postulated mechanisms of action involve both neural and humoral systems.[37] A few non-randomized and poorly controlled studies of the use of acupuncture in labour show that the efficacy of the technique for pain relief is hugely variable, but the women receiving acupuncture claim to feel calmer and more in control of their labour.[38]

Waterblocks

This technique, which is popular in the Scandinavian countries, involves the intradermal injection of approximately 0.1 ml of sterile water in four spots overlying the sacrum. There follows an initial burning sensation for 20–30 s and its mechanism of action has been suggested to be similar to TENS. Ader et al[39] and Trolle et al[40] conducted double-blind randomized controlled studies that showed a reduction in labour pain after water blocks. However, a survey in Finland by Ranta et al[41] found that parturients did not rate waterblocks as effective as other methods of pain relief.

OTHER COMPLEMENTARY THERAPIES

- Aromatherapy
- Homeopathy
- Herbalism.

Aromatherapy

Aromatherapy uses the essential oils of plants and flowers for therapeutic effect. Aromatherapy is thought to work by assisting in the relaxation and uplifting of mental and emotional state. It is standard practice for the aromatherapist to test out the oils for use with the individual parturient, as smell is an individual sensation. Lavender oil is claimed to have a relaxing effect reducing anxiety and relaxing uterine contractions.

Clary sage is used to hasten labour by relieving stress as well as having a humoral effect. Peppermint oil is used for nausea and vomiting. There are however no randomized trials on the use of aromatherapy.

Homeopathy

Homeopathy works on the principle that a minute amount of a substance that in larger quantities would cause symptoms, can be used to alleviate the same symptoms. Remedies include arnica, which is supposed to reduce pain, inflammation and promote healing; caulophyllum to strengthen contractions and hypericum to promote healing and reduce tissue damage.

Herbalism

Herbalists utilize raw extracts of plants or herbal remedies for individual needs. A combination of extracts are used to strengthen the reproductive organs for labour and delivery, increase stamina, relieve pain and calm the parturient. To date, there are no controlled trials to validate or refute the efficacy of complementary therapies for the relief of pain during childbirth.

IMPLICATIONS FOR THE ANAESTHETIST

There are important reasons why anaesthetists should be aware of non-pharmacological methods of pain relief. Firstly, these methods are being utilized by a large number of women in labour. Secondly, although there is insufficient scientific evidence to support the efficacy of a large number of non-pharmacological methods of pain relief, they do provide a choice for the woman and this itself is an important factor. It is vitally important that anaesthetists are involved in the provision of good information, which allows women to form realistic expectations and increase their awareness of the limitations of certain methods of analgesia. Equally, it is also important to have available regional analgesia when a request is made for it. Understanding the complex multi-facet nature of labour pain and the ability to communicate effectively with the parturient and her carers is a primary role of an obstetric anaesthetist.

REFERENCES

1. Melzack R. The myth of painless childbirth. *Pain* 1984; **19**: 321–337.

2. Melzack R, Taenzer P, Feldman P et al. Labour is still painful after prepared childbirth training. *Can Med Assoc J* 1981; **125**: 357–363.

3. Chamberlain G, Wraight A, Steer P (eds) *Pain and its relief in childbirth: the results of a national survey conducted by the National Birthday Trust*. Edinburgh: Churchill Livingstone, 1993.

4. Morgan BM, Bullpitt CJ, Clifton P et al. Analgesia and satisfaction in childbirth (the Queen Charlotte's 1000 mother survey). *Lancet* 1982a; **ii**: 808–810.

5. Rickford WJK, Reynolds F. Expectations and experiences of pain relief in labour. In: *Society for obstetric anaesthesia and perinatology (Abstracts)*. Halifax: Nova Scotia, 1987, p 163.

6. Capogna G, Alahuta S, Celleno D et al. Maternal expectations and experiences of labour pain and analgesia: a multicentre study of nulliparous women. *Int J Obstet Anesth* 1996; **5**: 229–235.

7. Morgan BM, Bullpitt CJ, Clifton P et al. Effectiveness of pain relief in labour. *Br Med J* 1982b; **285**: 689–690.

8. Seguin L, Therrien R, Champagne F et al. The components of women's satisfaction with maternity care. *Birth* 1989; **16**(3): 109–113.

9. Green JM, Coupland VA, Kitzinger JV. *Birth* 1990; **17**(1): 15–24.

10. Wee M, Gande R, Longhorn R et al. A pain relief in labour algorithm for the delivery suite. *Poster presentation at the annual meeting of the Obstetric Anaesthetists Association*, Liverpool, 1999.

11. Skibsted L, Lange AP. The need for pain relief in uncomplicated deliveries in an alternative birthing centre compared to an obstetric delivery ward. *Pain* 1992; **48**: 183–186.

12. Waldenstrom U, Nilsson C-A. Experience of childbirth in birth centre. *Acta Obstet Gynecol Scand* 1994; **73**: 547–554.

13. Morgan BM, Bullpitt CJ, Clifton P et al. The consumers' attitude to obstetric care. *Br J Obstet Gynecol* 1984; **91**: 624–628.

14. Kennell J, Klaus M, McGrath S et al. Continuous emotional support during labor in a US hospital. *JAMA* 1991; **265**(17): 2197–2201.

15. Keirse MJNC, Enkin M, Lumley J. Support from caregivers during childbirth. In: *The cochrane pregnancy and childbirth database*. The Cochrane Collaboration and Update Software, Issue 1, 1995.

16. Dick-Read G. *Natural childbirth*. London: Heinemann, 1933.

17. Dick-Read G. *Childbirth without fear*. New York: Harper & Brothers, 1944.

18. Leboyer F. *Birth without violence*. New York: Alfred A Knof, 1975.

19. Lamaze F. *Painless childbirth*. London: Burke, 1958.

20. St. James-Roberts I, Chamberlain G, Haran FJ et al. Use of electromyographic and skin-conductance biofeedback relaxation training to facilitate childbirth in primiparae. *J Psychosom Res* 1982; **26**: 455–462.

21. Simkin P. Biofeedback in prenatal class attenders. In: *The cochrane pregnancy and childbirth database*. The Cochrane Collaboration and Update Software, Issue 1, 1995.

22. Fee FA, Reilley RR. Hypnosis in obstetrics: a review of techniques. *J Am Soc Psychosom Dent Med* 1982; **29**: 17–29.

23. Wickelstein LB. Routine hypnosis for obstetrical delivery. An evaluation of hypnosuggestion in 200 consecutive cases. *Am J Obstet Gynecol* 1958; **76**: 152–160.

24. Spiegel H. An eye-roll test for hypnotisability. *Am J Clin Hypn* 1972; **15**: 25–28.

25. Freeman RM, McAulay AJ, Eve L et al. Randomised trial of self-hypnosis for analgesia in labour. *Br Med J* 1986; **292**: 657–658.

26. Wahl CW. Contraindications and limitations of hypnosis in obstetric analgesia. *Am J Obstet Gynecol* 1962; **84**: 1869–1872.

27. *Changing childbirth*. Report of the Expert Maternity Group, Department of Health. London: HMSO, 1993.

28. Stewart DE. Psychiatric symptoms following attempted natural childbirth. *Can Med Assoc J* 1982; **127**: 713–716.

29. House of Commons Health Committee. *Maternity services*, 2nd report. London: HMSO, 1992.

30. Nikodem VC. Immersion in water during pregnancy, labour and birth. In: *Cochrane review*. The Cochrane Library, Issue 2. Oxford: Update Software, 1999.

31. Steer P. The availability of pain relief and the methods of pain relief used. In: Chamberlain G, Wraight A, Steer P (eds) *Pain and its relief in childbirth*. Edinburgh: Churchill Livingstone, 1993, pp 45–67.

32. Melzack R, Wall PD. Pain mechanisms: a new theory. *Science* 1965; **150**: 971–979.

33. Sjolund B, Terenius L, Eriksson M. Increased cerebrospinal fluid levels of endorphins after electroacupuncture. *Acta Physiol Scand* 1977; **100**: 382–384.

34. Carroll D, Tramer M, McQuay H et al. Transcutaneous electrical nerve stimulation in labour pain: a systematic review. *Br J Obstet Gynaecol* 1997; **104**: 169–175.

35. Yelland S. *Acupuncture in midwifery*, Vol. 10. Hale: Books for Midwives Press, 1996.

36. Chapman CR, Gehrig JD, Wilson ME. Acupuncture compared with 33 percent nitrous oxide for dental analgesia: a sensory decision theory evaluation. *Anesthesiology* 1975; **42**: 532–537.

37. Cheng RSS, Promeranz B. Electroacupuncture analgesia could be mediated by at least two pain-relieving mechanisms: endorphin and non-endorphin systems. *Life Sci* 1979; **25**: 1957–1962.

38. Skelton IF, Flowerdew MW. Acupuncture in labour – a summary of the results. *Midwives Chronicle* 1988; **101**: 134–137.

39. Ader L, Hansson B, Wallin G. Parturition pain treated with intracutaneous injections of sterile water. *Pain* 1990; **41**: 133–138.

40. Trolle B, Moller M, Kronborg et al. The effect of sterile water blocks on low back labor pain. *Am J Obstet Gynecol* 1991; **164**: 1277–1281.

41. Ranta P, Jouppilla P, Spalding M et al. Parturients' assessment of water blocks, pethidine, nitrous oxide, paracervical and epidural blocks in labour. *Int J Obstet Anesth* 1994; **3**: 193–198.

5

NON-REGIONAL ANALGESIA II: PHARMACOLOGICAL METHODS

Mike Wee

SYSTEMIC ANALGESICS

Systemic analgesics can be subdivided into parenteral opioids, other pharmacological agents and inhalational analgesia. Systemic analgesics are widely used despite being significantly less efficacious than epidural analgesia.

REASONS FOR CONTINUED USAGE OF SYSTEMIC ANALGESICS

- Widely available
- Relatively inexpensive
- Simple to administer
- Often used early on in the analgesia ladder
- Perceived (by parturients) to be less invasive and less risk than epidurals
- Epidurals may not be appropriate or contraindicated.

Hughes and Cohen[1] discussed in an editorial the moral and ethical dilemmas of the provision and withdrawal of epidural analgesia. Hawkins[2] published the results of anaesthetic practice in the United States, which showed that systemic medications remained the most frequent used form of analgesia, despite the increase in epidural analgesia. It is also a popular form of analgesia in Europe and around the world. In a survey of 17 European countries, intramuscular pethidine was the most common method of systemic analgesia.[3]

PARENTERAL OPIOIDS

Opioids have been used for the relief of labour pain for centuries by ancient civilizations. In the early 20th century twilight sleep, induced by a combination of morphine and hyoscine, gained popularity. Unfortunately, this caused sedation and amnesia as well as unpleasant side effects among the women who used it. The 1930s heralded the introduction of pethidine in Germany, probably because morphine was unavailable there at the time. Pethidine was also mistakenly perceived to be safer and more potent than morphine in labour. Pethidine was made legally available to midwives for independent use in the United Kingdom in 1950. It remains the most widely available, used and investigated opioid in labour. The NBT survey of 1990 found pethidine to be available in 98% of maternity units in the United Kingdom and used by 37% of parturients.[4] The survey also showed that midwives overrated the efficacy of pethidine when compared to parturients' own experiences.

PETHIDINE (MEPERIDINE OR DEMEROL)

Pethidine is a synthetic opioid; a weakly basic phenylpiperidine derivative, related to fentanyl and sufentanil. It is approximately 28 times more lipid soluble than morphine. The dose of pethidine commonly used by midwives is 1 mg/kg up to 150 mg intramuscularly. The intramuscular route is not dependable and absorption may be variable.[5] Intravenous administration is more reliable. In a randomized controlled study Isenor and Penny-MacGilliray[6] compared intramuscular and intravenous pethidine limited to a maximum total dose of 200 mg. The intravenous group reported significantly lower pain scores with no differences in maternal or neonatal complications.

Patient controlled analgesia (PCA) with pethidine

Scott[7] first raised the concept of patient controlled analgesia for systemic opioids. Patient controlled analgesia (PCA) using pethidine have shown conflicting results, when compared to intramuscular pethidine[8] or nurse administered pethidine.[9] However, Sharma et al[10] in a large randomized study of Caesarean delivery outcomes comparing epidural analgesia and PCA pethidine, found that although women receiving epidurals reported lower pain scores, out of 259 women randomized to receive PCA pethidine, only five requested epidural analgesia because of ineffective pain relief. The pethidine PCA regime they used was 50 mg pethidine plus 25 mg promethazine loading dose, 10 mg bolus dose with 10 min lockout during the first hour, and thereafter, 15 mg bolus, 10 min lockout until delivery. Additional 'top-up' doses of 25 mg pethidine was allowed so long as the total dose did not exceed 100 mg every 2 h. There were no significant differences in the Apgar scores and umbilical pHs of neonates in the two groups. However, significantly more neonates in the pethidine PCA group required treatment with naloxone (13 vs 3 in the epidural group). Sedation was also significantly higher in the pethidine PCA group, but 70% of parturients who received it said that they would be happy to use it again at a future labour and delivery.

Potential benefits of PCA

- Provides a degree of control (psychological benefit)
- Ease of administration
- May be less demanding of staff attention
- Can be continued for the duration of the labour
- Can be used when epidural analgesia is contraindicated.

Efficacy

Although pethidine continues to be widely used, its efficacy as an analgesic in labour has been questioned. Holdcroft and Morgan[11] showed that pethidine provided satisfactory analgesia in less than 25% of women, compared to almost 50% of women using Entonox. Harrison et al[12] in a comparative study of TENS, Entonox, pethidine with promazine and epidural analgesia found that the pethidine–promazine combination provided partial relief to only 54% of women compared to 90% using Entonox. The NBT survey of 1990[13] showed that of the women who received pethidine, 16% rated it as helpful but 25% rated it as unhelpful. Interestingly, pethidine was rated much higher by the midwife, than by the woman or her partner as an analgesic. The author, herself a midwife, surmised that sedation might have been confused with analgesia.

EFFECTS OF PETHIDINE ON THE PARTURIENT

Central nervous system

Steer[4] reported that women who used pethidine during labour complained of feelings of confusion, loss of control, sedation and poor pain relief. In parturients with severe pregnancy induced hypertension, pethidine is relatively contraindicated as the active metabolite norpethidine has proconvulsant properties.[14]

Gastrointestinal system

Pethidine given during labour decreased gastric emptying by at least 5 h in 70% of women.[15] Nimmo et al[16] clearly demonstrated that parenteral opioids delayed gastric emptying and Holdsworth[17] showed that the administration of pethidine in labour increased gastric volumes during labour. O'Sullivan et al[18] using a non-invasive impedance technique to measure gastric emptying during labour showed a significant difference between groups receiving pethidine and epidural analgesia. This has practical implications, should a general anaesthetic be required for the parturient who has received opioids. Parturients opting for systemic opioids with a high risk of operative delivery should therefore receive ranitidine and metoclopramide during labour, to reduce stomach contents and improve gastric emptying. Metoclopramide given before or at the same time as pethidine may improve gastric emptying[19] but is of little use in late labour.[16] Nausea and vomiting was made worse by pethidine.[20] An antiemetic such as metoclopramide should be used, but phenothiazine antiemetics should be avoided as it may not only exacerbate the sedative effect of pethidine but also antagonize the analgesia.[20]

Respiratory system

Pethidine, in common with all opioid analgesics, causes dose related respiratory depression and hypoventilation. Maternal hypoxic episodes are also more common with pethidine[21] than with epidural analgesia.[22] Maternal hyperventilation could be related to inadequacy of pain relief during contractions and periods of hypoventilation in between contractions. The combination of Entonox and pethidine tends to exacerbate maternal desaturation.[22–25]

Uterine contractility

Pethidine has no major effects on uterine contractility.[26] However, when given during painful labour associated with uterine incoordination, opioids may lead to more normal uterine activity.[27]

EFFECTS ON THE FETUS AND NEONATE

Pethidine is principally bound to alpha$_1$-acid glycoprotein but readily crosses the placenta by passive diffusion. It achieves equilibrium between the maternal and fetal compartments within 6 min.[28] The effects of opioids, including pethidine, are dependent mainly on the dose and timing of administration. After intramuscular administration, the highest fetal concentrations are likely to occur 2–3 h later.[29,30] However, when given within one hour of delivery the neonatal effects are minimal (Fig. 5.1). Despite this fact, it is a common misconception that giving pethidine during the late stages of labour is detrimental. This unfortunately may deprive the parturient of analgesia at a time when labour may be most painful. As a weak base, pethidine is more ionized in the acidic environment of the fetal circulation, trapping pethidine in the fetal compartment.[31] This effect is exaggerated in the compromised acidotic fetus with enhanced ion trapping. Inadequacy of analgesia may lead to hyperventilation and decrease of maternal P_aCO_2, and increasing maternal haemoglobin affinity for oxygen.[32] This will cause vasoconstriction and reduction of placental blood flow, as well as reducing oxygen availability to the fetus.

Cardiovascular system

Fetal heart rate variability may be reduced approximately 25 min after intravenous and 40 min after intramuscular administration of pethidine.[33,34] Other

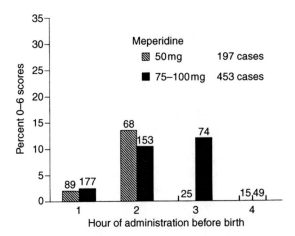

Figure 5.1 Correlation of the time of administrations of pethidine (meperidine) and neonatal depression according to Apgar scores (from Ref. 29, with permission from the publishers).

observed changes include reduced fetal movements,[35] altered fetal EEG activity[36] and reduced fetal scalp oxygen tension.[37] However, the clinical significance of the fetal changes is unknown. Changes in fetal heart rate variability may lead to unnecessary intervention.

Respiratory system

The respiratory depressant effects of pethidine at a given blood concentration is more pronounced in the neonate than in the parturient. This may be a reflection of the immaturity of the neonatal respiratory system and the presence of a higher concentration of free drug in the neonate, due to lower plasma protein binding or ion trapping.[31,38] The respiratory depression may result in lower Apgar scores,[29] depressed oxygen saturations[39] and increased carbon dioxide tensions.[40] The neonatal effects of pethidine are compounded by the production of its active metabolite norpethidine. Norpethidine has limited analgesic efficacy and causes prolonged sedation and respiratory depression. It also has proconvulsant properties. Furthermore, the half lives of pethidine and norpethidine in the parturient are approximately 4 and 20 h but in the neonate are approximately 13 and 62 h.[41,42] The long half-life of norpethidine is implicated in the late effects of the drug (see below). Hamza et al[43] reported that neonates from parturients who had received pethidine with normal Apgar scores demonstrated low SaO_2 levels (less than 90%) during active sleep when compared with neonates who had not received opioids.

Neurobehavioural changes and breastfeeding

There are a multitude of studies demonstrating abnormal neurobehavioural patterns and babies, who are sleepier, less attentive and less able to establish breast feeding in parturients who have received pethidine during labour.[44–47] These changes have occurred with normal Apgar scores at birth. The long-term significance of these behavioural changes remains unclear. A retrospective study of 200 drug addicts by Jacobson[48] found that children of mothers who had received pethidine in labour might be more liable to develop drug addiction problems later on in life. They postulated that imprinting of opioid usage in utero may be the cause, but the evidence is weak.

Antagonism of pethidine opioid side effects

The effects of pethidine and norpethidine can be reversed by intramuscular naloxone, a specific opioid antagonist. A large dose given intramuscularly at a dose of 60–100 µg/kg has long-acting effects and may have an effect for up to 48 h.[49,50] Naloxone reverses opioid depression of neonatal minute ventilation and increases the slope of the CO_2 response curve.[51] Naloxone should not be given to the neonate of an opioid dependent parturient, as withdrawal symptoms may result from this antagonism.

MORPHINE

The dose of morphine used for maternal analgesia is 2–5 mg intravenously or 5–10 mg intramuscularly. The onset of analgesia is within 5 min after intravenous administration, with peak effect at around 20 min. After intramuscular injection, the onset of analgesia is between 20 and 40 min with peak effect after 1–2 h.[52] Morphine has a low molecular weight and rapidly crosses the placenta. It is primarily bound to albumin and is approximately 35% protein bound in plasma. Gerdin et al[53] demonstrated rapid maternal clearance of morphine and a shorter elimination half-life of morphine, thereby decreasing the fetal exposure to morphine. The analgesic efficacy of morphine, for early labour pain, has been questioned by Olofsson et al.[54] However, a number of women with back pain experienced some benefit. In another prospective, double blind randomized study comparing intravenous morphine and pethidine in a small number of parturients in labour, Olofsson et al[55] recorded high pain scores on the visual analogue scale with sedation of the parturients. They concluded that neither drug is effective for pain relief and question the ethical and medical aspects of using systemically administered morphine or pethidine. The side effects of morphine are dose related and similar to pethidine. However, morphine is metabolized to morphine-3-glucuronide, which does not have analgesic efficacy or side effects unlike norpethidine.

DIAMORPHINE

Diamorphine is available for obstetric use in the United Kingdom and a few maternity units (less than 5% nationally) use it enthusiastically. In the NBT survey of 1990, both midwives and the parturients who used diamorphine graded it better than either Entonox or pethidine.[13] Unlike pethidine, diamorphine cannot be used independently by midwives. As it is more lipid soluble than morphine, this would suggest that its onset of action is faster but there are no controlled trials of its efficacy or side effect profile. Comparison of pethidine and diamorphine has been reported in an abstract.[56]

FENTANYL (SUBLIMAZE)

Fentanyl is a highly lipid-soluble, (approximately 50 times more soluble than morphine), phenypiperidine derivative and also highly protein, bound principally to albumin. Its analgesic potency is 75–100 times that of morphine and 800 times that of pethidine. Due to its lipid solubility, it has a rapid onset of action but its terminal half-life of approximately 8 h is longer than that of morphine or pethidine.[57] Its advantages for obstetric use include rapid onset and short duration of action, as well as lack of active metabolites. However, large doses of fentanyl will result in accumulation of the drug both in the parturient and fetus. Fentanyl rapidly crosses the placenta, appearing in the fetal circulation within 1 min, with peak fetal concentrations detected around 5 min.[58] After intravenous administration of 50–100 μg fentanyl, no effects on maternal or fetal cardiovascular function, uterine tone, uterine blood flow or maternal/fetal acid–base status were noted in pregnant ewes. Fentanyl 1 μg/kg given to women undergoing Caesarean section resulted in average umbilical/maternal fentanyl concentration ratio of 0.31.[59] Administration of fentanyl did not affect Apgar scores, umbilical cord blood gas or neurobehavioral scores at 4 and 24 h. Smith et al[60] investigated the effect of 50 μg fentanyl given intravenously during active labour in 24 (12 controls) fetuses at 37–41 weeks gestation. They found that fetuses that received fentanyl, had reduced body movements between contractions, breathing was abolished at 10 min post-dosing and fetal heart rate variability was reduced between contractions for 30 min in 8 out of 12 fetuses. None of the fetal heart rate changes

persisted for longer than 40 min. Apgar scores and umbilical gas were within normal limits at delivery. Rayburn et al[61] administered intravenous fentanyl in doses of 50–100 μg to 137 women in active labour as often as every hour on maternal request. The cumulative doses ranged from 50 to 600 μg and all parturients experienced transient analgesia. Onset of analgesia occurred within 5 min and with a duration of 45 min. Transient decrease in fetal heart rate variability was observed for 30 min after administration. There were no differences between the control group (112 women), and the fentanyl group, in Apgar scores, incidence of respiratory depression and neuroadaptive capacity scores at 4 and 24 h post-delivery. One neonate from each group received naloxone. In a randomized, non-blinded study, Rayburn et al[62] compared 105 healthy pregnant women at term receiving either intravenous fentanyl (50–100 μg/h) or pethidine (25–50 mg every 2–3 h). Pain scores were high with no significant differences in analgesic efficacy between the two drugs using those doses. However, maternal nausea, vomiting and sedation were worse in the pethidine group.

Fentanyl PCA during labour

Fentanyl PCA has been used in two case reports for parturients with thrombocytopaenia.[63,64] Nikkola et al[65] randomized 20 primiparous women to receive either fentanyl PCA or epidural. The fentanyl PCA regime consisted of a 50 μg loading dose, 20 μg bolus and a lock-out period of 5 min. The maximum dose allowed in 1 h was 240 μg. The dose range of fentanyl varied between 190 and 885 μg over a period of 43–418 min. Initially, epidural analgesia was more effective and 3 out of 10 parturients in the fentanyl PCA group opted for epidural analgesia. Overall satisfaction for the analgesia was similar in both groups. There were no differences in Apgar scores, umbilical blood pH or neuroadaptive capacity scores at 1 and 13 h. None required naloxone. However, oxygen saturations were generally lower in the fentanyl group neonates. The authors concluded that PCA fentanyl may have a role as a substitute for epidural analgesia, but the fetus and neonate require careful observation post-delivery. Morley-Foster et al[66] in a randomized blinded study compared PCA fentanyl and PCA alfentanil. A loading dose of 50 or 500 μg fentanyl or alfentanil was administered with bolus doses of 10 or 100 μg, lockout 5 min and background infusion of 20 or 200 μg fentanyl or alfentanil respectively. Parturients receiving fentanyl PCA were found to have significantly lower visual analogue pain scores during the later stages of labour at 7–10 cm cervical dilatation when compared to alfentanil PCA parturients.

Forty-two per cent of alfentanil PCA parturients described the analgesia as inadequate, as opposed to 9% of the fentanyl PCA parturients. There were no significant differences between the neonates in the two groups in Apgar scores, umbilical blood gases, neurobehavioural scores or requirement for naloxone.

Implications of fentanyl PCA on neonatal monitoring

Morley-Foster et al[67] retrospectively reviewed the outcome of 32 neonates whose mothers had received PCA fentanyl during labour. Fourteen (44%) of the neonates had a 1 min Apgar score of less than 6 but all had scores greater than 7 at 5 min. Three neonates received naloxone. Gestational age, birth weight, method of delivery, PCA duration, time from last dose to delivery, bolus dose and rate of fentanyl infusion were not predictive of low 1 min Apgar scores. However, the total dose of fentanyl received by parturients whose neonates required naloxone, were significantly higher (770 vs 298 μg). Nikkola et al[65] had also demonstrated that despite normal Apgar scores, umbilical pH and neuroadaptive capacity scores, neonates from parturients who received fentanyl had lower SpO_2 compared to the non-fentanyl neonates during the 12 h post-delivery. Respiratory rate was not affected. The authors recommended that when intravenous fentanyl is used for labour analgesia, the neonate should be monitored for a period post-delivery.

Summary of fentanyl PCA

- Not as effective but a useful substitute for epidural analgesia.
- The ideal loading dose, bolus dose, lockout time and maximum hourly dose is still unknown, due to lack of large randomized controlled trials.
- Both the parturient and neonate require careful monitoring during and post-delivery.
- Absence of active metabolites is an advantage.

REMIFENTANIL

Remifentanil is a relatively new, ultrashort-acting opioid derivative of fentanyl.[68] It is a pure mu agonist with rapid breakdown of the ester linkage by non-specific tissue and plasma esterases. Its metabolism is independent of hepatic or renal function. The speed of onset of remifentanil is similar to that of alfentanil and potency similar to fentanyl in non-obstetric surgical cases. Kan et al[69] evaluated the intravenous infusion of remifentanil during Caesarean section under epidural anaesthesia. They concluded that placental

transfer of remifentanil was rapid, coupled with rapid distribution and metabolism in the neonate. The authors speculated that the pharmacokinetics of remifentanil might lend itself as a systemic analgesic for labour. Brada et al[70] reported the use of intravenous remifentanil to facilitate placement of an epidural during labour. Jones et al[71] described the use of patient-controlled remifentanil analgesia for three parturients with thrombocytopaenia. The most successful regimen comprised a bolus dose of 0.5 μg/kg with a lockout period of 2–3 min. Analgesia was effective when the parturient learned to anticipate the next contraction and administered a bolus dose approximately 30 s before the next contraction. The range of remifentanil consumption was 426–1050 μg/h. There was one episode of excessive maternal sedation and fetal heart rate decelerations, when a larger bolus dose of 1 μg/kg, lockout 2 min was used over a period of 12 min. Thurlow and Waterhouse[72] described two parturients with thrombocytopaenia who were given remifentanil PCA. The authors used a bolus dose of 20 μg with lockout time of 3 min with no background infusion. Analgesia was reported as very good by the parturients and attending midwives. There were no adverse maternal or neonatal sequelae.

OTHER SYSTEMIC DRUGS

A Cochrane review of sixteen randomized controlled trials of types of intra-muscular opioids for maternal pain relief was conducted to assess their efficacy and side effects.[73] The reviewers found that there was no evidence of difference between tramadol and pethidine in terms of pain relief but there appeared to be more nausea and vomiting and drowsiness with tramadol, compared with pethidine. The dose of tramadol usually used is 50–100 mg four hourly. Maternal pain relief seemed almost identical between meptazinol and pethidine, but meptazinol gave rise to slightly more side effects. Maternal satisfaction for pain relief appeared similar for pentazocine and pethidine with more frequent nausea and vomiting with pethidine. A summary of the characteristics of these opioid partial agonist–antagonists are given in Table 5.1.

Sub-anaesthetic doses of ketamine, a pencyclidine derivative, provide a dissociative state of analgesia. Intravenous ketamine has a rapid onset of action with short duration of action of approximately 3–5 min. Ketamine may have a role during the second stage of labour or as an adjunct to regional analgesia, where a small dose of 10–20 mg repeated may provide sufficient

Table 5.1 Some characteristics of opioid agonists/antagonists used in labour

Opioid	Type	Usual dose	Onset	Efficacy	Other notes
Nalbuphine (Nubaine)	Agonist/antagonist with kappa agonist activity	10–20 mg i.m. every 4–6 h PCA dose 1–3 mg with 10 min lockout	Within 15 min or 2–3 min i.v.	Similar to 100 mg pethidine i.m.	Kappa mediated sedation may cause dysphoria
Meptazinol (Meptid)	Agonist/antagonist	100–150 mg i.m. every 2–4 h		1/10th potency of morphine, similar to pethidine	May cause dysphoric effects in high doses, increased nausea and vomiting
Pentazocine (Talwin)	Agonist/antagonist	40 mg i.m. every 2–4 h	Within 15–60 min after i.m. Within 10 min of i.v.	1/3rd potency of morphine, similar or slightly less potent than pethidine	May cause dysphoric effects in high doses but less nausea and vomiting
Butorphanol (Stadol)	Agonist/antagonist activity similar to pentazocine	1–2 mg i.m. or i.v.		5 times more potent than morphine 40 times more potent than pethidine	Ceiling effect of respiratory depression Lack of active metabolites

analgesia. The dose should not exceed 1 mg/kg as higher doses may lead to loss of consciousness, increased uterine tone and hallucinations.

INHALATIONAL ANALGESIA

Inhalational analgesia has a long history in obstetrics and the earliest form of patient controlled analgesia. It also has an enviable record of safety. The ideal inhalational analgesic should be potent, have rapid onset and offset, be simple to use as well as economical and have minimal side effects to mother and baby.

In 1847, James Young Simpson, professor of midwifery in Edinburgh was the first to use an inhalational agent, ether, for pain relief in labour. Later, he successfully used chloroform to aid childbirth. The royal seal of approval was obtained when John Snow administered chloroform to Queen Victoria in 1853 for the birth of Prince Leopold. Ether was pungent, irritant to the upper airways and a powerful emetic. Chloroform had a more pleasant odour, non-irritant, more potent and quicker onset. However, its side effects include cardiac arrhythmias and hepatic damage. Since the days of ether and chloroform, other inhalational agents including cyclopropane, trichloroethylene and methoxyflurane have been used for labour pain in obstetrics.

TRICHLOROETHYLENE (TRILENE)

Trichloroethylene was introduced in obstetrics in 1943. It is highly potent with good analgesic properties at concentrations of 0.35–0.5%, which provided similar analgesia to 50% nitrous oxide and 0.35% methoxyflurane.[74] Trichloroethylene was most popular and safe when used with calibrated, temperature compensated drawover vaporizers such as the Emotril and Tecota Mark 6. It has a high blood/gas partition coefficient

(9.0) which result in delayed onset and offset. This resulted in 'carry-over' of trichloroethylene to subsequent contractions, which not only improved its efficacy, but also caused increasing maternal sedation as well as neonatal depression.[75] It was also associated with a high incidence of nausea and vomiting. Trichloroethylene was used extensively by midwives, until the 1980s. Its approval for use by midwives was withdrawn by the Central Midwives Board in 1993.

METHOXYFLURANE (PENTHRANE)

Methoxyflurane is a potent halogenated ether (MAC 0.16), introduced in 1960. Like trichloroethylene, methoxyflurane has a high blood/gas partition coefficient displaying similar characteristics. Accumulation occurs with prolonged use, and the risk of renal damage due to inorganic fluoride ions from hepatic metabolism led to its withdrawal from clinical use in 1984. However, there was no evidence of renal damage in parturients or neonates.

Of the more recently introduced inhalational agents, enflurane, isoflurane and desflurane have made their debut in obstetrics, but the agent which has withstood the test of time as the inhalational analgesia for labour is nitrous oxide in oxygen. It was introduced into obstetric practice in 1880 by Klikovicz and has gained popularity since the 1930s.

ENTONOX (50% NITROUS OXIDE IN OXYGEN)

Entonox, is the most widely available inhalational analgesic in the United Kingdom, with availability in 99% of units, and used by 60% of parturients.[4] Tunstall[76] demonstrated that under a pressure of 2000 psi, oxygen would dissolve nitrous oxide in a gaseous phase producing a mixture. Nitrous oxide with its low blood/gas partition coefficient of 0.47 equilibrates rapidly with arterial concentration. Consequently, there is minimal accumulation with intermittent use during labour when nitrous oxide is washed out of the lungs. To achieve near-maximum effect, approximately 10 breaths or approximately 50 s are required.[77] This has important implications in the timing of administration of Entonox, so that peak concentration coincide with peak contraction. This may not be easy to achieve, as the first 30 s of a contraction may not be painful and therefore when the parturient starts inhaling Entonox in response to pain, the peak concentration of Entonox does not coincide with peak contraction pain. Careful coaching of the parturient is essential for successful use of Entonox. In an attempt to reduce the need for accurate timing, low concentrations of nitrous oxide has been administered via a nasal catheter in parturients[78,79] increasing the baseline concentration of nitrous oxide.

EFFICACY

The use of 50% nitrous oxide is a compromise between efficacy and safety. Jones et al[80] found that the optimum balance of analgesia and level of consciousness was achieved when a concentration of 41% was administered continuously, which translates to intermittent inhalation of 74% nitrous oxide. The Medical Research Council trials of 50%, 60% and 70% nitrous oxide with oxygen concluded that 50% nitrous oxide was safer than 70%, as the higher concentration caused loss of consciousness in 2.9% of women, compared to 0.4% in those receiving 50%.[81] Reports from trials and surveys gave mixed results, regarding the efficacy of intermittent nitrous oxide. Complete or satisfactory pain relief range from 75% to 50% and no or slight analgesia from 25% to 48%.[11,74,81] On the other hand, reports from surveys indicate that Entonox is generally more efficacious than pethidine and TENS.[11–13] In contrast, Carstoniu et al[82] in a randomized, double blind, crossover and placebo-controlled trial comparing Entonox with compressed air, in 26 women, could not distinguish between the two in terms of analgesic efficacy. However, the study was carried out in very early labour over a maximum of 10 contractions. Pain relief from inhalational anaesthetic agents may depend not only on reaching effective analgesic concentration, but also on other factors including distraction, relaxation and a sense of control derived from self-administration.

Side effects and complications

- General side effects – drowsiness, disorientation, nausea
- Potential for reduced fetal oxygenation
- Potential for reduced maternal oxygenation
- Methionine synthetase inhibition.

Nitrous oxide may cause drowsiness and light-headedness as well as nausea. With prolonged use, some parturients become disorientated and 0.4% unconsciousness.[81] As the efficacy of Entonox is variable, in an attempt to improve analgesia, some parturients may hyperventilate and use it continuously. This may ultimately lead to maternal hypocapnia, alkalosis and vasoconstriction, resulting in reduced uterine blood flow that can potentially reduce fetal oxygenation.[83]

Maternal oxygenation may be affected by the use of nitrous oxide particularly when inadequate analgesia results in maternal hypoventilation and diffusion hypoxia.[84,85] The combination of Entonox and pethidine[22–25] increases the frequency of desaturation. However, the picture is not so clear-cut. Episodes of hypoxaemia occur during painful labour[86] and also in those receiving epidural analgesia.[85] Furthermore, a well-conducted study by Carstoniu[82] and an earlier study by Davies et al[87] failed to demonstrate desaturation in parturients receiving Entonox alone. Despite the studies demonstrating significant episodes of maternal desaturation, particularly with the Entonox and pethidine combination, none have to date demonstrated adverse maternal or neonatal clinical outcome.

Nitrous oxide inhibits methionine synthase activity by inactivating co-factor vitamin B_{12}. This may theoretically cause bone marrow suppression with prolonged use and has also been implicated in teratogenicity. A recent editorial from Maze and Fujinaga[88] discussed the recent advances in understanding the actions and toxicity of nitrous oxide.

OTHER INHALATIONAL AGENTS AND ADJUVANTS TO ENTONOX

Both enflurane and isoflurane are halogenated ethers related to methoxyflurane but with blood/gas partition coefficients approximately 6 times less than methoxyflurane, but 3–4 times higher than Entonox. There is therefore a lower risk of accumulation and since they are biodegraded less than methoxyflurane, the risk of organ toxicity is less than methoxyflurane. Both 1% enflurane[89] and 0.75% isoflurane[90] have been administered intermittently for labour pain. Although analgesia was better compared to Entonox, this was at the expense of increased maternal sedation. Enflurane 0.25–1.25% and isoflurane 0.2–0.7% in oxygen have been administered continuously for the second stage of labour during normal vaginal delivery, but analgesic efficacy and patient satisfaction was no better than with Entonox.[91,92]

In an attempt to improve the efficacy of Entonox, Aurora et al[93] and Wee et al[94] added 0.2–0.25% isoflurane to Entonox. Pain relief scores and reduction in visual analogue pain scores as well as patient satisfaction were superior in those who received low dose isoflurane with Entonox as opposed to Entonox alone. Maternal sedation was not significantly increased, and maternal acceptance high. Isoflurane was administered using the drawover vaporizer in circuit with Entonox and an example is depicted in Fig. 5.2. Ross et al[95]

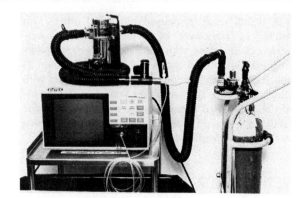

Figure 5.2   Set-up for low dose isoflurane with Entonox via the Isotec temperature compensated drawover vaporizer and agent monitor.

used premixed 0.25% isoflurane in Entonox for analgesia when Entonox failed to relieve labour pain in 221 parturients. Intolerance to the mixture was found in 7.7% of cases and 14.5% of parturients elected to have an epidural. The Apgar scores at 1 and 5 min were unaffected by the use of the isoflurane–Entonox mixture but a positive correlation between Apgar scores less than 8 was found in neonates whose mothers were given opioids in addition to the isoflurane–Entonox mixture. The authors suggest that low dose isoflurane–Entonox mixture may have a role when Entonox has failed, and epidural may not be a suitable option. Sub-anaesthetic doses of isoflurane have not been shown to exhibit analgesic properties in volunteers. One possible effect of sub-anaesthetic doses of isoflurane is that of sedation and relaxation. From personal observation over a number of years, of parturients inhaling low dose isoflurane–Entonox mixtures, respiratory rate is generally reduced, tidal volumes increased and parturients describe feeling more relaxed. This may lead to improved alveolar concentration of nitrous oxide with improved efficacy of Entonox; a form of reversible sedo-analgesia.

Desflurane has low blood-gas partition coefficient, (0.42), allowing rapid onset and offset of action. Abboud et al[96] has compared the use of desflurane 1–4.5% in oxygen for the second stage of labour comparing it with 30–60% nitrous oxide. Both agents were found to be effective, but 23% of women in receiving desflurane reported amnesia during usage.

ENVIRONMENTAL POLLUTION IN THE DELIVERY SUITE

Pollution is a concern despite the general opinion that the newer inhalational agents are safe. However, in the delivery suite high concentrations of inhalation agents in constant use may lead to chronic exposure, particularly to health care workers[97] and this may lead to adverse consequences.[98,99] In the United Kingdom, the Health and Safety Executive introduced occupational exposure standards limiting ambient concentrations of nitrous oxide not to exceed 100 ppm and isoflurane 50 ppm.[100] To achieve these standards, active scavenging will be required in all delivery suites and regular monitoring of exposure to health care workers.

REFERENCES

1. Hughes SC, Cohen SE. Labor analgesia makes the news: an introduction. Labor epidural analgesia: back to the dark ages or a potential win-win situation. *Int J Obstet Anesth* 1999; **8**: 223–225.

2. Hawkins JL, Gibbs CP, Orleans M et al. Obstetric anesthesia workforce survey 1981 versus 1992. *Anesthesiology* 1997; **87**: 135–143.

3. Rawal N, Allvin R. Management of obstetric pain in Europe – a 17 nation survey (Abstract). *Annual congress of European Society of Anesthesiologists*, London.

4. Steer P. The availability of pain relief and the methods of pain relief used. In: Chamberlain G, Wraight A, Steer P (eds) *Pain and its relief in childbirth*. Edinburgh: Churchill Livingstone, 1993, pp 45–67.

5. Lazebnik N, Kuhnert BR, Carr PC et al. Intravenous, deltoid or gluteus administration of meperidine during labor? *Am J Obstet Gynecol* 1989; **160**: 1184–1189.

6. Isenor L, Penny-MacGillivray T. Intravenous meperidine infusion for obstetric analgesia. *J Obstet Gynecol Neonat Nurs* 1993; **22**: 349–356.

7. Scott JS. Obstetric analgesia. A consideration of labor pain and a patient-controlled technique for its pain relief with meperidine. *Am J Obstet Gynecol* 1970; **106**: 959–978.

8. Robinson JO, Rosen M, Evans JM et al. Self-administered intravenous and intramuscular pethidine. A controlled trial in labour. *Anaesthesia* 1980; **35**: 763–770.

9. Rayburn WF, Leuschen MP, Earl M et al. Intravenous meperidine during labor: a randomised comparison between nurse and patient controlled administration. *Obstet Gynecol* 1989a; **74**: 702–706.

10. Sharma SK, Sidawi EJ, Ramin SM et al. A randomised trial of epidural versus patient-controlled meperidine analgesia during labor. *Anesthesiology* 1997; **87**(3): 487–494.

11. Holdcroft A, Morgan M. An assessment of the analgesic effect in labour of pethidine and 50% nitrous oxide in oxygen (Entonox). *J Obstet Gynaecol Br Commonw* 1974; **81**: 603–607.

12. Harrison RF, Shore M, Woods T et al. A comparative study of TENS, Entonox, pethidine+promazine and lumbar epidural for pain relief in labor. *Acta Obstet Gynecol Scand* 1987; **66**: 9–14.

13. Wraight A. Coping with pain. In: Chamberlain G, Wraight A, Steer P (eds) *Pain and its relief in childbirth*. Edinburgh: Churchill Livingstone, 1993, pp 79–92.

14. Pryl BJ, Grech H, Stoddard PA et al. The toxicity of norpethidine in sickle cell crisis. *Br Med J* 1992; **304**: 1478–1479.

15. La Salvia LA, Steffen EA. Delayed gastric emptying time in labor. *Am J Obstet Gynecol* 1950; **59**: 1075–1081.

16. Nimmo WS, Wilson J, Prescott LF. Narcotic analgesics and delayed gastric emptying during labour. *Lancet* 1975; **i**: 890–893.

17. Holdsworth JD. Relationship between stomach contents and analgesia in labour. *Br J Anaesth* 1978; **50**: 1145–1148.

18. O'Sullivan GM, Sutton AJ, Thompson SA et al. Non-invasive measurement of gastric emptying in obstetric patients. *Anesth Analg* 1987; **66**: 505–511.

19. Murphy DF, Nally B, Gardiner J et al. Effect of metoclopramide on gastric emptying before elective and emergency Caesarean section. *Br J Anaesth* 1984; **56**: 1113–1116.

20. Vella L, Francis D, Houlton P et al. Comparison of the antiemetics metoclopramide and promethazine in labour. *Br Med J* 1985; **290**: 1173–1175.

21. Huch A, Huch R, Lindmark G et al. Maternal hypoxaemia after pethidine. *J Obstet Gynaecol Br Commonw* 1974; **81**: 608–614.

22. Reed PN, Colquhoun A, Hanning CD. Maternal oxygenation during normal labour. *Br J Anaesth* 1989; **62**: 316–318.

23. Deckardt R, Fembacher PM, Schneider KTM et al. Maternal arterial oxygen saturation during labor and delivery: pain-dependent alterations and effects on the newborn. *Obstet Gynecol* 1987; **70**: 21–25.

24. Zelcher J, Owers H, Paull JD. A controlled oximetric evaluation of inhalational, opioid and epidural analgesia in labour. *Anaesth Intens Care* 1989; **17**: 418–421.

25. Griffin RP, Reynolds F. Maternal hypoxaemia during labour and delivery: the influence of analgesia and effect on neonatal outcome. *Anaesthesia* 1995; **50**: 151–156.

26. Petrie RH, Wu R, Miller FC et al. The effect of drugs on uterine activity. *Obstet Gynecol* 1976; **48**: 431–435.

27. De Voe SJ, De Voe Jr K, Rigsby WC et al. Effect of meperidine on uterine contractility. *Am J Obstet Gynecol* 1969; **105**: 1004–1007.

28. Shnider SM, Way EL, Lord MJ. Rate of appearance and disappearance of meperidine in fetal blood after administration of narcotic to the mother (Abstract). *Anesthesiology* 1966; **27**: 227–228.

29. Shnider SM, Moya F. Effect of meperidine on the newborn infant. *Am J Obstet Gynecol* 1964; **89**: 1009–1015.

30. Belfrage P, Boreus LO, Hartwig P et al. Neonatal depression after obstetrical analgesia with pethidine: the role of the injection-delivery time interval and of the plasma concentrations of pethidine and norpethidine. *Acta Obstet Gynaecol Scand* 1981; **60**: 43–49.

31. Benson DW, Kaufman JJ, Koski WS. Theoretic significance of pH dependence of narcotics and narcotic antagonists in clinical anaesthesia. *Anesth Anal Curr Res* 1976; **55**: 253–256.

32. Huch R. Maternal hyperventilation and the fetus. *J Perinat Med* 1986; **14**: 3–17.

33. Kariniemi V, Ammala P. Effects of intramuscular pethidine on fetal heart rate variability during labour. *Br J Obstet Gynecol* 1981; **88**: 718–720.

34. Petrie RH, Yeh S, Murata Y et al. The effect of drugs on fetal heart rate variability. *Am J Obstet Gynecol* 1978; **130**: 294–299.

35. Zimmer EZ, Divon MY, Vadasz A. Influence of meperidine on fetal movements and heart rate beat to beat variability in the active phase of labor. *Am J Perinat* 1981; **5**: 197–200.

36. Rosen MG, Scibetta JJ, Hochberg CJ. Human fetal EEG III: pattern changes in the presence of fetal heart rate alterations and after use of maternal medication. *Obstet Gynecol* 1970; **361**: 132–140.

37. Baxi LV, Petrie RH, James LS. Human fetal oxygenation (tcPO$_2$), heart rate variability and uterine activity following maternal administration of meperidine. *J Perinat Med* 1988; **16**: 23–30.

38. Nation RL. Meperidine binding in maternal and fetal plasma. *Clin Pharmacol Ther* 1981; **29**: 472–479.

39. Taylor ES, von Fumetti HH, Essig EL et al. The effects of demerol and trichloroethylene on arterial oxygen saturation in the newborn. *Am J Obstet Gynecol* 1955; **69**: 348–351.

40. Koch G, Wendel H. Effect of pethidine on the post natal adjustment of respiration and acid–base balance. *Acta Obstet Gynecol Scand* 1968; **47**: 27–37.

41. Kuhnert BR, Kuhnert PM, Tu ASL et al. Meperidine and normeperidine levels following meperidine administration in labor. I. Mother. *Am J Obstet Gynecol* 1979; **133**: 904–908.

42. Kuhnert BR, Kuhnert PM, Phillipson EH et al. Disposition of meperidine and normeperidine following multiple doses during labor. II. Fetus and neonate. *Am J Obstet Gynecol* 1985; **151**: 410–415.

43. Hamza J, Benlabed M, Orhant E et al. Neonatal pattern of breathing during active and quiet sleep after maternal administration of meperidine. *Pediatr Res* 1992; **32**: 412–416.

44. Brackbill U, Kane J, Manniello RL et al. Obstetric meperidine usage and assessment of the neonatal status. *Anesthesiology* 1974; **40**: 116–120.

45. Emde RN, Swedberg J, Suzudi B. Human wakefulness and biological rhythms after birth. *Arch Gen Psychiatr* 1975; **32**: 780–783.

46. Nissen E, Lilja G, Matthiesen AS et al. Effects of maternal pethidine on infants developing breast feeding behaviour. *Acta Paediatr* 1975; **84**: 140–145.

47. Weiner PC, Hogg MIJ, Rosen M. Neonatal respiration, feeding and neurobehavioural state. *Anaesthesia* 1979; **34**: 996–1004.

48. Jacobson B, Nyberg K, Gronbladh L et al. Opiate addiction in adult offspring through possible imprinting after obstetric treatment. *Br Med J* 1990; **301**: 1067–1070.

49. Weiner PC, Hogg MIJ, Rosen M. Effects of naloxone on pethidine induced neonatal depression. *Br Med J* 1977; **2**: 228–231.

50. Weiner PC, Wallace S. Effects of naloxone on pethidine induced neonatal depression (letter). *Br Med J* 1980; **280**: 252.

51. Gerhardt T, Bancalari E, Cohen H et al. Use of naloxone to reverse narcotic respiratory depression in the newborn infant. *J Pediatr* 1977; **90**: 1009–1012.

52. Stoelting RK. Opioid agonists and antagonists. In: *Pharmacology and physiology in anaesthetic practice*, 2nd edn. Philadelphia: JB Lippincott, 1991, pp 74–82.

53. Gerdin A, Salmonson T, Lindberg B et al. Maternal kinetics of morphine during labor. *J Perinat Med* 1990; **18**: 479–487.

54. Oloffson C, Ekblom A, Ekman-Ordeberg G et al. Analgesic efficacy of intravenous morphine in labour pain. A reappraisal. *Int J Obstet Anesth* 1996a; **5**: 176–180.

55. Oloffson C, Ekblom A, Ekman-Ordeberg G et al. Lack of analgesic effect of systemically administered morphine or pethidine on labour pain. *Br J Obstet Gynaecol* 1996b; **103**: 968–972.

56. Fairlie FM, Marshall L, Walker JJ. Pethidine compared with diamorphine for pain relief in labour. *Am J Obstet Gynecol* 1992; **166**: 394.

57. Shafer SL, Varvel JR. Pharmacokinetics, pharmacodynamics and rational opioid selection. *Anesthesiology* 1991; **74**: 53–63.

58. Craft JB, Coaldrake LA, Bolan JC et al. Placental passage and uterine effects of fentanyl. *Anesth Analg* 1983; **62**: 894–898.

59. Eisele JH, Wright R, Rogge P. Newborn and maternal fentanyl levels at caesarean section. *Anesth Analg* 1982; **61**: 179–180.

60. Smith CV, Rayburn WF, Allen KV et al. Influence of intravenous fentanyl on fetal biophysical parameters during labor. *J Matern Fetal Med* 1996; **5**: 89–92.

61. Rayburn WF, Rathke A, Leuschen P et al. Fentanyl citrate analgesia during labor. *Am J Obstet Gynecol* 1989b; **161**: 202–206.

62. Rayburn WF, Smith CV, Parriott JE et al. Randomized comparison of meperidine and fentanyl during labour. *Obstet Gynecol* 1989c; **74**: 604–606.

63. Kleiman SJ, Wiesel SW, Tessler MJ. Patient-controlled analgesia (PCA) using fentanyl in a parturient with platelet function abnormality. *Can J Anaesth* 1991; **38**(4): 489–491.

64. Rosaeg OP, Kitts JB, Koren G et al. Maternal and fetal effects of intravenous patient-controlled fentanyl analgesia during labour in a thrombocytopenic patient. *Can J Anaesth* 1992; **39**(3): 277–281.

65. Nikkola EM, Ekblad UU, Kero PO et al. Intravenous fentanyl PCA during labour. *Can J Anaesth* 1997; **44**(12): 1248–1255.

66. Morley-Foster PK, Reid DW, Vandeberghe H. A comparison of patient controlled analgesia fentanyl and alfentanil for labour analgesia. *Can J Anesth* 2000; **47**(2): 113–119.

67. Morley-Foster PK, Westphals J. Neonatal effects of patient-controlled analgesia using fentanyl in labour. *Int J Obstet Anesth* 1998; **7**: 103–107.

68. Thompson JP, Rowbotham DJ. Remifentanil – an opioid for the 21st century (Editorial). *Br J Anaesth* 1996; **76**(3): 341–342.

69. Kan RE, Hughes SC, Rosen MA et al. Intravenous remifentanil: placental transfer, maternal and neonatal effect. *Anesthesiology* 1998; **88**: 1467–1474.

70. Brada SA, Egan TD, Viscomi CM. The use of remifentanil infusion to facilitate epidural catheter placement in a parturient: a case report with pharmacokinetic simulations. *Int J Obstet Anesth* 1998; **7**: 124–127.

71. Jones R, Pegrum A, Stacey RGW. Patient-controlled analgesia using remifentanil in the parturient with thrombocytopaenia. *Anaesthesia* 1999; **54**: 461–465.

72. Thurlow JA, Waterhouse P. Patient-controlled analgesia in labour using remifentanil in two parturients with platelet abnormalities. *Br J Anaesth* 2000; **84**(3): 411–413.

73. Elbourne D, Wiseman RA. Types of intra-muscular opioids for maternal pain relief in labour. In: *Cochrane review*. The Cochrane Library, Issue 2. Update Software, Oxford.

74. Rosen M, Mushin WW, Jones PL et al. Field trial of methoxyflurane, nitrous oxide and trichlorethylene as obstetric analgesics. *Br Med J* 1969; **iii**: 263–267.

75. Phillips TJ, Macdonald RR. Comparative effect of pethidine, trichloroethylene and Entonox on fetal and neonatal acid–base and PO$_2$. *Br Med J* 1971; **iii**: 558–560.

76. Tunstall ME. Obstetric analgesia. The use of a fixed nitrous oxide and oxygen mixture from one cylinder. *Lancet* 1961; **ii**: 964.

77. Waud BE, Waud DR. Calculated kinetics of distribution of nitrous oxide and methoxyflurane during intermittent administration in obstetrics. *Anesthesiology* 1970; **32**: 306–316.

78. Davies JM, Willis BA, Rosen M. Entonox analgesia in labour. A pilot study to reduce the delay between demand and supply. *Anaesthesia* 1978; **33**: 545–547.

79. Arthurs GJ, Rosen M. Self-administered intermittent nitrous oxide analgesia for labour. Enhancement of effect with continuous nasal inhalation of 50 per cent nitrous oxide (Entonox). *Anaesthesia* 1979; **34**: 301–309.

80. Jones PL, Rosen M, Mushin WW et al. Methoxyflurane and nitrous oxide as obstetric analgesics. I. A comparison by continuous administration. *Br Med J* 1969; **iii**: 255–259.

81. Cole PV, Crawford JS, Doughty AG et al. Clinial trials of different concentrations of oxygen and nitrous oxide for obstetric analgesia. Report to the medical research council of the committee on nitrous oxide and oxygen analgesia in midwifery. *Br Med J* 1970; **i**: 709–713.

82. Carstoniu J, Levytam S, Norman P et al. Nitrous oxide in early labor. Safety and analgesic efficacy assessed by a double-blind, placebo-controlled study. *Anesthesiology* 1994; **80**: 30–35.

83. Levinson G, Shnider SM, DeLorimer AA et al. Effects of maternal hyperventilation on uterine blood flow and fetal oxygenation and acid–base status. *Anesthesiology* 1974; **40**: 340–347.

84. Lin DM, Reisner LS, Benumof J. Hypoxaemia occurs intermittently and significantly with nitrous oxide labor analgesia. *Anesth Analg* 1989; **68**: S167.

85. Arfeen Z, Armstrong PJ, Whitfield A. The effects of Entonox and epidural analgesia on arterial oxygen saturation of women in labour. *Anaesthesia* 1994; **49**: 32–34.

86. Griffin RP, Reynolds F. Maternal hypoxaemia during labour and delivery: the influence of analgesia and effect on neonatal outcome. *Anaesthesia* 1995; **50**: 151–156.

87. Davies JM, Hogg M, Rosen M. Maternal arterial oxygen tension during intermittent inhalation analgesia. *Br J Anaesth* 1975; **47**: 370–378.

88. Maze M, Fujinaga M. Editorial: recent advances in understanding the actions and toxicity of nitrous oxide. *Anaesthesia* 2000; **55**: 311–314.

89. McGuiness C, Rosen M. Enflurane as an analgesic in labour. *Anaesthesia* 1984; **39**: 24–26.

90. McCleod DD, Ramayya GP, Tunstall ME. Self-administered isoflurane in labour. A comparative study with Entonox. *Anaesthesia* 1985; **40**: 424–426.

91. Abboud TK, Shnider SM, Wright RG et al. Enflurane analgesia in obstetrics. *Anesth Analg* 1981; **60**: 133–137.

92. Abboud TK, Gangolly J, Mosaad P et al. Isoflurane in obstetrics. *Anesth Analg* 1989; **68**: 388–391.

93. Aurora S, Tunstall M, Ross J. Self-administered mixture of Entonox and isoflurane in labour. *Int J Obstet Anesth* 1992; **1**: 199–202.

94. Wee MYK, Hasan MA, Thomas TA. Isoflurane in labour. *Anaesthesia* 1993; **48**: 369–372.

95. Ross JAS, Tunstall ME, Campbell DM et al. The use of 0.25% isoflurane premixed in 50% nitrous oxide and oxygen for pain relief in labour. *Anaesthesia* 1999; **54**: 1166–1172.

96. Abboud TK, Swart F, Shu J et al. Desflurane analgesia for vaginal delivery. *Acta Anaesth Scand* 1995; **39**: 259–261.

97. Mills GH, Singh D, Longan M et al. Nitrous oxide exposure on the labour ward. *Int J Obstet Anaesth* 1996; **5**: 160–164.

98. Burning JE, Hennekens CH, Mayrent SL et al. Health experiences of operating room personnel. *Anesthesiology* 1985; **62**: 325–330.

99. Spence AA. Environmental pollution by inhalational anaesthetics. *Br J Anaesth* 1987; **59**: 96–103.

100. Health and Safety Executive. EH40/96. *Occupational exposure limits.* London: HMSO, 1996.

6

REGIONAL ANALGESIA FOR LABOUR

Roshan Fernando & C.M. Price

INTRODUCTION

Regional blockade unquestionably provides the most effective form of analgesia in labour. In the UK alone, more than 100 000 procedures are performed annually.[1]

In recent years, concern has been expressed over whether or not 'epidurals' influence the progress of labour itself. Mothers have also reported dissatisfaction with the intensity of motor blockade produced by using local anaesthetic alone. In order to address this and maintain standards of safety and efficacy, emphasis is now placed on providing good quality analgesia, and not anaesthesia, during the course of labour.

This goal has been easier to achieve due to a greater understanding of relevant anatomy and physiology together with a wider choice of opioid drugs and improved equipment. Technological advances include better microprocessors in infusion pumps to provide safer epidural infusions and spinal needles which are blunt yet fine in calibre and allow intrathecal injections with minimal risk of post-dural puncture headache.

ANATOMY OF THE EPIDURAL SPACE

In order to practice regional blockade safely for labour analgesia, it is important to understand the anatomy of this area. Techniques which have improved our knowledge of epidural anatomy include cadaveric dissection,[2] resin injection studies in cadavers,[3] epidurography (dye injection into the epidural space), CT epidurography[4] and epiduroscopy (using a fine fibreoptic endoscope).[5] More recently, magnetic resonance imaging (MRI) has provided detailed images of this area[6-9] without the injection of contrast media which itself may artificially distort the anatomy.

BASIC ANATOMY

- The spinal cord and its various coverings of dura lie within the bony vertebral canal.
- Within the vertebral canal lies the epidural space, which actually *begins* at the foramen magnum, where the bony periosteum and dural layers fuse, and *ends* at the level of the sacral hiatus (sacrococcygeal membrane).
- The vertebral bodies, intervertebral discs and the posterior longitudinal ligament lie anteriorly.
- The vertebral laminae and *ligamenta flava* lie posteriorly.
- The pedicles and the intervening intervertebral foramina lie laterally.

- In adults the spinal cord ends as the *conus medullaris* commonly but not invariably at the level of L1. Nerve roots from the spinal cord pass downwards, encased in dura – this leash of nerves is termed the *cauda equina*.
- The epidural space below the level of L1 contains nerve roots, blood vessels, lymphatics and fat.
- The spinal cord and its nerve roots are covered by *pia mater* and lie within a sac filled with cerebrospinal fluid (CSF).
- This outer dural sac consists of a thin internal *arachnoid mater* and a tougher external *dura mater*.
- The dural sac continues below the conus medullaris as the cauda equina, which contains tightly packed lower lumbar and sacral nerve roots lying within CSF. The cauda equina ends at the S2 level.
- The *filum terminale*, a continuation of the pia mater which originally covered the spinal cord, is a structure running within the cauda equina to end in the sacral region.
- The *subdural space* is an area lying between the arachnoid and dura mater membranes separated by serous fluid, which can potentially be entered by an epidural catheter leading to an atypical block (see later).

MAGNETIC RESONANCE IMAGING

MRI techniques have shown the epidural space to be divided into four compartments, a finding common to cadaveric studies – anterior, posterior and two laterally. The size of these compartments, vary segmentally. At each spinal level, two ligamenta flava meet on either side of the midline, at 90° or less.[10,11] Occasionally when they do not meet in the midline, the interspinous ligament fills the gap. The ligamentum flavum itself can be as much as 2–5 mm thick.[2,11]

On an MRI midline sagittal section the segmental shape of the posterior epidural space is obvious (Fig. 6.1) and is described as 'saw-toothed' in appearance. This posterior space is filled with fat but is not continuous since areas of contact with the rostral bony laminae separate it. It is actually the discontinuous nature of the epidural fat in the posterior epidural space on a sagittal MRI image, which gives the distinctive 'saw-toothed' shape. Axial MRI images on the other hand show that the posterior epidural space, filled with fat, is triangular in shape (Fig. 6.2). Hirabayashi et al have shown the antero-posterior dimensions of the posterior epidural space at L2–3 to be 7.1 mm.[8] The two lateral spaces surrounding the

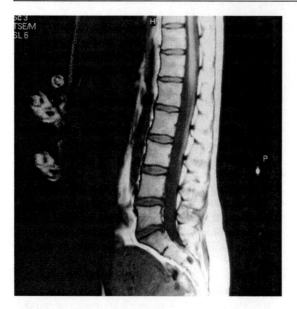

Figure 6.1 T1-weighted MRI midline sagittal section, showing the segmental shape of the posterior epidural space, described as 'saw-toothed' in appearance.

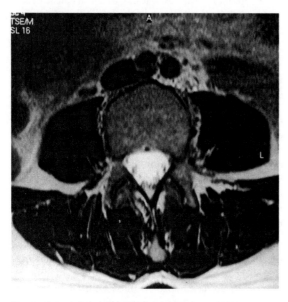

Figure 6.2 T2-weighted axial MRI image through the pedicle at L3, showing the posterior epidural space. (Central white area is the CSF, dark dots are the cauda equina nerves.)

nerve roots are widely open as they exit through the intervertebral foraminae. MRI has also shown that the distance from skin to epidural space correlates well with body weight.[9]

EPIDUROGRAPHY

This technique involves injecting a dye into the epidural space producing an epidurogram on radiography. The procedure may mimic how epidural drugs spread when injected. In an anteroposterior view 10–13 ml of contrast given through an indwelling epidural catheter spreads over six vertebral levels.[12] The characteristic appearance is a central contrast column with spilling around the intervertebral foraminae producing a Christmas tree distribution.[12] Maldistribution of contrast is also seen in some patients possibly due to an anatomical midline barrier, which may explain unilateral blocks or 'missed segments' during regional analgesia.[5,12] The epidural space becomes the paravertebral region within the vertebral foraminae.[12]

PHYSIOLOGY OF LABOUR PAIN

Pain transmission

Labour pain is made up of visceral and somatic components.[13] The *visceral* component involves distension of the cervix and the lower uterine segment (and possibly also the uterine body) during the first stage of labour contractions. The patient usually only feels pain if the intrauterine pressure exceeds 25 mmHg and experiences minimal discomfort below this pressure.[14] Myometrial and cervical ischaemia during contractions may also cause additional pain via other nerve afferents in uterine muscle fibres. Visceral pain is transmitted by Aδ and C fibres which run together with sympathetic fibres eventually passing through various nerve plexuses (e.g. cervical, hypogastric) into the main sympathetic chain which lies parallel to and either side of the vertebral bodies. From the sympathetic chain the pain fibres enter the white rami communicantes associated with T10–T12 and L1 spinal nerves and pass via their posterior nerve roots to synapse in the dorsal horn of the spinal cord.

Early labour pain is referred to T11–T12 dermatomes so that pain is felt in the lower abdomen and back. At this early stage of labour the pain is dull, predominantly C-fibre transmitted and sensitive to opioid drugs. As labour progresses to the active first stage (3–4 cm) and uterine contractions become more intense, the pain becomes sharper and spreads to the adjacent dermatomes (T10, L1). The sharper pain is thought to be predominantly Aδ fibre transmitted and more opioid resistant.[15] Stretching and distension of the pelvic floor, perineum and vagina during the late first stage and second stage of labour causes *somatic* pain, which is transmitted via the pudendal nerve (S2–4). This pain is also opioid resistant.

Knowing the anatomical labour pain pathways, it is clear how blocks such as paracervical, lumbar sympathetic, paravertebral, and pudendal can modify pain transmission at different levels. However an epidural block using an indwelling epidural catheter is the most flexible of all techniques and potentially the only one which can guarantee complete analgesia throughout labour, with the added bonus of being able to be extended for an emergency Caesarean section.

Uterine contractions

Uterine contractions also produce a widespread neuro-endocrine stress response including:

1. Increased oxygen consumption, hyperventilation and respiratory alkalosis.
2. Increased cardiac output, systemic vascular resistance and arterial blood pressure.
3. Delayed gastric emptying.

As labour progresses uterine perfusion diminishes and metabolic acidosis results. This is enhanced by anxiety, starvation and physical exertion. These physiological responses can potentially all be modified by regional analgesia.

EFFECTS OF REGIONAL BLOCKADE ON FETO-MATERNAL PHYSIOLOGY

Placental blood flow

In normal pregnancy at term, placental blood flow is 500–700 ml/min. Uterine artery perfusion pressure depends upon maternal arterial pressure. Hypotension can occur as a result of sympathetic blockade and/or aorto-caval compression and will lead to a decrease in placental blood flow. Therefore it is essential to monitor the fetus during any potential periods of hypotension, e.g. during establishment of regional blockade.

Relief of pain leads to a decrease in circulating catecholamines and an increase in placental blood flow. Lumbar epidural anaesthesia reduces maternal catecholamines possibly by eliminating the psychological and physical stress associated with painful uterine contractions or by denervating the adrenal medulla.[16] In summary, regional blockade in healthy patients does not influence resistance in uterine vessels, intervillous blood flow or flow velocity in the umbilical artery if maternal hypotension is avoided.[17]

Fetal outcome

As improved placental haemodynamics may occur, neonatal outcome may be better with epidural blockade compared to mothers who receive systemic medication.[18,19] However, prolonged fetal decelerations are seen more commonly with maternal hypotension, which may occur during epidural analgesia.[20]

Aorto-caval compression

It cannot be overemphasised that aorto-caval compression by the gravid uterus of both the inferior vena cava and the aorta should be avoided during the performance and maintenance of regional analgesia. Aorto-caval compression (ACC) can lead to reduced venous return and subsequently reduced cardiac output with obvious maternal and fetal consequences. Therefore a mother should never be placed supine under normal circumstances let alone after a regional block. Often minor degrees of ACC are compensated for by maintenance of venous return through vertebral and paraspinous veins draining into the azygous system. An increase in peripheral resistance can also maintain cardiac output. However sympathetic blockade during regional analgesia can abolish this physiological response.

Maternal body temperature

Maternal body temperature increases after epidural analgesia for labour.[21–23] The mechanisms are not well understood. In most cases the hyperthermia is mild and not associated with maternal shivering or fetal problems. In some cases, hyperthermia is more pronounced, associated with shivering and fetal tachycardia and difficult to distinguish from intrapartum infection. Mercier and Benhamou provide a review on the subject.[24]

PSYCHOLOGY OF LABOUR PAIN

The pain of labour is an interaction of physiological and psychological mechanisms. Whether labour is induced desirability of pregnancy and the support given during labour have been found to be predictors of the perception of pain.[25] In general, women who feel in control in labour have a more positive experience of it. Those that have positive expectations are more likely to feel better about the labour. Pre-existing anxiety or depression may cause or worsen the pain perceived.[26]

INDICATIONS AND CONTRAINDICATIONS FOR REGIONAL ANALGESIA

Although regional analgesia can be given for pain relief during any labour there are particular situations where it is useful. Indications can be divided into obstetric, anaesthetic and patient factors.

Obstetric indications

Pre-eclampsia is the most common obstetric indication for a regional blockade. It will also aid controlled delivery of a vaginal breech, multiple pregnancies and of the premature infant. It may also be of help in incoordinate uterine action.[27]

Anaesthetic indications

1. Morbidly obese parturients – in the morbidly obese there is a high incidence of ante-partum medical disease. Emergency Caesarean section is also a more frequent occurrence. Regional blockade although difficult, is usually feasible and should be attempted early, the block assessed frequently and provision made for alternative airway management.[28]
2. Potentially difficult airway – although total spinal anaesthesia and respiratory arrest is a possibility, it would seem sensible to provide careful epidural analgesia for labour so that the need for general anaesthesia is diminished.

Patient factors

- Patient request: the most common reason why regional blocks are administered on a labour ward.
- Regional blocks are medically indicated for cardio-respiratory disease since the haemodynamic effects of uterine contractions are reduced. On the other hand, a rapid sympathetic block caused by regional block may dramatically reduce cardiac output.

Contraindications

- Patient refusal
- Hypovolaemia
- Major coagulopathy
- Raised intracranial pressure–accidental dural puncture with an epidural needle may cause coning
- Localized skin infection
- Inadequate resuscitation facilities
- Lack of trained staff to care for the woman with the epidural.

SPECIAL CIRCUMSTANCES

Low platelets

An isolated platelet count above $80 \times 10^9/l$ is considered to be the lower limit of normal during pregnancy.[29] If the count is between 50 and $80 \times 10^9/l$, then senior haematology advice should be sought before considering a regional block. It should be remembered that a low platelet count gives no indication of platelet function. At our institution a thromboelastograph (TEG)[30] is performed to assess platelet function if the count is between 50 and $80 \times 10^9/l$. Before proceeding to site an epidural we establish that a normal maximum amplitude (MA) exists on a TEG, indicating adequate platelet function. The normal ranges for the MA are 58–78 mm in the 3rd trimester of pregnancy and 50–61 mm for non-pregnant subjects. A platelet count below $50 \times 10^9/l$ is regarded as a relative contraindication to an epidural block.

Aspirin

Aspirin therapy is not regarded as a contraindication to regional blockade.[31]

Low molecular weight heparin (e.g. dalteparin [Fragmin])

The use of low molecular weight heparins (LMWH) for effective venous thromboembolism prophylaxis has been shown in over 60 trials, which collectively have included more than 20 000 patients.[32] Many high risk obstetric patients who have had previous thrombo-embolism or with thrombotic tendencies, such as those with protein S, protein C and Factor V Leiden deficiencies, may present to the anaesthetist for regional analgesia on subcutaneous LMWH. Due to the extremely low risk of epidural haematoma associated with LMWH, many obstetric units have guidelines as to when regional blockade can safely be undertaken. Currently our local haematology department manage all obstetric patients receiving LMWH and routinely monitor the heparin effect during pregnancy by measuring plasma anti-Xa activity which is kept between 0.05 and 0.3 IU/ml by adjusting the dose of LMWH. Anti-Xa levels are measured in these patients 2 h after injection every 2–4 weeks together with the platelet count. Although anti-Xa activity peaks at 3–4 h after a subcutaneous injection of LMWH, 50% of peak levels are still present at 12 h.[33] Currently we recommend waiting a minimum of 12 h after a dose of LMWH before an epidural catheter is sited, or removed, in obstetric patients. If LMWH is to be given after administration of an epidural, then we advise waiting a minimum of 2 h as recommended by Horlocker and Heit.[33] Standard *in vitro* coagulation tests are unlikely to be affected by LMWH[34] and so have a minimum role in determining the timing of a regional block.

Maternal pyrexia

If a woman is pyrexial during a normal labour it may be a sign of incipient chorioamnionitis or other form of infection. If the patient is overtly septic the problems with epidural analgesia are severe hypotension due to pre-existing vasodilatation and concern that regional blockade may allow direct introduction of infected blood into the epidural space. Two large studies, which have included patients undergoing urological and gynaecological operations, (associated with bacteraemia), under spinal or epidural anaesthesia described no cases of CNS infection.[35,36] Bader et al observed no cases of CNS infection after 279 regional blocks in patients with chorioamnionitis.[37] Forty-three of these patients received antibiotics before an epidural was sited. Similarly Ramanathan et al observed no problems after 113 blocks in patients with chorioamnionitis.[38] Current opinion recommends the administration of antibiotics before placing an epidural in such patients.[39,40]

The HIV infected patient

Theoretically there may be a risk to performing epidural analgesia because of neuropathological changes. However, in practice, there have been no reported problems. HIV should not be considered a contraindication to epidural analgesia.[41]

TECHNIQUES OF EPIDURAL INSERTION

For labour analgesia epidural catheters are usually inserted at L2–3 or L3–4. Although epidural catheters can theoretically be placed in the low thoracic region for labour analgesia, apart from potential injury to the spinal cord, which terminates at L1–2, any perineal pain developing in late labour may be difficult to relieve.

POSITION

Placing the patient in either the lateral or sitting position makes no difference to complications such as dural puncture with the epidural needle or intravenous placement of the epidural catheter.[42] However in the full lateral position uteroplacental perfusion is better maintained since there is less risk of aorto-caval compression. In obese women it may be easier to identify the midline if the woman is sitting up.

APPROACH

The *midline approach* is favoured by the majority of anaesthetists.[43] It is relatively easy and for most patients will provide satisfactory access to the epidural space. During the midline approach the epidural needle passes through skin, subcutaneous fat, the supraspinous ligament, the interspinous ligament and the ligamentum flavum before entering the epidural space. With a *paramedian approach* the needle passes only through the paravertebral muscles before puncturing the ligamentum flavum. The paramedian approach is favoured by some anaesthetists for difficult patients as there is less risk of dural puncture and the catheter is more likely to pass straight upwards.[5,44] However, insertion is said to be more painful. It is not used routinely in labouring women as clinically the difference between the two approaches is small.[45] Rotation of the epidural needle is not recommended as this significantly reduces the force needed to produce a dural puncture.[46]

LOCATION OF THE EPIDURAL SPACE

Most anaesthetists now use the loss of resistance technique to locate the epidural space. Reynolds advocated that the medium used should be saline rather than air as the incidence of inadvertent dural puncture is lower.[47,48] However, this may make identification of an accidental dural puncture more difficult. Glucose testing of CSF alone may give false positive results due to CSF drainage into the epidural space. Current recommendations include the use of skin temperature, or protein testing if in doubt.[49,50] However no test is entirely reliable.

CATHETERS

Both single and multi-orifice catheters are available. There is contradictory evidence as to which is better.[51,52] Dye techniques show that single orifice catheters provide more even spread and better sacral distribution than multi-orifice catheters. Better analgesia would be expected as a result. Clinical experience, however, shows this not to be the case. Multi-orifice catheters are better in this respect. To counterbalance this argument, multi-orifice catheters are said to be less safe because they allow multi-compartment spread of local anaesthetic.[53]

FETAL MONITORING DURING ESTABLISHMENT OF REGIONAL BLOCKADE

Electronic fetal heart rate monitoring has become more commonplace during hospital deliveries despite its poor sensitivity in predicting fetal outcome. Continuous fetal monitoring in uncomplicated deliveries, therefore, can be called into question. There are, however, situations where continuous fetal monitoring is strongly recommended and administration of regional blockade is one of them. The prevention of aorto-caval compression can never be fully guaranteed even in the supine wedged position.[54,55]

Hypotension following sympathetic blockade may affect the fetus by reducing utero-placental flow. Fetal heart rate changes have been reported up to 1 h after administration of epidural bupivacaine or intrathecal sufentanil for labour analgesia.[56] Fetal monitoring is important during this time. After this period no difference in fetal outcome is observed whether monitoring is continuous or intermittent.[57] Clearly, however, fetal monitoring is essential if any subsequent intermittent epidural top-ups or continuous epidural infusions are given as hypotension may again occur.

FLUID MANAGEMENT

As described above, sympathetic blockade can result in hypotension due to vasodilatation. To avoid this, standard practice has been to give a form of fluid preload. Some studies have suggested that fluid preloading can be effective in reducing fetal heart rate abnormalities due to epidural analgesia.[58–60] However, a well-designed randomized controlled trial to examine this question has not been performed. Ephedrine, a combined alpha and beta-receptor agonist, is commonly used to counteract hypotension. Animal data suggests that ephedrine constricts both uterine and systemic vessels by actions on alpha adrenoreceptors and that ephedrine may spare uterine perfusion during pregnancy due to more selective constriction of systemic vessels compared to pure alpha agonists such as metaraminol.[61] Caesarean section studies using other alpha agonists, phenylephrine and methoxamine, indicate that these drugs may also be safe to use and that the choice of vasopressor drug may be of minor importance, compared to avoiding hypotension.[62,63]

TEST DOSE

The appropriateness of an epidural test dose has been the subject of debate. The object of a test dose is to check that the epidural catheter is correctly situated in the epidural space. The catheter may have entered CSF, a vein or the subdural space[64] instead of the epidural space. Care with injection, observing for signs of toxicity and production of the expected level of analgesia are probably more important than the test dose itself. The total test dose should be equivalent to an intrathecal dose of local anaesthetic used for Caesarean section. Suggested constituents of a test dose have been epinephrine, local anaesthetic, opioid, isoprenaline or even air.[65] Any dose in excess of a safe intrathecal dose should be avoided. A large volume test dose may rupture the subdural space if the epidural catheter has been accidentally placed there. The test dose would then enter the subarachnoid space. No technique is completely reliable[66] and the inclusion of epinephrine is not entirely sensitive.[67] Currently our unit's epidural test dose for labour analgesia is 10 ml of our epidural low dose mixture consisting of 0.1% bupivacaine and 2 μg/ml fentanyl. However every epidural dose administered should be regarded as a test dose and potential intrathecal or intravenous placement of the epidural catheter regauged a possibility at any point.

Epidural test doses for labour include:[68–73]

- Bupivacaine 7.5–12.5 mg
- Lidocaine 45–60 mg
- Local anaesthetic above with 15 μg epinephrine or isoprenaline 5 μg
- Fentanyl 100 μg
- 10 ml of low dose epidural mixture (e.g. 0.1% bupivacaine + 2 μg/ml fentanyl)
- 1–2 ml air.

A plan for administering a test dose is shown:

1. Insert the epidural catheter observing for blood or fluid.
2. Aspirate the epidural catheter before giving the test dose.
3. Observe patient for signs or symptoms of accidental intravenous or intrathecal injection.
4. Rapid onset of analgesia, high sensory block, maternal hypotension and motor block, especially of the S1 nerve root, are highly suggestive of intrathecal injection.
5. Maintain a low threshold for repeating the test dose.

DRUGS USED FOR EPIDURAL ANALGESIA

The main drugs used in the epidural space in labour are local anaesthetics and opioids. During the past few years although there has been evidence of an anti-nociceptive effect of alpha-2 adrenergic agonists, anticholinergics, GABA-A receptor agonists, calcium antagonists and NMDA receptor antagonists, few of these agents have provided clinically useful analgesia. Clonidine and epinephrine have been used in labour but, as discussed below, have limiting side effects. Many drugs used in the epidural space do not have a specific product licence:[74,75] For example, pre-packed Marcaine® (bupivacaine) 0.5% with 1:200 000 epinephrine and Naropin® (ropivacaine) 0.2% have distinct product licences for labour epidural analgesia. Certainly for pre-packed Marcaine® (bupivacaine) 0.5% with 1:200 000 epinephrine, the dense lower limb motor block it produces makes it unsuitable for routine labour analgesic use. Very few obstetric anaesthetists are likely to use this epidural solution in labour. In other words changing clinical practice has left a drug licensed for a clinically inappropriate indication. However, many drugs, especially the opioids, are widely used without a product licence. The lack of a product licence for a specific clinical indication does not imply that the drug is unsafe to use; more likely that the drug company has not sought a specific product licence for that application.

LOCAL ANAESTHETICS

Epidural requirements differ in pregnancy. The injection of a dose of local anaesthetic results in a 35% increase in segmental spread of analgesia compared with the non-pregnant state. This may be due to a decrease in the volume of the epidural space due to venous engorgement, increase in the pH of CSF or increased sensitivity to local anaesthetics due to the effect of progesterone.[76]

Local anaesthetics work by reversibly blocking transmission in nerve fibres subserving both slow (C-fibre) and pinprick (Aδ fibre) pain. They act by blocking nerve membrane depolarization and impulse transmission. This is achieved by plugging sodium channels so that sodium ions cannot enter a cell and thus depolarize it. The site at which they are applied determines the effect seen. Epidurally, local anaesthetics act by diffusing across the dura into the CSF

and then to the spinal cord and the adjacent nerve roots. Lipid solubility, protein binding and the dissociation constant (pKa) influence the pharmacological action of local anaesthetics.[77] Highly lipid soluble local anaesthetics are the most potent and have the longest duration of action. Protein binding also increases duration of action. Local anaesthetics are weak bases. Those with a pKa close to 7.40 have a greater amount in the unionized, lipid soluble, form that can quickly diffuse across nerve sheaths to act rapidly. Most amide local anaesthetics are chiral drugs, each possessing a single asymmetrical carbon atom and existing as two enantiomers. These are optically active stereoisomers, which are mirror images of each other. The isomers are called L and D (laevo and dextro) or S and R (sinister and rectus) – the more modern nomenclature. For example, a racaemic mixture will contain both R and S forms. Usually the R-isomer is responsible for the unwanted side effects and the S-isomer for the physiological effects. Interest in developing single isomer local anaesthetics has resulted in the recent introduction of ropivacaine and levobupivacaine.

The ideal local anaesthetic for labour analgesia would block sensory fibres without affecting motor fibres and also would have no side effects on the mother or the fetus. Although it is commonly thought that C pain fibres are more sensitive to the effects of local anaesthetic than the larger Aδ (proprioceptive, somatic motor) or Aβ (touch, pressure) fibres, this may not be true since the actual response of these nerves *in vivo* is less clear. It appears that the diffusional barrier (myelin) around C fibres compared to A fibres is much less, resulting clinically in a faster *rate* of C fibre block.[77]

The most common problems with epidural use of local anaesthetics are hypotension due to sympathetic blockade and motor blockade. Hypotension is made worse by aorto-caval compression. It can be avoided by the use of fluid and vasopressors and careful maternal positioning. Epidural local anaesthetics increase uteroplacental blood flow. This is probably secondary to a decrease in circulating catecholamines following analgesia.[16] If hypotension is avoided, then the blood supply to the fetus will improve. Although local anaesthetic agents cross the placenta there is little evidence to show any direct effect on the fetus in the absence of haemodynamic changes in the doses clinically used today. Motor blockade of the lower limbs can be reduced by using low dose mixtures of local anaesthetic and opioids. The physical properties of currently used local anaesthetics are illustrated in Table 6.1.

Table 6.1   Physicochemical characteristics of commonly used local anaesthetics in labour

	Lidocaine	Ropivacaine	Bupivacaine	L-bupivacaine
Molecular weight	234	274	288	325
pKa	7.7	8.0	8.2	8.1
Lipid solubility (N-heptane/buffer)	2.9	3	28	25
Mean tissue uptake ratio	1	1.8	3.3	?
Uv/Mv$_{tot}$ ratio	0.6	0.28	0.3	0.3
Protein binding (%)	65	94	95	98

Uv/Mv$_{tot}$: reflect the fetal/maternal concentration ratios of the total (protein bound + unbound) drug plasma concentrations of maternal and umbilical venous plasma.

MINIMUM LOCAL ANALGESIC CONCENTRATION

Minimum local analgesic concentration (MLAC) is a new way of comparing the potencies of local anaesthetic drugs used epidurally in a similar manner to the way the minimum anaesthetic concentration (MAC) is used to compare anaesthetic potencies of volatile agents. Until the use of MLAC, studies comparing the efficacies of epidural analgesics have been hindered by ignorance of the relative potencies of the agents concerned, whether alone or in combination with drugs such as opioids. An equianalgesic dose or concentration, or identical visual analogue pain scores (VAPS) for both single agents and drug combinations could potentially provide an epidural equivalent to MAC. One such equianalgesic measure is the MLAC of bupivacaine in labour.[78] This has provided a model, which allows estimation of potency, and permits the bupivacaine sparing effect of successive doses of epidural opioid to be measured.[79] The technique of measuring MLAC involves using an up down sequential allocation method. The results are analysed using the Dixon and Massey formula.[80] In a similar way, since the intrathecal effect of analgesic drugs depends on dose rather than concentration, the MLAD (the minimum local analgesic dose – the intrathecal equivalent to MLAC) of various drugs can also be determined.[81]

BUPIVACAINE

Bupivacaine is the most popular local anaesthetic in use as it has less motor blocking effect than other agents and has a relatively long duration of action. It is highly lipid soluble (see Table 6.1) and diffuses easily into the subarachnoid space and nerve roots when given epidurally. One major concern has been its cardiotoxicity. Bupivacaine produces arrhythmias of the re-entry type.[82] It is thought that bupivacaine's effect on the sodium channels of cardiac nerve fibres is enhanced in the presence of increased levels of progesterone although other studies have contradicted this finding.[83,84] The effect on sodium channels is thought to be stereo-selective with the R-isomer being more toxic. When used as the sole agent for production of epidural blockade at least 12.5 mg/h of bupivacaine is necessary. This eventually leads to significant motor blockade.[85]

LEVOBUPIVACAINE

Levobupivacaine is the S-enantiomer of bupivacaine. It has an improved cardiovascular safety profile compared to the racemate.[86,87] Lyons et al, studying the MLAC of levobupivacaine, have shown that with regard to commercial preparations, levobupivacaine is 2% less potent than racemic bupivacaine (Marcaine®).[88] This is unlikely to be of clinical significance.

However, in animal models L-bupivacaine appears more potent than bupivacaine. This may be because of its vasoconstrictor properties or other modes of action.

ROPIVACAINE

Ropivacaine is the S-enantiomer of the amide local anaesthetic propivacaine. For physical characteristics see Table 6.1. Like bupivacaine it produces less motor blockade than sensory blockade. It is said to be more specific for sensory than motor fibres, producing a so-called 'differential blockade'. It is also less cardio-toxic than bupivacaine when given intravenously.[89,90] Studies in labour have found that it produces the same quality analgesia and motor blockade as bupivacaine.[91,92]

Administration of 0.2% ropivacaine as an infusion set at 6–8 ml/h was found to be the optimum dose when used alone for labour anlagesia.[93] However, clinically when used in labour at a concentration of 0.25%, there is little to choose between the two drugs.[94] In a volunteer study comparing infusions of 0.1%, 0.2%, and 0.3% ropivacaine with 0.25% bupivacaine, Zaric et al observed a decrease in spread and progressive reduction in sensory blockade over time with all concentrations of ropivacaine.[95,96] This study demonstrates how the use of lower doses can reveal differences in local anaesthetic potency, not apparent at higher doses.[97] Studies comparing epidural ropivacaine to low dose bupivacaine/opioid combinations in labour are awaited. However there is growing clinical evidence that 0.2% ropivacaine used alone for labour provides inadequate analgesia. MLAC studies comparing epidural bupivacaine with ropivacaine have shown that ropivacaine is 40% less potent than racemic bupivacaine.[98,99] Capogna et al found that the MLAC in labour for ropivacaine was 0.156% compared to 0.093% for bupivacaine.[99] The molar potency ratio was estimated to be 0.57 making ropivacaine significantly less potent than bupivacaine. Therefore the differences in motor block claimed for ropivacaine are simply due to a lack of potency rather than any consequence of 'differential blockade'.

LIDOCAINE

Lidocaine has been used in labour but its higher degree of motor blockade has meant that it is less popular than bupivacaine. More drug passes to the acidotic fetus, although this would be true of any of the amide local anaesthetics as they are all weak bases.[100] There is also evidence that lidocaine may be neurotoxic in high doses and it is recommended that it be used in the lowest concentration possible.[101] Its use may include extending a pre-existing labour epidural block for emergency Caesarean section.[102,103]

ALKALINIZATION OF LOCAL ANAESTHETICS

The addition of sodium bicarbonate to a local anaesthetic increases the non-ionized lipid soluble form of local anaesthetic which are weak bases. This decreases the onset time of epidural blockade since the time taken to diffuse across the nerve cell membrane is reduced. This has been shown to be of clinical relevance. In the UK alkalinization of local anaesthetics is rarely used to improve the quality of epidural block during labour, but may be used more commonly for

Caesarean section.[104,105] Bupivacaine precipitates if the pH is greater than 7.0 and therefore only moderate alkalinization is possible.[106,107]

SIDE EFFECTS OF LOCAL ANAESTHETICS

HYPOTENSION

Local anaesthetics block conduction in preganglionic autonomic B fibres causing vasodilatation and reduced sweating. Subsequent venous pooling can also reduce cardiac output secondary to a reduced venous return. Any degree of aorto-caval compression occurring simultaneously while establishing a regional block will obviously further diminish cardiac output. Traditionally, fluid preloading is used to reduce the incidence of hypotension. Although incidences of hypotension in the region of 17% in labouring women without preloading have been described, the epidural technique consisted of 4–6 ml of 0.5% bupivacaine.[108] Clinical impressions with today's low dose epidural mixtures indicate a much lower incidence of hypotension although further evaluation is needed.[109,110]

ACCIDENTAL INTRAVENOUS INJECTION

Accidental intravenous injection occurs usually as a result of accidental placement of the epidural catheter in an epidural vein. These connect directly with the cerebral venous system and even a small dose can produce central nervous system effects. Care to avoid placement in the first place and care with subsequent top-ups should minimize the risk of giving a toxic dose (see Box 6.1 for management).

UNEXPECTED HIGH BLOCK (TOTAL SPINAL BLOCKADE/SUBDURAL BLOCKADE)

An unexpected high block is usually the result of the epidural catheter being placed unintentionally in the subarachnoid space, followed by the injection of an epidural dose of local anaesthetic through that catheter. Crawford reported six cases of high or total spinal block in a series of 27 000 lumbar epidurals for labour analgesia; an incidence of 1 in 4500.[111] If modern low dose local anaesthetic/opioid mixtures (e.g. 0.1% bupivacaine + fentanyl 2 μg/ml) are used for labour, an accidental intrathecal injection of

Toxicity effects
- Numbness
- Circumoral tingling
- Slurred speech
- Confusion
- Dizziness
- Tinnitus
- Loss of consciousness
- Convulsions
- Cardiovascular collapse.

Management
- Stop injecting drug
- Turn mother into lateral position
- Administer oxygen/support ventilation if necessary
- Summon help, resuscitation trolley
- Monitor airway, breathing, ECG, blood pressure
- Control seizures with diazepam 2–10 mg
- Correct hypotension with fluids, vasopressors as appropriate.

Cardiac arrest
- Start CPR, consider immediate delivery of fetus to facilitate resuscitation
- Correct ventricular dysrhythmias with DC shock
- Administer bretilyium 5–10 mg/kg for refractory arrhythmia (bupivacaine induced).

Box 6.1   Management of local anaesthetic toxicity.

- May be rapid or slow in onset
- Early warning signs – husky voice, agitation, dyspnoea
- Later – hypotension, loss of consciousness
- Avoid aorto-caval compression
- Administer 100% oxygen
- Call for help, maintain oxygenation/ventilation
- When help arrives, intubate and ventilate (i.v. induction agent may be required)
- Support circulation with intravenous fluids and ephedrine (epinephrine may be required)
- Consider urgent delivery of fetus.

Box 6.2   Management of total spinal blockade.

10–15 ml of such a solution will only produce a rapid dense lower limb motor block and not a total spinal. It is important to remember that as far as intrathecal effects are concerned, the total dose of drug injected is more important than the total volume in which it is injected[112,113] (see Box 6.2 for management).

Subdural block[114–116]

A high block may also result from a subdural block. The subdural space is a potential space between dura and arachnoid mater. The epidural space extends only to the foramen magnum, whereas the subdural space extends upwards. A subdural block may result from a breach of the dura mater and can theoretically occur at any time in labour. It should be recognized by an increase in level of anaesthesia. The usual features of a subdural block are slow onset, patchy blockade, minimal sacral analgesia, cranial nerve palsies and a relative lack of sympathetic blockade. Although previously, the subdural space was thought to be impossible to enter, MRI imaging has now demonstrated that it can occur.[117] Table 6.2 demonstrates the difference between epidural, subdural and intrathecal blockade. Subsequent injection of a large volume of local anaesthetic drug into the subdural space may rupture the arachnoid mater causing intrathecal effects.

Table 6.2   Distinguishing between epidural, subdural and subarachnoid blockade

	Epidural	Subdural	Subarachnoid
Onset time	Slow (20 min)	Slow	Rapid (5 min)
Spread	Predictable	Higher than expected; may extend intracranially	High; may extend intracranially
Sacral blockade	Usual; may be poor	Rarely present	Good
Nature of blockade	Segmental	Patchy	Dense
Motor block	Minimal	Minimal	Dense
Hypotension	Depends on extent of block	Depends on extent of block	Expected

OPIOIDS

Intrathecal or epidural opioids have become increasingly popular for labour regional analgesia. The effects of intrathecally administered opioids, are dependent on local action on opioid receptors within the spinal cord and on systemic uptake.[118–120] When an opioid is administered intrathecally, the effects (analgesia,[121–123] respiratory depression,[124–126] pruritus[125,127] and nausea and vomiting[125]) are caused by the drug gaining access to the spinal cord and brainstem from the CSF. When an opioid is administered epidurally, only a fraction of the drug crosses the meningeal layers and gains access to the CSF; it then exerts its pharmacological action in the same way as intrathecal opioids.[128–131] This fraction is dependent on its physio-chemical properties.[118,119,132,133] The remainder is absorbed systemically and gains access to the central nervous system from the blood. Therefore side effects such as respiratory depression, sedation, nausea and vomiting can also occur by this route.[134,135]

Epidural opioids in common use are shown in Table 6.3. Epidural opioids alone are sometimes effective in the early stages of labour for reasons discussed earlier, but usually need supplementation with local anaesthetic as labour progresses. *Morphine* has gradually fallen from favour as it is not very lipid soluble and so has a slow onset of action and higher incidence of side effects.[136] No more than 50% of patients obtain satisfactory analgesia during early labour when 2–10 mg epidural morphine is given.[137–139] It is also necessary to use preservative-free morphine. *Pethidine* results in sympathetic and motor blockade due to its local anaesthetic effect and thus has not been widely used in labour.[140] Epidural doses of pethidine for labour may also have a short duration of action.[141] *Fentanyl* used epidurally has a more rapid onset of action due to high lipid solubility, which also limits its duration of action. Epidural fentanyl of 150–200 μg provides adequate analgesia for approximately 60–90 min.[142,143] Epidural *sufentanil*[144] (no product licence available in the UK) and epidural *alfentanil* are other lipid soluble opioids which have been used in labour. Heytens et al using a continuous epidural infusion of 30 μg/kg/h of alfentanil observed neonatal hypotonia at delivery as well as poor second stage analgesia necessitating local anaesthetic use.[145]

The main advantage of using opioids is that they reduce the dose of local anaesthetic necessary to provide analgesia, improving maternal satisfaction and reducing side effects from the local anaesthetic.[146] They also improve quality of analgesia as the block is less segmentally dependent and can be used to treat a patchy block, or improve perineal analgesia.

SIDE EFFECTS OF OPIOIDS

Regardless of whether opioids are given intrathecally or epidurally, their side effect profile is similar.

Respiratory depression

Respiratory depression is more frequent after morphine than any of the other opioids.[147–149] It has been reported after fentanyl,[150] sufentanil,[151] and alfentanil.[152] The more lipid soluble opioids are associated with a rapid onset of respiratory depression (<2 h) at a time therefore when the women are still being monitored closely and thus can be considered marginally safer for this reason. Continuous pulse oximetry studies during labour suggest that minor degrees of maternal desaturation are more likely with epidural opioids compared to plain bupivacaine infusions, especially during the second stage of labour,[153] presumably because the response to hypercarbia is blunted, but this has no clinical effect on the mother or the baby.[154]

Urinary retention

Opioids have been associated with urinary retention, the possible mechanism being inhibition of sacral parasympathetic outflow and consequent detrusor muscle relaxation.[155,156] However, immobility, bladder

Table 6.3	Characteristics of commonly used opioids in labour				
	Fentanyl	Sufentanil	Pethidine	Morphine	Diamorphine
Lipid solubility	816	1727	39	1.4	280
Normal epidural doses	50–100 μg	5–10 μg	25–50 mg	3–5 mg	2.5–5 mg
Onset time (min)	5–10	5–10	5–10	30–60	9–15
Duration (h)	1–2	1–3	2–4	4–12	6–12

outlet obstruction by the presenting fetal part and local anaesthetic drugs may also contribute. It seems reasonable to assume that the more ambulant a woman is in labour the less the incidence of catheterization, but no controlled studies have yet demonstrated this.

Neonatal depression

Any opioid that reaches high enough concentration in the umbilical vein will cause respiratory depression in the fetus. An epidural bolus of fentanyl at a dose of 150–200 µg can produce respiratory depression and has been found to produce an umbilical artery concentration of 0.25 ng/ml.[157] Neither Apgar scores nor neonatal adaptive behavioural scores correlate well with umbilical vein fentanyl concentration in the doses used, suggesting that fentanyl has minimal effect.[158] Intramuscular pethidine has a longer, more profound effect.[159]

Pruritus

This is the most common symptom of intrathecal or epidural opioids. Although not life-threatening it can be very troublesome. It is thought to be due to interaction with the trigeminal nucleus and nerve roots via the anterior spinal artery.[160] Suggested treatments include opioid antagonists (naloxone 40–80 µg, i.v.), although they may reverse analgesia, antihistamines (chlorpheniramine 10 mg, i.v. or 4 mg p.o.), and subhypnotic doses of propofol (10–20 mg, i.v.),[161] although the efficacy of the latter treatment has been questioned.[162]

Gastric emptying

Systemic opioids are known to delay gastric emptying. Epidural analgesia with local anaesthetic alone has no effect. However, there is a dose dependent effect of epidural opioids on gastric emptying. Bolus doses of 50 and 100 µg fentanyl, 5 mg diamorphine and greater than 100 µg fentanyl in an epidural infusion all have an effect.[163–165] This should be considered when general anaesthesia is being undertaken.

LOCAL ANAESTHETIC AND OPIOID COMBINATIONS

Epidural or intrathecal opioids are often adequate for early labour analgesia, but are less effective in late labour. On the other hand, high doses of local anaesthetic alone can provide analgesia for the entire labour, but with the side effect of lower limb motor block. For these reasons, most obstetric anaesthetists combine a dilute mixture of local anaesthetic with a small opioid dose. Such solutions speed up the onset and prolong analgesia with fewer side effects than the administration of an equipotent dose of local anaesthetic or opioid alone. Laboratory studies suggest that such low dose mixtures act synergistically.[166]

The most commonly used combination is a low dose mixture of fentanyl (2–2.5 µg/ml) and bupivacaine (0.0625–0.1%).[167] Continuous infusions or intermittent boluses of these mixtures can be administered throughout labour,[168] once an initial loading dose (10–15 ml) of the same mixture has been used to initiate analgesia.[169] Large volumes may be needed to initiate analgesia, especially with very dilute solutions, however as labour progresses higher doses of local anaesthetic are required.[170] Other opioid drugs including sufentanil,[171–173] alfentanil[174] and diamorphine[175–177] have also been used in combination with low dose bupivacaine.

OTHER DRUGS USED IN LABOUR

Clonidine

Clonidine, an α_2 agonist, has been evaluated for epidural use in labour. It acts on α_2 receptors in the dorsal horn of the spinal cord to provide analgesia by modifying pain transmission pathways.[178] Its attractiveness for use in labour stems from a lack of motor blockade, respiratory depression, nausea or pruritus associated with its use. In addition, fentanyl and clonidine have been found to have a synergistic effect.[179] The dose of clonidine used has been 75–150 µg.[180]

Unfortunately, clonidine has undesirable side effects of its own including hypotension and sedation. Its use without a local anaesthetic agent is not entirely satisfactory and therefore additional local anaesthetic is often needed.[181] Its use has also been associated with significant fetal heart tracing abnormalities. Although there is complete absence of motor blockade which may be useful[182] it seems unlikely that its use will become widespread.

Epinephrine

Epinephrine is commonly used in North America in combination with local anaesthetics. Its α_2 agonist properties can be used to provide analgesia, and its α_1 vasoconstrictor properties can be used to decrease local anaesthetic absorption and prolong blockade. It is also used as part of the test dose because intravenous epinephrine will produce a tachycardia. A problem is that increased motor blockade is seen.

SIDE EFFECTS OF EPIDURAL ANALGESIA

Side effects can be classified as immediate or late and associated with the procedure or the drug injected. Drug related side effects are discussed under the relevant sections on those drugs. Scott and Tunstall examining complications after epidural blockade, found that the most common complications were neurological problems, high blockade, backache and urinary retention; the incidence of each was very small.[183]

IMMEDIATE COMPLICATIONS

Accidental dural puncture

This is one of the more troublesome and common problems with epidural analgesia in pregnant women. The incidence is 0.5–2.6%. The continued leak of CSF gives rise to a low pressure headache, (post dural puncture headache – PDPH), in at least 70% of women who have had an accidental dural puncture in labour with an epidural needle.[184] Symptoms include postural headache, photophobia and often neck stiffness. Dizziness, nausea and double vision through traction on the sixth cranial nerve may also occur. Long-term sequelae include cranial nerve palsies, unmasking of cerebral pathology, persistent CSF leak, epidural fistulae and subdural haematoma.[185] Although the traditional view is that the headache is due to traction on nerves secondary to low pressure, it has been postulated that a decrease in intracranial pressure causes reflex cerebrovascular dilatation.[186,187] Unpublished work, using cerebral doppler studies of women with PDPH, which shows a high degree of cerebral vasodilatation reduced after blood patch, supports this hypothesis.[188]

Since the onset of headache may occur several days after discharge from hospital, health workers outside hospital must be able to recognize it[189] (see Box 6.3). Failure to adequately treat PDPH may rarely cause subsequent problems such as subdural haemorrhage.[190]

---

1. Postural headache aggravated by a Valsalva manoeuvre
2. Frontal/occipital headache, may be accompanied by neck stiffness and photophobia
3. Onset within 0–48 h
4. Associated symptoms – visual, auditory disturbance, nausea, vomiting
5. Rarely cranial nerve palsies, blurred vision due to traction on VI cranial nerve.

Box 6.3   Symptoms and signs of PDPH.

Treatment

Caffeine,[191] sumatriptan[192,193] and ACTH[194,195] have all been reported as treatments but are not as effective as a blood patch since frequently the dural leak persists for several days. Caffeine produces cerebral vasoconstriction.[196] Its efficacy is only 25% and seizures have been reported with its use.[197] The standard technique is epidural blood patch. Although the blood patch involves another epidural injection, it provides relief in 61–75% of patients.[198] Alternatively blood may be administered 6–8 h after delivery through the existing, (resited), epidural catheter, which has been used for labour analgesia.[199] Occasionally another blood patch is necessary. As the headache may interfere with the mother's care of the baby treatment is essential. MRI scans of epidural blood patches have demonstrated the blood lies over the dural puncture hole.[200] Initially a large clot is seen which is then reabsorbed. Delayed MRI scans show decreased clot size with an adherent fibrin clot over the dural hole.

Technique of epidural blood patch

1. Take a history and examine patient looking for the above. Exclude local or systemic sepsis. Obtain consent for procedure.
2. Two operators, aseptic conditions (procedure should ideally be conducted in theatre).
3. Establish i.v. access.
4. Position of the patient: lateral – usually the sitting position is impossible because of the headache.
5. First operator locates the epidural space.
6. Second operator withdraws 20 ml blood under aseptic conditions and transfers syringe to first operator.
7. First operator injects 15–20 ml blood into the epidural space. Epidural needle removed.
8. Advise patient to lie flat for 1–2 h.
9. Advise patient to avoid straining for 4–5 h.
10. If headache free at 12–24 h, discharge with advice to return if symptoms recur.
11. Obtain patient contact details and arrange further follow-up appointment in 2–4 weeks.

Management of an epidural after dural puncture

From a practical point of view, if accidental dural puncture occurs when siting the epidural needle, the anaesthetist has two choices. Either the epidural can be resited at a different interspace or the epidural catheter can be threaded into the subarachnoid space and subsequently used as an intrathecal catheter. The first option requires considerable care, since

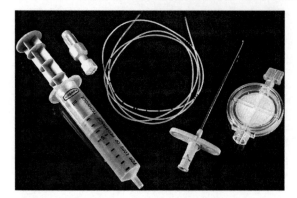

Figure 6.3   Standard epidural kit with Tuohy needle, loss of resistance syringe, filter and catheter.

accidental injection of 'epidural' doses can still occur through this catheter into the subarachnoid space. If an 'intrathecal catheter' management plan is adopted, intermittent top-ups of 2–3 ml of low dose epidural mixture (e.g. bupivacaine 0.1% + fentanyl 2 μg/ml) can be given by the anaesthetist. It is unknown whether the introduction of a subarachnoid catheter and the use of spinal analgesia under these circumstances reduces the incidence of PDPH.[201]

Catheter migration

Epidural catheters may migrate at any time during labour. Migration into the subarachnoid space is most likely when the dura has been partially breached by the Tuohy needle (Fig. 6.3) but has gone unrecognized. Intravenous catheter migration may also occur. Although anaesthetists are very aware of the dangers of large doses of local anaesthetic in the subarachnoid space or intravenous injections of local anaesthetic and are able to deal with the consequences, this is less true of other staff. Increased awareness that this may occur at any time is essential.

Unilateral blockade/partial blockade

As discussed above unilateral blockade is due to either a midline anatomical barrier, spinal deformity or epidural catheter malfunction. If delivery is imminent, it is probably best to resite the epidural catheter immediately. If time allows, assess the block carefully in terms of pinprick or loss of cold sensation to ethyl chloride spray. Touching the patient's feet and assessing foot temperature may also give useful information on the spread of the sensory block.[202] If one foot or both feet are cold and clammy, this gives an indication that all is not well with the epidural block.[203] Partial withdrawal of the catheter and/or an injection of a large

volume (20 ml) of dilute local anaesthetic with opioid may solve the problem. Failing that, the epidural must be resited.

Shivering

Women have frequently been observed to shiver during epidural analgesia. The mechanisms remain obscure – it may be multifactorial and relate to abnormal thermoregulation and abnormal perception of the thermal environment.[204] Injection of cold or warm saline epidurally has not been shown to affect shivering in volunteers.[205] Shivering during labour has been estimated at 33–66% with an epidural and 10% without. It is generally regarded as a nuisance although it may increase maternal oxygen consumption. Pethidine, fentanyl and sufentanil are all effective treatments given epidurally.[206]

LATE COMMON COMPLICATIONS

Backache

Backache is common in pregnancy, occurring in more than 50% of women. Unfortunately, if a patient has received an epidural during labour, backache during the post-partum period is likely to be attributed to the epidural. Two large retrospective studies suggested that the incidence of long-term backache was higher in women receiving epidural analgesia.[207,208] It was postulated that epidurals caused backache during labour secondary to motor block of the lower limbs, leading to the adoption of 'stressed postures'. However, recall bias may have contributed strongly to this association. Prospective studies have now demonstrated that backache is not increased amongst women receiving epidural analgesia.[209–212] The degree of motor blockade has not been found to be a factor in the development of backache.[209] Weight gain, short stature and back pain during pregnancy are all associated with increased risk of backache. MRI imaging of women after delivery has demonstrated considerable lower lumbar superficial tissue oedema regardless of whether epidurals had been used during labour.[213] In this study, women who had epidurals exhibited similar amounts of tissue oedema in the lumbar region as those receiving other forms of analgesia, suggesting that epidurals are unlikely to cause significant tissue damage in the lower back. Another interesting fact is the presence, on MRI scans, of asymptomatic lumbar disc degeneration in 30% of pregnant women and women of childbearing age.[214] The influence of labour in women with lumbar disc problems is unknown, but potentially may influence postpartum back problems. In conclusion, it appears that backache is a common symptom during pregnancy and epidural analgesia does not appear to affect its development.

Long-term headaches

In the same study of backache as above[207] headaches were found to be more common in women receiving epidurals. However, this was the same group that were suffering from backache. Prospectively, there was no difference found.[209]

Long-term neurological sequelae

Neurological problems after epidural analgesia are uncommon. Holdcroft et al estimated the incidence as 1 in 13 000 deliveries.[215] Neurological deficits, which range from minor sensory impairment in the lower limbs to foot drop and paraplegia may occur in any labour. However, they may be mistakenly attributed to an epidural. Post-partum nerve palsy often results from mild cephalopelvic disproportion or from forceps blades[216] – the lumbosacral trunk may get compressed as it crosses the pelvic brim. The common peroneal nerve may also be damaged in the lithotomy position. In a post-mortem study Lazorthes et al demonstrated that the blood supply to the conus medullaris of the spinal cord may arise from the internal iliac vessels in 15% of the population instead of the upper aorta via the artery of Adamkiewicz.[217] Compression of these vessels in such a population may potentially occur during delivery resulting in ischaemia and ultimately paraplegia. Interestingly in a large survey in a Nigerian teaching hospital, Bademosi et al reported 34 cases of postpartum neurological problems of which the most common injury was unilateral or bilateral foot drop. Results of electromyographic examination and determinations of conduction velocities were consistent with proximal neuropraxia of the lumbosacral trunk in 88% of these patients. Five (15%) patients in this series suffered permanent paraplegia.[218] None of these obstetric patients with neurological problems had received epidural analgesia!

Although non-anaesthetic problems may lead to neurological sequelae during delivery this should not however, mitigate the need for good anaesthetic practice to minimize the risk of neurological problems occurring. The use of low dose anaesthetic mixtures and a brief neurological examination have been advocated[219] but the latter is probably impractical in a labour ward setting. If a patient has severe pain on insertion of the epidural needle or epidural catheter, the anaesthetist should withdraw the needle and avoid that interspace.

SPINAL MICROCATHETERS

Spinal microcatheters of 28–32G have been associated with cauda equina syndrome due to the possibility of pooling of hyperbaric 5% lidocaine.[220] Of more concern the use of intrathecal lidocaine itself, regardless of baricity and unassociated with microspinal catheters, has been associated with transient nerve symptoms.[221–227]

METHODS OF ADMINISTRATION (TABLE 6.4)

The epidural solutions for labour may need to be administered over 12 h or so. Therefore the ability

Table 6.4 Suggested regimens for maintenance of epidural blockade during labour			
Drug	Intermittent top-up	Continuous epidural infusion (ml/h)	Patient controlled analgesia
Bupivacaine 0.25%	10 ml every 2 h	5	Bolus 3 ml Lockout 10 min
Bupivacaine 0.125%	10–15 ml every hour	8–15	Bolus 5 ml Lockout 20 min
Fentanyl 2 µg/ml + bupivacaine 0.1%	10–15 ml every hour	8–15	Bolus 5 ml Lockout 20 min
Sufentanil 0.25 µg/ml + bupivacaine 0.0625%	10–15 ml every hour	10–12	

to give repeat injections is provided via a catheter. The methods of providing continued analgesia are:

Continuous epidural infusion

Potential benefits of continual epidural infusion (CEI) include a stable level of analgesia, cardiovascular stability and less need for bolus injections. Analgesia is maintained by varying the infusion rate to provide an upper sensory level to T10. Low dose local anaesthetic/opioid infusions are commonly started at 10–12 ml/h with rates being increased or supplementary top-ups administered for breakthrough pain. Migration of the epidural catheter into an epidural vein is more likely to show itself by regression of the sensory block rather than systemic toxicity. Migration of the catheter into the subdural space is likely to result in a slowly evolving dense motor block, secondary to tearing of the delicate arachnoid mater and subsequent infusion into the subarachnoid space.

The disadvantages of CEI are that changes in analgesia occur slowly, increased doses of local anaesthetic tend to be required compared to an intermittent top-up technique, leading to the increased likelihood of motor blockade and as there is less need to assess analgesia a midwife may spend less time with the mother.

Typical doses for continuous infusion are given in Table 6.4. Supervision should be regular and the block assessed at frequent intervals. Guidelines as to what to assess should be clear. The infusion pump may malfunction and ideally should differ from that used to give other infusions on the labour ward.

Intermittent epidural boluses (Top-ups)

When using an intermittent technique, top-ups should be given immediately pain sensation returns following the initial epidural loading dose, since it takes several minutes for subsequent epidural top-ups to act. In the UK, midwives usually give increments of epidural drugs and may indeed give the first epidural dose (usually low dose epidural mixture following the spinal component of a combined spinal-epidural technique), although this is not common practice. One survey found that only 3/100 000 midwife top-ups lead to life-threatening complications and all were appropriately managed.[228] Of prime importance is that midwives should be properly trained, follow strict guidelines and anaesthetic help should be available within 5 min. Problems can occur at any time in labour. Suggested guidelines recommend that any top-up should be given in a divided dose with a 5 min interval between increments, and that should any complications arise, the mother should be turned to the left lateral position, oxygen administered and help immediately summoned.

Patient controlled epidural analgesia

Patient controlled epidural analgesia (PCEA) was first suggested for use in labour in 1988.[229] The claimed advantages over CEI or intermittent top-ups are flexibility, minimization of drug dosage and a reduced demand on staff time. Safety is still paramount. Eisenach concluded that PCEA should be administered with very dilute amounts of bupivacaine and reasonable hourly limits prescribed with periodic assessments by anaesthetists.[230] When compared with CEI, PCEA has been found to produce similar levels of satisfaction with a lower use of bupivacaine and a lower need for supplemental analgesia.[231] When compared to intermittent boluses there is little difference found, although greater maternal satisfaction has been reported.[232] Bupivacaine is the main local anaesthetic agent that has been evaluated for PCEA. Fentanyl and sufentanil are the opioids that have been used in doses of 8–25 µg/h. Lockout should be of moderate length with at least a 10–15 min interval to await onset of effect. No serious adverse effects have been reported. Not all women are suitable for PCEA – these include those who do not want to use it and those who are exhausted.[233] Supervision should be as for top-up administration. Pumps need to be lightweight yet able to carry large volumes. The cost of the technology may represent a significant deterrent to its use.

Combined-spinal epidural anaesthesia

A combined-spinal epidural (CSE) technique is a combination of both a spinal and epidural blockade.[234–236] A CSE for labour analgesia allows the anaesthetist the flexibility of both techniques, i.e. a rapid onset spinal blockade together with further epidural boluses when the spinal block regresses. The advantages and disadvantages of the three techniques are compared in Table 6.5.

A CSE is commonly performed nowadays as a single interspace, needle through needle technique, using a standard epidural needle and a longer pencil point spinal needle (e.g. a 27G, 119 mm Whitacre needle) inserted through it (Fig. 6.4). Although when first used for labour analgesia, 5 mg bupivacaine alone was used for the intrathecal component,[237] it is more usual today in the UK to inject a low dose combination of bupivacaine and fentanyl, not only to provide rapid analgesia but also to reduce lower limb motor block to allow ambulation.[238–240] Analgesia is continued

Table 6.5 Characteristics of epidural, spinal and CSE blockade

	Spinal	Epidural	CSE
Onset time	Rapid	Slow	Rapid
Blockade characteristics	Dense	Less dense	Dense
Top-up facility	No	Yes	Yes
Headache risk	Yes	Yes	Yes
Technical difficulty	+	++	+++

Table 6.6 Modified Bromage score

1 – Complete block
2 – Able to move feet
3 – Knee flexion
4 – Hip flexion weak
5 – Full flexion of hips and knees
6 – Ability to perform a partial knee bend whilst standing

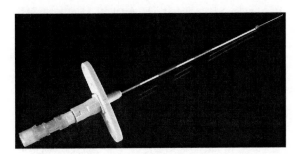

Figure 6.4 Standard Tuohy needle with a 119 mm 27G Whitacre spinal needle placed through it for CSE analgesia.

via the epidural catheter after the spinal block has regressed, again using low dose mixtures. It may actually be convenient and safer to use a small dose of pre-mixed low dose epidural solution intrathecally.[241]

Intrathecal doses used for CSE in labour include:

- 2.5 mg bupivacaine + 25 µg fentanyl (original Queen Charlotte's Hospital regimen[239])
- 2.5 mg bupivacaine + 5 µg fentanyl (2.5 ml of pre-mixed epidural solution: 0.1% bupivacaine + 2 µg/ml fentanyl, is our own current standard[254])
- 10 µg sufentanil[242]
- 2.5 mg bupivacaine + 10 µg sufentanil.[243]

The disadvantages of the technique include:

- Headache – multiple passages of the spinal needle to detect CSF may increase the incidence
- Pruritus
- Meningitis[244]
- Respiratory depression[245,246]
- Falls during walking.[247,248]

Low doses of local anaesthetic/opioid mixtures whether given intrathecally, epidurally or in combination may allow women to mobilize if they are carefully monitored. There may be advantages to this in that this avoids the recumbent position. Maternal satisfaction is also high with minimal lower limb motor blockade.[240] These women should be carefully assessed prior to walking and throughout labour as proprioception may be altered increasing the chance of falling while ambulating.[247] It has been recommended that the modified Bromage score (Table 6.6), a Romberg's test or a supervised walk be used to minimize the chances of falling while ambulating.[249] Several recent studies from our institution using standard clinical tests as well as somatosensory evoked potentials[250] and computerized dynamic posturography[251] to assess balance after low dose CSE analgesia have endorsed the safety of ambulatory epidurals.[252–254]

CONCLUSION

Over the past 10 years or more, labour regional analgesic techniques have become inherently safer primarily due to the increasing use of low dose local anaesthetic/opioid combinations. Their added advantage of reducing motor block has led to many units permitting low risk mothers to ambulate for short periods after receiving labour epidural analgesia. The fairly recent introduction of low dose CSE analgesia for labour with its distinct advantage of providing rapid pain relief has added a useful technique to the obstetric anaesthetist's armamentarium. Low dose CSEs can also permit ambulation again due to a reduction in lower limb motor block. However there are still many unanswered questions regarding CSEs. Should its use be restricted to late labour or for extremely distressed mothers and more importantly do potential complications associated with the technique outweigh any benefits? Also does ambulation after low dose regional block confer any obstetric advantage to the mother and is it really safe to allow patients to walk after analgesia is established?

The recent introduction of two local anaesthetics ropivacaine and levobupivacaine offers interesting possibilities. But are they any better than those what we are currently using for labour? The use of MLAC studies, to assess local anaesthetic potencies, provide a truly scientific way in which to answer such questions. Ultimately, regardless of various advantages to some of these new drugs, an element of cost/benefit will naturally come into the equation influencing local hospital policies.

What of the future? Is there a revolutionary new drug around the corner poised to significantly influence labour regional analgesia? Probably not. Certainly for the foreseeable future, obstetric anaesthetists will most likely use the same type of drugs they are currently using for regional blockade, with increasing emphasis on finding the combination which will optimize analgesic benefits while simultaneously reducing unwanted side effects.

REFERENCES

1. Chamberlain G, Wraight A, Steer P (eds) *Pain and its relief in childbirth.* (Report of the 1990 NBT Survey.) Edinburgh: Churchill Livingstone, 1993.

2. Parkin IG, Harrison GR. The topographical anatomy of the lumbar epidural space. *J Anat* 1985; **141**: 211–217.

3. Harrison GR, Parkin IG, Shah JL. Resin injection studies of the lumbar extradural space. *Br J Anaesth* 1985; **57**: 333–336.

4. Reynolds AF, Roberts PA, Pollay M, Stratemeier PH. Quantative anatomy of the thorocolumbar epidural space. *Neurosurgery* 1985; **17**: 905–907.

5. Blomberg RG. The technical advantages of the paramedian approach for lumbar epidural puncture and catheter introduction. A study using epiduroscopy in autopsy subjects. *Anaesthesia* 1988; **43**: 837–843.

6. Westbrook JL, Renowden SA, Carrie LES. Study of the anatomy of the extradural region using magnetic resonance imaging. *Br J Anaesth* 1993; **71**: 495–498.

7. Hirabayashi Y, Shimizu R, Fukuda H, Saitoh K, Igarashi T. Soft tissue anatomy within the vertebral canal in pregnant women. *Br J Anaesth* 1996; **77**: 153–156.

8. Hirabayashi Y, Saitoh K, Fukuda H, Igarashi T, Shimizu R, Seo N. Magnetic resonance imaging of the extradural space of the thoracic spine. *Br J Anaesth* 1997; **79**: 563–566.

9. Capogna G, Celleno D, Simonetti C, Lupoi D. Anatomy of the lumbar epidural region using magnetic resonance imaging: a study of dimensions and a comparison of two postures. *Int J Obstet Anesth* 1997; **6**: 97–100.

10. Hogan QH. Lumbar epidural anatomy. A new look by cyromicrotome section. *Anesthesiology* 1991; **75**: 767–775.

11. Zarzur E. Anatomic studies of the human lumbar ligamentum flavum. *Anesthesia and Analgesia* 1984; **63**: 499–502.

12. Collier CB. Why obstetric epidurals fail: a study of epidurograms. *Int J Obstet Anesth* 1996; **5**: 19–31.

13. Cheek TG, Gutsche BB, Gaiser RR. The pain of childbirth and its effect on the mother and fetus. In: Chestnut DH (ed) *Obstetetric anesthesia: principles and practice.* St Louis: Mosby Year Book 1994, pp 314–329.

14. Bonica JJ. *Principles and practice of obstetric analgesia and anesthesia,* vol 1. Philadelphia: FA Davis, 1967.

15. Mather LE. Opioid analgesic drugs. In: Nimmo WS, Rowbotham DJ, Smith G (eds) *Anaesthesia* 2nd edn. Oxford: Blackwell, 1994, pp 132–165.

16. Shnider SM, Abboud TK, Artal R, Henriksen EH, Stefani SJ, Levinson G. Maternal catecholamines decrease during labor after lumbar epidural anesthesia. *Am J Obstet Gynecol* 1983; **147**: 13–15.

17. Hollmen AI. The effects of regional anaesthesia on utero- and feto-placental blood flow. In: Reynolds F (ed) *Effects on the baby of maternal analgesia and anaesthesia.* London: Bailliere Tindall, 1993, pp 67–87.

18. Dailey PA, Baysinger CL, Levinson G, Shnider SM. Neurobehavioural testing of the newborn infant: effects of obstetric anesthesia. *Clin Perinatol* 1982; **9**: 191–214.

19. Hodgkinson R, Marx GF, Kim SS, Miclat NM. Neonatal neurobehavioral tests following vaginal delivery under ketamine, thiopental, and extradural anesthesia. *Anesth Analg* 1977; **56**: 548–553.

20. Armand S, Jasson J, Talafre M-L, Amiel-Tison C. The effects of regional analgesia on the newborn. In: Reynolds F (ed) *Effects on the baby of maternal analgesia and anaesthesia.* London: Bailliere Tindall, 1993, pp 191–220.

21. Larue F, Labaille Th, Mazoit X, Mezzaroba Ph, Benlabed M, Benhamou D. Anesthésie péridurale et surveillance de la température au cours du travail. *Annales Francaises d'Anesthesie et de Réanimation* 1987; **6S**: R163.

22. Fusi L, Steer PJ, Maresh MJA, Beard RW. Maternal pyrexia associated with the use of epidural analgesia in labour. *Lancet* 1989; **I**: 1250–1252.

23. Camann WR, Hortvet LA, Hughes N, Bader AM, Datta S. Maternal temperature regulation during extradural analgesia for labour. *Br J Anaesth* 1991; **67**: 565–568.

24. Mercier FJ, Benhamou D. Hyperthermia related to epidural analgesia during labor. *Int J Obstet Anesth* 1997; **6**: 19–24.

25. Dannenbring D, Stevens MJ, House AE. Predictors of childbirth pain and maternal satisfaction. *J Behav Med* 1997; **20**: 127–142.

26. Slade P, MacPherson SA, Hume A, Maresh M. Expectations, experiences and satisfaction with labour. *Br J Clin Psychol* 1993; **32**: 469–483.

27. Moir DD, Willocks J. Management of incoordinate uterine action under continuous epidural analgesia. *BMJ* 1967; **3**: 396–400.

28. Hood DD, Dewan DM. Anesthetic and obstetric outcome in morbidly obese parturients. *Anesthesiology* 1993; **79**: 1210–1218.

29. Letsky EA. Haemostasis and epidural anaesthesia. *Int J Obstet Anesth* 1991; **1**: 51–54.

30. Mallett SV, Cox DJ. Thromboelastography. *Br J Anaesth* 1992; **69**: 307–313.

31. Orlikowski CEP, Payne AJ, Moodley J, Rocke DA. Thromboelastography after aspirin ingestion in pregnant and non-pregnant subjects. *Br J Anaesth* 1992; **69**: 159–161.

32. Hirsh J, Levine MN. Low molecular weight heparin: laboratory properties and clinical evaluation. *Eur J Surg* 1994; **571**(suppl): 9–22.

33. Horlocker TT, Heit JA. Low molecular weight heparin: biochemistry, pharmacology, perioperative prophylaxis regimens, and guidelines for regional anaesthetic management. *Anesth Analg* 1997; **85**: 874–885.

34. Nelson-Piercy C, Letsky EA, de Swiet M. Low molecular weight heparin for obstetric thromboprophylaxis: experience of sixty-nine pregnancies in sixty-one women at high risk. *Am J Obstet Gynecol* 1997; **176**: 1062–1068.

35. Dripps RD, Vandan LD. Long-term follow-up of patients who received 10 098 spinal anaesthetics. *J Am Med Assoc* 1954; **156**: 1486–1491.

36. Phillips OC, Ebner H, Nelson ATY, Black MH. Neurological complications following spinal anesthesia with lidocaine; a prospective review of 10 440 cases. *Anesthesiology* 1969; **30**: 284–289.

37. Bader AM, Gilbertson L, Kirz L, Datta S. Regional anesthesia in women with chorioamnionitis. *Region Anesth* 1992; **17**: 84–86.

38. Ramanathan J, Vaddadi A, Mercer BM, Sibai B, Angel JJ. Epidural anesthesia in women with chorioamnionitis. *Anesthesiol Rev* 1992; **19**: 35–40.

39. Carp H, Chestnut DH. Fever and infection. In: Chestnut DH (ed) *Obstetric anesthesia: principles and practice*. St Louis: Mosby Year Book 1994, pp 686–698.

40. Swanson L, Madej T. The febrile patient. In: Russell IF, Lyons G (eds) *Clinical problems in obstetric anaesthesia*. London: Chapman and Hall Medical, 1997.

41. Gershon RY, Manning-Williams D. Anesthesia and the HIV-infected parturient: a retrospective study. *Int J Obstet Anesth* 1997; **6**: 76–81.

42. Stone PA, Kilpatrick AWA, Thorburn J. Posture and epidural catheterisation. The relationship between skill, experience and maternal posture on the outcome of epidural catheter insertion. *Anaesthesia* 1990; **45**(11): 920–923.

43. Davies MW, Harrison JC, Ryan TDR. Current practice of epidural analgesia during normal labour – a survey of maternity units in the United Kingdom. *Anaesthesia* 1993; **48**: 63–65.

44. Blomberg RG, Jaanivald A, Walther S. Advantages of the paramedian approach for lumbar epidural analgesia with catheter technique. *Anaesthesia* 1989; **44**: 742–746.

45. Griffin RM, Scott RPF. A comparison between the midline and paramedian approach to the extradural space. *Anaesthesia* 1984; **39**: 584–586.

46. Meiklejohn BH. The effect of rotation of an epidural needle. The effect of an *in vitro* study. *Anaesthesia* 1987; **42**: 1180–1182.

47. Stride PC, Cooper GM. Dural taps revisited. A 20 year survey from the Birmingham Maternity Hospital. *Anaesthesia* 1993; **48**: 247–255.

48. Reynolds F. Dural puncture and headache. *Br Med J* 1993; **306**: 874–876.

49. Waters JH, Ramanathan S, Chuba JV. Glucose in extradural catheter aspirate. *Anesth Analg* 1993; **76**: 546–548.

50. El Behesy BAZ, James D, Koh KF, Hirsch N, Yentis SM. Distinguishing cerebrospinal fluid from saline used to identify the extradural space. *Br J Anaesth* 1977; **6**: 784–786.

51. Magides AD, Sprigg A, Richmond MN. Lumbar epidurography with multiorifice and single orifice catheters. *Anaesthesia* 1996; **51**: 757–763.

52. Beck H, Brassow F, Doehn M, Bause H, Dziadzka A, Schulte am Esch J. Epidural catheters of the multiorifice type: dangers and complications. *Acta Anaesth Scand* 1986; **30**: 549–555.

53. Dickson MA, Moores C, McClure JH. Comparison of single, end-holed and multi-orifice extradural catheters when used for continuous infusion of local anaesthetic during labour. *Br J Anaesth* 1997; **79**: 297–300.

54. Kinsella SM, Whitwam JG, Spencer JAD. Aortic compression by the uterus: identification with the Finapres digital arterial pressure instrument. *Br J Obstet Gynaecol* 1990; **97**: 700–705.

55. Kinsella SM, Whitwam JG, Spencer JAD. Reducing aortocaval compression: how much tilt is enough. *Br Med J* 1992; **305**: 539–540.

56. Nielsen PR, Erickson JR, Aboulish EI, Perriatt S, Sheppard C. Fetal heart changes after intrathecal sufentanil v. epidural bupivacaine for labor analgesia incidence and clinical significance. *Anesth Analg* 1996; **83**(4): 742–746.

57. White AO, Moore CH, Bless NH. Plasma concentration profile of epidural alfentanil. Bolus followed by continuous infusion technique in the parturient. Effect of epidural alfentanil and fentanyl on fetal heart rate. *Region Anesth* 1994; **19**(3): 164–168.

58. Collins KM, Bevan DR, Beerd RV. Fluid loading to reduce abnormalities of fetal heart rate and maternal hypotension during epidural analgesia in labour. *Br Med J* 1978; **2**: 1460–1461.

59. Ramanathan S, Masih A, Rock I, Chalon J, Turndorf H. Maternal and fetal effects of prophylactic hydration with crystalloids or colloids before epidural anesthesia. *Anesth Analg* 1983; **62**: 673–678.

60. Umstad MP, Ross A, Rushford DD, Permezel M. *Aust NZ J Obstet Gynaecol* 1993; **33**: 269–272.

61. Tong C, Eisenach JC. The vascular mechanism of ephedrine's beneficial effect on uterine perfusion during pregnancy. *Anesthesiology* 1992; **76**: 792–798.

62. Ramanathan S, Grant GJ. Vasopressor therapy for hypotension due to epidural anesthesia for cesarean section. *Acta Anaesth Scand* 1988; **32**: 559–565.

63. Wright PM, Iftikhar M, Fitzpatrick KT, Moore J, Thompson W. Vasopressor therapy for hypotension during epidural anesthesia for cesarean section: effects on maternal and fetal flow velocity ratios. *Anesth Analg* 1992; **75**: 56–63.

64. Reynolds F, Speedy HM. The subdural space: the third place to go astray. *Anaesthesia* 1990; **45**: 120–123.

65. Leighton BL, Gross JB. Air: an effective indicator of intravenously located epidural catheters. *Anesthesiology* 1989; **71**: 848–851.

66. McLean BY, Rottman RL, Kotelko DM. Failure of multiple test doses and techniques to detect intravascular migration of an epidural catheter. *Anesth Analg* 1992; **74**: 454–456.

67. Leighton BL, Norris MC, Sosis M, Epstein R, Chayen B, Larijani GE. Limitations of epinephrine as a marker of intravascular injection in laboring women. *Anesthesiology* 1987; **66**: 688–691.

68. Abraham RA, Harris AP, Maxwell LG, Kaplow S. The efficacy of 1.5% lidocaine with 7.5% dextrose and epinephrine as an epidural test dose for obstetrics. *Anesthesiology* 1986; **64**: 116–119.

69. Prince GD, Shetty GR, Miles M. Safety and efficacy of a low volume extradural test dose of bupivacaine in labour. *Br J Anaesth* 1989; **62**: 503–508.

70. Moore DC, Batra MS. The components of an effective test dose prior to epidural block. *Anesthesiology* 1981; **55**: 693–696.

71. Leighton BL, DeSimone CA, Norris MC, Chayen B. Isoproterenol is an effective marker of intravenous injection in laboring women. *Anesthesiology* 1989; **71**: 206–209.

72. Yoshii WY, Miller M, Rottman RL, Kotelko DM, Wright WC, Stone JJ, Rasmus KT, Rosen PJ. Fentanyl for epidural intravascular test dose in obstetrics. *Region Anesth* 1993; **18**: 296–299.

73. Gieraerts R, Van Zundert A, De Wolf A, Vaes L. Ten ml bupivacaine 0.125% with 12.5 micrograms epinepherine is a reliable epidural test dose to detect inadvertent intravascular injection in obstetric patients: a double blind study. *Acta Anaesth Scand* 1992; **36**: 656–659.

74. Eisenach JC. It's all in how you read the label. *Int J Obstet Anesth* 1999; **8**: 1–2.

75. Howell PR, Madej TH. Administration of drugs outside of product licence: awareness and current practice. *Int J Obstet Anesth* 1999; **8**: 30–36.

76. Conklin KA. Physiologic changes of pregnancy. In: Chestnut DH (ed) *Obstetric anesthesia: principles and practice*. St Louis: Mosby Year Book 1994, pp 17–42.

77. Wildsmith JAW. Peripheral nerve and local anaesthetic drugs. *Br J Anaesth* 1986; **58**: 692–700.

78. Columb MO, Lyons G. Determination of the minimum local analgesic concentrations of epidural bupivacaine and lidocaine in labour. *Anesth Analg* 1995; **81**: 833–837.

79. Lyons G, Columb M, Hawthorne L, Dresner M. Extradural pain relief in labour: bupivacaine sparing by extradural fentanyl is dose dependent. *Br J Anaesth* 1997; **78**: 493–497.

80. Dixon WJ, Massey FJ. *Introduction to statistical analysis*, 4th edn. New York: McGraw-Hill, 1983, pp 428–439.

81. Stocks GM, Hallworth SP, Fernando R, England AJ, Columb MO, Lyons G. The minimum local analgesic dose (MLAD) of intrathecal bupivacaine in labor and the effect of intrathecal fentanyl. *Anesthesiology* 2001; **94**: 593–598.

82. McClure JH. Ropivacaine. *Br J Anaesth* 1996; **76**: 300–307.

83. Moller RA, Covino BG. Effect of progesterone on the cardiac electrophysiological alterations produced by ropivaccaine and bupivacaine. *Anesthesiology* 1992; **77**: 735–741.

84. Santos AC, Arthur GR, Wlody D, DeArmas P, Morishima HO, Finster M. Comparative systemic toxicity of ropivacaine and bupivacaine in non-pregnant and pregnant ewes. *Anesthesiology* 1995; **82**: 734–740.

85. Lysach JC, Dobson CE. Patient controlled epidural analgesia during labor: a comparison of three solutions with a continuous infusion control. *Anesthesiology* 1990; **72**: 44–49.

86. Gristwood R, Bardsley H, Baker H, Dickens J. Reduced cardiotoxicity of laevobupivacaine compared with racaemic bupivacaine (Marcain): new clinical evidence. *Expert Opin Inv Drug* 1994; **3**: 1209–1212.

87. Mazoit JX, Boico O, Samii K. Myocardial uptake of bupivacaine. *Anesth Analg* 1993; **77**: 477–482.

88. Lyons G, Columb M, Wilson RC, Johnson RV. Epidural pain relief in labour: potencies of levobupivacaine and racemic bupivacaine. *Br J Anaesth* 1998; **81**: 899–901.

89. Scott DB, Lee A, Fagan D, Bowler GMR, Bloomfield P, Lundh R. Acute toxicity of ropivacaine compared with that of bupivacaine. *Anesth Analg* 1989; **69**: 563–569.

90. Knudsen K, Beckman M, Blomberg S, Sjövall J, Edvardsson N. Central nervous and cardiovascular effects of i.v. infusions of ropivacaine, bupivacaine and placebo in volunteers. *Br J Anaesth* 1997; **78**: 507–514.

91. Sientra R, Jonker TA, Bourderez P, Kuijpers JC, Van Kleef JW, Lundberg U. Ropivacaine 0.25% v.

Bupivacaine 0.25% for continous epidural use in labor: a double blind comparison. *Anesth Analg* 1995; **80**: 285–289.

92. McCrae AF, Jourion H, McClure JH. Comparison of ropivacaine and bupivacaine for extradural analgesia for the relief of pain in labour. *Br J Anaesth* 1995; **74**: 261–265.

93. Benhamou D, Hamza J, Eledjam J-J, Dailland P, Palot M, Seebacher J, Milon D, Heeroma K. Continuous extradural infusion of ropivacaine 2 mg/ml for pain relief during labour. *Br J Anaesth* 1997; **78**: 748–750.

94. McCrae AF, Westerling P, McClure JH. Pharmacokinetic and clinical study of ropivacaine and bupivacaine in women receiving extradural analgesia in labour. *Br J Anaesth* 1997; **79**: 558–562.

95. Zaric D, Nydahl PA, Adel SO, Enbom H, Magnusson M, Philipson L, Axelsson K. The effect of continuous epidural infusion of ropivacaine (0.1%, 0.2% and 0.3%) on nerve conduction velocity and postural control in volunteers. *Acta Anaesth Scand* 1996; **40**: 342–349.

96. Zaric D, Nydahl PA, Philipson L, Samuelsson L, Heierson A, Axelsson K. The effect of continuous lumbar epidural infusion of ropivacaine (0.1%, 0.2%, 0.3%) and 0.25% bupivacaine on sensory and motor block in volunteers: a double blind study. *Region Anesth* 1996; **21**: 14–25.

97. Reynolds F. Does the left hand know what the right hand is doing? Appraisal of single enantiomer local anaesthetics. *Int J Obstet Anesth* 1997; **6**: 257–269.

98. Polley LS, Columb MO, Naughton NN, Wagner DS, Van de Ven CJM, Dorantes DM. Relative potencies of ropivacaine and bupivacaine for epidural analgesia in labor. *Anesth Analg* 1998; **86**: S384.

99. Capogna G, Celleno D, Lyons G, Columb M. Determination of the minimum local analgesic concentration (MLAC) of epidural ropivacaine in labour. *Br J Anaesth* 1998; **80**: 148.

100. Biehl D, Schnider SM, Levinson G, Callender K. Placental transfer of lidocaine. *Anesthesiology* 1978; **48**: 409–412.

101. Douglas MJ. Neuro toxicity of lidocaine: does it exist? *Can J Anaesth* 1995; **42**: 181–185.

102. Price ML, Reynolds F, Morgan BM. Extending epidural blockade for emergency caesarean section: evaluation of 2% lignocaine with adrenaline. *Int J Obstet Anesth* 1991; **1**: 13–18.

103. Gaiser RR, Cheek TG, Gutshe BB. Epidural lidocaine versus 2-chloroprocaine for fetal distress requiring urgent cesarean section. *Int J Obstet Anesth* 1994; **3**: 208–210.

104. Fernando R, Jones HM. Comparison of plain and alkalinized local anaesthetic mixtures of lignocaine and bupivacaine for elective extradural caesarean section. *Br J Anaesth* 1991; **67**: 699–703.

105. Patel M, Craig R, Laishley R. A comparison between epidural anaesthesia using alkalinized solution and spinal (combined spinal/epidural) anaesthesia for elective caesarean section. *Int J Obstet Anesth* 1996; **5**: 236–239.

106. Capogna G, Celleno D, Laudano D, Giunta F. Alkalinisation of local anesthetics: which block, which local anesthetic? *Region Anesth* 1995; **20**: 369–377.

107. Morison DH. Alkalisation of local anaesthetics. *Can J Anaesth* 1995; **42**: 1076–1079.

108. Hollmén A, Jouppila A, Pihlajaniemi R, Karvonen P, Sjostedt E. Selective lumbar epidural block in labour: a clinical analysis. *Acta Anaesth Scand* 1977; **21**: 174–181.

109. Shennan A, Cooke V, Lloyd-Jones F, Morgan B, de Swiet M. Blood pressure changes during labour and whilst ambulating with combined spinal epidural analgesia. *Br J Obstet Gynaecol* 1995; **102**: 192–197.

110. Slaymaker A, Bamber J, Hawthorne L, Dresner M. Is a fluid preload necessary with low-dose epidural analgesia in labour? *Int J Obstet Anesth* 1998; **7**: 197–198.

111. Crawford JS. Some maternal complications of epidural analgesia for labour. *Anaesthesia* 1985; **40**: 1219–1225.

112. Van Zundert AA, De Wolf AM, Vaes L, Soetens M. High volume spinal anaesthesia with bupivacaine 0.125% for caesarean section. *Anesthesiology* 1988; **69**: 998–1003.

113. Russell IF. Cesarean section and spinal anesthesia with dilute solutions of bupivacaine: the relationship between infused volume and spread. *Region Anesth* 1991; **16**: 130–136.

114. Lee A, Dodd KW. Accidental subdural catheterisation. *Anaesthesia* 1986; **41**: 847–849.

115. Boys JE, Norman PF. Accidental subdural analgesia: a case report, possible clinical implications and relevance to 'massive extradurals'. *Br J Anaesth* 1975; **47**: 1111–1113.

116. Abouleish E, Goldstein M. Migration of an extradural catheter into the subdural space. *Br J Anaesth* 1986; **58**: 1194–1197.

117. Ralph CJ, Williams MP. Subdural or epidural? Confirmation with magnetic resonance imaging. *Anaesthesia* 1996; **51**: 175–177.

118. Cousins MJ, Mather LE. Intrathecal and epidural administration of opioids. *Anesthesiology* 1984; **61**: 276–310.

119. Sjostrom S, Hartvig P, Perrson P, Tansen A. Pharmacokinetics of epidural morphine and meperidine in humans [a]. *Anesthesiology* 1987; **67**: 877–888.

120. Sjostrom S, Hartvig P, Perrson P, Hartvig P. Pharmacokinetics of intrathecal morphine and meperidine in humans [b]. *Anesthesiology* 1987; **67**: 889–898.

121. Wang JK, Nauss LE, Thomas JE. Pain relief by intrathecally applied morphine in man. *Anesthesiology* 1979; **50**: 149–151.

122. Baraka A, Noveihid R, Hajj S. Intrathecal injection of morphine for obstetric analgesia. *Anesthesiology* 1981; **54**: 136–140.

123. Nordberg G, Hedner T, Mellstrand T, Dahlstrom B. Pharmacokinetic aspects of intrathecal morphine analgesia. *Anesthesiology* 1984; **60**: 448–454.

124. Davies GK, Tolhurst-Cleaver JTL. Respiratory depression after intrathecal narcotics. *Anaesthesia* 1980; **35**: 1080–1083.

125. Mok MS, Tsai SK. More experience with intrathecal morphine for obstetric analgesia. *Anesthesiology* 1981; **55**: 481.

126. Abouleish E. Apnoea associated with intrathecal administration of morphine in obstetrics. *Br J Anaesth* 1988; **60**: 592–594.

127. Scott PV, Fisher HB. Intraspinal opiates and itching: a new reflex? *Br Med J* 1982; **284**: 1015–1016.

128. Chauvin M, Samii K, Schermann JM, Sandouk P, Bouden R, Viars P. Plasma pharmacokinetics of morphine after i.m., extradural and intrathecal administration. *Br J Anaesth* 1981; **54**: 843–847.

129. Bromage PR, Camporesi E, Durant PAC, Neilsen CH. Rostral spread of epidural morphine. *Anesthesiology* 1982; **56**: 431–436.

130. Bromage PR, Camporesi E, Durant PAC, Neilsen CH. Non-respiratory side-effects of epidural morphine. *Anesth Analg* 1982; **61**: 490–495.

131. Youngstrom PC, Cowan RI, Sutheimer C, Eastwood DW, Yu JCM. Pain relief and plasma concentrations from epidural and intramuscular morphine in post-Caesarean patients. *Anesthesiology* 1982; **57**: 404–409.

132. Moore RA, Bullingham RSJ, McQuay HJ, Hand CW, Aspel JB, Allen MC, Thomas D. Dural permeability to narcotics: *in vitro* determination and application to extradural administration. *Br J Anaesth* 1982; **54**: 1117–1128.

133. Bernards CM, Hill HF. Physical and chemical properties of drug molecules governing their diffusion through the spinal meninges. *Anesthesiology* 1992; **77**: 750–756.

134. Scott DB, McClure J. Selective epidural analgesia. *Lancet* 1979; **1**: 1410–1411.

135. Yaksh TL. Spinal opiate analgesia: characteristics and principles of action. *Pain* 1981; **11**: 293–346.

136. Hughes SC, Rosen MA, Shnider SM, Abboud TK, Stefani SJ, Norton M. Maternal and neonatal effects of epidural morphine for labour and delivery. *Anesth Analg* 1984; **63**: 319–324.

137. Husemeyer R, O'Connor M, Davenport H. Failure of epidural morphine to relieve pain in labour. *Anaesthesia* 1980; **35**: 161–163.

138. Booker P, Wilkes R, Bryson T, Beddard J. Obstetric pain relief using epidural morphine. *Anaesthesia* 1980; **35**: 377–379.

139. Crawford J. Experiences with epidural morphine in obstetrics. *Anaesthesia* 1981; **36**: 207–209.

140. Skjoldebrand A, Garle M, Gustafsson LL, Johansson H, Lunell NO, Rane A. Extradural pethidine with and without adrenaline during labour: wide variation in effect. *Br J Anaesth* 1982; **54**: 415–420.

141. Husemeyer RP, Cummings AJ, Rosenkiewicz JR, Davenport HT. A study of pethidine kinetics and analgesia in women in labour following intravenous, intramuscular and epidural administration. *Br J Clin Pharmacol* 1982; **13**: 171–176.

142. Justins D, Francis D, Houlton P, Reynolds F. A controlled trial of extradural fentanyl in labour. *Br J Anaesth* 1982; **54**: 409–414.

143. Carrie L, O'Sullivan G, Seegobin R. Epidural fentanyl in labour. *Anaesthesia* 1981; **36**: 965–969.

144. Steinberg RB, Powell G, Hu X, Dunn S. Epidural sufentanil for analgesia for labor and delivery. *Region Anesth* 1989; **14**: 225–228.

145. Heytens L, Cammu H, Camu F. Extradural analgesia during labour using alfentanil. *Br J Anaesth* 1987; **59**: 331–337.

146. Murphy JD, Henderson K, Bowden MI, Lewis M, Cooper GM. Bupivacaine versus bupivacaine plus fentanyl for epidural analgesia: effect on maternal satisfaction. *Br Med J* 1983; **302**: 564–567.

147. Rawal N, Arner S, Gustafsson L, Allvin R. Present state of extradural and intrathecal opioid analgesia in Sweden. *Br J Anaesth* 1987; **59**: 791–799.

148. Christensen V. Respiratory depression after extradural morphine. *Br J Anaesth* 1980; **52**: 841.

149. Davies G, Tolhurst-Cleaver C, James T. CNS depression from intrathecal morphine. *Anesthesiology* 1980; **52**: 280.

150. Brockway MS, Noble DW, Sharwood-Smith GH, McClure JH. Profound respiratory depression after extradural fentanyl. *Br J Anaesth* 1990; **64**: 243–245.

151. Streinstra R, Van Poorten F. Immediate respiratory arrest after caudal epidural sufentanil. *Anesthesiology* 1989; **71**: 993–994.

152. Krane B, Kreutz J, Johnson D, Mazuzan J. Alfentanil and delayed respiratory depression: case studies and review. *Anesth Analg* 1990; **70**: 557–561.

153. Griffin RP, Reynolds F. Maternal hypoxaemia during labour and delivery: the influence of analgesia and effect on neonatal outcome. *Anaesthesia* 1995; **50**: 151–155.

154. Porter JS, Bonello E, Reynolds F. The effects of epidural opioids on maternal oxygenation and delivery. *Anaesthesia* 1996; **51**: 899–903.

155. Dray A. Epidural opiates and urinary retention: new models provide new insights. *Anesthesiology* 1988; **68**: 323–324.

156. Durrant PAC, Yaksh TL. Drug effects on urinary bladder tone during spinal morphine induced inhibition of micturition reflex in unanaesthetised rats. *Anesthesiology* 1988; **68**: 325–334.

157. Carrie LE, O'Sullivan GM, Seegobin R, Epidural fentanyl in labour. *Anaesthesia* 1981; **36**: 965–969.

158. Fernando R, Bonello E, Gill P, Urquhart J, Reynolds F, Morgan B. Neonatal welfare and placental transfer of fentanyl and bupivacaine during ambulatory combined spinal epidural analgesia for labour. *Anaesthesia* 1997; **52**: 517–524.

159. Reynolds F, Crowhurst JA. Opioids in labour – no analgesia effect. *Lancet* 1997; **349**: 4–5.

160. Ballantyne JC, Loach AB, Carr DB. Itching after epidural and spinal opiates. *Pain* 1988; **33**: 149–160.

161. Kam PCA, Tan KH. Pruritis. Itching for a cause and relief? *Anaesthesia* 1996; **51**: 1133–1138.

162. Beilin Y, Bernstien HH, Zucker-Pinchoff B, Zahn J, Zenzen WJ. Subhypnotic doses of propofol do not relieve pruritus induced by intrathecal morphine after cesarean section. *Anesth Analg* 1998; **86**: 310–313.

163. Ewah B, Yau K, King M, Reynolds F, Carson RJ, Morgan B. Effect of epidural opioids on gastric emptying in labour. *Int J Obstet Anaesth* 1993; **2**: 125–128.

164. Wright PMC, Allen RW, Moore J, Donnelly JP. Gastric emptying during lumbar extradural analgesia in labour: effect of fentanyl supplementation. *Br J Anaesth* 1992; **68**: 248–251.

165. Porter JS, Bonello E, Reynolds F. The influence of epidural administration of fentanyl infusion on gastric emptying in labour. *Anaesthesia* 1997; **52**: 1151–1156.

166. Maves TJ, Gebhart GF. Antinociceptive synergy between intrathecal morphine and lidocaine during visceral and somatic nociception in the rat. *Anesthesiology* 1992; **76**: 91–99.

167. Chestnut DH, Owen CL, Bates JN, Ostman LG, Choi WW, Geiger MW. Continuous infusion epidural analgesia during labor: a randomized, double blind comparison of 0.0625% bupivacaine/0.0002% fentanyl versus 0.125% bupivacaine. *Anesthesiology* 1988; **68**: 754–759.

168. Lamont RF, Pinney D, Rodgers P, Bryant TN. Continuous versus intermittent epidural analgesia. *Anaesthesia* 1989; **44**: 893–896.

169. Russell R. Maintenance and monitoring. In: Reynolds F (ed) *Pain relief in labour*. London: BMJ Publishing Group, 1997, pp 209–219.

170. Capogna G, Celleno D, Lyons G, Columb M, Fusco P. Minimum local analgesic concentration of extradural bupivacaine increases with progression of labour. *Br J Anaesth* 1998; **80**: 11–13.

171. Russell R, Reynolds F. Epidural infusions for nulliparous women in labour: a randomized double blind comparison of fentanyl/bupivacaine with sufentanil/bupivacaine. *Anaesthesia* 1993; **48**: 856–861.

172. Cohen S, Amar D, Pantuck CB, Pantuck EJ, Goodman EJ, Leung DH. Epidural analgesia for labour and delivery: fentanyl or sufentanil? *Can J Anaesth* 1996; **43**: 341–346.

173. Van Steenberge A, DeBroux H, Noorduin H. Extradural bupivacaine with sufentanil for vaginal delivery: a double blind trial. *Br J Anaesth* 1987; **59**: 1518–1522.

174. Bader AM, Ray N, Datta S. Continuous epidural infusion of alfentanil and bupivacaine for labor and delivery. *Int J Obstet Anaesth* 1992; **1**: 187–190.

175. Lowson SM, Eggers KA, Warwick JP, Moore WJ, Thomas TA. Epidural infusions of bupivacaine and diamorphine in labour. *Anaesthesia* 1995; **50**: 420–422.

176. Hill DA, McCarthy G, Bali IM. Epidural infusion of alfentanil or diamorphine with bupivacaine in labour – a dose finding study. *Anaesthesia* 1995; **50**: 415–419.

177. Enever GR, Noble HA, Kolditz D, Valentine S, Thomas TA. Epidural infusion of diamorphine with bupivacaine in labour: a comparison with fentanyl and bupivacaine. *Anaesthesia* 1991; **46**: 169–173.

178. Eisenach J, Detweiler D, Hood D. Hemodynamic and analgesic actions of epidurally administered clonidine. *Anesthesiology* 1993; **78**: 277–287.

179. Celleno D, Capogna G, Costantino P, Zangrillo A. Comparison of fentanyl with clonidine adjuvants for epidural analgesia with 0.125% bupivacaine in the first stage of labour. *Int J Obstet Anesth* 1995; **4**: 26–29.

180. Chassard D, Mathon L, Dailler F, Golfier F, Tournadre JP, Bouletreau P. Extradural clonidine combined with sufentanil and 0.0625% bupivacaine for analgesia in labour. *Br J Anaesth* 1996; **77**: 4458–4462.

181. O'Meara ME, Gin T. Comparison of 0.125% bupivacaine with 0.125% bupivacaine with clonidine as extradural analgesia in the first stage of labour. *Br J Anaesth* 1993; **71**: 651–656.

182. Husaini SW, Russell IF. Epidural clonidine-fentanyl combination for labour analgesia. A comparison with bupivacaine-fentanyl. *Int J Obstet Anesth* 1995; **4**: 150–154.

183. Scott DB, Tunstall ME. Serious complications associated with epidural spinal blockade in obstetrics – A 2 year prospective study. *Int J Obstet Anesth* 1995; **4**: 133–139.

184. Gutsche BB. Lumbar epidural analgesia in obstetrics: taps and patches. In: Reynolds F (ed) *Epidural and spinal blockade in obstetrics*. London: Balliere Tindall, 1990, pp 95–106.

185. MacArthur C, Lewis M, Knox EG. Accidental dural puncture in obstetric patients and long term symptoms. *Br Med J* 1993; **306**: 883–885.

186. Hattingh J, McCaldoon TA. Cerebrovascular effects of cerebrospinal fluid removal. *S Afr Med J* 1978; **54**: 780–781.

187. Grant R, Condon B, Patterson J, Wyper DJ, Hadley MD, Teasdale GM. Changes in cranial CSF volume during hypercapnia and hypocapnia. *J Neurol, Neurosurg Psychiat* 1989; **52**: 218–222.

188. Alvarado M, Vadhera R, Suresh M, Cruz A, Gayathri Y, Belfort M. The relation of cerebral blood flow to postdural puncture headache. *Proceedings of the 26th meeting of SOAP, Philadelphia, 1994.*

189. Maclean AR, Raju S. The management of postdural puncture headache (PDPH) in patients discharged before the onset of headache. *Int J Obstet Anesth* 1995; **4**: 184–185.

190. Reynolds F. Dural puncture and headache. *Br Med J* 1993; **306**: 874–876.

191. Camann WR, Murray RS, Mushlin PS, Lambert DH. Effects of oral caffeine on postdural puncture headache: a double-blind, placebo-controlled trial. *Anesth Analg* 1990; **70**: 181–184.

192. Carp H, Singh PJ, Vadhera R, Jayaram A. Effects of the serotonin-receptor agonist sumatriptan on postdural puncture headache: report of six cases. *Anesth Analg* 1994; **79**: 180–182.

193. Lhuissier C, Mercier FJ, Dounas M, Benhamou D. Sumatriptan: an alternative to epidural blood patch? *Anaesthesia* 1996; **51**: 1078.

194. Collier BB. Treatment for post dural puncture headache. *Br J Anaesth* 1994; **72**: 366–367.

195. Foster P. ACTH treatment for post-lumbar puncture headache. *Br J Anaesth* 1994; **73**: 429.

196. Matthew RJ, Wilson WH. Caffeine induced changes in cerebral circulation. *Stroke* 1985; **16**: 814–817.

197. Cohen SM, Laurito CE, Curran MJ. Grand mal seizure in a post-partum patient following intravenous infusion of caffeine sodium benzoate to treat persistent headache. *J Clin Anesth* 1992; **24**: 48–51.

198. Duffy PJ, Crosby ET. The epidural blood patch. Resolving the controversies. *Can J Anaesth* 1999; **46**: 878–886.

199. Lowenwirt I, Cohen S, Zephyr J, Hamer R, Hronkova B, Rovner JS. Treatment of accidental dural puncture in obstetric patients: prohylactic vs. therapeutic blood patch. *Anesthesiology* 1998; A38.

200. Beards SC, Jackson A, Griffiths AG, Horsman EL. Magnetic resonance imaging of extradural blood patches: appearances from 30 min to 18 h. *Br J Anaesth* 1993; **71**: 182–188.

201. Norris MC, Leighton BL. Continuous spinal analgesia after unintentional dural puncture in parturients. *Region Anesth* 1990; **15**: 285–287.

202. Griffin RP, Reynolds F. The association between foot temperature and asymmetrical epidural blockade. *Int J Obstet Anesth* 1994; **3**: 132–136.

203. Reynolds F. They think it's all over. In: Reynolds F (ed) *Pain relief in labour*. London: BMJ Publishing Group, 1997, pp 209–219.

204. Hynson JM, Sessler DI, Glosten B, McGuire J. Thermal balance and tremor patterns during epidural anesthesia. *Anesthesiology* 1991; **74**: 680–690.

205. Ponte J, Sessler DI. Extradurals and shivering: effects of cold and warm extradural saline injections in volunteers. *Br J Anaesth* 1990; **64**: 731–733.

206. Crossley AW. Peri-operative shivering. *Anaesthesia* 1992; **47**: 193–195.

207. McArthur C, Lewis M, Knox EG, Crawford JS. Epidural anaesthesia and long term backache after childbirth. *Br Med J* 1990; **301**: 9–12.

208. Russell R, Groves P, Taub N, O'Dowd J, Reynolds F. Assessing long-term backache after childbirth. *Br Med J* 1993; **306**: 1299–1302.

209. Russell R, Dundas R, Reynolds F. Long term backache after childbirth: prospective search for causative factors. *Br Med J* 1996; **312**: 1384–1388.

210. Breen TW, Ransil BJ, Groves PA, Oriol NE. Factors associated with back pain after childbirth. *Anesthesiology* 1994; **81**: 29–34.

211. Macarthur A, Macarthur C, Weeks S. Epidural anaesthesia and long term back pain after delivery: a prospective cohort study. *Br Med J* 1995; **311**: 1336–1339.

212. Patel M, Fernando R, Gill P, Urquhart J, Morgan B. A prospective study of long-term backache after childbirth in primigravidae – the effect of ambulatory epidural analgesia during labour. *Int J Obstet Anesth* 1995; **4**: 187.

213. Holdcroft A, Baudouin C, Fernando R, Samsoon G, Oatridge A. Post-partum magnetic resonance imaging: lumbar tissue changes are unrelated to epidural analgesia or mode of delivery. *Int J Obstet Anesth* 1995; **4**: 201–206.

214. Powell MC, Wilson M, Szypryt P, Symonds EM, Worthington BS. Prevalence of lumbar disc degeneration observed by magnetic resonance in symptomless women. *Lancet* 1986; **2**: 1366–1367.

215. Holdcroft A, Gibberd FB, Hargrove RL, Hawkins DF, Dellaportas CI. Neurological complications associated with pregnancy. *Br J Anaesth* 1995; **75**: 522–526.

216. Hill EC. Maternal obstetric paralysis. *Am J Obstet Gynecol* 1962; **83**: 1452–1460.

217. Lazorthes G, Gouazé A, Bastide G, Soutoul JH, Zadeh O, Santini JJ. La vascularisation artérielle du renflement lombaire: études des variations et des suppléances. *Revue Neurologique* 1966; **114**: 109–122.

218. Bademosi O, Osuntokun BO, Van de Werd HJ, Bademosi AK, Ojo OA. Obstetric neuropraxia in the Nigerian African. *Int J Gynaecol Obstet* 1980; **17**: 611–614.

219. Bromage PR. Neurological complications of labor, delivery, and regional anesthesia. In: Chestnut DH (ed) *Obstetric anesthesia: principles and practice*. St Louis: Mosby Year Book 1994, pp 621–639.

220. Rigler M, Drasner K, Krejcie T, Yelich SJ, Scholnick FT, DeFontes J, Bohner D. Cauda equina syndrome after continuous spinal anesthesia. *Anesth Analg* 1991; **72**: 275–281.

221. Schneider M, Ettlin T, Kaufmann M, Schumacher P, Urwyler A, Hampl K, von Hochstetter A. Transient neurologic toxicity after hyperbaric subarachnoid anesthesia with 5% lidocaine. *Anesth Analg* 1993; **76**: 1154–1157.

222. Hampl KF, Schneider MC, Ummenhofer W, Drewe J. Transient neurologic symptoms following spinal anesthesia. *Anesth Analg* 1995; **81**: 1148–1153.

223. Tarkkila P, Huhtala J, Tuominen M. Transient radicular irritation after spinal anaesthesia with hyperbaric 5% lignocaine. *Br J Anaesth* 1995; **74**: 328–329.

224. Pollock JE, Neal JM, Stephenson CA, Wiley CE. Prospective study of the incidence of transient radicular irritation in patients undergoing spinal anesthesia. *Anesthesiology* 1996; **84**: 1361–1367.

225. Hampl KF, Schneider MC, Thorin D, Ummenhofer W, Drewe J. Hyperosmolarity does not contribute to transient radicular irritation after spinal anesthesia with hyperbaric 5% lidocaine. *Region Anesth* 1995; **20**: 363–368.

226. Hampl KF, Schneider MC, Thorin D, Ummenhofer W, Kindler C. Comparison of low dose hyperbaric 0.5% bupivacaine with 5% hyperbaric lidocaine for short gynecological procedures. *Anesthesiology* 1994; **81**: A1032.

227. Hampl KF, Schneider MC, Pargger H, Drasner K, Gut J, Drewe J. A similar incidence of transient neurologic symptoms after spinal anesthesia with 2% and 5% lidocaine. *Anesth Analg* 1996; **83**: 1051–1054.

228. Crawford JS. Some maternal complications of epidural analgesia in labour. *Anaesthesia* 1985; **40**: 1219–1225.

229. Gambling GR, Yu P, Cole C, McMorland GH, Palmer L. A comparitive study of patient controlled epidural analgesia (PCEA) and continuous infusion epidural analgesia (CIEA) during labour. *Can J Anaesth* 1988; **35**: 249–254.

230. Eisenach JC. Patient controlled epidural analgesia. *Int J Obstet Anesth* 1995; **2**: 53–64.

231. Purdie J, Reid J, Thorburn J, Asbury AJ. Continuous extradural analgesia: comparison of midwife top-ups, continuous infusion and patient controlled administration. *Br J Anaesth* 1992; **68**: 580–584.

232. Gambling DR, McMorland GH, Yu P, Lazlo C. Comparison of patient controlled epidural analgesia and conventional 'top-up' injections during labour. *Anesth Analg* 1990; **70**: 256–261.

233. Paech MJ. Patient-controlled epidural analgesia in obstetrics. *Int J Obstet Anesth* 1996; **5**: 115–125.

234. Carrie LES. Extradural, spinal or combined block for obstetrical surgical anaesthesia. *Br J Anaesth* 1990; **765**: 225–233.

235. Rawal N, Schollin J, Wesstrom G. Epidural versus combined spinal epidural block for cesarean section. *Acta Anaesth Scand* 1988; **32**: 61–66.

236. Rawal N, Van Zundert A, Holmström B, Crowhurst JA. Combined spinal-epidural technique. *Region Anesth* 1997; **22**: 406–423.

237. Stacey RGW, Watt S, Kadim MY, Morgan BM. Single space combined spinal extradural technique for analgesia in labour. *Br J Anaesth* 1993; **71**: 499–502.

238. Morgan BM, Kadim MY. Mobile regional analgesia in labour. *Br J Obstet Gynaecol* 1994; **101**: 839–841.

239. Collis RE, Baxandall ML, Srikantharajah ID, Edge G, Kadim MY, Morgan BM. Combined spinal epidural (CSE) analgesia: technique, management, and outcome of 300 mothers. *Int J Obstet Anesth* 1994; **3**: 75–81.

240. Collis RE, Davies DWL, Aveling W. Randomized comparison of combined spinal-epidural and standard epidural analgesia in labour. *Lancet* 1995; **345**: 1413–1416.

241. Vercauteren M, Bettens K, Van Springel G, Schols G, Van Zundert J. Intrathecal labor analgesia: can we use the same mixture as is used epidurally? *Int J Obstet Anesth* 1997; **6**: 242–246.

242. Cohen SE, Cherry CH, Holbrook H, El Sayed YY, Gibson RN, Jaffe RA. Intrathecal sufentanil for labor analgesia-sensory changes, side effects and fetal heart rate changes. *Anesth Analg* 1993; **77**: 1155–1160.

243. Campbell DC, Camann WR, Datta S. The addition of bupivacaine to intrathecal sufentanil for labor analgesia. *Anesth Analg* 1995; **81**: 305–309.

244. Harding SA, Collis RE, Morgan BM. Meningitis after combined spinal-extradural anaesthesia in obstetrics. *Br J Anaesth* 1994; **73**: 545–547.

245. Hays RL, Palmer CM. Respiratory depression after intrathecal sufentanil during labor. *Anesthesiology* 1994; **81**: 511–512.

246. Hamilton CL, Cohen SE. High sensory block after intrathecal sufentanil for labor analgesia. *Anesthesiology* 1995; **83**: 1118–1122.

247. Buggy D, Hughes N, Gardiner J. Posterior column sensory impairment during ambulatory epidural analgesia in labour. *Br J Anaesth* 1994; **73**: 540–542.

248. Breen TW, Shapiro T, Glass B, Foster-Payne D, Oriol NE. Epidural anesthesia for labor in an ambulatory patient. *Anesth Analg* 1993; **77**: 919–924.

249. Elton CD, Ali P, Mushambi MC. 'Walking extradurals' in labour: a step forward? *Br J Anaesth* 1997; **79**: 551–554.

250. Loughman BA, Fenelly ME, Henley M, Hall GM. The effects of differing concentrations of bupivacaine on the epidural somatosensory evoked potential after posterior tibial nerve stimulation. *Anesth Analg* 1995; **81**: 147–151.

251. Nashner LM. Computerized dynamic posturography: clinical applications. In: Jacobson GP, Newman CW, Kartush JM (eds) *Handbook of balance function testing*. Chicago: Mosby Year Book 1993, pp 308–334.

252. Bell R, Parry MG, Fernando R, Hallworth S, Jethwa N, Harling B, Sherrratt RM. Assessment of dorsal column function using somatosensory evoked potentials (SEPs) after ambulatory combined spinal epidural analgesia (CSE) for labour. *Int J Obstet Anesth* 1997; **6**: 199–200.

253. Parry MG, Fernando R, Bawa GPS, Poulton BB. Dorsal column function after epidural and spinal blockade: implications for the safety of walking following low dose regional analgesia for labour. *Anaesthesia* 1998; **53**: 382–403.

254. Pickering AE, Parry MG, Ousta B, Fernando R. Effect of combined spinal-epidural ambulatory labor analgesia on balance. *Anesthesiology* 1999; **91**: 436–441.

7

AMBULATORY ANALGESIA IN LABOUR

Felicity Plaat

INTRODUCTION

A woman who lies in bed, with a dense motor and sensory block from T10 to S5, unable to move her legs, and therefore physically unaware of her labour, has not received analgesia. She is anaesthetized. Such a clinical scenario has become less common over the past decade, as the dose of local anaesthetic used to produce labour analgesia has gradually been reduced. Pain-relief can now be achieved with preservation of sensation and minimal or absent motor blockade. The possibility of labouring whilst mobilizing out of bed with regional analgesia has become a reality.

THE SIGNIFICANCE OF MOTOR BLOCK

Motor block is an unwanted side effect, which is disliked by women.[1] In a survey of women's experiences of childbirth, 40% of women felt that motor block was unhelpful and 10% felt it contributed to their inability to relax. Women and their partners believed that being able to move might have shortened the labour.[2]

Motor block results in the need for more intensive nursing care and can thus 'medicalize' the experience of labour. Mothers with severe motor block have to be turned and moved and this can potentially increase physical injury amongst staff.

Post-partum backache does not appear to be caused by epidural analgesia in labour,[3] but many pregnant women have backache that is exacerbated by immobility. It is possible that frequent changes in position, which is possible with low-dose epidurals, may reduce this type of back strain.

AMBULATION

'NATURAL' ACTIVITY IN LABOUR

What do women in labour do? If we could answer this question, the effect of position, mobility and ambulation on the process of labour, the mother and the fetus might be easier to understand.

There is little data concerning the kind of activity associated with 'normal' labour. Women in the latent phase and early labour are often seen walking up and down the corridor, pausing to lean against the wall or their companions when a contraction occurs.

When active labour begins the majority of women, at least in Western Europe and the USA, retire to bed:

- But is this 'natural behaviour'?
- What is most advantageous behaviour?

Such behaviour patterns almost certainly reflect what the woman's carers believe to be the right thing to do; women may have been told to 'go for a walk until labour gets going/to get things going'. When things do get going many women are obliged to return to bed because monitoring, examinations and analgesia all require it. Anthropological data shows that such behaviour is not universal.

Amongst western obstetricians there has been debate about the correct position for labour for over a century. Mauriceau introduced the horizontal position, for women in the first stage of labour in the 18th century, to facilitate the obstetrician's activities.[4]

It was not however long before the wisdom of this was challenged. In 1903 the obstetrician J Williams wrote 'During the first stage of labour the patient usually prefers to move about her room, and is frequently more comfortable when occupying the sitting position. During this period, therefore, she should not be compelled to take to her bed unless so inclined'.[5]

In 1976 Peter Dunn, a paediatrician made a plea to obstetricians to 'regain confidence in the normality of the great majority of women and leave them in the care of midwives and husbands'. He identified the posture (recumbent/semi-recumbent) women are obliged to adopt during labour as the main reason why 'in the wake of "civilization" labour has always appeared to become more protracted and more painful.'

He argues that, based on the study of the anthropology of childbirth, women left to their own devices are driven by pain rather than instinct, to adopt different positions during labour, which are not just the least uncomfortable, but are also those which will most enhance the progress of labour. Recumbency is not usually one of the positions that the mother naturally adopts, and the ability to change position and to remain mobile is essential to enhance labour. Complete analgesia produced by neuraxial blockade is detrimental, because the woman no longer has the pain to drive them to adopt these optimal positions.[6]

A large, well designed study by Bloom and colleagues for the first time attempted to quantify ambulation, using a pedometer. The study group, who were instructed to 'walk as desired in the first stage of labour', spent a mean time of 56 ± 46 min ambulating with the number of recorded steps taken 553 ± 801. The authors found that there appeared to be no effect of walking on labour or delivery but it was not harmful to mother or baby.[7] In this study the effect of ambulating in the absence of pain was not investigated as women in the study group were instructed to return to bed when intravenous or epidural analgesia was required.

THE EFFECT OF AMBULATION ON THE OUTCOME OF LABOUR WITHOUT REGIONAL ANALGESIA

In a systematic review of studies found on the Cochrane pregnancy and childbirth database, a total of 26 randomized controlled trials were reviewed to assess the upright versus recumbent position in the first or second stages of labour.[8] None of these studies include women using regional analgesia and all were performed before the introduction of low-dose epidural regimes.

The effects of ambulation *per se* could not be analysed: in the studies in which it was mentioned, ambulation was not differentiated from other forms of non-recumbency. The 'upright' position included ambulation, sitting in chairs and being propped up in bed. Recumbency involved lying in bed either in the lateral position or supine.

The methodology of the majority of these trials was considered poor (see Table 7.1). A problem encountered in the majority of trials was that a varying proportion of women in the upright groups did not remain allocation compliant.

The reviewers concluded that in the first stage of labour, being upright was associated with less pain and reduced analgesic requirements. The need for labour augmentation, (either artificial rupture of membranes or syntocinon), was also less. Position in the first stage of labour did not appear to influence neonatal well-being. Only one trial reported a significantly lower rate of fetal heart rate abnormalities in the study group.[9] Maternal well-being and mode of delivery did not appear to be influenced by posture in the first stage.

Of the 16 trial looking at posture in the second stage of labour, eight used the birthing chair for the upright group, a device now rarely used due to its association with increased perineal trauma and blood loss. The remaining eight trials suggested that the upright position might be advantageous in this stage of labour: there was less pain and increased ease of 'bearing down', which was associated with fewer assisted deliveries and less perineal or vulval trauma. The only improvement in neonatal outcome was suggested by a higher proportion of 1 min Apgar scores of greater than 7.

In the majority of studies there was enthusiastic acceptance of the upright position. Patients felt that they were contributing something to their labour, it relieved the boredom of lying strapped to a monitor and they felt it was more 'normal'.[10]

The studies included nulliparae and/or multiparae and because management protocols for labour were so different between studies the value of meta-analysis is questionable.

Unlike other workers, Flynn's group found that not only did ambulation decrease the need for analgesia, but also significantly reduced the duration of labour.[9] This is the only study where radiotelemetry enabled continuous fetal monitoring in both groups. Those in the ambulant group were given free choice as to where they went; they could go to the TV room, to the ward kitchen, etc. This is in contrast to the majority of other studies where 'ambulation was much more limited'.[11] For example, Mendez-Bauer required women to alternate between the standing and supine positions at 30 min intervals thus serving as their own controls.[12] In Flynn's study ambulation was only allowed in the first stage of labour and 'intravenous therapy' was an indication to return to bed – no women in this group had regional analgesia, although women who received pethidine were allowed to continue to ambulate. In the study group, women spent 50% of the duration of the first stage ambulating – a much greater proportion of time than in similar studies. It may be that ambulation as opposed to the upright position, for a large proportion of labour, does have beneficial effects. In order to encourage this level of activity the fetus needs continuous telemetry monitoring if indicated and women need to be given the freedom to do something

Table 7.1   Methodology of studies of upright versus recumbent positions for labour

	First stage studies $n = 10$	Second stage studies $n = 16$
Randomization with sealed envelopes	2	8
Principal outcome defined	0	5
Power calculation	0	4
Exclusions after randomization	3	7
Blinded assessment	2	1

interesting with their ability to mobilize. Alternatively it has been suggested that an easy labour encourages mobility rather than mobility enhancing the progress of labour.[13]

THE EFFECT OF AMBULATION ON THE OUTCOME OF LABOUR WITH REGIONAL ANALGESIA

Nageotte randomly assigned nulliparae to continuous epidural analgesia, combined spinal–epidural (CSE) analgesia or CSE analgesia with ambulation. They found that the 'absence of ambulation' was a risk factor for Caesarean section for dystocia. However ambulation was defined as little as 5 min walking per hour.[14] Olofsson found that compared with bupivacaine 0.25% with epinephrine, a lower dose of bupivacaine with sufentanil resulted in significantly fewer assisted deliveries and shorter labours amongst multiparae. Twice as many women in the low-dose group ambulated during labour (30%) but an equal number in both groups remained in bed for delivery. Ambulation was not associated with more spontaneous deliveries.[15] Collis and colleagues found no differences in duration or outcome of labour, analgesia requirements or neonatal well-being between women with CSE analgesia encouraged to ambulate for 20 min/h during the first stage of labour and those who remained in bed.[16] In common with others, Collis found that women viewed ambulating positively: 99% of women asked in the Bloom study stated they would prefer to ambulate in subsequent labours.

Little work has been done on the effect of ambulation in the second stage of labour. A small study suggested a trend towards more spontaneous vaginal deliveries in mothers who stand in the second stage of labour.[17] An audit of mode of delivery over a period when mobile neuraxial analgesia was introduced showed that whereas the 'epidural' rate increased substantially, this was not associated with an increase in obstetric intervention.[18] A similar impact study in another centre found similar results when low-dose epidural analgesia was introduced.[19]

Women with and without regional analgesia appear to appreciate being able to ambulate but it is still unclear whether doing so influences the process or outcome of labour. Arguably the greatest benefit of ambulation in labour is that prolonged periods of recumbency are avoided. Not only does this seem prudent amongst patients known to be at increased risk of thromboembolic complications but also the effects of supine hypotension on the mother and fetus due to aortocaval compression are minimized, as only

the extremes of lateral tilt in the recumbent position will abolish this.[20] A mother frequently adopts the semi-recumbent position whether she has an epidural or not. She is slumped on two or three pillows with her legs straight out in front of her and in effect is almost lying on her back. The standing position has been found to be associated with improvements in fetal heart rate patterns and a better maintenance of maternal blood pressure.[21]

COMPLIANCE – DO WOMEN WISH TO AMBULATE?

In all the above studies there was a significant degree of non-compliance: 22% of Bloom's study group failed to ambulate at all and only 66% of women achieved the 5 min/h required by Nageotte. Although 86% of Collis' study group got out of bed only 46% achieved the goal of ambulation for one third of the time. This group found that fatigue was the most commonly sited reason for non-compliance. In an earlier study, McManus found that multigravid parturients were much more keen 'to be up and about' than primagravidae: the latter had labours which, on average, were twice as long and presumably the mothers were more tired in consequence.[22] Bloom on the other hand found that non-compliers had significantly shorter labours than those who walked. As these women had no analgesia, pain during a faster first stage may have precluded ambulation: indeed the idea of women ambulating and in pain, was seen as distasteful by one reviewer.[23]

Nageotte found no differences between women who walked and those who did not, but suggested that the 'Labour Management Team' might have a critical role in defining response to pain and levels of activity. Collis found that nearly 20% of non-compliers had been told not to ambulate by their attending midwife.[16] In our institution we found that when 'mobile epidurals' were first introduced, few mothers mobilized and were frequently advised not to: after this initial period, more than 80% of women leave their beds at some time and this is seen as beneficial by obstetric and midwifery staff. Another group found that the incidence of Caesarean section was lower amongst women with ambulatory CSE analgesia compared with conventional epidural analgesia. All the patients in the first group were reported to ambulate at some time during labour compared with none in the second, but the amount or timing of the ambulation was not specified.[24] A common finding of these studies was that women appreciated the ability to choose and change position during labour even if they do not want to walk.

AMBULATORY NEURAXIAL ANALGESIA – CHARACTERISTICS

Effective analgesia without loss of all sensation

This is achieved through a combination of local anaesthetic (bupivacaine, levobupivacaine or ropivacaine) and an opioid (fentanyl or sufentanil). The drugs may be administered epidurally or as part of a CSE.

A barely perceptible, sensory block

When the initial dose is intrathecal, a demonstrable diminution in touch and temperature sensation may or may not be present: if present it does not necessarily correlate with analgesic efficacy. Proprioceptive block is minimal at all joints with either a low-dose epidural or the CSE technique,[25] allowing more than 95% women to ambulate normally,[26] as long as a traditional test-dose is not used.[27]

Minimal sympathetic block

Intrathecal or epidural low-dose bupivacaine with an opioid, or epidural opioids alone, will usually produce minimal sympathetic blockade. After an initial intra-thecal dose of bupivacaine 2.5 mg with fentanyl 25 μg, although rapid analgesia is usually obtained, there may be no change in foot temperature.

There is however an incidence of hypotension, especially after the initial dose. Shennan found that there was a 12% incidence of significant maternal hypotension within 30 min of the initial spinal injection after low-dose CSE analgesia, but this did not recur after subsequent top-ups.[28] When compared with 25 mg epidural bupivacaine Collis, showed this intrathecal dose was associated with a trend towards more maternal hypotension in the subsequent 20 min.[29] Other workers have found no difference.[30] Hypotension is not a problem even when low-dose top-ups are given in the upright position, once analgesia has been established.[21,28]

Absent motor block

Motor blockade may be avoided either through the use of the CSE technique or by using a low-dose epidural. If the former technique is used there will be a period of approximately 30–45 min following the initial dose when motor block will be present in about 10% of women, precluding ambulation.[26] After this initial period, more than 90% of women demonstrate no deficit and are able to ambulate[31] and 80% retain this ability throughout the first stage.[16,29] Work by

Price et al suggests that this period of motor blockade is less profound when the initial (low) dose is given epidurally.[32] However in advanced labour, 17% of women required an additional top-up within half an hour of the initial low epidural dose,[33] opposed to fewer than 5% following CSE, to achieve effective pain-relief.[31] The effect of this increased local anaesthetic usage initially may affect the ability to maintain mobility at a later point during the labour.

Although the ability to ambulate is not affected, it is interesting to note that the pelvic floor is blocked early and profoundly by low-dose CSE,[30] this is in contrast with epidural analgesia where there is gradual, slow onset of sacral blockade.[34]

AMBULATORY NEURAXIAL ANALGESIA – UNDERLYING PRINCIPLES

The means of achieving regional analgesia without dense sensory and motor block is to reduce the amount of local anaesthetic required to achieve and maintain analgesia:

- Avoid a conventional epidural test-dose.
- Injecting the initial dose intrathecally (i.e. using a CSE technique).
- Using a combination of local anaesthetic and opioid.
- Maintaining analgesia using intermittent top-ups and not continuous infusions.

AVOID A CONVENTIONAL TEST-DOSE

There is no reason why the initial 'test-dose' should be separate from the first 'analgesic dose': the low-dose top-ups now commonly used (10 mg bupivacaine diluted to 10 ml), should not endanger the patient if the catheter has migrated. Gieraerts et al gave 12.5 mg bupivacaine (10 ml 0.125% solution), with epinephrine intravenously[35] and Van Zundert et al gave the same solution intrathecally[36] to simulate a positive test-dose. This dose was found to give a high degree of sensitivity and specificity and to be safe. Accidental intravascular injection of 10 or 12.5 mg of bupivacaine intravascularly would produce no analgesic effect. This approach will minimize the initial total dose and therefore reduce motor block, compared to giving a conventional test-dose of 3 ml bupivacaine 0.5% followed by a low-dose top-up to achieve analgesia.[27]

It is known that epidural catheters can migrate and it has been estimated that approximately one third of unexpectedly high blocks are preceded by 'negative' test-doses.[37] There is therefore a strong case to suggest that when low-dose epidural analgesia is used, (either as part of the CSE technique or alone), each and every 'top-up' should be regarded as a test-dose and the use of the conventional test should be abandoned as unnecessary.

COMBINED SPINAL EPIDURAL

Concerns of the technique

Headache

There is an increased risk of headache amongst labouring women who undergo deliberate dural puncture with an incidence of 0–2.5%.[29,31,38] In comparison the risk of PDPH after spinal injection varies between 1% and 40%.[39] Interestingly Norris et al found that women receiving epidural analgesia were significantly more likely to have unintended dural puncture than those with CSE.[38]

Meningitis

Infection is theoretically one of the greatest risks of breaching the dura during labour and subsequently siting an epidural catheter near the site of puncture. The majority of reports of meningitis following CSE involved multiple needling of the back[40,41] and there are few details of the aseptic precautions taken. At present, data is lacking to support an increased risk of this complication after CSE, but strict asepsis must be maintained and the practice of 'at the bedside' mixing of drug solutions for neuraxial blockade has been condemned.[42]

Neurological trauma

There is no evidence that the risk of neurological damage is increased compared to simple spinal insertion for other procedures, although the occurrence of dysasthesia should be an absolute contraindication to continuing the procedure. The level of the intrathecal injection must always be below the termination of the spinal cord.

Positive aspects of the CSE

Despite these concerns, a survey of more than 4000 CSE blocks for labour analgesia found a decreased failure rate with no increase in complications, compared with epidural or single shot spinal techniques.[43] There is evidence to suggest that after an initial intrathecal dose, the subsequent analgesia throughout labour is more reliable and requires less anaesthetic input than after an epidural first dose.[44]

The intrathecal route is particularly appropriate if an opioid is used, as the drug is deposited close to its site of action. Analgesia produced by the intrathecal route compared with the epidural one is more efficacious, more reliable and longer lasting.[45] The most commonly used opioids are fentanyl[46] and sufentanil.[47] However intrathecal sufentanil has been associated with hypotension, sedation, respiratory depression and adverse fetal heart rate changes. All intrathecal opioids cause pruritus in a large proportion of cases and opioids alone do not provide adequate analgesia for the second stage of labour.

By using the intrathecal route with an opioid/local anaesthetic combination rather than the epidural route, even those mothers in extreme pain/in advanced labour can achieve rapid relief with doses of bupivacaine of 2.5 mg or less, with minimal motor block after 20–30 min. In contrast 25 mg of bupivacaine, given epidurally will result in 30% of women developing significant motor block.[29] If 25 mg of bupivacaine is given without an opiate, only 50% of mothers will have satisfactory pain-relief in advanced labour[48] with distressing rectal pressure, the most common complaint.

DRUG COMBINATIONS

Opioids

The synergism between local anaesthetics and opioids is well described.[49] In clinical practice the addition of opioids significantly reduces local anaesthetic required to produce labour analgesia.[50–52] A lower local anaesthetic use results in less motor block.[16] The local anaesthetic effect of pethidine makes it less than ideal in the context of mobile analgesia, as hypotension and sedation have been found to be a problem with its use.[46]

Other drug combinations

Epinephrine has been added to local anaesthetic–opioid mixtures. Whilst it appears to enhance analgesia,[53] it also increases the intensity of motor block.[54]

Clonidine: The alpha-2 adrenergic receptor agonist has been used to produce analgesia without motor block or the side effects of the opioids. It has been combined with low-dose bupivacaine and sufentanil and the duration of analgesia was found to be prolonged, but it was associated with a fall in mean arterial pressure.[55] Another undesirable side effect of clonidine, particularly in relation to ambulation, is one of sedation.[56]

INTERMITTENT TOP-UPS

Continuous epidural infusions, although popular, have been consistently shown to result in higher bupivacaine usage with less efficacious analgesia, (demonstrated by an increased requirement for physician interventions), and more motor block.[57–59] Collis et al found that increased bupivacaine usage was associated not only with more motor block after 6 h when a continuous infusion was used, but more women in this group reported problems with mobility (Table 7.2).[60]

Intermittent top-ups can be administered by midwives or by the parturient herself, (patient controlled epidural analgesia: PCEA). A comparison of these techniques found that when midwives administered top-ups, drug usage was significantly less and there was a trend towards less motor block as labour progressed.[60] The equipment used for PCEA may malfunction, is expensive[32] and the equipment required for either continuous infusion or PCEA may in itself inhibit the mother's ability to ambulate. The use of PCEA may however reduce any delays in the midwives giving top-ups and being in control of her own analgesia may improve maternal satisfaction.

ASSESSMENT OF NEUROLOGICAL FUNCTION

SYMPATHETIC FUNCTION

Blood pressure monitoring in the recumbent and upright positions is mandatory. Accurate oscillometric wrist monitors to measure blood pressure are now available. They are portable and have been shown to produce fewer posture-related errors, making them useful for monitoring during ambulatory analgesia.[61] With minimal sympathetic blockade, the need for intravenous fluids either during initiation of the block or continuing throughout labour may be unnecessary.[62]

PROPRIOCEPTIVE FUNCTION

A routine test of proprioception such as Romberg's sign has been recommended.[63] Some authors believe however that as long as vision and the vestibular apparatus are intact, proprioception is not essential for ambulation,[64] but ascertaining that the women subjectively feels able to walk is essential.[26,62]

MOTOR POWER

There are two fundamental problems when attempting to assess motor function:

- The tests in widespread use were designed to test the effect of local anaesthetics administered epidurally not intrathecally. Differences in the concentration of drugs to which the neural tissues are exposed and differences in the anatomy within these compartments result in different patterns of motor blockade. It may not matter that an assessment used in the context of *epidural* blockade omits the test of L5/S1 function, because the motor component of these nerve roots are usually spared.[34] This is because the concentration of local anaesthetic in the cerebrospinal fluid (CSF) that can be achieved with epidural injection is not high enough to allow penetration to the core (motor) fibres of these – the largest of the nerve roots (the phenomenon of 'S1 escape').[65] If the intrathecal route is used these fibres will be more vulnerable.
- These tests were not designed to measure the motor function required for ambulation. In order to ambulate the minimal requirements in terms of motor function are intact movements of the lower limb (Fig. 7.1). To maintain an upright posture the function of the musculature of the anterior abdominal wall must be intact (rectus abdominis; T5–T12, internal and external obliques; T12 and transversalis; T7–T12) and the muscles of the back must be functioning (C2–S1).

Table 7.2 Local anaesthetic usage, motor block and mobility: a comparison of midwife top-ups (MW) and continuous infusions (CI)			
	MW	CI	p
Bupivacaine usage mg/h (mean (SD))	7.59 (3.13)	11.5 (3.25)	<0.001
Percentage of women with motor block at 6 h	16.7	53.4	0.015
Percentage of women retrospectively reporting problems with mobility	55	79.9	0.05
From Collis 1999.			

Movement	Muscles	Spinal innervation									
		L1	L2	L3	L4	L5	S1	S2	S3	S4	S5
Hip flexion	Psoas major, Iliacus, Rectus femoris, Pectineus, Sartorius		▓	▓	▓						
Hip extension	Gluteus maximus, Hamstrings				▓	▓	▓	▓			
Adduction	Pectineus, Adductors, Gracilis		▓	▓	▓		▓	▓			
Abduction	Gluteus medius and minimus, Piriformis				▓	▓	▓	▓			
Lateral rotation	Gluteus maximus, Medius, Minimus					▓	▓	▓			
Medial rotation	Iliopsoas, Pectineus, Adductus longus	▓	▓	▓							
Knee flexion	Hamstrings, Gracilis, Sartorius, Popliteus		▓	▓			▓				
Knee extension	Quadriceps femoris		▓	▓	▓						
Ankle dorsi-flexion	Tibialis anterior				▓	▓	▓				
Ankle plantar-flexion	Gastrocnemius, Soleus						▓	▓			

Figure 7.1 Movements of the lower limb.

The Bromage scale

This is the most widely used test of motor function in obstetric anaesthesia.[66] This scale was designed to test motor function in the lower limbs 30–40 min after administration of epidural lidocaine or prilocaine. Movements are graded on a four-point scale (Fig. 7.2). A score of IV denotes no blockade and requires full flexion of the knees and feet. However because the assessment is made with the subject sitting in bed, as Russell has pointed out, knee flexion will passively follow hip flexion in this position.[67] Thus Bromage grade IV does not test active knee flexion and therefore can still allow significant motor weakness. The illustration in Bromage's article appears to show ankle dorsi-flexion but not plantar-flexion. Dorsi-flexion is a function of L5 root and plantar-flexion the S1 root. Thus no movements involving S1 (hip extension, abduction lateral rotation and plantar-flexion), are tested in this classic description, although loss of power involving both these movements occur at a similar rate. Whilst the motor component of S1 is rarely blocked by epidural administration of low dose local anaesthetics it may be when the intrathecal route is used.

Breen's modification

Breen and colleagues modified the scale in the context of ambulation by adding two categories: The first was

Intensity of motor block
(with sensory block to S5)

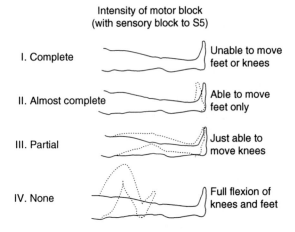

I. Complete — Unable to move feet or knees

II. Almost complete — Able to move feet only

III. Partial — Just able to move knees

IV. None — Full flexion of knees and feet

Figure 7.2 Bromage scale for assessment of motor blockade (from *Acta Anaesthesiologica Scandinavica*, 1965; Supplement XVI. Reproduced with permission from Munksgaard International Publishers Ltd, Copenhagen, Denmark).

'no detectable weakness of hip flexion with full flexion of the knees'; 17% of women with no block using the unmodified scale, (grade IV), demonstrated weakness in this new category, which precluded ambulation. A second category was added after one woman suffered a fall. This test requires the ability to flex the knees whilst standing; three subjects were unable to perform this although they had no demonstrable weakness of hip flexion.[68] In the sitting position hip flexion is advanced through the action of quadriceps (L2–L4) whereas flexion of this joint when the pelvis and trunk are unsupported (i.e. standing), requires iliopsoas (L1–L2). A partial knee bend also requires dorsi-flexion of the ankle (L4–L5) during bending and plantar-flexion (S1–S2) during straightening. Thus this movement tests all the nerve roots from L1 to S2.

Rectus abdominis muscle test

Van Zundert and colleagues using the rectus abdominis muscle test (RAM test) have assessed the musculature of the anterior abdominal wall. This test requires the subject to raise the trunk from fully supine with the legs extended to the sitting position with the spine flexed (in effect a 'sit-up').[69] Although this does undoubtedly test the anterior abdominal muscles it is a manoeuvre difficult to perform in an advanced state of pregnancy and requires the parturient to adopt a fully supine position initially, which is undesirable.

The straight leg raise test

The test of motor power popularized by Queen Charlotte's is the 'straight leg raise (SLR)' test.[31] The parturient sits in bed with the back supported and is required to raise each leg off the bed with the knee fully extended. This requires hip flexion (quadriceps and iliopsoas; L2–L4 and L1–L2), and knee extension (quadriceps L2–4), with contraction of the muscles of the anterior abdominal wall (T5–T12). Movements at the ankle joint are not tested.

The most comprehensive test in the context of ambulation would therefore be the combination of the SLR and deep knee bend. The woman must also feel confident in her ability to ambulate. Whilst ambulating, her midwife or partner should continuously accompany the mother, and a safe environment should be ensured (uneven flooring and stairs should be avoided and appropriate footwear worn). Although of great concern, falling during ambulatory analgesia has not been found to be a hazard.[16] It has been shown that women with ambulatory analgesia, who feel confident to walk, mobilize as safely as any pregnant woman.[70]

MATERNAL AND FETAL MONITORING

There is debate about the degree of monitoring required by the parturient with regional blockade in labour. In the context of normal labour and previously normal fetal heart rate patterns, it is no longer universally considered that this form of analgesia is an indication for continuous monitoring of the fetal heart. If there are obstetric indications for continuous monitoring, the appropriate form of monitoring which would allow ambulation is radiotelemetry, although this is costly and not widely available.

CONCLUSION

Ambulatory analgesia in labour is possible, and seems to be safe for mother and fetus, but analgesia without any motor block has not yet been achieved. Work to date does not suggest that the use of new local anaesthetics such as ropivacaine and levobupivacaine or alpha-2 agonists is the solution. Improvements may come not from new drugs but from new methods of drug delivery. The use of indwelling intrathecal catheters would allow a further reduction in the use of local anaesthetics; their safety is open to question and it is not known if the ability to ambulate would be enhanced. The use of epidural saline to extend the intrathecal block has allowed reduced doses of local anaesthetic to be used for Caesarean anaesthesia. This technique needs to be evaluated in the context of analgesia.

The benefits of pain free ambulation have still to be fully elucidated. The introduction of 'mobile epidurals' may increase demand for regional analgesia in labour, to the extent that difficulties with anaesthetic manpower have been anticipated.[62] This may be because ambulatory regional analgesia is associated with greater maternal satisfaction than non-mobile techniques, even if the mother chooses to stay in bed. Since straightforward pain-relief in labour has little purpose other than patient satisfaction, it is irrational to dismiss this form of analgesia on the grounds of difficulty or expense. There has been a significant change in practice for the provision of regional analgesia in labour[71,72] and in our consumer led society it is likely that ambulatory labour analgesia is here to stay.

PRACTICAL GUIDELINES FOR PROVISION OF AMBULATORY LABOUR ANALGESIA

These are based on those used at Queen Charlotte's hospital in London where CSEs are routinely used for analgesia in labour.

ANTENATAL EDUCATION

Women need to be informed about the potential for this type of regional analgesia and its limitations.

Having an anaesthetist to run these classes has the advantage of providing women with the opportunity to discuss in depth specific concerns. All women should be given written information in this period.

EDUCATION OF OBSTETRICIANS AND MIDWIVES

Care of parturients with low-dose regional analgesia is fundamentally different from that of women with high-dose regional analgesia. The use of low-doses means that particular vigilance is required to prevent breakthrough pain. Analgesia may suddenly become inadequate during the second stage of labour, and this may inhibit rather than enhance pushing. If instrumental vaginal delivery is necessary the anaesthetist must assess the block even if it appears satisfactory, as the low-dose top-ups may be inadequate for surgical delivery.

Midwives must be taught how to test for motor blockade and understand when mobility should or should not be allowed.

PROCEDURE

- Prior to regional blockade the mother is encouraged to empty her bladder and maternal blood pressure and the fetal heart rate monitored.
- Intravenous access is established but a routine fluid pre-load may not be required.
- Because of the vulnerability of the intrathecal space to infection, full aseptic precautions must be undertaken when a CSE is performed. The anaesthetist wears cap, mask, gown and gloves. In our unit, the anaesthetist's assistant also wears a cap and mask and if the block is performed with the mother sitting, she also wears a cap.
- Spirit based skin preparation is sprayed on the back by the anaesthetist's assistant.

THE INITIAL DOSE

The needle through needle combined spinal-epidural technique

This should be performed at the L3/4 interspace or below.

After location of the epidural space with a 16G Tuohy needle, a 119 mm long 27G Whitacre needle is inserted through the Tuohy needle into the intrathecal compartment. The characteristic 'click' as the dura is punctured should be sought. Gentle aspiration may be necessary to identify CSF especially if the lateral position is used.

When CSF is observed at the hub of the Whitacre needle, 1 ml 0.25% bupivacaine (2.5 mg) + 25 μg fentanyl are injected. Lower doses of either local anaesthetic or opioid may be used. The spinal needle is then removed and the epidural catheter inserted 3–4 cm into the epidural space. If dural puncture is unsuccessful no further attempt to puncture the dura is made unless urgent delivery is required. The woman should be warned of the increased risk of postural headache if there is the possibility of more than one hole made in the dura.

Epidural initial dose

If an initial epidural dose is used, the starting dose is 10–15 mg bupivacaine with 50 μg fentanyl made up to 15 ml with normal saline.

An alternative to this bedside mixing is to use a pre-made solution containing 0.1% bupivacaine and fentanyl 2 μg/ml; 2.5–4 ml of this mixture may be used for the initial intrathecal dose. When the epidural route is used 10 ml of this solution can be given every 10–15 min until the mother is satisfied with her analgesia.[73] Using a pre-made solution may decrease error associated with drug mixing. In order to maintain sterility for intrathecal injection the solution must be taken from an ampoule that can be snapped open or squirted from a syringe, not from a bag or other container, which requires a membrane to be pierced.

MONITORING

Following the initial dose, the mother will sit up in bed or lie in the full lateral position and maternal blood pressure and pulse monitored at 5 min intervals for 30 min. During this period there is continuous CTG monitoring. At the end of this period if analgesia and monitored parameters are satisfactory, the intravenous infusion and infusion set may be disconnected. Further intravenous fluids are not required during subsequent top-ups unless clinically indicated. The ability to mobilize is first tested by the SLR test and then by a positive response to the question 'do you feel you could walk?' If analgesia is adequate, there is full motor power and no postural hypotension, the mother is encouraged to get out of bed and under close supervision perform a deep knee bend. If the mother has significant proprioceptive loss she will not want to walk. If intermittent fetal monitoring is appropriate the mother may leave her labour room. She is encouraged to attempt to empty her bladder (but warned not to strain) at two hourly intervals. She must be accompanied by her partner or midwife at all times.

If labour augmentation and/or continuous fetal monitoring are required, the mother may stand by the bed or sit in a rocking chair.

During the second stage of labour the woman is encouraged to adopt different positions. Maternal blood pressure and fetal heart rate should be monitored at least every 30 min and at 5 min intervals for 20 min after each epidural top-up.

TOP-UPS

The top-up solution is prepared by the hospital pharmacy to minimize 'at the bedside' mixing of drugs. The solution used is bupivacaine 0.1% + fentanyl 0.0002% (2 µg/ml). The midwife may give 10 ml of this mixture at half hourly intervals if required. Only qualified midwives who have undergone specified training may give top-ups. Prior to each top-up the midwife will test foot temperature to detect the development of a one-sided block. No separate test-dose is used but all top-ups are given slowly to detect catheter misplacement or migration. The woman is required to return to her labour room for top-ups, but she does not have to return to bed but should sit in a chair; 20–30 min after each top-up tests of motor power are repeated. The woman is advised to request a top-up before pain recurs. If the first dose was intrathecal she is warned that subsequent top-ups will have a slower onset of action.

Following delivery the ability to ambulate and absence of postural hypotension must be confirmed before the mother is allowed to get up.

REFERENCES

1. Murphy JD, Henderson K, Bowden MI, Lewis M, Cooper GM. Bupivacaine versus bupivacaine plus fentanyl for epidural analgesia: effect on maternal satisfaction. *Br Med J* 1991; **302**: 564–567.

2. Chamberlain G, Wraight A, Steer P (eds) *Pain and its relief in childbirth*. Edinburgh: Churchill Livingstone, 1993.

3. Russell R, Dundas R, Reynolds F. Long term backache after childbirth: prospective search for causative factors. *Br Med J* 1996; **312**: 1384–1388.

4. Liu YC. Position during labour and delivery: history and perspective. *J Nurs Midwifery* 1979; **24**: 23.

5. Williams JW. *Obstetrics: a text-book for the use of students and practitioners.* New York: D Appleton, 1903, p 282.

6. Dunn PM. Obstetric delivery today – for better or for worse? *Lancet* 1976; **10**: 790–793.

7. Bloom SL, McIntyre DD, Kelly MA et al. Lack of effect of walking on labor and delivery. *New Engl J Med* 1998; **339**: 76–79.

8. Nikodem VC. Upright vs recumbent position during first stage of labour. In: Enkin MW, Keirse MJNC, Renfrew MJ, Neilson JP (eds) *Pregnancy and childbirth module.* Cochrane database of systematic reviews, disk issue 2, 1995.

9. Flynn AM, Kelly J, Hollins G, Lynch PF. Ambulation in labour. *Br Med J* 1978; **2**: 591–593.

10. Williams RM, Thom MH, Studd JWW. A study of the benefits and acceptability of ambulation in spontaneous labour. *Br J Obstet Gynaecol* 1980; **87**: 122–126.

11. Mitre I. The influence of maternal position on duration of the active phase of labor. *Int J Obstet Gynaecol* 1974; **12**: 181–183.

12. Mendez-Bauer C, Arroyo C, Garcia-Ramos C et al. Effects of standing position on spontaneous uterine activity and other aspects of labor. *J Perinat Med* 1975; **3**: 89–100.

13. Stewart P, Calder AA. Posture in labour: patient's choice and its effect on performance. *Br J Obstet Gynaecol* 1984; **91**: 11.

14. Nageotte MP, Larson D, Rumney PJ, Sidhu M, Hollenbach K. Epidural analgesia compared with combined spinal–epidural analgesia during labour in nulliparous women. *New Engl J Med* 1997; **337**: 1715–1719.

15. Olofsson CH, Ekblom A, Ekman-Ordeberg G, Irestedt L. Obstetric outcome following epidural analgesia with bupivacaine–adrenaline 0.25% or bupivacaine 0.125% with sufentanil – a prospective randomized controlled study in 1000 parturients. *Acta Anaesthesiol Scand* 1998; **42**: 284–292.

16. Collis RE, Harding SA, Morgan BM. Effect of maternal ambulation on labour with low-dose combined spinal–epidural analgesia. *Anesthesia* 1999; **54**: 535–539.

17. Golara M, Plaat F, Shennan AH. Upright versus recumbent position in the second stage of labour in women with combined spinal-epidural analgesia. *Int J Obstet Anesth* 2002; **11**: 19–22.

18. Shennan A, Almulfti R. Introducing mobile combined spinal extradural analgesia: effect on extradural rates and obstetric outcome. *Br J Anaesth* 1996; **76**(S2): 102.

19. Norman B, Jenkins G. The effect on obstetric outcome of introducing low-dose epidurals for obstetric analgesia. *Int J Obstet Anesth* 1997; **6**: 211–212.

20. Kinsella SM, Whitwam JG, Spencer JAD. Reducing aortocaval compression: how much tilt is enough. *Br Med J* 1992; **305**: 539–540.

21. Al-mufti R, Morey R, Shennan A, Morgan BM. Blood pressure and fetal heart rate changes with patient-controlled combined spinal epidural analgesia while ambulating in labour. *Br J Obstet Gynaecol* 1997; **102**: 192–197.

22. McManus TJ, Calder AA. Upright posture and the efficiency of labour. *Lancet* 1978; **14**: 72–74.

23. Cefalo RC, Bowes WA. Never walk alone (editorial). *New Engl J Med* 1998; **339**: 117–118.

24. May AE, Elton CD. Ambulatory extradural analgesia in labour reduces the risk of Caesarean section. *Br J Anaesth* 1996; **77**: 692–693.

25. Parry MG, Fernando R, Bawa GPS, Poulton BB. Dorsal column function after epidural and spinal blockade: implications for the safety of walking following low-dose regional analgesia for labour. *Anaesthesia* 1998; **53**: 382–387.

26. Plaat F, Singh R, Alsoad SM, Crowhurst JA. Selective sensory blockade with low-dose combined spinal–epidural allows safe ambulation in labour: a pilot study. *Int J Obstet Anesth* 1996; **5**: 220.

27. Buggy D, Hughs N, Gardiner J. Posterior column sensory impairment during ambulatory extradural analgesia in labour. *Br J Anaesth* 1994; **73**: 540–542.

28. Shennan AH, Cook V, Lloyd-Jones F, Morgan BM, DeSwiet M. Blood pressure changes during labour with mobile combined spinal epidural analgesia whilst ambulating in labour. *Br J Obstet Gynaecol* 1995; **102**: 192–197.

29. Collis RE, Davies DWL, Aveling W. Randomised comparison of combined spinal epidural and standard epidural analgesia in labour. *Lancet* 1995; **345**: 1413–1416.

30. Mumtaz T, Shawe A, Crowhurst JA, Plaat F. Low-dose CSE analgesia for labour: influence of cephalad/caudad Whitacre needle orientation. *Int J Obstet Anesth* 1999; **8**: 215–216.

31. Collis RE, Baxandell ML, Srikantharajah ID, Edge G, Kadim MY, Morgan BM. Combined spinal–epidural (CSE) analgesia: technique, management, and outcome in 300 mothers. *Int J Obstet Anesth* 1994; **3**: 75–81.

32. Price C, Lafreniere L, Brosnan C, Findley I. Regional analgesia in early active labour: combined spinal epidural vs. epidural. *Anaesthesia* 1998; **53**: 951–955.

33. Plaat FS, Royston P, Morgan BM. Comparison of 15 mg and 25 mg of bupivacaine both with 50 µg fentanyl as initial dose for epidural analgesia. *Int J Obstet Anesth* 1996; **5**: 240–243.

34. Yarnell RW, Ewing DA, Tierney E, Smith Mh. Sacralization of epidural block with repeated doses of 0.25% bupivacaine during labour. *Reg Anaesth* **15**: 275–279.

35. Gieraerts R, Van Zundert A, De Wolf AM, Vaes L. Ten ml bupivacaine 0.125% with 12.5 µg epinephrine is a reliable epidural test dose to detect inadvertent intravascular injection in obstetric patients. A double-blind study. *Acta Anaesthesiol Scand* 1992; **36**: 656–659.

36. Van Zundert A, De Wolf AM, Vaes L, Soetens M. High volume spinal anesthesia with bupivacaine 0.125% for cesarean section. *Anesthesiology* 1988; **69**: 998–1003.

37. Morgan BM. Is an epidural test dose mandatory? *Eur J Obstet Gynaecol* 1995; **59**: 559–560.

38. Norris MC, Grieco WM, Borkowski M. Complications of labor analgesia: epidural versus combined spinal–epidural techniques. *Anesth Analg* 1995; **79**: 529–537.

39. Shnider SM, Levinson G. Anaesthesia for Caesarean section. In: Shnider SM, Levinson G (eds) *Anaesthesia for obstetrics.* Baltimore: Williams and Wilkins, 1987, pp 159–178.

40. Harding SA, Collis RE, Morgan BM. Meningitis after combined spinal–extradural anaesthesia in obstetrics. *Br J Anaesth* 1994; **73**: 545–547.

41. Stallard N, Barry P. Another complication of the combined extradural–subarachnoid technique *Br J Anaesth* 1995; **73**: 370–371.

42. Rawal N. *The combined spinal–epidural technique.* Mallorca Permanyer Publications, 1997.

43. Albright GA, Forster RM. The safety and efficacy of combined spinal and epidural analgesia/anesthesia (6002 blocks) in a community hospital. *Reg Anesth Pain Med* 1999; **24**(2): 117–125.

44. Bedson CR, Crowhurst JA, Plaat F. Audit of inadequate analgesia in labour. *European Society of Obstetric Anesthesia annual meeting,* Dublin 1999.

45. Camman WR, Denney RA, Holby ED, Datta S. A comparison of intrathecal, epidural, and intravenous sufentanil for labor analgesia. *Anesthesiology* 1992; **77**: 884–887.

46. Honet JE, Arkoosh VA, Norris MC, Huffnagle JH, Silverman NS, Leighton BL. Comparison among intrathecal fentanyl, meperidine and sufentanil for labour analgesia. *Anesth Analg* 1991; **75**: 734–739.

47. Cohen SE, Cherry CM, Holbrook RH, El-Sayed YY, Gibson RN, Jaffe RA. Intrathecal sufentanil for labour analgesia: sensory changes, side effects and fetal heart rate changes. *Anesth Analg* 1993; **77**: 1155–1160.

48. Capogna G, Celleno D, Lyons G, Columb M, Fusco P. Minimum local analgesic concentration of extradural bupivacaine increases with progression of labour. *Br J Anaesth* 1998; **80**: 11–13.

49. Solomon RE, Gebhart GF. Synergistic antinociceptive interaction among drugs administered to the spinal cord. *Anesth Analg* 1994; **78**: 1164–1172.

50. Phillips GH. Combined epidural sufentanil and bupivacaine for labour analgesia. *Reg Analg* 1987; **121**: 165–168.

51. Phillips GH. Continuous infusion epidural analgesia in labor: effect of adding sufentanil to 0.125% bupivacaine. *Anaesthesia* 1988; **67**: 462–465.

52. Vertommen JD, Vandermeulen Aken AV et al. The effect of the addition of sufentanil to 0.1255 bupivacaine on the quality of analgesia during labour and the incidence of instrumental deliveries. *Anesthesiology* 1991; **74**: 809–814.

53. Eisenach JC, Grice SC, Dewan DM. Epinephrine enhances analgesia produced by epidural bupivacaine during labour. *Anesth Analg* 1987; **66**: 447–451.

54. Lysak SZ, Eisenach JC, Dobson II. Patient controlled epidural analgesia during labor: a comparison of three solutions with continuous epidural infusion (CEI) control. *Anesthesiology* 1988; **69**: A690.

55. Chassard D, Mathon L, Dailler F, Golfier F, Tournadre JP, Bouletreau P. Extradural clonidine combined with sufentanil and 0.0625% bupivacaine for analgesia in labour. *Br J Anaesth* 1996; **77**: 458–462.

56. Nishikawa T, Dohi S. Clinical evaluation of clonidine added to lidocaine solution for labor analgesia. *Anesthesiology* 1990; **73**: 853–859.

57. Bogod DG, Rosen M, Rees GAD. Extradural infusion of 0.125% bupivacaine at 10 ml/h to women during labour. *Br J Anaesth* 1987; **59**: 325–330.

58. Purdie J, Reid J, Thorburn J, Ashbury AJ. Continuous epidural analgesia; comparison of midwife top-ups, continuous infusions and patient controlled administration. *Br J Anaesth* 1992; **68**: 580–584.

59. Tan S, Reid J, Thorburn J. Extradural analgesia in labour: complications of three techniques of administration. *Br J Anaesth* 1994; **73**: 619–623.

60. Collis RE, Plaat F, Morgan BM. Comparison of midwife top-ups, continuous infusion and patient-controlled epidural analgesia for maintaining mobility after a low-dose combined spinal–epidural. *Br J Anaesth* 1999; **82**: 233–236.

61. Sudunagunta S, Shennan A, Plaat F. Evaluation of an oscillometric wrist blood pressure monitor for use in labour. *Int J Obstet Anesth* 1998; **7**: 198.

62. Morgan BM, Kadim MY. Mobile regional analgesia in labour. *Br J Obstet Gynaecol* 1994; **101**: 839–841.

63. Elton CD, Ali P, Mushambi MC. 'Walking extradurals' in labour: a step forward? *Br J Anaesth* 1997; **79**: 551–554.

64. Fernando R, Price CM. Letter. *Br J Anaesth* 1995; **74**: 349–350.

65. Galindo A, Hernanadez J, Benavides O, Ortegon DE, Munoz S, Bonica JJ. Quality of spinal extradural anaesthesia: the influence of spinal nerve root diameter. *Br J Anaesth* 1975; **47**: 41–47.

66. Bromage PR. A comparison of the hydrochloride and carbon dioxide salts of lidocaine and prilocaine in epidural analgesia. *Acta Anaesthesiol Scand* 1965; **16**(S): 55–69.

67. Russell R. Assessment of motor blockade during epidural analgesia in labour. *Int J Obstet Anesth* 1992; **1**: 230–234.

68. Breen TW, Shapiro T, Glass B, Foster-Payne D, Oriol NE. Epidural anesthesia for labor in an ambulatory patient. *Anesth Analg* 1993; **77**: 919–924.

69. Van Zundert A, Vaes L, Soetens M, De Vel M, Maesen F. Measuring motor block during lumbar epidural analgesia for vaginal delivery. *Obstet Anesth Dig* 1984; **4**: 31–34.

70. Fernando R. Opposer to the motion 'ambulation during regional analgesia for labour should be discouraged'. *Int J Obstet Anesth* 1998; **8**: 180–183.

71. Davies MW, Harrison JC, Ryan TD. Current practice of epidural analgesia during normal labour. A survey of maternity units in the United Kingdom. *Anaesthesia* 1993; **48**: 63–65.

72. Burnstein R, Buckland R, Pickett JA. A survey of epidural analgesia for labour in the United Kingdom. *Anaesthesia* 1999; **7**: 634–640.

73. Vercauteren M, Bettens K, Van Springel G, Schols G, Van Zundert J. Intrathecal labor analgesia: can we use the same mixture as is used epidurally? *Int J Obstet Anesth* 1997; **6**: 242–246.

8

ANAESTHESIA FOR CAESAREAN SECTION: GENERAL ANAESTHESIA

Rachel E. Collis

INTRODUCTION

It has been estimated that around 75% of Caesareans could be done using a regional technique.[1] A recent survey of anaesthetic techniques used for Caesarean section in the United Kingdom, found that general anaesthesia was indeed used for 25% of cases overall. The clinical rationale for the reduction in general anaesthetic rates is compelling, considering the number of deaths directly related to general anaesthesia and the problems of airway management and aspiration. Although it is widely believed that general anaesthesia is more dangerous than regional, deaths associated with general anaesthesia have usually been ascribed to substandard care, and have therefore been considered avoidable. A well-conducted general anaesthetic is safe for both mother and baby, and may be the better option in some circumstances. General anaesthesia over the past four decades has evolved into a safe option, as long as maternal and fetal physiology is understood and recommendations for the safe practice of general anaesthesia are followed.

HISTORY

The introduction in the early 1950s of 'balanced anaesthesia' for Caesarean section completely changed anaesthetic practice. Up until then, anaesthesia for elective and emergency Caesarean sections had been performed using an open breathing system with gauze and cyclopropane, ether or chloroform. Such techniques resulted in at least 100 deaths per year in the United States. The incidence of vomiting at Caesarean section was as high as 6.3% with an open breathing system and a spontaneously breathing patient.[2] Mendelson in his classic paper of 1946 suggested that aspiration was common, although not necessarily lethal, and regurgitation of particulate material could lead to asphyxia and death. He concluded that it was dangerous to allow ingestion of food 6–12 h prior to delivery and recommended that feeding, even in early labour, should be restricted.[3]

By the mid-1950s the use of tubocurarine to facilitate intubation became common practice. Use of muscle relaxants was initially restricted by the fear that they would paralyse the baby. Suxamethonium became popular after its introduction because of the dangers associated with the delay in intubating the trachea when tubocurarine was used alone. A thiopentone–suxamethonium induction became an accepted technique in 1959. It is interesting to note that it is the rapid onset of action, rather than the short duration of action that made suxamethonium the drug of choice at this time. In the report on maternal mortality of 1964–1966 however, the number of anaesthetic related deaths doubled, as a result of difficulties during intubation in the apnoeic mother. Lessons learned from these early days lead to the practice of pre-oxygenation, the use of cricoid pressure and the use of a logical failed intubation drill. The result has been a decline in the number of deaths associated with general anaesthesia.

Mendelson in his seminal paper came to several conclusions that are interesting not least because, despite the passage of time and changes in many aspects of anaesthetic practice, many of his recommendations are still followed. He suggested that

- aspiration of stomach contents into the lungs is preventable;
- withholding oral feeds during labour and substituting with parental administration is necessary;
- emptying the stomach and alkinalization of the contents must be performed prior to general anaesthesia;
- competent administration of general anaesthesia, with full appreciation of the dangers of aspiration, especially at induction and recovery is mandatory;
- there should be adequately equipped delivery rooms containing tables which could be tilted, with transparent anaesthetic masks, suction, laryngoscopes and bronchoscopes available;
- local anaesthesia should be used whenever possible (at this time it was common practice to give a general anaesthetic for an instrumental vaginal delivery).

As a result of improved training in regional techniques and better communication with obstetric staff, regional anaesthesia is now used in 75% of emergency Caesareans. In some units the general anaesthetic rate for Caesarean section has been reduced to 3%.[4] There may now be less than one general anaesthetic performed per week, even in large delivery units, and it may well be outside daytime hours. This has given rise to concerns about reduced training opportunities in general anaesthesia for Caesarean section for anaesthetists, anaesthetic assistants and midwifery staff. The obstetric anaesthetist must know how to rapidly assess the pregnant woman prior to general anaesthesia and to understand the physiological changes of pregnancy that can make it more difficult and dangerous. Nowadays, urgent delivery is most often the indication for general anaesthesia, and the anaesthetist may have little time to make his pre-operative assessment. Although the teaching of principles is essential, anaesthesia depends very much on the acquisition of practical skills. In other words 'it is the sheer lack of skill that kills'.[5]

INDICATIONS FOR GENERAL ANAESTHESIA

MATERNAL REQUEST

Maternal request remains a frequent indication for general anaesthesia. The reasons for wanting a general anaesthetic are varied and include anxiety about the possibility of hearing or seeing the operation, dislike of needles and fear of developing backache or becoming paralysed after the anaesthetic.[6] Good communication and explanation will allay most concerns but there will be some mothers who will not consider a regional technique. In the elective setting, if there are no contraindications to general anaesthesia (e.g. obesity or anticipation of a difficult airway), then general anaesthesia is a safe option.

OBSTETRIC INDICATIONS

Extreme urgency

Extreme urgency, (e.g. placental abruption, cord prolapse with fetal compromise), may make general anaesthesia the most appropriate technique to choose. General anaesthesia remains the most reliable technique for anaesthesia and, in most hands, the quickest. Administering a high concentration of oxygen to the mother may improve fetal oxygenation.[7] In cases of placental abruption a coagulopathy can develop rapidly with no time to measure and correct clotting abnormalities.

Low platelets

Low platelets are associated with pre-eclampsia, HELLP syndrome and other rare complications of pregnancy such as thrombotic thrombocytopenic purpura (TTP). A cut-off value below which a regional technique is contraindicated remains controversial, but a figure between 80 and 100×10^9/l is widely used.

Severe haemorrhage

Severe haemorrhage is an indication for general anaesthesia, especially if it is ongoing, as it can provide better cardiovascular stability than regional techniques, because sympathetic blockade is avoided. Hypovolaemia will amplify the hypotension associated with sympathetic blockade, making hypotension difficult to interpret.

Placenta previa

Placenta previa as an indication for general anaesthesia is hotly debated. In the elective setting many obstetric anaesthetists will consider a regional technique for a posterior placenta previa. Many choose a general anaesthetic for an anterior placenta previa, especially when there has been a previous Caesarean section, which increases the risk of placenta accreta.[8] Invasion of myometrium by an anterior, low lying placenta is estimated to occur in 65% of cases in which there are two previous scars. Haemorrhage can be torrential necessitating Caesarean hysterectomy. General anaesthesia may offer better haemodynamic stability and be more acceptable to the mother if surgery is prolonged.

MATERNAL INDICATIONS

Cardiac pathology

Cardiac pathology may be a contraindication to regional anaesthesia. In severe pulmonary or aortic out-flow obstruction, the sudden changes in after-load arising from sympathetic blockade may cause cardiovascular de-compensation. Likewise in cyanotic congenital heart disease, reduction in after-load will increase a right to left shunt thereby worsening central cyanosis.

Anatomical abnormalties

Anatomical abnormalties may make regional anaesthesia impossible, for example, severe kyphoscoliosis, (often with Harrington rod fixation), abnormal lumbar vertebra and spina bifida.

EQUIPMENT FOR CAESAREAN SECTION UNDER GENERAL ANAESTHESIA

The extreme haste with which general anaesthesia may have to be given makes regular checking of anaesthetic equipment, by a trained designated person, mandatory. Minimum monitoring equipment should include non-invasive blood pressure monitor with a 1 min repeat cycle, ECG, pulse oximetry, end tidal carbon dioxide analyser, ventilator disconnection alarm and an oxygen analyser.[9] General anaesthesia should be induced only where all this is available, and if an anaesthetic room is not so equipped, then induction should take place in the operating theatre itself. An operating department assistant or specifically trained anaesthetic nurse should be available to assist the anaesthetist. If a registered nurse or midwife is asked to perform this task then they should have an equivalent qualification, assist the anaesthetist on a regular basis and, very importantly, have no other duties in the operating theatre during the anaesthetic.

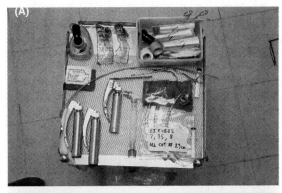

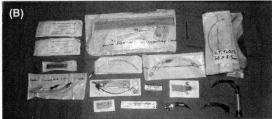

Figure 8.1 Equipment required on the obstetric intubation trolley. (A) Immediately available: short and long blade Macintosh laryngoscope, McCoy laryngoscope, choice of Guedel airways, cut tracheal tubes sizes 6–8, bougie and tube stilete. (B) Also available usually on a shelf under the intubation trolley: laryngeal mask, polio blade laryngoscope, mini-tracheostomy kit and uncut tracheal tubes.

EQUIPMENT FOR AIRWAY MANAGEMENT

As many of the life-threatening complications of general anaesthesia are associated with airway management, a wide range of equipment must be readily available, (the anaesthetist will usually only have one assistant who is applying cricoid pressure and is therefore not available to go searching for such equipment). All aids for a difficult intubation should be on a designated intubation trolley and regularly checked (Fig. 8.1).

It is recommended that there should be[10]

- one standard and one long bladed laryngoscope;
- a short handled laryngoscope or polio blade laryngoscope, which may be useful when there are difficulties in inserting the laryngoscope blade;
- a McCoy levering laryngoscope, which can improve intubating conditions when the view at laryngoscopy is poor;
- a gum-elastic bougie and tube introducer;
- tracheal tubes cut to the required length, in a range of sizes from 6 to 8 mm;

- oral airways;
- a size 3 laryngeal mask;
- a mini-tracheostomy set or the equivalent.

The McCoy laryngoscope

This has a levering tip operated by a mechanism in the handle.[11] The epiglottis may be lifted forward by the levering tip, making visualization of the arytenoids or vocal cords more likely, during a difficult intubation. The McCoy blade seems not to behave identically with a Macintosh blade in its neutral position, because of the overall shape of the blade and the handle can be awkward to hold. It should not be used routinely in obstetric practice unless its use is widely practiced during non-obstetric anaesthesia. When the vocal cords cannot be visualized with a Macintosh blade, however, the McCoy improve the view of the vocal cords or pharynx and therefore may aid a difficult intubation.[12]

The laryngeal mask

The laryngeal mask has entered into everyday anaesthetic practice: most anaesthetists are very familiar with its use; an advantage during the emergency management of a difficult airway in obstetrics. Unfortunately there are also disadvantages to its use in obstetrics. It does not prevent regurgitation of gastric contents into the oropharynx.[13] The application of effective cricoid pressure can make correct placement of the laryngeal mask more difficult than usual, and if correct placement is achieved, there may be inadequate ventilation through the mask. The position of the laryngeal mask during properly applied cricoid pressure has been investigated using a fibreoptic intubating laryngoscope. The grilles of the mask were frequently found not to be over the laryngeal opening.[14] Therefore if cricoid pressure is removed to allow placement of a laryngeal mask, subsequent ventilation may be impaired when it is reapplied.[15] This is particularly so if cricoid pressure is provided with one hand without counter-pressure to the back of the neck. These findings provide an explanation for anecdotal evidence of ventilation problems encountered when the laryngeal mask has been used during emergency management of the airway at Caesarean section. It follows that the use of a laryngeal mask to aid insertion of either an uncut size 5 tracheal tube or the fibreoptic scope may not be successful under these conditions.

Cricoid pressure prevents gastric insufflation with a laryngeal mask in place in the non-pregnant population, therefore theoretically a laryngeal mask may not make the risk of regurgitation in a pregnant woman worse. Faced with failure to secure the airway with a tracheal tube, then the laryngeal mask may be useful. Repeated attempts at insertion may however be counter-productive, and other methods of airway management should be considered early.

Cricothyrotomy

Cricothyrotomy should be considered in an extreme emergency when oxygenation can be maintained in no other way. A mini-tracheostomy set is most suitable, as the tube is relatively easy to insert and the standard 15 mm connector can be used with a conventional breathing circuit. Oxygenation can be maintained through the 4 mm internal diameter of the tube, although ventilation with an adequate expiratory phase is not possible in the face of complete upper airway obstruction.

Fibreoptic intubation

Fibreoptic intubation has no place in obstetric practice during a failed intubation. It should be used if intubation difficulties are anticipated or when it has been necessary to wake a mother up after failed intubation. There is some controversy over the best method of anaesthetising the upper airway in a patient who is at risk of regurgitation. If the anaesthetist is very skilled then the intubating scope can be used when the mother is unconscious and paralysed with cricoid pressure applied. In the majority of hands it is safer to use the intubating scope with the mother awake in a slightly head up position using a minimal 'spray as-you-go' local anaesthetic technique.

ASSESSMENT OF THE AIRWAY

A retrospective review found that failed intubation occurred in 1/280 in the obstetric population compared with 1/2230 in the general population.[16] In a series of 1500 general anaesthetics, with a general anaesthetic rate for Caesarean sections of 93%, there were two failed intubations; a rate of 1/750.[17] It would seem that even in experienced hands the rate of failed intubation is very much higher than in the non-obstetric population. The reasons for this may be related to the changes associated with pregnancy such as breast enlargement, general weight gain and laryngeal oedema. The latter may be present even when pre-eclampsia is not.

There are numerous methods for assessing the airway, which may help in predicting a difficult intubation.

Mallampati scoring[18] is easy to carry out at the bedside. It should be performed with the mother in a sitting position with her head in a neutral position and her tongue protruding. An increase in Mallampati score may occur during normal pregnancy[19] and increases have been noted during normal labour.[20] Rocke demonstrated the relationship between Mallampati score and view at laryngoscopy,[17] and he also found a correlation between high scores and a short neck, obesity, missing maxillary incisors, protruding maxillary incisors and a receding mandible. These anatomical features are significant because difficulty or failure at intubation did not necessarily occur with a grade 4 view at laryngoscopy.[21]

Wilson[22] examined the anatomy and movement of the bony structures of the head and neck. He found that there was a good correlation between limited head extension, a small thyromental distance and difficulties at intubation, but found that some patients with these features were not difficult to intubate. Whilst these studies may have considerable relevance to obstetric practice some methods may be impractical in the clinical setting when very rapid assessment of the airway may be needed.

Harmer has suggested a checklist for obstetrics.[10] It is pragmatic, readily learned and is easy to apply.

- Mouth opening; is there an inter-incisor gap of at least 5 cm (3 finger breadth)?
- Is the Mallampati score less than 3?
- Temporo-mandibular joint mobility; can the lower incisors be moved in front of upper incisors?
- Is 90° flexion of head on neck possible?
- Was the weight no greater than 90 kg at booking?
- Is there low risk for airway oedema?

The questions require a yes/no answer. If two or more are answered in the negative then a regional technique or awake fibreoptic intubation should be considered.

The rate of desaturation in the apnoeic term mother may contribute to the high failed intubation rate. A fully pre-oxygenated mother prior to induction will desaturate rapidly because there is a 20% reduction in her functional residual capacity at term and increased oxygen consumption. This is particularly marked in labour. In the face of a rapidly desaturating mother it is imperative that attempts at intubation are not prolonged and a failed intubation drill be rapidly instituted. Anxiety on the part of the inexperienced anaesthetist during induction may contribute to the high rate of failed intubation. Attempting intubation before full muscle relaxation has taken place can also create problems.

REDUCING THE RISK OF PULMONARY ASPIRATION OF GASTRIC CONTENTS

The physiological changes, which occur during pregnancy increase the likelihood of regurgitation. The woman who requires an emergency section in labour is at greater risk than one undergoing surgery pre-labour.

The physiological changes that increase the risk of regurgitation and the risk of acid aspiration syndrome in a pregnant woman are:

- a reduction in lower oesophageal tone, a progesterone effect that occurs early in pregnancy;
- a delay in gastric emptying with a tendency for higher gastric volumes and reduced gastric pH; this may be due to gastrin production from the placenta;
- increase incidence of reflux, due to increased intra-abdominal pressure by the enlarging uterus.

Heartburn is a very common symptom in pregnancy and is closely associated with demonstrable gastric reflux. Many women who do not complain of heartburn also have considerable reflux,[23] therefore its presence or absence should not be used to determine the degree of risk of regurgitation.

FEEDING IN LABOUR AND PRIOR TO CAESAREAN SECTION

Elective Caesarean section

Fasting before an elective Caesarean section is mandatory. It has been found that even a light breakfast of tea and toast taken 4 h before general anaesthesia, is associated with a higher intragastric volume and more acidic contents, than when a 6 h fast has been observed.[24] Although gastric emptying may not be significantly delayed even in the third trimester,[25] it would seem prudent to insist on at least a 6 h fast before an elective Caesarean section because of the high incidence of reflux and lowered pH of gastric contents in pregnancy.

Emergency Caesarean section

Withholding food in labour is much more controversial, because although nowadays a minority of women will require surgical delivery under general anaesthesia, this group cannot be identified with any certainty. However, many women who are at risk of requiring Caesarean section will have regional analgesia in labour, which if well managed, can be converted to anaesthesia for delivery. The dehydration and ketosis which may develop during severely prolonged labour will have a detrimental effect on the parturient, the fetus and the progress of labour. Prolonged periods of fasting, especially withholding fluids, can also be very unpleasant for the mother. Midwives and maternal pressure groups have demanded a more liberal approach to eating in labour. Many delivery units have a non-selective policy allowing most mothers to eat and drink. In other units either food or food and fluids are withheld, depending on a number of criteria relating to the risk of obstetric intervention.[26]

The administration of opioids either systemically or epidurally does result in profound slowing of gastric emptying: using ultrasound imaging it was shown that solid food could be detected in the stomach of labouring mothers with an opiate containing epidural 8–24 h after ingestion.[27] Dehydration and ketosis severe enough to be detrimental are rarely allowed to develop with modern management of labour; delay is promptly treated with oxytocin, which requires the administration of intravenous fluids. A labouring mother who has ingested food within the last 6–8 h and has received an opiate, will almost certainly have large gastric volume with a low pH which is particulate in nature. It is therefore highly dangerous if aspirated and thus the decision whether to allow feeding in labour remains controversial.

NASOGASTRIC TUBES

Pre-induction

The use of a nasogastric tube prior to induction, to enable physical emptying of the stomach has been suggested, particularly if a mother has had opiates in labour and is therefore most likely to have a full stomach. However, this is not only unpleasant for the awake mother, but it may delay induction of anaesthesia in an emergency. The majority of units in the UK do not routinely follow this recommendation.[28] Physical removal of gastric contents will reduce the volume by a greater degree than pharmacological methods, but the remaining volume may still make the mother vulnerable to aspiration. Brock-Utne et al appreciated the unpleasant nature of the routine use of a nasogastric tube, but recommend that pre-operative emptying be carried out if a recent meal has been ingested.[29] If a nasogastric tube is passed, some mothers have been found to have a large volume low pH residue despite full antacid prophylaxis.[28] The authors of this paper continue to recommend the routine use of a nasogastric tube in the emergency setting.

Post-induction

In a mother at high risk of aspiration, it may be more practical to insert a nasogastric or orogastric tube after induction of anaesthesia, once the airway is secured. As the risk of aspiration continues into the recovery period, this may be a logical approach and one that is more acceptable to the mother.

ANTACID PROPHYLAXIS

It is generally believed that the volume, pH and nature of aspirated material effects the severity of the pneumonitis that may develop. The published research that supports this is however largely based on animal experiments. The critical volume of aspirate is said to be between 0.4 ml/kg (25 ml)[30] and 0.8 ml/kg (50 ml)[31] with a pH of less than 2.5. These figures are used as a benchmark for the adequacy of therapeutic manoeuvres.

A survey revealed that in the early 1980s it was common practice to give all labouring mothers routine antacid prophylaxis.[32] This prophylaxis consisted of magnesium tricilicate, sodium citrate or a H_2 antagonist. The cost of this policy was significant, especially considering that the absolute rate of serious gastric aspiration is very low. About a third of units which did not have such a policy, gave antacids to mothers perceived as being at high risk for Caesarean section. The majority of delivery suites followed a different regime before elective and emergency surgery. Although the authors did not comment on the relative numbers of regional and general anaesthetics given in each unit, the reduction in the number of general anaesthetics which are now given makes it logical to give antacid treatment only when Caesarean section is planned or seems likely.

Magnesium trisilicate

Magnesium trisilicate was the first widely used antacid to be used in labour and before Caesarean delivery. Although it effectively reduces gastric pH it mixes only slowly with gastric contents and its particulate nature is potentially hazardous.[33]

Sodium citrate

Sodium citrate is an unpalatable antacid with a short shelf life. When sodium citrate (30 ml of 0.3 M solution) was given 10–60 min before elective surgery, it was found to increase the pH of gastric contents above 2.5 in a predictable manner.[34] After 60 min the results were less predictable. However, the pH values in the study group were still higher than those of the controls none of whom had a pH of 2.5 or above. Giving sodium citrate does not seem to increase the intragastric volume (in fact only 5% of mothers given 30 ml of sodium citrate were found to have an intragastric volume greater than 25 ml or a pH of less than 2.5).[35] Such studies suggest that sodium citrate is an effective antacid, which will reliably reduce the risk of acid pneumonitis, at least at induction of anaesthesia. Problems of aspiration may occur however during emergence of anaesthesia, when the effect of sodium citrate is much less predictable.

H_2 antagonists (cimetidine and ranitidine)

These are effective at reducing gastric pH and gastric volume,[36] especially when administered with metaclopramide. Ranitidine is now used in preference to cimetidine because the latter may cause haemodynamic instability when given parenterally and has been associated with changes in liver function. If an oral dose of ranitidine 150 mg is given at least 60 min before Caesarean section, then it is effective.[37] This is the preferred route of administration for elective surgery and during labour, when Caesarean section is anticipated. Intravenous ranitidine is effective within half an hour of administration. In the event of an extreme emergency, it is still useful to give intravenous ranitidine at induction because it will be effective by the time the mother emerges from anaesthesia, when sodium citrate is unreliable.

Omeprazole

Omeprazole is a H^+ ATPase proton-pump inhibitor. It has been in use since 1989. A single oral dose of 80 mg has been found to be effective at reducing intragastric volume and increasing pH in the majority of mothers.[38,39] It is well tolerated and seems to be free of fetal side effects. Intravenous omeprazole 40 mg is also effective at increasing pH and reducing gastric volume if given at least 30 min before induction. It does not however appear to have any advantages over ranitidine, and is more expensive.

Metoclopramide

Metoclopramide is a dopamine antagonist which may be used to accelerate gastric emptying and increase lower oesophageal tone. This is particularly useful in the mother who suffers from heartburn.[40] The delay in gastric emptying, which occurs in labour and after opiate administration, can be partially reversed with metoclopramide.[41] It is most effective when used in conjunction with other drugs such as ranitidine or omeprazole.[35] The anti-emetic effect is an added bonus.[42] This, in conjunction with the low incidence of maternal or fetal side effects, can justify its routine use.

STANDARDS OF CARE DURING INDUCTION OF GENERAL ANAESTHESIA

POSITIONING

The 'supine hypotension syndrome' or aorto-caval compression can occur from the second trimester of pregnancy. There is a reduction in venous return and cardiac output leading to a fall in systemic blood pressure. The woman may feel light-headed and nauseous and she will tend to automatically adopt a position that relieves the compression. During natural sleep in pregnancy, women have been found to lie in the right, or more commonly the left, lateral position.[43] When the supine position is adopted vasoconstriction may compensate for the reduction in venous return.

The effect of aorto-caval compression is perceived to be a greater problem during regional than general anaesthesia, because of the presence of sympathetic blockade. However, any parturient may have concealed aorto-caval compression and it is mandatory to position the woman to minimize this risk using a 15° left lateral tilt.[44,45] During general anaesthesia, the effects of the anaesthetic drugs will partially obtund compensatory vasoconstriction. Positive pressure ventilation will further reduce venous return and therefore blood supply to the fetus.

PRE-OXYGENATION

There is an increase in oxygen consumption at term of 20%, compared with non-pregnant controls. In early labour, oxygen consumption increases by a further 20% and in the second stage it may be 100% greater than in the pre-pregnancy state.[46]

In the healthy non-pregnant patient, careful pre-oxygenation will allow at least 3 min to elapse during apnoea before haemoglobin oxygen saturation begins to fall. This period is markedly reduced in the labouring mother at term, even with adequate denitrogenation.

The mask must be tightly applied to the face otherwise 20% of room air can be entrained despite a 10 ml/min oxygen flow.[47,51] The traditional method of taking tidal breaths for 3 min will effectively reduce alveolar nitrogen to 1%. The alternative method of taking four deep breaths reduces this to 5%.[48] The traditional method will increase safe apnoea time by 15 s.

In an extreme emergency, capacity breaths may benefit the fetus requiring rapid delivery by reducing time to delivery by a few minutes. This technique may also be beneficial to those mothers who cannot tolerate a close fitting facemask for 3 min.

A traditional 3-min pre-oxygenation, however, has the advantage of giving the anaesthetist more time to check patient, drugs and equipment before induction, and therefore has much to recommend it.

RAPID SEQUENCE INDUCTION

During induction of anaesthesia, cricoid pressure is applied. Sellick first described the technique in 1961.[49] It consists of firm pressure applied to the cricoid cartilage by the index finger. The thumb and middle finger are placed either side of the cricoid to prevent lateral movement of the cartilagenous ring which could make intubation difficult. The backward pressure compresses the oesophagus on the vertebral column and causes it to be occluded, whilst the airway remains patent because the cricoid is a complete ring of cartilage. A constant backward pressure of 44 N will prevent the passive regurgitation of stomach contents.[50] If active vomiting occurs, cricoid pressure with oesophageal occlusion could lead to rupture and should be abandoned.

It is important to establish cricoid pressure before induction of anaesthesia. Pressures above 20 N, are poorly tolerated by the awake patient[51] but during loss of consciousness pressure should be rapidly increased. This manoeuvre needs to be carefully taught. Most untrained personnel apply too little force or do not maintain the force over a sufficient period of time.[52] It seems particularly difficult to maintain cricoid pressure for more than 5 min[53] even when 30 N are applied, as has been recently recommended.

In Sellick's original description the assistant also places his left hand behind the neck; bi-manual cricoid pressure (Fig. 8.2). This positions the head in the 'sniffing position' and stretches the oesophagus, making it easier to occlude. Bi-manual cricoid pressure also stabilizes the head and reducing the tendency for the pressure to distort the larynx. It has been suggested that the forward pressure of the posterior hand may push the larynx into a more anterior position. When firm backward pressure is required to bring the larynx into view, the two-handed technique may make intubation more difficult.[54]

Perhaps the major disadvantage of the two handed technique is that the anaesthetist's assistant no longer has a hand free to reach for any additional equipment that may be required. If a second assistant is not available to help the anaesthetist, the one handed technique has much to commend it and one handed cricoid pressure is widely used.[55]

Although cricoid pressure has become a mandatory part of general anaesthesia for Caesarean delivery in

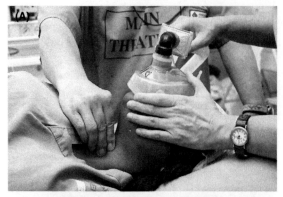

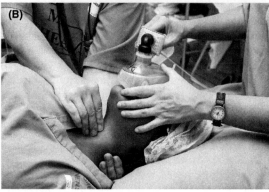

Figure 8.2   (A) One handed cricoid pressure.
(B) Two handed cricoid pressure, showing improved extension at the atlanto-occipital joint and stability of backwards pressure.

the UK, its use has not been universally accepted in Europe. Badly applied cricoid pressure probably does increase the risk of failed intubation.

FAILED INTUBATION

It is the dread of the obstetric anaesthetist to have a failed intubation, especially when there is fetal distress. It is important to remember that failure to intubate a mother will cause no harm as long as oxygenation is maintained. Repeated attempts at intubation often associated with the administration of a second dose of suxamethonium, will increase the chances of aspiration.[56] Unrecognized oesophageal intubation is a major hazard of a difficult intubation and has lead to maternal deaths. End tidal CO_2 monitoring is now mandatory in the obstetric theatre.

Correct positioning of the mother is very important to reduce the risk of intubation problems. In obstetric practice in the UK, it is usual for induction to be undertaken in theatre, on the operating table. This allows the height of the patient to be adjusted to optimize intubating conditions. The woman should have a pillow placed to produce good neck support, whilst allowing head extension. This is especially important if she has a lot of braided or platted hair, which can make it difficult for her to adopt the 'sniffing the morning air' position. For the large breasted mother, insertion of the laryngoscope can be made more difficult if her arms are folded across her chest. Positioning the arms out of the way of the surgical field is best left until after intubation.

FAILED INTUBATION DRILL

Following induction of anaesthesia, if the anaesthetist fails to intubate the trachea after trying a gum elastic bougie, smaller tracheal tubes and/or a McCoy laryngoscope then a failed intubation drill should be instituted. If difficulties have been encountered during intubation, then the position of the tube must be checked using capnography.

A failed intubation drill is most readily taught using an algorithm (Fig. 8.3).[10] These algorithms are complex and should be committed to memory prior to starting as an obstetric anaesthetist. A 'fire drill' using a mannequin is a useful exercise.

The next section has been reproduced with the kind permission of Prof. M. Harmer.

- A second dose of suxamethonium should not be given as this may precipitate profound bradycardia, especially in the presence of hypoxaemia, and it is illogical to assume that intubating conditions will be improved.
- It is no longer recommended that the mother is turned to the lateral position, but rather cricoid pressure should be maintained with the mother supine, with left lateral tilt. This is because of the difficulty associated with safely turning a large patient on a narrow operating table. It is also more difficult to ventilate using a facemask in the lateral position, because a second hand is needed to give counter pressure on the occiput and a third hand is then needed to squeeze the reservoir bag. Furthermore operating on a patient in the lateral position is technically difficult.
- Maintaining cricoid pressure: when faced with a failed intubation, the anaesthetist must quickly answer two questions:

  1. Is it possible to maintain oxygenation either through a laryngeal mask or facemask?
  2. How urgent is the Caesarean section?

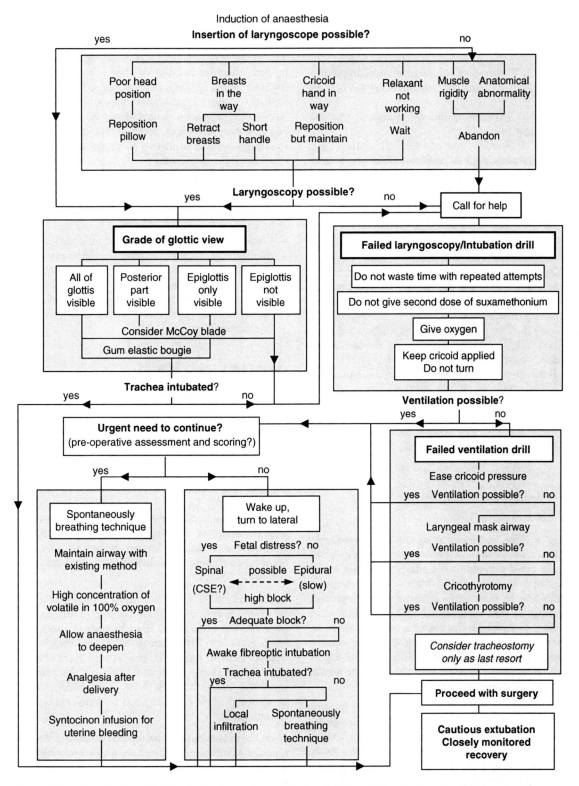

Figure 8.3   Algorithm for failed intubation taken from obstetric guidelines University Hospital of Wales, Cardiff.

The urgency of the Caesarean section can be graded and if oxygenation can be maintained, the need to continue surgery can be evaluated:

- *Grade 1*: The mother's life depends on completion of surgery, e.g. massive haemorrhage or cardiac arrest.
- *Grade 2*: Maternal pathology makes a regional technique unsuitable.
- *Grade 3*: Sudden and severe fetal distress, e.g. placental abruption or prolapsed cord necessitates surgery to save the baby.
- *Grade 4*: There is longer standing fetal distress, which shows signs of recovery between contractions.
- *Grade 5*: The procedure is elective.

- *Grade 1*: Surgery should continue under almost any circumstances.
- *Grade 2*: The safest option, even if oxygenation is adequate, is to wake the mother up and proceed with an awake fibreoptic intubation if equipment and expertise allows.
- *Grade 3*: If oxygenation can be maintained with good cricoid pressure, then to save the life of the fetus, anaesthesia may continue, although this type of anaesthetic even in the most skilled hands can be very difficult. If the mothers life is at risk because of continuing difficulties with airway management the mother should be woken.
- *Grades 4 and 5*: The safer option is to wake the mother and proceed with a regional technique.

SAFE ANAESTHESIA AFTER A FAILED INTUBATION

There is some argument as to the best anaesthetic technique to use in these circumstances. A spinal will provide rapid anaesthesia, an advantage when speed is a priority because of fetal distress. Haemodynamic stability may be more easily achieved with an epidural technique. A slow incremental epidural technique is advisable to minimize the risk of a total spinal block. A combined spinal epidural may give a more reliable regional technique with a reduced dose of local anaesthetic. If expertise and equipment allow, an awake fibreoptic intubation is probably the safest option.

If anaesthesia is continued in a spontaneously breathing mother, then depth of anaesthesia should be increased rapidly to allow surgery. The inhalational agent must be increased in increments to three times MAC, as surgery in a poorly anaesthetized patient may precipitate breath holding, coughing and vomiting. Once the patient is fully anaesthetized then the inhalational agent may be reduced to provide better

haemodynamic stability and greater uterine contraction after delivery.

Traditionally, halothane has been the agent of choice in this situation, because of the ease of induction without breath holding and coughing. Sevoflurane is probably a more logical agent to use, if available. It has similar properties to halothane in the spontaneously breathing patient, depth of anaesthesia is easier to control because of its low blood gas solubility and it is less cardio-depressant.[57]

- A gastric tube should not be passed: cricoid pressure would be very difficult to maintain during this procedure and additional instrumentation of the airway can lead to coughing and vomiting.
- Once the operation is finished and anaesthesia discontinued, then the mother should be turned to the left lateral position with a little head down tilt.
- The anaesthetist must remain with the mother until she is fully recovered. She must be fully informed and counselled about the problems encountered.

INDUCTION AND MAINTENANCE OF ANAESTHESIA

PREVENTING AWARENESS

Awareness during general anaesthesia for Caesarean section is more common than in general anaesthetic practice. The incidence of awareness may be as great as 0.4–1.3%.[58] In the un-premedicated, anxious mother, an induction dose of thiopentone, which may be adequate in other situations, can result in awareness soon after induction, before an adequate brain concentration of the inhalational agent has been achieved.

In the past, after delivery, nitrous oxide was used alone to maintain unconsciousness because of the fear of poor uterine contraction if an inhalation agent was used. However, 70% nitrous oxide in oxygen has a MAC value of only 0.65. Following a spate of cases of awareness in the 1970s and 1980s[59,60] this practice has been abandoned. At least 0.5% MAC of an inhalational agent must be used to supplement 60% nitrous oxide.[61]

With the newer inhalational agents; isoflurane, desflurane and sevoflurane, which have much lower blood/gas partition coefficients, anaesthesia can be induced more rapidly, reducing the risk of awareness immediately after induction. The rate at which a sleep concentration of the inhalational agent can be achieved at the start of anaesthesia can be increased by raising the initial concentration of the agent, (over-pressure). The time required to do so will depend on the inhalational agent used, and is best monitored by measuring the MAC value of the exhaled gas.

As many of the signs of light anaesthesia are obscured by the physiological changes of pregnancy, the use of an agent analyser to monitor inspiratory and expiratory concentrations during general anaesthesia should be used, to reduce the risk of awareness.

REDUCTION OF MAC DURING PREGNANCY

Awareness results from inadequate depth of anaesthesia, but it is recognized that there is a reduction in the amount of anaesthetic required during pregnancy. This, conversely, can result in the administration of relative overdoses. In animal studies the reduction of MAC was related to elevated progesterone concentrations in plasma and cerebrospinal fluid. In pregnant women at 8–12 weeks gestation, the MAC of isoflurane is reduced by 28% compared to non-pregnant controls.[62] This is caused by the phenomenon of pregnancy-induced analgesia, which may be produced by increased endorphin levels in pregnancy;[63] the reduction in MAC can be reversed by naloxone.[64]

INDUCTION-DELIVERY INTERVAL

The length of time between induction of general anaesthesia and delivery may affect the baby in two ways:

- Firstly the baby may become progressively acidotic during this period. This can be minimized if aorto-caval compression and hypotension are avoided. A high maternal FiO_2 of 60–70% may also improve the condition of the baby. High concentrations of nitrous oxide may result in diffusion hypoxia and fetal acidosis. In the 1960s it was recommended that the induction–delivery interval be limited to 4 min, which lead to the practice of draping the mother before induction. Crawford however suggested that an interval of up to 30 min should not adversely affect the fetal acid–base status[65] if the above precautions were taken.
- The second problem of a prolonged induction–delivery interval is that it allows the progressive uptake of lipid-soluble anaesthetic agents by the fetus, whilst a gradient exists between the maternal and fetal circulations. Intravenous induction agents that cause unconsciousness in the mother do not affect the baby, because of rapid maternal redistribution, which limits placental exposure. However,

during a prolonged induction–delivery interval, the maternal–fetal transfer of thiopentone may continue for 40 min, eventually resulting in a higher concentration in the fetus than the mother. The fetal liver probably protects the fetal brain from very high concentrations and the baby is usually born in a vigorous state.

- Inhalational agents have a more detrimental effect during a prolonged interval because maternal levels are constant and therefore a maternal–fetal gradient is maintained.
- A prolonged uterine incision to delivery is more dangerous to the fetus. Intervals in excess of 180 s are associated with low Apgar scores and fetal acidosis.[66] It is thought that uterine manipulation may cause maldistribution of placental blood flow and enhance aorto-caval compression.

MATERNAL VENTILATION DURING GENERAL ANAESTHESIA

OXYGEN

During anaesthesia for Caesarean delivery a high inspired oxygen concentration is not only necessary because of the woman's increased metabolic requirements, but it will also improve the condition of the baby at birth. Early work in this field, which was carried out with patients in the supine position, suggested that fetal well-being was improved with an inspired oxygen concentration of 66% compared to 33%.[7] With the mother in the left lateral tilt position, an inspired oxygen concentration of 50% appears optimal.[65]

CARBON DIOXIDE

At term the P_aCO_2 is reduced to 4.1 kPa. This reduction allows elimination of CO_2 by the fetus to the mother down a concentration gradient. If the woman is ventilated, the maternal CO_2 must not be allowed to rise or this gradient will be abolished. An excessive fall must also be avoided as a P_aCO_2 below 3.6 kPa causes vasoconstriction of the umbilical vessels and results in fetal acidosis and increased time to sustained respiration after birth.[67] Fetal acidosis is associated with a left shift of the oxygen-dissociation curve; oxygen becomes more tightly bound and is less readily available.[68]

MECHANICAL PRESSURE

Mechanical hyperventilation can cause an increase in intra-thoracic pressure. This may reduce maternal venous return, cardiac output and compound the effects of aorto-caval compression.[69]

ANAESTHETIC AGENTS

INTRAVENOUS INDUCTION AGENTS

There is a wide variety of intravenous induction agents used for anaesthesia in the non–pregnant population. All can and have been used for induction of anaesthesia in the obstetric patient but thiopentone still represents the gold standard.

Thiopentone

When thiopentone is given in a dose of 4 mg/kg it can be detected in the umbilical vein within seconds of induction, but the baby is protected from excessive sedation because of the fetal circulation through the liver. At a dose of 8 mg/kg fetal depression will occur.[70] There have been reports of subtle changes in behaviour patterns in babies even when the lower dose is used. These changes appear to persist for several days after delivery, despite normal acid–base status and Apgar scores at birth.[71] The major advantage of thiopentone is that anaesthesia can be reliably produced in the mother, because of its relatively long duration of action, whilst the baby is not severely compromised.

Propofol

Propofol has become a very popular induction agent in non-obstetric practice. It has been extensively investigated in the obstetric setting because of the possible advantage to the mother and baby of rapid recovery due to redistribution and elimination of the drug. Propofol rapidly crosses the placenta, but after an induction dose of 2.5 mg/kg does not cause excessive neonatal depression compared with thiopentone.[72] A number of studies have investigated the effects of propofol infusions to maintain anaesthesia. At a relatively low maintenance dose of 6 mg/kg/h the condition of the neonate was found to be good.[73] Doses in excess of 2.5 mg/kg can cause neonatal depression and lower doses may increase the incidence of maternal awareness. The evidence suggests that although the mother may be less sedated during emergence from anaesthesia if propofol is used, any advantage to the baby is minimal and there is a risk of rapid maternal waking occurring before adequate inhalational anaesthesia is achieved. Propofol does not have a clear role during the induction of anaesthesia for Caesarean section.[74]

Ketamine and etomidate

Ketamine and etomidate are commonly used for induction when maintenance of blood pressure and cardiovascular stability is important. Although neither are routinely used for Caesarean section, and both have drawbacks, they have a role in specific circumstances.

Ketamine is indicated in the presence of hypovolaemia following haemorrhage. Its powerful sympathomimetic action can help to maintain cardiovascular stability. This action may also be beneficial during an asthma attack. Ketamine tends to cause delirium and hallucinations especially in the un-premedicated patient, which makes it unsuitable for routine obstetric use.

Ketamine can be rapidly detected in the fetus, but in a dose of 1 mg/kg the condition of the baby at birth compares favourably with that of thiopentone.[75] A lower dose, which is associated with light anaesthesia, will make adverse dreams more likely. An induction dose of 2 mg/kg is associated with neonatal depression and low Apgar scores.[76]

Etomidate may also be useful for induction in the haemodynamically compromised woman. It causes less myocardial depression than thiopentone and less histamine release, (making it useful for the asthmatic). In a dose of 0.3 mg/kg; its rapid metabolism produces rapid awakening in the mother and good fetal Apgar scores with early sustained respiration in the baby.[77] Etomidate is partially hydrolysed to an inactive metabolite by cholinesterase, which is found in high concentrations in the placenta. Etomidate can be measured in the fetal circulation after induction of anaesthesia, but its concentration does not increase as rapidly as the other induction agents, which may be due to this placental metabolism.

Etomidate has the disadvantage of being associated with increased post-operative vomiting, pain on injection and myoclonic rigidity with involuntary movements. These movements can make a rapid sequence technique difficult. It also significantly reduces plasma cortisol concentrations, 1 h post delivery, in the baby.[78] The significance of this is unclear but in an already stressed baby this is a potential disadvantage.

Benzodiazepines

Benzodiazepines have been used for induction for Caesarean delivery. Their slow onset of action compared with the other agents, makes them less appropriate under normal circumstances, increasing the interval during which aspiration can occur. An induction dose of 0.2 mg/kg of midazolam also doubles the time to sustained respiration, compared to thiopentone in the fetus.[79] These drugs have limited use because they cause neonatal hypothermia, hypotonia, jaundice, lethargy, respiratory depression and poor feeding.[80] Induction with benzodiazepines does allow haemodynamic stability to be maintained, and therefore they may have a role when this is critical.

NEUROMUSCULAR BLOCKING AGENTS

Neuromuscular blocking drugs are used to facilitate intubation and maintain muscle relaxation. They are all ionized compounds at physiological pH and contain at least one quaternary ammonium group. Placental transfer of ionized compounds is minimal and the fetus is unaffected under normal circumstances. One case report did describe neonatal paralysis after tubocurarine was given in ten times the normal dose[81] and in another, a baby was born with weakness after suxamethonium was used in a mother with pseudocholinesterase deficiency – the baby was found to have the same abnormality.[82]

DEPOLARIZING NEUROMUSCULAR BLOCKERS

Suxamethonium – (succinyl choline)

Suxamethomium remains the drug of choice in obstetric anaesthesia allowing intubation within 90 s.[83] It is used as part of a rapid sequence induction in a dose of 1–1.5 mg/kg. It is the only drug commonly available which is metabolized rapidly enough to enable spontaneous respiration to return within 1–5 min. In pregnancy, due to dilution, pseudocholinesterase concentrations are lower than in the non-pregnant population. The effect of this is of doubtful clinical significance. Despite the side effects of suxamethonium, which have lead to the reduction of its use in other fields of anaesthesia, the use of suxamethonium in obstetrics has remained almost universal. When it was first introduced, it was the rapid onset of action that was attractive. It is the early return of spontaneous respiration after a failed intubation, allowing the mother to be woken with the return of her laryngeal reflexes, which has maintained its popularity.

There are however a number of situations when suxamethonium must be avoided:

- 0.3% of the population have pseudocholinesterase deficiency. If a woman suffers from this condition suxamethonium may cause prolonged paralysis requiring post-operative ventilation.
- Hyperkalemia can result from the use of suxamethonium after burns and recent cord transection.
- Hyperkalemia may also arise from its use if the patient has a severe demyelinating neurological condition.

- Severe rigidity, making intubation impossible, may result from the use of suxamethonium in a patient with myotonia.
- Suxamethonium may trigger malignant hyperthemia in a susceptible patient.

NON-DEPOLARIZING NEUROMUSCULAR BLOCKERS

Rocuronium

Rocuronium is a drug of intermediate duration. It can produce rapid intubating conditions and is useful when suxamethonium is contraindicated. Adequate conditions can be achieved with a dose of 0.6 mg/kg after 70 s.[84] Conditions are not usually as good as with suxamethonium, except when thiopentone is supplemented with alfentanil.[85] The disadvantage of all the non-depolarizing muscle relaxants is that after a dose adequate to produce rapid intubating conditions, paralysis will last for 50 min.[86]

Vecuronium and atracurium

Vecuronium and atracurium are both widely used and have replaced pancuronium and D-tubocurarine because of their predictable intermediate duration of action. After recovery from suxamethonium, vecuronim 0.05 mg/kg or atracurium 0.25 mg/kg can be safely used to provide 20–30 min of muscle relaxation. Their effects are easily reversed with glycopyrrolate or atropine and neostigmine, allowing the mother to rapidly regain control of her airway.

MAGNESIUM SULPHATE

Magnesium sulphate recently become popular for both the control and treatment of pre-eclampsia and to prevent recurrent seizures in eclampsia. Women who require magnesium for pre-eclampsia also have an increased risk of surgical intervention. Interactions of magnesium with anaesthetic drugs, particularly neuromuscular blockers, have been reported.

Interaction with suxamethonium

The fasciculations that are normally seen following suxamethonium may not occur. This can lead to concerns that the suxamethonium had not worked, although its action is actually unaffected by magnesium.[87]

Interaction with non-depolarizing muscle relaxants

The interaction of magnesium sulphate with the non-depolarizing blocking drugs may lead to enhanced or prolonged neuromuscular blockade.[88] Monitoring of neuro-muscular blockade is essential before reversal is attempted. Magnesium sulphate can cause recurarization in women previously given neuromuscular blocking drugs. Mothers must be monitored closely for several hours after anaesthesia, to detect signs of increasing muscle weakness. This is especially important when magnesium sulphate infusions are continued into the post-operative period.[89]

INHALATIONAL ANAESTHESIA

Nitrous oxide

Nitrous oxide has a low lipid solubility and is used, mixed with oxygen, as a carrier gas for other inhalational agents. It freely crosses the placenta and fetal concentrations rise during the first 15–19 min of maternal administration.[90] If more than 50% nitrous oxide is used, then it may cause depressed neonatal Apgar scores. With higher concentrations there is also a risk of diffusion hypoxia in the neonate, resulting in a deteriorating acid–base status. Nitrous oxide used alone with oxygen produces unacceptably light anaesthesia and a high incidence of maternal awareness. Even if the mother has no recall, high maternal catecholamine release causes vasoconstriction in the placental vascular bed, which will also have a detrimental effect on neonatal acid–base status.

Nitrous oxide does not cause uterine muscle relaxation and does not interfere with oxytocin induced uterine contraction. It therefore continues to be a useful carrier gas during Caesarean section, reducing the amount of other inhalational agents required.

The volatile anaesthetic agents

The halogenated anaesthetic agents halothane, enflurane and isoflurane have all been successfully used for Caesarean section. All cause dose and time dependent neonatal depression. If any are used at a one MAC equivalent with nitrous oxide and the induction-delivery interval is kept below 11 min, excessive neonatal depression is avoided. All the volatile agents cause dose dependent uterine relaxation and reduced sensitivity to oxytocin. If their use is restricted to a 0.5% MAC equivalent, then excessive bleeding is not usually a problem.[91]

The potential advantage of sevoflurane or desflurane is the low blood solubility, allowing very rapid induction of anaesthesia and reducing time to full recovery. Using the standard MAC equivalents, both drugs have been shown to be safe for mother and baby.[92] Neither have been shown to have any specific benefits over isoflurane, which has become a well established drug for Caesarean section.

Sevoflurane metabolism is associated with the production of fluoride ions. Serum fluoride concentrations have been found to be elevated in babies 24 h after delivery following sevoflurane anaesthesia. The consequences of this are unknown and to date there have been no reports of renal or hepatic toxicity.[93]

OPIATES

Opiates are not routinely used as part of a standard rapid sequence induction in obstetrics: these drugs rapidly cross the placenta to the baby, as well as potentially delaying the return of spontaneous respiration in the mother. They can however be used to obtund the hypertension and tachycardia associated with laryngoscopy when this is considered undesirable. A modest dose of fentanyl 1 μg/kg is safe for the neonate, but higher doses result in high fetal blood levels within 5 min, potentially causing respiratory depression.

Once the baby is delivered it is very important that the mother is given an adequate dose of an opiate to allow her to wake reasonably pain free after her operation. 100–200 μg of fentanyl or 10 mg of morphine are appropriate.

POST-OPERATIVE ANALGESIA

Mothers who have a Caesarean section under general, rather than regional anaesthesia, suffer more pain in the post-operative period. This has been found in non-randomized Caesarean section studies and after non-obstetric operations.[94,95]

After general anaesthesia it is usual to have to rely on intramuscular or intravenous opiates to provide analgesia. It is very important that mothers are given frequent and regular access to these drugs. Drugs such as pethidine or morphine may be administered by intramuscular injection, at up to one hourly intervals, with appropriate sedation and respiratory monitoring[96] or via a patient controlled pump.[97]

A non-steroidal anti-inflammatory such as diclofenac 100 mg rectally or tenoxicam 20 mg intravenously will enhance the analgesic efficacy of opiates and thereby produce an opiate sparing effect.[98,99] Non-steroidal anti-inflammatory drugs have been very widely used after Caesarean section without adverse effect to mother or baby. The usual contraindications, such as sensitive asthma and renal failure, must be observed.

STANDARDS OF CARE IN THE POST-OPERATIVE PERIOD

Poor standards of post-operative care have lead to deaths after Caesarean section. The mother after her Caesarean section is often recovered in an isolated unit. This requires the duplication of adequate monitoring equipment and expertise in recovery staff. In the majority of delivery suites in the UK, midwives are asked to recover mothers after Caesarean section. The majority of them do so infrequently and many are confused about the monitoring equipment available.[100] If midwives are asked to recover patients, then there should be a local policy of teaching and updating of skills.

REFERENCES

1. Davis AG. Anaesthesia for Caesarean section. The potential for regional block. *Anaesthesia* 1982; **37**(7): 748–753.

2. Balanced anaesthesia for Caesarean section: a review of 614 cases 1948–1956. William Bingham. *Anaesthesia* 1957; **12**: 435–452; *Anaesthesia* 1995; **50**: 623–632.

3. Mendelson CL. The aspiration of stomach contents into the lungs during obstetric anaesthesia. *Am J Obstet Gynecol* 1947; **52**: 191–205.

4. Morgan B. Controversies in obstetric anaesthesia. *Int J Obstet Anesth* 1996; **5**: 64–67.

5. Morgan M. Anaesthetic contribution to maternal mortality. *Br J Anaesth* 1987; **59**: 842–855.

6. Gajraj NM et al. A survey of obstetric patients who refuse regional anaesthesia. *Anaesthesia* 1995; **50**(8): 740–741.

7. Marx GF, Mateo CV. Effects of different oxygen concentrations during general anaesthesia for elective Caesarean section. *Can Anaesth Soc J* 1971; **18**(6): 587–593.

8. Bonner SM, Haynes SR, Ryall D. The anaesthetic management of Caesarean section for placenta praevia: a questionnaire survey (see comments). *Anaesthesia* 1995; **50**(11): 992–994.

9. Association of Anaesthetists and Obstetric Anaesthetist Association. *Guidelines for obstetric anaesthetic services.* 1998; The Association of Anaesthetists.

10. Harmer M. Difficult and failed intubation in obstetrics. *Int J Obstet Anesth* 1997; **6**(1): 25–31.

11. McCoy EP, Mirakhur RK. The levering laryngoscope (see comments). *Anaesthesia* 1993; **48**(6): 516–519.

12. Cook TM, Tuckey JP. A comparison between the Macintosh and the McCoy laryngoscope blades (see comments). *Anaesthesia* 1996; **51**(10): 977–980.

13. Akhtar TM, Street MK. Risk of aspiration with the laryngeal mask (see comments). *Br J Anaesth* 1994; **72**(4): 447–450.

14. Asai T et al. Cricoid pressure impedes placement of the laryngeal mask airway and subsequent tracheal intubation through the mask (see comments). *Br J Anaesth* 1994; **72**(1): 47–51.

15. Asai T et al. Cricoid pressure applied after placement of the laryngeal mask prevents gastric insufflation but inhibits ventilation. *Br J Anaesth* 1996; **76**(6): 772–776.

16. Samsoon GL, Young JR. Difficult tracheal intubation: a retrospective study. *Anaesthesia* 1987; **42**(5): 487–490.

17. Rocke DA et al. Relative risk analysis of factors associated with difficult intubation in obstetric anesthesia. *Anesthesiology* 1992; **77**(1): 67–73.

18. Mallampati SR et al. A clinical sign to predict difficult tracheal intubation: a prospective study. *Can Anaesth Soc J* 1985; **32**(4): 429–434.

19. Pilkington S et al. Increase in Mallampati score during pregnancy (see comments). *Br J Anaesth* 1995; **74**(6): 638–642.

20. Farcon EL, Kim MH, Marx GF. Changing Mallampati score during labour. *Can J Anaesth* 1994; **41**(1): 50–51.

21. Cormack RS, Lehane J. Difficult tracheal intubation in obstetrics. *Anaesthesia* 1984; **39**(11): 1105–1111.

22. Wilson ME et al. Predicting difficult intubation. *Br J Anaesth* 1988; **61**(2): 211–216.

23. Hey VM et al. Gastro-oesophageal reflux in late pregnancy. *Anaesthesia* 1977; **32**(4): 372–377.

24. Lewis M, Crawford JS. Can one risk fasting the obstetric patient for less than 4 hours? *Br J Anaesth* 1987; **59**(3): 312–314.

25. Macfie AG et al. Gastric emptying in pregnancy (see comments). *Br J Anaesth* 1991; **67**(1): 54–57.

26. Michael S, Reilly CS, Caunt JA. Policies for oral intake during labour. A survey of maternity units in England and Wales. *Anaesthesia* 1991; **46**(12): 1071–1073.

27. Carp H, Jayaram A, Stoll M. Ultrasound examination of the stomach contents of parturients. *Anesth Analg* 1992; **74**(5): 683–687.

28. Rhodes A, Hughes KR, Cohen DG. An argument for orogastric tubes during Caesarean section. *Int J Obstet Anesth* 1996; **5**(3): 156–159.

29. Brock-Utne JG et al. Influence of preoperative gastric aspiration on the volume and pH of gastric contents in obstetric patients undergoing Caesarean section. *Br J Anaesth* 1989; **62**(4): 397–401.

30. Roberts RB, Shirley MA. Reducing the risk of acid aspiration during cesarean section. *Anesth Analg* 1974; **53**(6): 859–868.

31. Raidoo DM et al. Critical volume for pulmonary acid aspiration: reappraisal in a primate model. *Br J Anaesth* 1990; **65**(2): 248–250.

32. Greiff JMC et al. Acid aspiration prophylaxis in 202 obstetric anaesthetic units in the UK. *Int J Obstet Anesth* 1994; **3**(3): 137–142.

33. Gibbs CP et al. Antacid pulmonary aspiration in the dog. *Anesthesiology* 1979; **51**(5): 380–385.

34. Dewan DM et al. Sodium citrate pretreatment in elective cesarean section patients. *Anesth Analg* 1985; **64**(1): 34–37.

35. Stuart JC et al. Acid aspiration prophylaxis for emergency Caesarean section. *Anaesthesia* 1996; **51**(5): 415–421.

36. Rout CC, Rocke DA, Gouws E. Intravenous ranitidine reduces the risk of acid aspiration of gastric contents at emergency cesarean section. *Anesth Analg* 1993; **76**(1): 156–161.

37. Escolano F et al. The efficacy and optimum time of administration of ranitidine in the prevention of the acid aspiration syndrome. *Anaesthesia* 1996; **51**(2): 182–184.

38. Moore J et al. Effect of single-dose omeprazole on intragastric acidity and volume during obstetric anaesthesia (see comments). *Anaesthesia* 1989; **44**(7): 559–562.

39. Rocke DA, Rout CC, Gouws E. Intravenous administration of the proton pump inhibitor omeprazole reduces the risk of acid aspiration at emergency cesarean section (see comments). *Anesth Analg* 1994; **78**(6): 1093–1098.

40. Hey VM, Ostick DG. Metoclopramide and the gastro-oesophageal sphincter. A study in pregnant women with heartburn. *Anaesthesia* 1978; **33**(5): 462–465.

41. Murphy DF et al. Effect of metoclopramide on gastric emptying before elective and emergency Caesarean section. *Br J Anaesth* 1984; **56**(10): 1113–1116.

42. Lussos SA et al. The antiemetic efficacy and safety of prophylactic metoclopramide for elective cesarean delivery during spinal anesthesia. *Reg Anesth* 1992; **17**(3): 126–130.

43. Mills GH, Chaffe AG. Sleeping positions adopted by pregnant women of more than 30 weeks gestation. *Anaesthesia* 1994; **49**(3): 249–250.

44. Crawford JS, Burton M, Davies P. Time and lateral tilt at Caesarean section. *Br J Anaesth* 1972; **44**(5): 477–484.

45. Eckstein KL, Marx GF. Aortocaval compression and uterine displacement. *Anesthesiology* 1974; **40**(1): 92–96.

46. Archer GW Jr, Marx GF. Arterial oxygen tension during apnoea in parturient women. *Br J Anaesth* 1974; **46**(5): 358–360.

47. McGowan P, Skinner A. Preoxygenation – the importance of a good face mask seal (see comments). *Br J Anaesth* 1995; **75**(6): 777–778.

48. Norris MC et al. Denitrogenation in pregnancy. *Can J Anaesth* 1989; **36**(5): 523–525.

49. Sellick BA. Cricoid pressure to control regurgitation of stomach contents during induction of anaesthesia. *Lancet* 1961; **ii**: 404–406.

50. Wraight WJ, Chamney AR, Howells TH. The determination of an effective cricoid pressure. *Anaesthesia* 1983; **38**(5): 461–466.

51. Vanner RG. Mechanisms of regurgitation and its prevention with cricoid pressure. *Int J Obstet Anesth* 1993; **2**(4): 207–215.

52. Ashurst N et al. Use of a mechanical simulator for training in applying cricoid pressure. *Br J Anaesth* 1996; **77**(4): 468–472.

53. Meek T, Vincent A, Duggan JE. Cricoid pressure: can protective force be sustained? (see comments). *Br J Anaesth* 1998; **80**(5): 672–674.

54. Cook TM. Cricoid pressure: are two hands better than one? (see comments). *Anaesthesia* 1996; **51**(4): 365–368.

55. Cook TM, McCrirrick A. A survey of airway management during induction of general anaesthesia in obstetrics. Are the recommendations in the Confidential Enquiries into Maternal Deaths being implemented? *Int J Obstet Anesth* 1994; **3**(3): 143–145.

56. King TA, Adams AP. Failed tracheal intubation (see comments). *Br J Anaesth* 1990; **65**(3): 400–414.

57. Smith I, Nathanson M, White PF. Sevoflurane – a long-awaited volatile anaesthetic (see comments). *Br J Anaesth* 1996; **76**(3): 435–445.

58. Lyons G, Macdonald R. Awareness during Caesarean section (see comments). *Anaesthesia* 1991; **46**(1): 62–64.

59. Payne JP. Awareness and its medicolegal implications. *Br J Anaesth* 1994; **73**(1): 38–45.

60. Crawford JS. Awareness during operative obstetrics under general anaesthesia. *Br J Anaesth* 1971; **43**(2): 179–182.

61. Aitkenhead AR. Awareness during anaesthesia: when is an anaesthetic not an anaesthetic? (editorial). *Can J Anaesth* 1996; **43**(3): 206–211.

62. Gin T, Chan MT. Decreased minimum alveolar concentration of isoflurane in pregnant humans. *Anesthesiology* 1994; **81**(4): 829–832.

63. Abboud TK et al. Effects of induction of general and regional anesthesia for cesarean section on maternal plasma beta-endorphin levels. *Am J Obstet Gynecol* 1983; **146**(8): 927–930.

64. Iwasaki H et al. Naloxone-sensitive, pregnancy-induced changes in behavioral responses to colorectal distention: pregnancy-induced analgesia to visceral stimulation. *Anesthesiology* 1991; **74**(5): 927–933.

65. Crawford JS et al. A further study of general anaesthesia for Caesarean section. *Br J Anaesth* 1976; **48**(7): 661–667.

66. Bader AM et al. Maternal and fetal catecholamines and uterine incision-to-delivery interval during elective cesarean. *Obstet Gynecol* 1990; **75**(4): 600–603.

67. Peng AT, Blancato LS, Motoyama EK. Effect of maternal hypocapnia v. eucapnia on the fetus during Caesarean section. *Br J Anaesth* 1972; **44**(11): 1173–1178.

68. Ralston DH, Shnider SM, DeLorimier AA. Uterine blood flow and fetal acid-base changes after bicarbonate administration to the pregnant ewe. *Anesthesiology* 1974; **40**(4): 348–353.

69. Levinson G et al. Effects of maternal hyperventilation on uterine blood flow and fetal oxygenation and acid–base status. *Anesthesiology* 1974; **40**(4): 340–347.

70. Kosaka Y, Takahashi T, Mark LC. Intravenous thiobarbiturate anesthesia for cesarean section. *Anesthesiology* 1969; **31**(6): 489–506.

71. Hodgkinson R et al. Neonatal neurobehavioral tests following cesarean section under general and spinal anesthesia. *Am J Obstet Gynecol* 1978; **132**(6): 670–674.

72. Moore J et al. A comparison between propofol and thiopentone as induction agents in obstetric anaesthesia (see comments). *Anaesthesia* 1989; **44**(9): 753–757.

73. Gregory MA et al. Propofol infusion anaesthesia for Caesarean section. *Can J Anaesth* 1990; **37**(5): 514–520.

74. Capogna G, Calleno D, Sebastiani M. Propofol and thiopentone for Caesarean section revisited. Maternal effect and neonatal outcome. *Int J Obst Anesth* 1991; **1**: 19–23.

75. Peltz B, Sinclair DM. Induction agents for Caesarean section. A comparison of thiopentone and ketamine. *Anaesthesia* 1973; **28**(1): 37–42.

76. Meer FM, Downing JW, Coleman AJ. An intravenous method of anaesthesia for Caesarean section. II. Ketamine. *Br J Anaesth* 1973; **45**(2): 191–196.

77. Downing JW et al. Etomidate for induction of anaesthesia at Caesarean section: comparison with thiopentone. *Br J Anaesth* 1979; **51**(2): 135–140.

78. Reddy BK, Pizer B, Bull PT. Neonatal serum cortisol suppression by etomidate compared with thiopentone, for elective Caesarean section. *Eur J Anaesth* 1988; **5**(3): 171–176.

79. Bland BA et al. Comparison of midazolam and thiopental for rapid sequence anesthetic induction for elective cesarean section. *Anesth Analg* 1987; **66**(11): 1165–1168.

80. Ravlo O et al. A randomized comparison between midazolam and thiopental for elective cesarean section anesthesia: II. Neonates. *Anesth Analg* 1989; **68**(3): 234–237.

81. Older PO, Harris JM. Placental transfer of tubocurarine. Case report. *Br J Anaesth* 1968; **40**(6): 459–463.

82. Cherala SR, Eddie DN, Sechzer PH. Placental transfer of succinylcholine causing transient respiratory depression in the newborn. *Anaesth Intens Care* 1989; **17**(2): 202–204.

83. Baraka A et al. Pseudocholinesterase activity and atracurium v. suxamethonium block. *Br J Anaesth* 1986; **58**(suppl 1): 91S–95S.

84. Abouleish E et al. Rocuronium (Org 9426) for Caesarean section (see comments). *Br J Anaesth* 1994; **73**(3): 336–341.

85. Sparr HJ et al. Influence of induction technique on intubating conditions after rocuronium in adults: comparison with rapid-sequence induction using thiopentone and suxamethonium. *Br J Anaesth* 1996; **77**(3): 339–342.

86. McCourt KC et al. Comparison of rocuronium and suxamethonium for use during rapid sequence induction of anaesthesia. *Anaesthesia* 1998; **53**(9): 867–871.

87. Stacey MR et al. Effects of magnesium sulphate on suxamethonium-induced complications during rapid-sequence induction of anaesthesia. *Anaesthesia* 1995; **50**(11): 933–936.

88. Fuchs-Buder T et al. Interaction of magnesium sulphate with vecuronium-induced neuromuscular block. *Br J Anaesth* 1995; **74**(4): 405–409.

89. Fuchs-Buder T, Tassonyi E. Magnesium sulphate enhances residual neuromuscular block induced by vecuronium. *Br J Anaesth* 1996; **76**(4): 565–566.

90. Marx GF, Joshi CW, Orkin LR. Placental transmission of nitrous oxide. *Anesthesiology* 1970; **32**(5): 429–432.

91. Warren TM et al. Comparison of the maternal and neonatal effects of halothane, enflurane, and isoflurane for cesarean delivery. *Anesth Analg* 1983; **62**(5): 516–520.

92. Abboud TK et al. Desflurane: a new volatile anesthetic for cesarean section. Maternal and neonatal effects. *Acta Anaesthesiol Scand* 1995; **39**(6): 723–726.

93. Gambling DR et al. Use of sevoflurane during elective cesarean birth: a comparison with isoflurane and spinal anesthesia. *Anesth Analg* 1995; **81**(1): 90–95.

94. Morgan BM et al. Anaesthetic morbidity following Caesarean section under epidural or general anaesthesia. *Lancet* 1984; **1**(8372): 328–330.

95. Shir Y, Raja SN, Frank SM. The effect of epidural versus general anesthesia on postoperative pain and analgesic requirements in patients undergoing radical prostatectomy (see comments). *Anesthesiology* 1994; **80**(1): 49–56.

96. Harmer M, Davies KA. The effect of education, assessment and a standardised prescription on postoperative pain management. The value of clinical audit in the establishment of acute pain services. *Anaesthesia* 1998; **53**(5): 424–430.

97. James KS, Davidson IT, McGrady E. Patient-controlled analgesia following Caesarean section: a comparison of morphine and meptazinol. *Int J Obstet Anesth* 1997; **6**(2): 93–96.

98. Dennis AR, Leeson-Payne CG, Hobbs GJ. Analgesia after Caesarean section. The use of rectal diclofenac as an adjunct to spinal morphine. *Anaesthesia* 1995; **50**(4): 297–299.

99. Elhakim M, Nafie M. I.v. tenoxicam for analgesia during Caesarean section (see comments). *Br J Anaesth* 1995; **74**(6): 643–646.

100. Fairfield MC, Bland D, Mushambi MC. Post-anaesthesia recovery care on the labour ward. *Int J Obstet Anesth* 1997; **6**(3): 153–155.

REGIONAL ANAESTHESIA FOR CAESAREAN SECTION

Rachel E. Collis

INTRODUCTION

Over the past 10–15 years, there has been a large increase in the number of Caesarean sections[1] performed under regional rather than general anaesthesia. This has coincided with a reduction in the number of maternal deaths directly attributed to anaesthesia. It is tempting to conclude from this that a regional technique should be used whenever possible, but it is important to understand that a badly conducted regional technique can be dangerous both to mother and baby. It has recently been suggested that because of the general increase in the total number of Caesarean sections performed, the actual number of general anaesthetics for Caesarean section may have remained relatively static. The implication of this is that improved teaching in maternal physiology and standards of care in the obstetric theatre has caused the reduction in maternal mortality, rather than the type of anaesthetic used. Whatever the real answer, it is crucial not to be lulled into believing that if a regional technique is used for Caesarean section, then standards of care can be lower than for general anaesthesia.

The mother having an elective or emergency Caesarean must have the same pre-anaesthetic work up if the plan is regional or general anaesthesia. This must include pre-operative starvation if possible and pre-operative preparation of gastric contents with appropriate antacids. There must be the same level of pre-operative checking of theatre equipment, availability of special equipment such as a difficult intubation trolley and appropriate monitoring. The anaesthetist must have the same level of help and recovery facilities for both techniques.[2]

BENEFITS OF REGIONAL ANAESTHESIA FOR CAESAREAN SECTION

BENEFITS OF REGIONAL ANAESTHESIA TO THE MOTHER

Safety

If regional anaesthesia is performed with care, with clear understanding of maternal physiology and in appropriate circumstances, then it is probably safer than general anaesthesia for Caesarean section. The hazards of a difficult airway associated with weight gain and oedema can be avoided, along with the problems of gastric regurgitation. The pregnant woman however is prone to supine hypotension, the effects of which are exaggerated during regional blockade. Poor management of this can result in severe hypotension, vomiting and unconsciousness, which in itself can increase the risk of acid aspiration. There are fundamental differences in the spread of local anaesthetic in the epidural and intrathecal spaces in pregnancy, which can result in unacceptably high blockade with poor respiratory function and unconsciousness from total spinal anaesthesia. There are also a number of medical conditions where rapid changes in after-load, associated with regional blockade, can result in a marked reduction in cardiac output, e.g. aortic stenosis and worsening of venous shunting, e.g. cyanotic congenital heart disease. Sympathetic blockade may also make hypotension associated with significant blood loss more difficult to treat. The increased benefits and safety of a regional technique will only be maintained if used in the correct circumstances.

Blood loss

There appears to be less bleeding at the time of Caesarean delivery when a regional technique is used.[3] A prospective, randomized study has not been performed, but several studies where non-randomized groups have been compared, have showed a reduced transfusion requirement in the regional groups.[4] The major criticism of these studies is that cases, where blood loss may have been anticipated, were preferentially performed under general anaesthesia e.g. placenta previa. Blood loss at Caesarean section for placenta previa appears less if carried out under regional anaesthesia, although this data may again be skewed by general anaesthesia being selected for the most difficult cases.

The reason for the apparent reduction in bleeding when regional techniques are used may be:

- The avoidance of volatile anaesthetic agents, which are associated with uterine relaxation and bleeding.
- Reduced peri-operative venous bleeding from pelvic venous plexuses.[5]

Although there is a traditionally held view that regional anaesthesia is contraindicated during major haemorrhage, haemodynamic stability can be maintained with aggressive blood and colloid replacement under these circumstances.

Post-operative recovery

From simple observation, it is apparent that the mother who has had a regional technique recovers more rapidly from her Caesarean section. She is more likely to be mobile the following day, feeling hungry and thirsty, breast-feeding and caring for her baby. She is likely to develop fewer post-operative complications such as pyrexia and chest infections and feel less depressed both immediately and after one week.[6] This may be because she avoids the complications as stated, but also being awake may improve her attitude towards the birth making it easier to develop early bonding with her baby.

Post-operative pain

Post-operative pain is a major factor in the rate of recovery after an operation. Access to the intrathecal and epidural space makes it possible to use this route for administration of opioids. Before axial opioids were regularly used, post-operative opioid requirements were noted to be fewer after regional anaesthesia. This is also seen after non-obstetric surgery.[7] It has also been shown that after the same epidural opioids in labour, mothers who have their epidural topped up for her Caesarean get better post-operative pain relief than those receiving a general anaesthetic.[8] Laboratory work suggests that there is a reduction of centrally transmitted pain after regional techniques. Whatever the underlying mechanism, rapid pain-free recovery, which is characteristic of regional anaesthesia, is important for mother and baby after Caesarean section.

REGIONAL ANAESTHESIA AND THE BABY

Lipophilic general anaesthetic drugs rapidly cross the placenta causing sedation in the newborn. Although acid–base status is maintained with a good general anaesthetic technique, low Apgar scores associated with sedation, which are characteristically seen after general anaesthesia, can be caused by placental transfer of these drugs. It must be advantageous to the newborn to be vigorous at birth, which is a characteristic of regional anaesthesia. The lack of drug effect seen after regional anaesthesia means that the infant requires less intervention; can feed earlier and maternal-infant bonding may be encouraged. Caesarean delivery where there is the likelihood of a long pre-delivery phase, such as a redo Caesarean, makes a regional technique even more advantageous to the baby.

Poor condition of the baby after a regional technique is associated with a prolonged uterine incision to delivery time and maternal hypotension. This is important because, unlike general anaesthesia where low Apgar scores are usually a result of sedation, low Apgar scores after regional anaesthesia are associated with acidosis and asphyxia. This is particularly relevant when the Caesarean is for the delivery of an already distressed and acidotic baby. A good technique with meticulous avoidance of aorto-caval compression and maternal hypotension is therefore essential for the safety of the baby.

PROBLEMS ASSOCIATED WITH REGIONAL ANAESTHESIA FOR CAESAREAN SECTION

There are a number of conditions that make general anaesthesia more suitable than a regional technique. These include maternal choice, coagulopathy, low platelet count, anticipated or actual severe haemorrhage, local infection, anatomical problems and certain medical conditions.

Lack of time

The most common reason for choosing a general anaesthetic over a regional technique is lack of time, because of urgent delivery of a compromised baby. Although in some hands a spinal anaesthetic may be as rapid as a general anaesthetic, this is not universally so. Calling the anaesthetist early, will increase the number of Caesareans than can be performed under a regional technique. With good communications, some units report a general anaesthetic rate of 2–3%. The anaesthetist must know how to assess and top-up an epidural block, which was in place for labour analgesia. If an epidural is working well for labour analgesia then the anaesthetist can top-up most in around 10 min, which is rapid enough in the majority of circumstances.

Pain during surgery

Fear of pain during surgery is a potent reason for mothers to request a general anaesthetic. Without a full understanding of the physiology of the regional blockade, the mother's fears may not be unfounded. The rate at which additional analgesia required during surgery varies enormously from 5% to 60–70%. A mother may wish to be awake during the birth of her baby, even if she feels some pain, whilst another would prefer a general anaesthetic even if her pain were not severe. The anaesthetist must determine the quality of the block before surgery, and judge how able or motivated an individual mother is able to cope with discomfort or pain if the block is not perfect. Complaints of pain during Caesarean section under regional blockade are an increasing cause of litigation against anaesthetists. If the regional blockade is adequate, then the mother can be assured that a Caesarean section can be performed without pain.

Cardiovascular effects

Unlike regional blockade for labour analgesia, the rate of onset and extent of blockade required for Caesarean section makes the mother vulnerable to hypotension. Simultaneous blockade of the sympathetic nerves with sensory and motor blockade required for Caesarean section cause peripheral vasodilatation, venous pooling followed by a potential reduction in cardiac output and blood pressure. Blood pressure is well maintained during a high sympathetic block if venous return is maintained and the mother's heart rate not allowed to slow. A common problem of regional blockade for Caesarean section is blockade of the cardiac sympathetic nerves. There can be a very sudden fall in pulse rate, characteristically from 100 to 60 beats/min associated with the sudden on-set of maternal hypotension. These problems are treated with manoeuvres to maintain venous return, intravenous ephedrine and occasionally intravenous atropine. If venous return is not adequate, because of aorto-caval compression, cardiac output cannot be maintained by increasing stroke volume to compensate for a reduced heart rate. The placental-fetal unit is pressure dependent and therefore the baby is very sensitive to the effects of low maternal blood pressure. The extent of the sympathetic blockade can be several dermatomes higher than the measured sensory extent of the block. The rate at which the sympathetic block develops will affect the incidence of hypotension. The highest rate of hypotension is as much as 80% and is seen after a spinal block is established *de novo*, when the mother is not in labour. During elective Caesarean section at 38–39 weeks, the combination of a large fetus and maximal liquor volume, will make aorto-caval compression and poor compensation for rapid high sympathetic block, more likely. There is a much lower rate of hypotension associated with topping up an epidural used for labour, where rupture of membranes with reduced liquor volume and maternal physiological adjustments have already taken place.

SYSTEMIC SUPPLEMENTATION OF REGIONAL ANAESTHESIA

Intravenous sedatives

Intravenous sedatives may help a very anxious mother, e.g. 2.5 mg of diazepam. Fear of pain and being awake in an operating theatre is the usual causes of this type of anxiety. A positive rapport with the mother and an adequate block is more important than pharmacological supplementation. Partial sedation with non-analgesics, as a treatment for an inadequate block, is not advised. The mother will become confused, her perception of pain may be heightened, she risks respiratory depression and she is likely to complain after the surgery.

Analgesic drugs

Analgesic drugs may be used for the treatment of pain during Caesarean section. These include 50% nitrous oxide, intravenous ketamine 0.25 mg/kg and fentanyl 1 μg/kg. All have been shown to be effective, although sedation must be monitored. It becomes a matter of good judgement when intravenous supplementation has failed and a general anaesthesia is required.

PREVENTING MATERNAL HYPOTENSION

AORTO-CAVAL COMPRESSION

The importance of uterine displacement, from compression of the venacava, was first noted in the late 60s by Marx and colleagues. Further published work in 1974 looked at the relative importance of uterine displacement and volume pre-load. With no pre-load or uterine displacement the incidence of hypotension was 92% and with uterine displacement and pre-load 53%.[9] The relative importance of the two manoeuvres were not assessed, but it was noticed that hypotension in the mother led to acidosis in the baby and uterine displacement and pre-load, was adopted as standard practice.

UTERINE DISPLACEMENT

The full lateral position

The uterus is fully displaced from the great vessels. This is reflected by the lateral position that women in the third trimester choose to adopt whilst sleeping.[10] If the mother is turned from the full left lateral position to her right side with a firm pillow under her shoulders and head (so-called Oxford position) the final height of a subarachnoid block is more predictable and there is greater haemodynamic stability.[11] Predicting those mothers who are most likely to develop hypotension would be ideal, because the supine position, even with tilt could then be avoided. Kinsella found that mothers who developed a tachycardia in the supine position prior to spinal blockade and also bent their knees to improve venous return, were more likely to become hypotensive. There were few false positives, but there were more false negatives, making it a useful but unreliable test.[12] The full lateral position remains the safest position to establish a regional blockade if the mother is prone to aorto-caval compression or optimal haemodynamic stability is required.

Lateral tilt

By tilting the operating table by 15 degrees to the left, the uterus is displaced from the venocava and aorta. There is still a high incidence of hypotension in this group because venous compression may only be partly relieved. Increasing the lateral tilt from 15 to 30 degrees may need to be considered,[13] although there are practical difficulties, as the mother feels unsafe and not all operating tables tilt this far. The exact degree of tilt required has not been fully evaluated.

Wedge

This can be a purpose made wedge, a firm pillow or a large infusion bag filled with air.[14] This tilts the pelvis and displaces the uterus whilst the mother is supine. The mother's spine is twisted, which may not be ideal if the mother has pre-existing back problems and the degree of tilt is fixed.

Manual displacement

The uterus can be lifted and displaced by hand or device. There is a tendency with displacement systems to push the uterus laterally rather than lifting. Although this is partially effective at reducing venacava pressure, obstruction of the uterine artery can occur, with reduced blood flow to the baby.[15] This method should be used only when displacement is needed for a short time.

With all these manoeuvres (Fig. 9.1) it is important to actually see the displaced uterus. If the uterus is very large, e.g. twins or polyhydramnious, then aorto-caval compression can be a problem with conventional techniques. The mother may need to stay in the full lateral position until immediately before surgery; the table may need to be tilted more than 15 degrees or a combination of the above methods.

VOLUME PRELOADING

Crystalloid preloading

Crystalloids have been traditionally used for preloading. They are inexpensive and do not cause allergic reactions. The effectiveness of these measures has mostly been studied in association with spinal blockade, where the incidence of hypotension is highest. The use of crystalloid pre-load was established by Marx[16] in the late 1960s and had not been questioned until recently. The routine use of 1000 ml of a crystalloid solution does not reliably eliminate hypotension, with 40–60% of mothers developing hypotension and requiring treatment with vasopressors.[17,18] Increasing the volume of the crystalloid infusion also has little effect on the incidence of hypotension. When a pre-load of 10, 20 and 30 ml/kg was investigated, the incidence of hypotension was around 50% and the amount of ephedrine used was similar between the groups.[19] A rapid infusion of a large volume of fluid can cause an unpredictable and rapid rise in CVP, producing pulmonary oedema in some predisposed pregnant women.[19] These effects are generally short lived, however, with CVP readings returning to pre-infusion levels after the spinal blockade. If continuing intravenous fluids are used rather than a vasopressor to

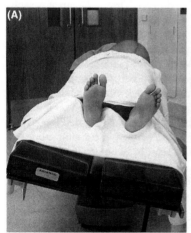 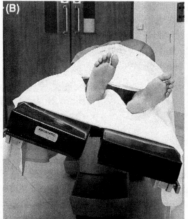 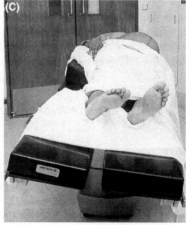

Figure 9.1   (A) Uterine displacement with 15 degrees of lateral tilt. (B) Uterine displacement with 20 degrees of lateral tilt-the mother feels unsafe with this tilt. (C) Uterine displacement with 15 degrees of lateral tilt and wedge under hip. The uterus is maximally displaced but she feels unsafe and her spine is twisted.

correct hypotension then 40–50 mg/kg of fluid may have to be used.[20] Such large volumes may have a significant effect on maternal packed cell volume already reduced by the physiological anaemia of pregnancy.

Colloid infusions

The colloid solutions have been studied, as crystalloids are known to be rapidly redistributed and are unreliable at preventing hypotension. There is some evidence that colloids reduce the incidence of hypotension. When 5% albumin at 15 ml/kg was used there was no maternal hypotension and the condition of the baby was better than in the crystalloid group.[21] When crystalloid solutions were combined with colloid solutions, with a total preload volume of 2000 ml, then the incidence of hypotension was lower than if a smaller colloid infusion was used alone.[22,23] With all these regimes substantial increases in CVP should be anticipated.

VASOPRESSORS

Ephedrine

Rout et al first questioned the practice of routine preloading. They compared no preload and 20 ml/kg and found no difference in the incidence of hypotension between the groups. When 1000 ml of crystalloid was compared to 200 ml crystalloid pre-load, the incidence of hypotension was also the same. The use of ephedrine with the smaller preload volumes was however greater, at around 50 mg compared to 6–10 mg, when larger preloads were used.[17,18] There may be little benefit in giving routine ephedrine prophylaxis to reduce the incidence of hypotension, compared to giving ephedrine as required.[24–26] It seems, that it is the avoidance of hypotension, rather than use of ephedrine, that is important to the baby when assessed by Apgar, cord pH and NACS scores.

Phenylephrine

Although this drug is a pure α-agonist, and may have a direct vaso-constrictive effect on the placental vasculature, it has been used in bolus doses of 25–100 μg to safely control hypotension.[27] It has not been studied as an infusion at Caesarean section, and excessive use could cause extreme hypertension and umbilical vasoconstriction. Although ephedrine is generally seen as the vasopressor of choice, phenylephrine is a useful drug when tachycardia is undesirable.

By avoiding large preloads, less time is required to initiate a spinal block, an advantage when rapid anaesthesia is required. Minimal preload will also avoid the

risk of excessive fluid use, high CVP, pulmonary oedema and dilutional anaemia.

RESPIRATORY EFFECTS OF REGIONAL ANAESTHESIA

Regional anaesthesia for Caesarean section requires sensory blockade extending high into the thoracic dermatomes. The density of the block requires that abdominal and thoracic respiratory muscles will be at least partially paralysed. Studies have shown that under epidural and spinal anaesthesia, base-line respiratory measurements and the ability to give a strong cough will decrease by 25–35% after regional blockade.[28,29] This reduction is maintained after the sensory and motor component of the block has worn off, and a further reduction has been measured 4 h after a spinal anaesthetic.[30,31] This secondary drop is presumably the result of atelectasis, which is established at the time of the block and will not resolve until the mother is encouraged to sit up and cough in the post-operative period.

The importance of this is probably limited, except when dealing with mothers who have limited respiratory reserve, due to co-existing medical disorders. The differences between the respiratory effects of epidural and spinal anaesthesia have not been evaluated in these mothers, but spinal anaesthesia with its shorter duration of action, followed by active chest physiotherapy, may be beneficial.

The routine use of oxygen therapy, during Caesarean section under regional anaesthesia, has been recommended. If pre-operative respiratory function is normal, then despite a drop in respiratory reserve, this is not reflected in a drop in arterial oxygenation. The use of around 35% oxygen will not improve oxygenation in the normal neonate,[31] although higher percentages have been recommended. The baby will however benefit from additional oxygen given to the mother if uterine incision–delivery time is prolonged.[32]

LEVEL OF BLOCK FOR CAESAREAN SECTION

THE MINIMUM BLOCK

When epidural blockade was first used for Caesarean section, a bilateral sensory block from S1 to T8 was suggested, accompanied by some lower limb weakness.[33] The authors however noted a 25% incidence of pain. Thorburn and Moir[34] made assessments of the sacral elements of the block and concluded that without a sacral block, pain was experienced during manipulation of the pelvic organs, but 25% of mothers in his study continued to experience pain even with sacral blockade. Crawford,[35] felt the block must extend to T6 and reduced the incidence of failure to less than 10%. A bilateral sensory block to T4, including the sacral roots, accompanied by motor block, became accepted as necessary for Caesarean section,[36] although an exact description of the spread and quality was not described.

Russell[37] showed that if the block extended to T5 to light touch, then the mother had no pain during surgery. He noted that there was a 20% incidence of pain during surgery if the regional block was lower than this. Interestingly, there were no differences between spinal and epidural blockade if the block spread equally. The observed difference in achieving pain free surgery between the two techniques is probably that a well-spread dense block is easier to achieve during spinal anaesthesia.

DIFFERENTIAL ZONES OF BLOCKADE

The apparent spread of a regional block is determined by the method used for assessment. There are zones of differential blockade at the upper and lower edges of a regional block. When assessing spinal and epidural blockade[38,39] it has been found that absence of cold sensation is two dermatomes higher than lack of pinprick sensation, which in turn is at least two dermatomes higher than lost sensation to light touch, (touching with a soft tissue or fine nylon filament) (Fig. 9.2).

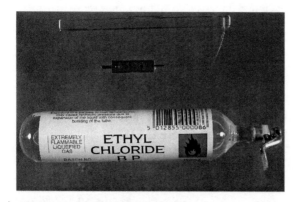

Figure 9.2 The sensation of cold (ice or ethyl chloride spray), pin prick (neurological pin) and light touch (nylon filament-Von Frey hair) to test the differential spread of a regional block for Caesarean section.

HOW TO TEST A BLOCK

Russell found testing a regional block with light touch is the most sensitive measure of block adequacy for Caesarean section,[37] but it is the least reproducible and most difficult for the mother and anaesthetist to understand.

Light touch assesses the pressure sensitive sensory fibres, which are the largest and most difficult to block, especially during epidural anaesthesia. An easier assessment of the intensity of the block is assessment of motor block, which mirrors that of light touch. With complete absence of hip flexion and ankle doriflexion movement, it is unusual, although possible to find a block that has an inadequate spread of anaesthesia to light touch. I personally use the corner of a tissue or nylon filament to lightly touch the skin in the thoracic and sacral dermatomes to confirm this.

I have found that absence of light touch is necessary from S1 to at least T8–6 with dense motor block of hips and ankles. The exact way this is measured and assessed, however, is very dependent on the individual anaesthetist. The exact level at which the mother feels sensation will depend on how the tissue or nylon filament is applied to the skin: a dabbing, stroking or flicking action will alter the mother's perception by around two dermatomes. I do not think that the exact technique is important, but the anaesthetist must always use the same technique. It is very unusual, in my experience, to find a block with measured absence of light touch to at least T8, if the absence of cold sensation is below T4 and it is more often accompanied by absence of cold sensation to T2.

Measuring the block must be bilateral as a common cause of intra-operative pain in an inadequate block on one side, (personal audit). Measuring the thoracic dermatomes must be assessed about 5 cm lateral to the midline. If a more lateral approach is made the height of the block can be over estimated because of the steeply sloping dermatomes, the slope of which is exaggerated by pregnancy.

ONSET AND REGRESSION OF THE BLOCK

The rate of block onset and regression differs between spinal and epidural blockade. Alahuhta[40] compared epidural and spinal blockade using pinprick. Spinal blockade rose quickly to T5 by 10 min and was maximal at T3 by 20 min. Spinal blockade also completely anaesthetized the sacral roots. Epidural blockade reached a maximal height at 30 min but some epidurals never completely anaesthetized the sacral roots. Spinal blockade remained at T3 for a short period of time and within 1 h began to regress rapidly. By 90 min the height of the block in this study was T9. In contrast, the epidural blockade regressed slowly and remained at T6 after 2 h. Pain was noted to be associated with block regression in the spinal group and inadequate sacral spread in the epidural group. The rate of regression of a spinal block will depend on the amount of bupivacaine that is initially injected. Some spinal blocks will provide anaesthesia for under 1 h. This may be important if there is a delay between spinal infection and start of surgery.

EPIDURAL ANAESTHESIA

Epidural blockade for elective Caesarean section has become increasingly uncommon because spinal blockade is quicker and more reliable. Most research has been conducted at elective surgery under epidural anaesthesia, although the majority of Caesareans where epidurals are used are now emergencies. There tends to be an assumption that initiating an epidural *de novo* is similar to topping up a partially established block from labour analgesia which is probably erroneous. What we know even less about is how the introduction of the low dose 'mobile' epidural for labour has affected the anaesthetist's ability to top-up an epidural rapidly for an emergency Caesarean.

Plain bupivacaine

Plain bupivacaine 0.5% was first used in 5–10 ml incremental boluses. The time to establish blockade was long, 25–183 min, 30–40 ml of 0.5% bupivacaine was often required and the resulting anaesthesia unpredictable.[34,35,41] Moir developed his technique by using a two-stage top-up of 10 + 10 ml of 0.5% bupivacaine, but still found it took an average block completion time of 42 min with 35% of mother's required intra-operative supplementation.[42] Techniques using a test dose followed by 18 ml of 0.5% bupivacaine reduced time to establish a block to 30 min, but supplementation was still required in 30–50% of cases.[40,43]

Lidocaine

Lidocaine was initially used with caution after infants born to mothers, who had received epidural analgesia with lidocaine for labour, were floppy and depressed.[44] Lidocaine 2% used as a one off bolus for Caesarean section compared favourably with bupivacaine from the neonatal point of view,[45,46] but was associated with a higher incidence of inadequate block compared to bupivacaine alone.

Epinephrine/bicarbonate

The addition of epinephrine (1 : 200 000) enhances the effect of lidocaine[47] and a single bolus technique increases the speed of onset. Alkanization with 2 ml of 8.4% bicarbonate in a 50 : 50 mixture of lidocaine and bupivacaine with epinephrine reduces onset time by nearly 50%, compared to the plain solution, and considerably improves the quality of the block with a reduction of intra-operative supplementation.[36] It has been suggested that warming lidocaine with epinephrine to 38 degrees may speed onset of anaesthesia, but the same effect is not seen with warm bupivacaine.[48]

TOPPING UP AN EPIDURAL DURING LABOUR FOR EMERGENCY CAESAREAN

The volume of epidural top-up which is needed to convert epidural analgesia for labour into a block for Caesarean section, is variable. Lucus[49] used 20 ml of whatever the pre-existing block had been established with, with rapid, complete results in the majority of mothers. Milne[50] used 16 ml of bupivacaine 0.5% and Dickson[51] used 10 ml of bupivacaine with variable results, after a low dose bupivacaine infusion for labour. In Dickson's study a third of the mothers had unsatisfactory blocks after the initial top-up and giving additional top-ups doubled the time it took before surgery could start. The major problem with Dickson's technique was that all the pre-existing blocks were similar and the authors were unable to predict when the larger dose was needed. The concern is that giving an initial large top-up after labour analgesia may produce an unacceptably high block. None of the studies however reported problems with high blocks, although loss of sensation to cold extended into the lower cervical dermatomes in some cases. There were no reports of respiratory difficulties in these studies, presumably because dense motor block occurs at least four dermatomes lower than the measured sensory block. If the sensory block appears high then good motor function can be verified if the mother has full strength in her hands. If surgery is urgent, a large initial bolus of local anaesthetic is required for rapid reliable onset of anaesthesia. Lucas found that, after a low dose epidural for labour,[49] 20 ml 0.5% bupivacaine took a median duration of 4 min longer (14 min 11–19) than a 50 : 50 mixture of bupivacaine and lidocaine with epinephrine (12 min 8.8–17) or lidocaine with epinephrine (10 min 9–18). The blocks in which only bupivacaine was used, were the most reliable in terms of onset time and requiring least supplementation. This study supports my own clinical observations that lidocaine containing solutions can fail

- Have a carefully assessed and well spread epidural block in labour.
- Early inclusion of the anaesthetist if Caesarean section is possible, before the actual decision is made.
- Top-up the epidural as early as possible if time is limited.
- Unless a very recent top-up in labour has been given, then 20 ml of solution (see above) is generally required.
- Topping-up in the delivery room is controversial but saves a lot of time. Once a top-up is given, stay with the mother at all times, be able to measure her blood pressure and have ephedrine mixed and immediately available. Staying with the mother is essential if the top-up is given in the delivery room or theatre.
- The safest position during transfer of the mother is the full lateral position.
- If there is any inequality in the spread of the block on initial assessment then put the mother in the full lateral position on that side and then give the top-up.
- Transfer her to the operating theatre as early as possible.

Box 9.1   Rapid conversion of an epidural for labour to anaesthesia for emergency Caesarean section.

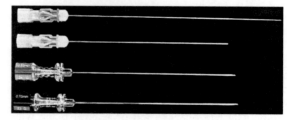

Figure 9.3   Spinal needles for Caesarean section: Top to bottom 119 mm 27G Whitacre; 90 mm 25G Whitacre; 90 mm 24G Sprotte; 90 mm 22G Sprotte.

Intrathecal bupivacaine

The dose of bupivacaine which produces a reliable block, may depend on patient height, although evidence for this is lacking. Unless the mother is very tall or very short, other factors have a greater influence on the spread of the anaesthetic, such as patient positioning and size of the pregnancy. By reducing the dose of intrathecal bupivacaine to less than 10 mg, without an opioid, the risk of an inadequate block increases, with 70% of mothers complaining of intra-operative pain.[56]

Patient position

Patient position does not have a major impact on the final block height, but does influence the rate of onset and spread of the block. The sitting position is commonly used because many anaesthetists can perform the injection more quickly. Ingis found that[57] although the cephalic spread of the block occurred more quickly in the lateral position, the time from start of injection to completed block was similar between the sitting and lateral groups, because there was quicker identification of CSF in the sitting group. When plain bupivacaine was investigated, which is slightly hypobaric to CSF, the right lateral position was preferable because the block spreads more evenly after the mother was placed in the supine position with left lateral tilt. The final height of the block is again similar between the right and left lateral position after postural manipulation.[58] The right lateral position is also acceptable when hyperbaric solutions are used because the right dermatomes are anaesthetized initially followed by the left side, once the mother is placed in the supine left wedge position.

unexpectedly and that bupivacaine 0.5% remains a good choice for Caesarean section. It is not known if levo-bupivacaine is equally effective in this situation, but as it seems to work in a similar way to bupivacaine, there is a theoretical safety advantage in its use for emergency Caesarean, where large boluses are given rapidly.

SPINAL ANAESTHESIA

Spinal anaesthesia is popular because of its relative simplicity, reliability and quick onset time[52] compared to epidural anaesthesia. When spinal anaesthesia was first investigated in the early 1980s its potential was recognized[53] but it seemed unlikely that it would become popular, with post-dural puncture headache rates of 13–24%.[54] With smaller needles and atraumatic pencil point tips, headache rates have declined to less than 1%[55] (Fig. 9.3).

Plain or hyperbaric solutions

Plain and hyperbaric solutions are thought to behave differently when injected into the CSF. Plain solutions tend to spread further, last for a shorter time and are less reliable in the non-pregnant patient. In pregnancy, subarachnoid injection of 12.5 mg of both solutions reliably and equally reach the upper thoracic dermatomes.[54] If a small dose of bupivacaine is used, e.g. 6.6 mg, with intrathecal sufentanil, the plain solutions seemed less reliable than an equal amount of heavy bupivacaine.[59] Small doses of intrathecal bupivacaine followed by epidural top-ups are becoming popular as part of the CSE technique (see later).

Volume of injectate

The spread of intrathecal bupivacaine is related to the mass or mg of the drug rather than the volume of its dilutent. Thus 0.25% bupivacaine has been used safely[60] not were there any significant differences either in rate of onset or final block height when 12 ml of 0.125% bupivacaine was compared to 3 ml of 0.5% bupivacaine.[61] Smaller volumes tend to be used because they are more convenient.

Pregnant versus non-pregnant

The dose of bupivacaine required for spinal anaesthesia in pregnancy is less than in similar non-pregnant women.[62] Women needed 25% more spinal anaesthetic to achieve similar blocks for post-partum tubal ligation compared to Caesarean section. This effect is at least partly the result of engorged epidural veins due to venocaval obstruction, which reduces epidural and CSF volume.[63] This effect is seen from the second trimester of pregnancy[64] and is more pronounced with twin pregnancies.[65]

COMBINED SPINAL EPIDURAL ANAESTHESIA

There are several different techniques for combined spinal-epidural anaesthesia. Different authors recommend their own technique, quoting different failure rates. In 1992 Lyons used a 30G spinal needle and found a 16% failure rate in the needle through needle group compared with 4% in the sequential group. He went on to recommend the separate approach, although the mothers did not like having two injections.[66] Westbrook used a 26G needle and identified the dura in 93% of cases using the needle through needle technique. Although the technique was said to be technically perfect in 88% of cases, 26% needed epidural supplementation before start of surgery.[67] In the sitting position, because of the time it took to insert, flush and fix the epidural catheter, the heavy bupivacaine resulted in a low block, which had to be extended in 74% of cases with the epidural catheter.[68] Randalls showed however that if the lateral position was used then the spinal component was satisfactory in all cases.[69]

Different spinal needles and different levels of expertise result in different failure rates for a CSE.[70] Feeling the dural puncture as a slight give or 'click' with a conical tipped needle improves success, as does choosing a needle with a low internal resistance to CSF. A failure rate of less than 5% can be achieved.[71,72]

Despite some technical difficulties, the CSE demands attention because it both increases the reliability of the epidural[73] and improves the flexibility of the spinal anaesthesia. Spinal anaesthesia produces reliable anaesthesia for Caesarean section for about 90 min and sometimes barely an hour. For routine surgery this may be adequate, but in many situations this is not so. The CSE technique is therefore particularly useful for emergency trial of instrumental vaginal delivery with possible Caesarean section or potentially prolonged elective Caesarean, i.e. repeat Caesarean, or Caesarean with tubal ligation.

THE TECHNIQUE OF NEEDLE THROUGH NEEDLE CSE

- A spinal needle that is about 20 mm longer than a Tuohy needle is required. A 119 mm low resistance 25G or 27G whitacre needle is ideal.
- The sitting position is acceptable.
- The inter-vertebral space must be chosen with care. The L3–4 inter-space is the best choice, as it is easy to be inaccurate by one space. If the L2–3 space is chosen then it may be L1–2 and therefore the conus of the cord is in danger. If a very low inter-space is used, then in my experience, the technique fails more often.
- The epidural space is ideally found by using saline.
- Remove the stylet of the spinal needle before use. CSF can then immediately appear at its hub, confirming correct placement in the CSF.
- The spinal needle is then passed through the Tuohy needle. If the needle is held like a pencil then the subtle feelings of the needle as it passes through the hubber tip of the Tuohy needle and through the dura can be felt most easily.
- If saline has been used to identify the epidural space, a small amount remains at the end of the Tuohy needle. As the spinal needle indents the dura, the saline is drawn into the needle and as the dura is pierced and springs back, one drop of saline comes back from the end of the Tuohy needle. Feeling the dural 'click' followed by a saline drop from the Tuohy needle is the best way to assess accurate placement of the spinal needle. It is also possible that air can be drawn into the CSF by the springing back of the dura, if air has been used to identify the epidural space.

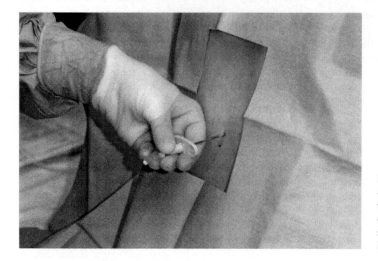

Figure 9.4   The operator's hand resting on the patients back with thumb and forefinger pinching the long spinal needle as it emerges from the Tuohy needle will stabilize the spinal needle during intrathecal injection.

- The spinal needle should not be advanced further, once placement has been confirmed by the appearance of CSF.
- Advancing the spinal needle unnecessarily to its full extent may increase failure due to crossing of the dural sac or increase the risk of neural damage.
- By resting the inner or outer aspect of the operator's hand against the patients back, the spinal and Tuohy needle can be held together by thumb and forefinger (Fig. 9.4). This prevents the spinal needle from moving in relation to the Tuohy needle. Various ratchet or holding devices can be used at this stage if a specially designed CSE kit is used.
- Once the spinal injection is given, the epidural catheter should be placed as quickly as possible. Once the epidural catheter is sited and the Tuohy needle removed, the mother should be put on her side if she was initially sitting. The catheter can then be withdrawn to an appropriate length, flushed and fixed.

The sequential block

Increasing the intrathecal dose of bupivacaine increases the reliability of the final block but at the expense of more haemodynamic instability. The sequential block, where a smaller initial spinal dose is given first and then supplemented by injection into the epidural space, may reduce the incidence and severity of hypotension. The size of the initial spinal dose, preload, ephedrine use and positioning the patient will also influence the incidence of hypotension. Thoren[74] found no difference between sequential CSE and full dose spinal injection in either recorded episodes of hypotension or ephedrine usage

but Rawal,[68] Patel[75] and Vercauteren[59] found a lower incidence of hypotension.

Squeezing effect of epidural injection on subarachnoid block

Injecting fluid into the epidural space can influence the height of the spinal block. Ten to Twenty minutes after a spinal injection, 10 ml of epidural fluid (either saline or bupivacaine 0.5%) can influence the cephalad spread of the block.[76] This is due to a volume effect; squeezing the dural sac. As little as 5 ml of saline can compress the CSF volume by 40%.[77] A large volume of saline injected into the epidural space, 80 min after spinal injection, has caused a rapid total spinal. The concept of early fixing of bupivacaine to spinal tissues may be incorrect.

Advantage

This squeezing effect with saline can be used to enhance a subarachnoid block without the use of further bupivacaine. A low dose spinal of less then 10 mg bupivacaine with an opioid, has been used as part of a CSE technique with good effect. The advantage of the technique is that the length of time the mother is blocked after her Caesarean is reduced, which the mothers prefer.[59] The anaesthetist can also extend the spinal block without changing the mother's position.

Disadvantage

A standard epidural dose injected after a subarachnoid injection can lead to rapid total spinal block. A safe approach to take is that after a CSE an initial epidural injection should not be made within 10 min of the spinal injection and then the volume should not exceed 5 ml every 5 min for the next 20 min. There must also be careful assessment of the block between each top-up.

SPINAL INJECTION AFTER EPIDURAL INJECTION

An exaggerated response to a spinal injection has been reported after failed epidural top-up for Caesarean section.[78–80] A volume effect is thought to be the mechanism (as above).

Although there is an increased risk of high spinal block after failed epidural top-up, even if a reduced spinal dose is used, i.e. 10 mg, the risk has not been quantified. In an audit of 72 spinal blocks after failed epidural, there were no reports of high blocks.[81] Over half of these women received the standard spinal dose of 12.5 mg bupivacaine.

If the spinal block is necessary because the epidural has not been topped up, or has fallen out, then a standard dose should be used. If the problem is a good epidural block that has either failed to spread to the sacral dermatomes or high enough into the thoracic dermatomes for Caesarean, then reduce the dose of heavy bupivacaine by 25%. The mother should then be carefully positioned with several pillows behind shoulders and head, which will control the height of the block.

INTRATHECAL AND EPIDURAL OPIOIDS

Intrathecal and epidural opioids can be added to the local anaesthetic solution, to reduce intra-operative discomfort and give prolonged post-operative pain-relief.

FENTANYL

Epidural fentanyl is a good adjunct to local anaesthetic solutions because it improves intra-operative comfort for the mother.[82,83] Noble used 100 μg and found the effect good, but two mothers had respiratory depression within a short time of the injection. Although respiratory depression has been reported, it occurs early when the mother is likely to be under close observation. Naulty[84] studied doses of fentanyl between 0 and 100 μg. He found that doses above 50 μg improved intra-operative comfort compared to placebo, and 50, 75 and 100 μg were equally effective at reducing intra-operative discomfort and provided about 4 h of post-operative pain relief. His recommended 50 μg as the optimal dose.

Intrathecal fentanyl has been studied in doses of 6.25–25 μg; 15 and 12.5 μg have been used to good effect.[69] Hunt[85] found 6.25 μg to be effective and increasing the dose to 12.5, 25, 37.5 or 50 μg did not significantly reduce intra-operative pain or increase post-operative pain-relief beyond 4 h.

The addition of fentanyl to morphine is more controversial. The theoretical advantage is that the onset of fentanyl is rapid, giving good intra-operative conditions, whilst morphine takes 60 min to have maximal effect.[86] Connelly[87] found the mixture of 10 μg fentanyl with 100 μg morphine reduced intra-operative pain, especially if the uterus was exteriorized. Sibilla[88] could not confirm these findings and felt that morphine alone gave good intra-operative pain-relief and prolonged post-operative pain-relief.

MORPHINE

Epidural morphine 3 mg is effective when given epidurally for the treatment of post-operative pain[89] but increasing the dose increases the side effects without improving the quality or duration of analgesia.

Intrathecal morphine 0.2 mg is effective when given intrathecally.[90] In a comparison of 0.1 and 0.2 mg intrathecal morphine, the lower dose gave equal post-operative analgesia with less nausea and vomiting.

DIAMORPHINE

Diamorphine 0.25 mg intrathecally and 5 mg epidurally produces similar quality and duration of analgesia,[91] although these investigators found a reduced problem of nausea and vomiting in the intrathecal group. Graham[92] found that 0.3 mg intrathecally was effective and in a dose finding study Kelly[93] found that 0.125, 0.25 and 0.375 mg were all effective and safe, but analgesia and side effects were dose dependant. Skilton[94] came to a similar conclusion that 0.3 mg was superior to the smaller doses with an acceptable increase in side effects.

Diclofenac

Many of the above studies have used intrathecal or epidural opioids in conjunction with rectal diclofenac 100 mg given at the end of surgery. Diclofenac has a marked morphine sparing effect[95] and the above regimes are considerably less effective when given without a non-steroidal anti-inflammatory. Diclofenac and a single dose of diamorphine 3 mg resulted in 92% of mothers with pain scores of 30 or less and nobody required additional opioids other than oral co-dydramol.

SAFETY

The use of intrathecal or epidural opioids has reduced the incidence of intra-operative pain for the mother, and may give her a prolonged period of excellent post-operative analgesia, which is superior to that of intravenous opioids.[96,97] The safety of using long acting spinal opioids without high dependency facilities has been questioned. Amongst obstetric patients, the incidence of respiratory depression with these doses of morphine or diamorphine, is very low. As long as systemic opioids are avoided, we use routine post-operative observations, for all types of opioid administration. During the first 2 h, observations are made half hourly, then hourly for 2 h, then 4 hourly for the rest of that 24 h. As well as blood pressure and pulse we observe and record pain and sedation scores as well as respiratory rate.

REFERENCES

1. Brown GW, Russell IF. A survey of anaesthesia for caesarean section. *Int J Obstet Anesth* 1995; **4**(4): 214–218.

2. Association T.A.o.A.o.G.B.a.I.a.T.O.A. *Guidelines for obstetric anaesthetic services.* The Association of Anaesthetists, 1998.

3. Morgan BM et al. Anaesthesia for caesarean section. A medical audit of junior anaesthetic staff practice. *Br J Anaesth* 1983; **55**(9): 885–889.

4. Lao TT, Halpern SH, Crosby ET. Anesthesia and blood loss in preterm cesarean section: comparison between general and regional anesthesia. *Int J Obstet Anesth* 1993; **2**(2): 85–88.

5. Shir Y et al. Postoperative morbidity is similar in patients anesthetized with epidural and general anesthesia for radical prostatectomy. *Urology* 1994; **44**(2): 232–236.

6. Morgan BM et al. Anaesthetic morbidity following caesarean section under epidural or general anaesthesia. *Lancet* 1984; **1**(8372): 328–330.

7. Shir Y, Raja SN, Frank SM. The effect of epidural versus general anesthesia on postoperative pain and analgesic requirements in patients undergoing radical prostatectomy (see comments). *Anesthesiology* 1994; **80**(1): 49–56.

8. Asantila R et al. Epidural analgesia with 4 mg of morphine after caesarean section: modulating effect of epidural block compared to general anaesthesia. *Int J Obstet Anesth* 1995; **4**(2): 89–92.

9. Eckstein KL, Marx GF. Aortocaval compression and uterine displacement. *Anesthesiology* 1974; **40**(1): 92–96.

10. Mills GH, Chaffe AG. Sleeping positions adopted by pregnant women of more than 30 weeks gestation. *Anaesthesia* 1994; **49**(3): 249–250.

11. Stoneham M et al. Oxford positioning technique improves haemodynamic stability and predictability of block height of spinal anaesthesia for elective caesarean section. *Int J Obstet Anesth* 1999; **8**(4): 242–248.

12. Kinsella SM, Norris MC. Advance prediction of hypotension at cesarean delivery under spinal anesthesia. *Int J Obstet Anesth* 1996; **5**(1): 3–7.

13. Kinsella SM, Whitwam JG, Spencer JAD. Aortic compression by the uterus: identification with the Finapres digital arterial pressure instrument. *Br J Obstet Gynecol* 1990; **97**: 700–705.

14. Carrie LE. An inflatable obstetric anaesthetic 'wedge'. *Anaesthesia* 1982; **37**(7): 745–747.

15. Alahuhta S et al. Uteroplacental haemodynamics during spinal anaesthesia for caesarean section with two types of uterine displacement. *Int J Obstet Anesth* 1994; **3**(4): 187–192.

16. Marx GF, Mateo CV. Effects of different oxygen concentrations during general anaesthesia for elective caesarean section. *Can Anaesth Soc J* 1971; **18**(6): 587–593.

17. Rout CC et al. A reevaluation of the role of crystalloid preload in the prevention of hypotension associated with spinal anesthesia for elective cesarean section. *Anesthesiology* 1993; **79**(2): 262–269.

18. Jackson R, Reid JA, Thorburn J. Volume preloading is not essential to prevent spinal-induced hypotension at caesarean section (see comments). *Br J Anaesth* 1995; **75**(3): 262–265.

19. Park GE et al. The effects of varying volumes of crystalloid administration before cesarean delivery on maternal hemodynamics and colloid osmotic pressure. *Anesth Analg* 1996; **83**(2): 299–303.

20. Norris MC. Hypotension during spinal anesthesia for cesarean section. Does it affect neonatal outcome. *Reg Anesth* 1987; **12**: 191–193.

21. Mathru M et al. Intravenous albumin administration for prevention of spinal hypotension during cesarean section. *Anesth Analg* 1980; **59**(9): 655–658.

22. Murray AM, Morgan M, Whitwam JG. Crystalloid versus colloid for circulatory preload for epidural caesarean section (see comments). *Anaesthesia* 1989; **44**(6): 463–466.

23. Vercauteren MP et al. Hydroxyethylstarch compared with modified gelatin as volume preload before spinal anaesthesia for Caesarean section. *Br J Anaesth* 1996; **76**(5): 731–733.

24. Rout CC et al. Prophylactic intramuscular ephedrine prior to Caesarean section (see comments). *Anaesth Intens Care* 1992; **20**(4): 448–452.

25. Chan WS et al. Prevention of hypotension during spinal anaesthesia for caesarean section: ephedrine infusion versus fluid preload. *Anaesthesia* 1997; **52**(9): 908–913.

26. Kang YG, Abouleish E, Caritis S. Prophylactic intravenous ephedrine infusion during spinal anesthesia for cesarean section. *Anesth Analg* 1982; **61**(10): 839–842.

27. Hall PA et al. Spinal anaesthesia for caesarean section: comparison of infusions of phenylephrine and ephedrine. *Br J Anaesth* 1994; **73**(4): 471–474.

28. Conn DA et al. Changes in pulmonary function tests during spinal anaesthesia for caesarean section. *Int J Obstet Anesth* 1993; **2**(1): 12–14.

29. Harrop-Griffiths AW et al. Regional anaesthesia and cough effectiveness. A study in patients undergoing Caesarean section. *Anaesthesia* 1991; **46**(1): 11–13.

30. Gamil M. Serial peak expiratory flow rates in mothers during caesarean section under extradural anaesthesia. *Br J Anaesth* 1989; **62**(4): 415–418.

31. Kelly MC, Fitzpatrick KTJ, Hill DA. Peak now rates during and after caesarean section under spinal anaesthesia and the need for supplementary oxygen. *Int J Obstet Anesth* 1995; **4**(3): 180–181.

32. Bassell GM, Marx GF. Optimization of fetal oxygenation. *Int J Obstet Anesth* 1995; **4**(4): 238–243.

33. Milne MK, Lawson JI. Epidural analgesia for Caesarean section. A review of 182 cases. *Br J Anaesth* 1973; **45**(12): 1206–1210.

34. Thorburn J, Moir DD. Epidural analgesia for elective Caesarean section. Technique and its assessment. *Anaesthesia* 1980; **35**(1): 3–6.

35. Crawford JS. Experiences with lumbar extradural analgesia for caesarean section. *Br J Anaesth* 1980; **52**(8): 821–825.

36. Fernando R, Jones HM. Comparison of plain and alkalinized local anaesthetic mixtures of lignocaine and bupivacaine for elective extradural caesarean section. *Br J Anaesth* 1991; **67**(6): 699–703.

37. Russell IF. Levels of anaesthesia and intraoperative pain at caesarean section under regional block. *Int J Obstet Anesth* 1995; **4**(2): 71–77.

38. Brull SJ, Greene NM. Zones of differential sensory block during extradural anaesthesia. *Br J Anaesth* 1991; **66**(6): 651–655.

39. Rocco AG et al. Differential spread of blockade of touch, cold, and pinprick during spinal anesthesia. *Anesth Analg* 1985; **64**(9): 917–923.

40. Alahuhta S et al. Visceral pain during caesarean section under spinal and epidural anaesthesia with bupivacaine. *Acta Anaesthesiol Scand* 1990; **34**(2): 95–98.

41. Crawford JS, Burton M, Davies P. Anaesthesia for section: further refinements of a technique. *Br J Anaesth* 1973; **45**(7): 726–732.

42. Dutton DA et al. Choice of local anaesthetic drug for extradural caesarean section. Comparison of 0.5% and 0.75% bupivacaine and 1.5% etidocaine. *Br J Anaesth* 1984; **56**(12): 1361–1368.

43. Laishley RS, Morgan BM. A single dose epidural technique for Caesarean section. A comparison between 0.5% bupivacaine plain and 0.5% bupivacaine with adrenaline. *Anaesthesia* 1988; **43**(2): 100–103.

44. Scanlon JW et al. Neurobehavioral responses of newborn infants after maternal epidural anesthesia. *Anesthesiology* 1974; **40**(2): 121–128.

45. Kileff ME et al. Neonatal neurobehavioral responses after epidural anesthesia for cesarean section using lidocaine and bupivacaine. *Anesth Analg* 1984; **63**(4): 413–417.

46. Abboud TK et al. Epidural bupivacaine, chloroprocaine, or lidocaine for cesarean section – maternal and neonatal effects. *Anesth Analg* 1983; **62**(10): 914–919.

47. Norton AC, Davis AG, Spicer RJ. Lignocaine 2% with adrenaline for epidural caesarean section. A comparison with 0.5% bupivacaine (see comments). *Anaesthesia* 1988; **43**(10): 844–849.

48. Clark V et al. Speed of onset of sensory block for elective extradural caesarean section: choice of agent and temperature of injectate (see comments). *Br J Anaesth* 1994; **72**(2): 221–223.

49. Lucas DN, Ciccone GK, Yentis SM. Extending low-dose epidural analgesia for emergency Caesarean section. A comparison of three solutions (see comments). *Anaesthesia* 1999; **54**(12): 1173–1177.

50. Milne MK et al. The extension of labour epidural analgesia for Caesarean section. *Anaesthesia* 1979; **34**(10): 992–995.

51. Dickson MA, Jenkins J. Extension of epidural blockade for emergency caesarean section. Assessment of a bolus dose of bupivacaine 0.5% 10 ml following an infusion of 0.1% for analgesia in labour. *Anaesthesia* 1994; **49**(7): 636–638.

52. Helbo-Hansen S et al. Subarachnoid versus epidural bupivacaine 0.5% for caesarean section. *Acta Anaesthesiol Scand* 1988; **32**(6): 473–476.

53. Russell IF. Spinal anaesthesia for caesarean section. The use of 0.5% bupivacaine. *Br J Anaesth* 1983; **55**(4): 309–314.

54. Russell IF, Holmqvist EL. Subarachnoid analgesia for caesarean section. A double-blind comparison of plain and hyperbaric 0.5% bupivacaine. *Br J Anaesth* 1987; **59**(3): 347–353.

55. Hopkinson JM et al. A comparative multicentre trial of spinal needles for Caesarean section. *Anaesthesia* 1997; **52**(10): 1005–1011.

56. Pedersen H et al. Incidence of visceral pain during cesarean section: the effect of varying doses of spinal bupivacaine. *Anesth Analg* 1989; **69**(1): 46–49.

57. Inglis A, Daniel M, McGrady E. Maternal position during induction of spinal anaesthesia for caesarean section. A comparison of right lateral and sitting positions (see comments). *Anaesthesia* 1995; **50**(4): 363–365.

58. Russell IF. Effect of posture during the induction of subarachnoid analgesia for caesarean section. Right v. left lateral. *Br J Anaesth* 1987; **59**(3): 342–346.

59. Vercauteren MP et al. Small-dose hyperbaric versus plain bupivacaine during spinal anesthesia for cesarean section. *Anesth Analg* 1998; **86**(5): 989–993.

60. Chung CJ et al. Spinal anaesthesia with 0.25% hyperbaric bupivacaine for Caesarean section: effects of volume (see comments). *Br J Anaesth* 1996; **77**(2): 145–149.

61. Vucevic M, Russell IF. Spinal anaesthesia for Caesarean section: 0.125% plain bupivacaine 12 ml compared with 0.5% plain bupivacaine 3 ml. *Br J Anaesth* 1992; **68**(6): 590–595.

62. Abouleish EI. Postpartum tubal ligation requires more bupivacaine for spinal anesthesia than does cesarean section. *Anesth Analg* 1986; **65**(8): 897–900.

63. Hirabayashi Y et al. Soft tissue anatomy within the vertebral canal in pregnant women. *Br J Anaesth* 1996; **77**(2): 153–156.

64. Hirabayashi Y et al. Spread of subarachnoid hyperbaric amethocaine in pregnant women. *Br J Anaesth* 1995; **74**(4): 384–386.

65. Jawan B et al. Spread of spinal anaesthesia for caesarean section in singleton and twin pregnancies. *Br J Anaesth* 1993; **70**(6): 639–641.

66. Lyons G, Macdonald R, Mikl B. Combined epidural/spinal anaesthesia for caesarean section. Through the needle or in separate spaces? (see comments). *Anaesthesia* 1992; **47**(3): 199–201.

67. Westbrook JL, Carrie LE. Combined spinal/epidural anaesthesia for caesarean section (letter; comment). *Anaesthesia* 1993; **48**(2): 172–173.

68. Rawal N, Schollin J, Wesstrom G. Epidural versus combined spinal epidural block for cesarean section (see comments). *Acta Anaesthesiol Scand* 1988; **32**(1): 61–66.

69. Randalls B et al. Comparison of four subarachnoid solutions in a needle-through-needle technique for elective caesarean section. *Br J Anaesth* 1991; **66**(3): 314–318.

70. Westbrook JL, Renowden SA, Carrie LE. Study of the anatomy of the extradural region using magnetic resonance imaging. *Br J Anaesth* 1993; **71**(4): 495–498.

71. Swami A et al. Combined spinal and epidural anaesthesia for caesarean section: use of small dose subarachnoid injection. *Int J Obstet Anesth* 1993; **2**(1).

72. Patel M, Swami A. Combined spinal-extradural anaesthesia for caesarean section (letter; comment). *Anaesth* 1992; **47**(11): 1005–1006.

73. Davies SJ et al. Maternal experience during epidural or combined spinal-epidural anaesthesia for cesarean section: a prospective, randomized trial. *Anesth Analg* 1997; **85**(3): 607–613.

74. Thoren T et al. Sequential combined spinal epidural block versus spinal block for cesarean section: effects on maternal hypotension and neurobehavioral function of the newborn (see comments). *Anesth Analg* 1994; **78**(6): 1087–1092.

75. Patel M, Craig R, Laishley R. A comparison between epidural anaesthesia using alkalinized solution and spinal (combined spinal/epidural) anaesthesia for elective caesarean section. *Int J Obstet Anesth* 1996; **5**(4): 236–239.

76. Blumgart CH et al. Mechanism of extension of spinal anaesthesia by extradural injection of local anaesthetic. *Br J Anaesth* 1992; **69**(5): 457–460.

77. Takiguchi T et al. The effect of epidural saline injection on analgesic level during combined spinal and epidural anesthesia assessed clinically and myelographically (see comments). *Anesth Analg* 1997; **85**(5): 1097–1100.

78. Kick O, Bohrer H. Unexpectedly high spinal anaesthesia following failed extradural anaesthesia for caesarean section (letter; comment). *Anaesthesia* 1993; **48**(3): 271.

79. Dell RG, Orlikowski CE. Unexpectedly high spinal anaesthesia following failed extradural anaesthesia for caesarean section (letter; comment). *Anaesthesia* 1993; **48**(7): 641.

80. Gupta A et al. Spinal anaesthesia for caesarean section following epidural analgesia in labour: a relative contraindication. *Int J Obstet Anesth* 1994; **3**(3): 153–156.

81. Simpson DS, McGrady E. Spinal anaesthesia following failed epidural anaesthesia for instrumental or operative delivery. *Int J Obstet Anesth* 1999; **8**: 211.

82. Noble DW et al. Adrenaline, fentanyl or adrenaline and fentanyl as adjuncts to bupivacaine for extradural anaesthesia in elective caesarean section. *Br J Anaesth* 1991; **66**(6): 645–650.

83. Gaffud MP et al. Surgical analgesia for cesarean delivery with epidural bupivacaine and fentanyl. *Anesthesiology* 1986; **65**(3): 331–334.

84. Naulty JS et al. Epidural fentanyl for postcesarean delivery pain management. *Anesthesiology* 1985; **63**(6): 694–698.

85. Hunt CO et al. Perioperative analgesia with subarachnoid fentanyl-bupivacaine for cesarean delivery. *Anesthesiology* 1989; **71**(4): 535–540.

86. Leighton BL et al. Intrathecal narcotics for labor revisited: the combination of fentanyl and morphine intrathecally provides rapid onset of profound, prolonged analgesia. *Anesth Analg* 1989; **69**(1): 122–125.

87. Connelly NR et al. The use of fentanyl added to morphine-lidocaine-epinephrine spinal solution in patients undergoing cesarean section. *Anesth Analg* 1994; **78**(5): 918–920.

88. Sibilla C et al. Perioperative analgesia for caesarean section: comparison of intrathecal morphine and fentanyl alone or in combination. *Int J Obstet Anesth* 1997; **6**(1): 43–48.

89. Hanson AL, Hanson B, Matousek M. Epidural anesthesia for cesarean section. The effect of morphine-bupivacaine administered epidurally for intra and postoperative pain relief. *Acta Obstet Gynecol Scand* 1984; **63**(2): 135–140.

90. Abouleish E et al. Combined intrathecal morphine and bupivacaine for cesarean section. *Anesth Analg* 1988; **67**(4): 370–374.

91. Hallworth SP et al. Comparison of intrathecal and epidural diamorphine for elective caesarean section using a combined spinal-epidural technique. *Br J Anaesth* 1999; **82**(2): 228–232.

92. Graham D, Russell IF. A double-blind assessment of the analgesic sparing effect of intrathecal diamorphine (0.3 mg) with spinal anaesthesia for elective caesarean section. *Int J Obstet Anesth* 1997; **6**(4): 224–230.

93. Kelly MC, Carabine UA, Mirakhur RK. Intrathecal diamorphine for analgesia after caesarean section. A dose finding study and assessment of side-effects. *Anaesthesia* 1998; **53**(3): 231–237.

94. Skilton RWH et al. Dose response study of subarachnoid diamorphine for analgesia after elective caesarean section. *Int J Obstet Anesth* 1999; **8**(4): 231–235.

95. Luthman J, Kay NH, White JB. The morphine sparing effect of diclofenac sodium following caesarean section under spinal anaesthesia. *Int J Obstet Anesth* 1994; **3**(2): 82–86.

96. Rapp-Zingraff N et al. Analgesia after caesarean section: patient-controlled intravenous morphine vs epidural morphine. *Int J Obstet Anesth* 1997; **6**(2): 87–92.

97. Sibilla C et al. Pain relief after caesarean section: comparison of different techniques of morphine administration. *Int J Obstet Anesth* 1994; **3**(4): 203–207.

10

ANAESTHESIA FOR THE DISTRESSED FETUS AND MAJOR OBSTETRIC HAEMORRHAGE

Stephanie Watts & Rachel E. Collis

INTRODUCTION

Anaesthetists have four points to consider when deciding on the method of anaesthesia for emergency Caesarean section, in the presence of fetal distress:

- How urgent is the Caesarean section?
- Maternal safety
- Fetal well-being
- Available anaesthetic skill.

In order to determine 'how urgent is urgent' the labour ward anaesthetist needs to be familiar with intrapartum fetal monitoring and its interpretation, and to understand the relationship between maternal and fetal factors which lead to the decision to operate. Maternal safety is of paramount importance and takes priority over all other factors, when deciding anaesthetic technique, but fetal well-being is also important as we wish to deliver a baby in the best possible condition given the circumstances.

Fetal distress is usually the result of a number of factors, some of which are predictable. Surveys of fetal distress in labour have shown that the sudden onset of fetal distress without previous warning signs is unusual. It has been shown that approximately 13% of fetal distress is of truly sudden onset. This means that more than 80% of emergency Caesarean sections for fetal distress, occur in mothers who could have had contact with an anaesthetist before their operative delivery. Team work is essential on the labour ward to ensure that both obstetricians and anaesthetists provide optimum care (Fig. 10.1).

FETAL DISTRESS AND ITS ORIGINS

The distressed fetus receives an inadequate oxygen supply for its needs, leading to an accumulation of lactate (metabolic acidosis). This in turn triggers the release of neurotoxic compounds, namely excitatory amino acids (glutamine) and oxygen radicals, leading to neurone damage. Increasing hypoxia and metabolic acidosis causes fetal heart rate changes, but the important measurement is the base deficit with the figure of $-11\,ml/l$, taken as the threshold for cerebral dysfunction.

The normal fetus develops a stress response during labour, releasing catecholamines, which help it withstand hypoxia during contractions and periods of asphyxia. This stress response helps maintain blood flow to the brain, heart, adrenal glands and placenta and also causes fetal bradycardia. Fetal catecholamines also contribute to neonatal adaptation post-delivery,

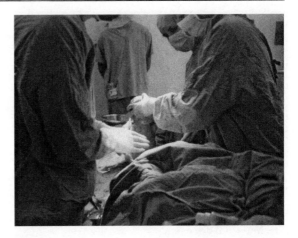

Figure 10.1

by increasing cardiac output, lung liquid absorption, release of surfactant, glucose and fatty acids and activating non-shivering thermogenisis. Preservation of this stress response is advantageous especially in the distressed fetus.

Detection of fetal distress in labour currently relies on CTG monitoring and fetal scalp blood sampling. The CTG may show non-reassuring heart rate patterns, such as tachycardia greater than 160 beats/min or type I or II bradycardia. In situations of non-reassuring CTG patterns, fetal blood sampling can be used and the fetal scalp pH measured. A pH of less than 7.20 is generally taken as the cut off point for delivery. The use of sequential sampling to show increasing acidosis, in combination with other factors, may lead to delivery before the pH reaches 7.2. Evidence of severe distress, i.e. unrecoverable bradycardia of less than 80 beats/min, or pH less than 7.0 needs immediate delivery.

By identifying mothers with a fetus at increased risk of distress, anaesthetic intervention at an early stage can be facilitated. This will decrease the need for emergency general or subarachnoid anaesthesia for immediate delivery in a patient unknown to the anaesthetist.

MATERNAL PROBLEMS CONTRIBUTING TO FETAL DISTRESS

Any maternal conditions which lead to decreased placental blood flow can lead to fetal distress. The commonest causes are shown in Box 10.1.

PLACENTAL PROBLEMS CONTRIBUTING TO FETAL DISTRESS

Placental insufficiency may be acute or chronic. Acute insufficiency is usually due to interruption of placental

- **Age:** at the extremes of reproductive life. The young mother is more likely to develop pre-eclampsia and intra-uterine growth restriction. The older mother may have other maternal disease associated with poor placental flow.
- **Parity:** the first and fourth or greater are associated with higher risk. This may be age related.
- **Socio-economic factors:** higher risk of maternal problems in the lower socio-economic groups.
- **Cigarette smoking:** can lead to chronic placental insufficiency.
- **Maternal disease:**
  — previous hypertension,
  — renal disease,
  — diabetes mellitus,
  — cardiac disease,
  — chronic anaemia.

Box 10.1

blood flow, and chronic is the result of placental tissue inadequacy.

During a uterine contraction, placental blood flow decreases, even in a healthy placenta. As contractions start, the myometrial veins are occluded, decreasing venous outflow. As the contractions become stronger, inflow decreases as uterine pressure exceeds arterial inflow pressure. This normal decrease in fetal oxygen supply becomes significant if other factors decrease the fetus's ability to cope with hypoxia, i.e. prematurity, infection, congenital anomaly, etc.

ACUTE PLACENTAL INSUFFICIENCY

ANTEPARTUM HAEMORRHAGE

Moderate to severe haemorrhage from the placenta leads to acute insufficiency. Bleeding occurs from the maternal circulation, but 25–30% of the mother's intravascular volume can be lost before significant changes in maternal vital signs are noticed. Fetal heart rate changes usually occur before the mother becomes hypotensive.

Placenta previa

Twenty per cent of antepartum haemorrhage is due to placenta previa. It presents as painless bright red vaginal

bleeding with vaginal clots. The bleeding can start suddenly and without provocation, but 25% will be associated with uterine contractions. The highest incidence occurs between 32 and 34 weeks gestation and if haemorrhage is not severe, tocolysis may be used to suppress contractions, if the bleeding settles.

Vasa previa

This is where there is a velementos insertion of the cord with the vessels lying in the membranes covering the internal os in front of the presenting part. Rupture of the membrane in labour leads to a rupture of the vessels and massive fetal and maternal blood loss. Severe fetal distress or even fetal death can rapidly occur.

Placental abruption

This is separation of part of the placenta before delivery. This disrupts the fetal blood supply at the placental implant site and leads to rapid maternal blood loss. Abruption may be concealed, with blood clot behind the placenta or in the broad ligament, or revealed with blood loss per vagina. Risk factors for abruption include:

- maternal hypertension,
- previous history of abruptions,
- abdominal wall trauma,
- smoking,
- increasing maternal age,
- uterine fibroids.

Patients with abruption present with pain (tender uterus) and strong uterine contractions with or without a dark red vaginal blood loss. The uterus may also appear larger than gestational age. The strong uterine contractions may force placental tissue into the maternal circulation, activating the coagulation cascade leading to disseminated intravascular coagulation. Placental abruption is potentially life threatening for both mother and fetus. A 30% placental separation leads to fetal compromise and a 50% separation leads to fetal death.

UMBILICAL CORD PROLAPSE

Any factor that interferes with the close association of the presenting part to the lower uterine segment can allow the umbilical cord to prolapse through the internal os. The commonest causes are as follows:

- Malpresentation of the fetus especially a footling breech, extended breech, transverse lie, brow and compounded face presentations. Twenty per cent occur with a transverse lie and 15% with footling breeches.

- The premature fetus of less than 34 weeks gestation.
- The abnormal fetus.
- Multiple pregnancy.
- Polyhydramnios.
- Premature ruptured membranes.
- High fetal head secondary to pelvic tumours, such as fibroids.

Cord prolapse also occurs during obstetric procedures:

- rotational forceps,
- external cephalic version.

Peri-natal mortality secondary to cord prolapse can be high, with detection and urgent delivery essential. As neonatal prognosis is related to detection to delivery time, the decision as to whether the baby is viable or not needs to be made quickly. Delivery by immediate Caesarean section is usually required, but manoeuvres to relieve cord compression should continue. These include pushing up the presenting part either manually or by filling the bladder, replacing the cord into the vagina to reduce vasospasm secondary to cold and placing the mother head down either in the knees to chest or lateral position.

UTERINE RUPTURE

This usually occurs during labour or induction of labour, but may occur spontaneously in late pregnancy. The commonest site of rupture is in a uterine scar from either a previous Caesarean section, uterine perforation (after termination of pregnancy, evacuation of retained products of conception, D&C) or other uterine surgery. Other factors include obstructed labour, intra-uterine manipulations, i.e. external version, forcible dilation of the cervix and injudicious use of oxytocic drugs. The higher the scar on the uterus, the greater the risk of rupture, e.g. classical Caesarean section scars. Rupture may also occur in pregnancy as a result of direct trauma or perforating injury to the abdomen (especially road traffic accidents).

Uterine rupture presents with sudden onset of severe abdominal pain, maternal shock, fetal distress and sometimes vaginal bleeding. Uterine rupture can lead to maternal and fetal death, especially if it goes unrecognized. With the increasing number of women having uterine surgery and subsequent pregnancies, the incidence may increase.

CHRONIC PLACENTAL INSUFFICIENCY

Chronic placental insufficiency results in the fetus having an inadequate oxygen and nutrition supply because the placenta does not act efficiently as an organ of transfer. Placental insufficiency may be due to placental infarct, small amounts of placental separation with a retro-placental bleed, pre-eclampsia, inadequate placental implantation and increasing age of the placenta (i.e. post-term; greater than 42 weeks). The consequence of chronic placental insufficiency is intra-uterine growth retardation in the fetus. If pregnancy is prolonged, the placenta may become inadequate for fetal needs making the fetus more vulnerable to the hypoxia which occurs during normal uterine contractions.

FETAL PROBLEMS CONTRIBUTING TO FETAL DISTRESS

The fetus itself may have problems which decrease its capacity to cope with the hypoxia of normal contractions. Fetal problems which lead to an increased chance of fetal distress include: congenital abnormalities, previous ante-natal hypoxic episodes, prematurity and intra-uterine growth retardation.

Intra-uterine growth retarded babies show an increased risk of intrapartum fetal distress, hypoxia, acidemia, abnormal CTG, passage of meconium and intra-uterine death. The second British peri-natal mortality survey showed that these infants have a five-fold increase in the stillbirth rate, so close supervision in labour and early intervention is essential.

Fetal pyrexia and fetal sepsis decrease the fetus' ability to cope with the normal hypoxia of labour, thereby increasing the chances of acidosis leading to abnormal fetal heart rate changes. Risk factors for fetal sepsis include prolonged rupture of membranes, maternal infection and reduced liquor volume. Maternal pyrexia is also a contributory factor to fetal pyrexia. Mothers may become pyrexial without infection during labour, and epidural anaesthesia can contribute to this, which can lead to confusion in the assessment of fetal well-being.

CHOICE OF ANAESTHETIC

There are three methods of anaesthesia available for an emergency Caesarean section:

- extending existing regional blockade,
- establishing subarachnoid blockade,
- general anaesthesia.

The choice of anaesthesia is the anaesthetist's not the obstetrician's.

Table 10.1		
	Contraindications	Caution in
General anaesthesia for emergency Caesarean section	Maternal refusal Known difficult intubation Known allergy to anaesthetic drugs	Predicted difficult intubation Known suxamethonium apnoea Hypertensive disease of pregnancy Uncorrected maternal hypovolaemia
Regional anaesthesia for emergency Caesarean section	Maternal refusal Low maternal platelet count Known maternal clotting abnormality Known allergy to local anaesthetics	Potential clotting abnormality Anatomical back problems Maternal sepsis Uncorrected maternal hypovolaemia

MATERNAL FACTORS

Table 10.1 shows maternal factors which influence the choice of anaesthetic in the emergency situation.

TIME FACTORS

The Royal College of Obstetricians and Gynaecologists have recommended that the maximum time from decision to delivery, in emergency Caesarean sections for fetal distress, should be no longer than 30 min. This time is echoed by the American College of Obstetricians and Gynaecologists and endorsed by the Obstetric Anaesthetists' Association. There are some situations, however, where a shorter time would be desirable. This has led to a further classification of non-elective Caesarean sections:

- *Grade 1*: immediate threat to life of fetus or mother. Delivery as soon as possible.
- *Grade 2*: maternal or fetal compromise which is not immediately life threatening.
- *Grade 3*: no maternal or fetal compromise but needing early delivery.

Thirty minutes is not long, but should allow the anaesthetist time to make a decision and achieve adequate anaesthesia. The anaesthetist must consider whether a general anaesthetic is quicker than a regional technique. This is a difficult question to answer as it depends on the circumstances and the type of regional anaesthesia used. In a previously unseen patient who requires a general anaesthetic, the anaesthetist needs to talk to the patient and take a relevant anaesthetic history, (allergies, etc.), to site an IVI, give antacid prophylaxis and then perform a rapid sequence induction,

before surgery can commence. If this is compared to a patient with a working epidural in labour, whom the anaesthetist knows and requires only a top up to achieve analgesia before surgery, the time taken is probably very similar. This is especially so if the epidural can be topped up in the labour room before transferring the mother to theatre. However, the time to establish a new subarachnoid block depends on the skill of the anaesthetist and rate of spread of block to give adequate anaesthesia. Subarachnoid blockade may be achieved either with a single shot spinal or a combined spinal-epidural technique. Whichever technique is chosen, the anaesthetic time includes aseptic preparation, insertion and an onset time. Thus it takes approximately 15 min from the time of entering theatre to the time the block is adequate for surgery. A *de-nova* epidural has the slowest onset time of any method and is not appropriate in the emergency situation, where fetal distress is involved.

Comparing the time courses of the different methods of anaesthesia is difficult but work done indicates that a general anaesthetic and an extended epidural have a very similar speed of onset. Price et al showed that the maximum time to extend an epidural was 12½ min. However, other factors can play a part in the delay between decision to operate and delivery of the fetus. These include transfer of the mother to the operating theatre, consent form signing, shaving the mother, catheterization, scrubbing and opening surgical packs, etc. A personal audit carried out at Queen Charlotte's showed that the average anaesthetic time was 11 min but waiting for surgeons and theatre staff to be ready prolonged this time considerably.

FETAL FACTORS

The effects of general and regional anaesthesia on the fetus have been investigated, but there is very little work on their effects on the distressed fetus. Any decrease in placental blood flow or oxygen availability will further distress an already acidotic fetus. Placental blood flow will be decreased by maternal hypotension and increasing uteroplacental vasoconstriction. Fetal oxygen availability is improved by increasing maternal blood oxygen tension and content and decreased by shifting the haemoglobin–oxygen dissociation curve to the left.

General anaesthesia

Two factors can affect fetal acid–base status during general anaesthesia. Light anaesthesia, often associated with standard general anaesthesia for Caesarean section, does not suppress maternal epinephrine and norepinephrine surges associated with intubation and surgical manipulation. The resulting vasoconstriction may decrease uterine blood flow. Intermittent positive pressure ventilation may decrease venous return leading to a reduction in cardiac output and a decrease in placental perfusion. If hypocapnia and alkalosis result from over ventilation, further fetal effects occur. Hypocapnia causes uteroplacental vasoconstriction and alkalosis shifts the oxygen dissociation curve to the left decreasing fetal oxygen availability.

Regional anaesthesia

Studies on the normal fetus, during regional anaesthesia, have shown that neonatal acidosis results from maternal hypotension. The commonest causes of maternal hypotension are aorto-caval compression and sympathetic blockade. Aorto-caval compression should be avoided at all costs in the distressed fetus, by the use of uterine displacement (only full left lateral tilt relieves the caval component). Hypotension, secondary to vasodilatation, can be obtunded by increasing maternal circulating volume by using intravenous fluids (at least 20–25 ml/kg body weight), and/or the use of an intravenous pressor agent. Current evidence would suggest that pre-loading is not essential if adequate vasopressor prophylaxis is used.

Extrapolation of these results would indicate that regional anaesthesia has no detrimental effect on the distressed fetus, providing maternal hypotension is prevented and that general anaesthesia properly conducted, without aorto-caval compression, and with a high (greater than 50%) inspired oxygen, is a useful alternative in situations where regional anaesthesia is contraindicated.

ANAESTHETIC SKILL

The anaesthetist must be honest when faced with the decision of which anaesthetic to choose:

- Can a subarachnoid block be established as quickly as required?
- Is the anaesthetist confident that the woman about to be anaesthetized can be intubated?
- Is the epidural *in situ* working adequately to allow a top up to produce surgical anaesthesia quickly and reliably?

It is essential that the trainee anaesthetist has exposure to all forms of anaesthesia and becomes competent in all techniques. It is also essential that the trainee is taught to think for himself and to make appropriate decisions, without allowing undue influence from obstetricians and midwives. Personal experience has taught most senior anaesthetists how to best handle 'panic' situations, which often exist at the time. It is something that trainees may not appreciate until they experience one in the middle of the night. The ability to be the 'island in the storm' is an under-rated skill. It must be remembered the priority, however difficult it may seem, is the mother. An anaesthetist should not unnecessarily endanger the mother in order to deliver a distressed fetus.

PRACTICAL PROCEDURES

BUYING SOME TIME

Attention to a few simple things may buy some time:

- Correct aorta-caval compression by putting the mother in the left (or right) lateral position or use tilt with uterine displacement.
- Treat hypotension with fluids and or vasopressors as appropriate.
- Stop all oxytocic infusions.
- Consider giving tocolytics either GTN or intravenous $\beta2$ agonists such as salbutamol if uterine spasm is contributing to the fetal distress. The dose of intravenous salbutamol is 25 μg (dilute 500 μg salbutamol into 20 ml normal saline and give 1 ml at a time) or intravenous GTN 0.5 mg (dilute 10 mg into 20 ml of normal saline and give 1 ml at a time).
- Increase maternal oxygen as this may increase available oxygen to the hypoxic fetus improving its acid–base status.

- Inflate the bladder with normal saline via a urinary catheter. This pushes the fetal head away from a compressed umbilical cord.
- Talking to and calming the mother in what is often a stressful situation can be beneficial, as decreasing natural maternal catecholamines will improve placental blood flow.

EXTENDING AN EXISTING EPIDURAL

The success of this technique is improved if the woman already has a good bilateral working epidural for analgesia in labour with bilateral sympathetic blockade. Adequate blockade for Caesarean section requires an upper level to at least T6 (light touch) or T4 (cold) and as importantly a lower level to S2–4. The block should always be tested carefully before commencing surgery. Some anaesthetists will allow surgery to start with the assumption that the block will carry on extending to reach adequate levels, this is not generally good practice unless very experienced.

The choice of top-up solution and the amount to be given can differ with each individual situation. The aim is, not only to get a higher dermatomal level of block, but to increase the density of the block. The level of blockade should be assessed before the top up is given. The top up may be given by the anaesthetist in the delivery suite to prevent any time delay, but there has to be established IV access, the ability to measure the blood pressure, available ephedrine and the anaesthetist must remain with the woman throughout. The commonly used local anaesthetic solutions are listed below:

- 2% lidocaine with 1:200 000 epinephrine and bicarbonate 2 ml 8.4% solution.
- 2% lidocaine, 0.5% bupivacaine 50/50 mix ± epinephrine 1:200 000.
- 0.5% bupivacaine ± epinephrine 1:200 000. (Ropivacaine 0.5% or levo-bupivacaine can be substituted for bupivacaine 0.5% but bicarbonate must not be used.)

SUBARACHNOID BLOCKS

In the presence of fetal distress, the most important aspects of this technique are as follows:

- avoiding maternal hypotension,
- speed of onset.

Preventing maternal hypotension relies on adequate maternal blood volume and the use of vasopressors. Fetal distress can be due to concealed abruption or maternal hypovolaemia, which is unmasked by sympathetic blockade, leading to severe maternal hypotension. The anaesthetist must be confident that hypovolaemia is corrected before embarking on this technique. Concerning vasopressors; evidence shows that ephedrine given by dilute continuous infusion has no significant effect on uterine artery resistance, whereas bolus doses can increase resistance, thus decreasing placenta blood flow. In the healthy fetus, mild uterine artery vasoconstriction is well tolerated, but the high risk or distressed fetus may be further compromised so ephedrine should be given as an infusion whenever possible.

Improving speed of onset and quality of subarachnoid blockade

- Speed of onset of spinal anaesthetic can be increased by the injection of fluid into the epidural space, which gives the combined spinal-epidural technique a theoretical advantage in this situation. Rapid extension of a block is not advised unless familiar with this technique in the non-urgent situation.
- Inserting the subarachnoid injection in the left or right lateral position gives improved spread compared to sitting.
- Cephalad positioning of the bevel at the time of injection.
- The addition of 25 μg of fentanyl to the subarachnoid injection has also been shown to reduce the need for intra-operative supplementation.

SUPPLEMENTATION OF REGIONAL BLOCKADE DURING SURGERY

The need for supplementary analgesia should be low, if the regional block is adequate at the start of surgery. If the mother is prepared well and informed of the type of sensations, especially pulling and tugging that she may feel, then she is less likely to complain of discomfort during the surgery. However, any complaint by the mother of pain or discomfort, must be taken seriously and every attempt made to alleviate the problem. A good rapport between the anaesthetist and the mother makes the situation easier to handle and reassurance may be all that is required. If supplemental analgesia is required then there are many different techniques that can be used, but if all these prove inadequate then a general anaesthetic should be offered.

GENERAL ANAESTHESIA

Points to remember to reduce the possibility of further fetal compromise are; avoid aorto-caval compression, increase maternal oxygen, maintain maternal carbon dioxide within normal limits and ensure adequate anaesthesia to minimize the maternal stress response.

POST-OPERATIVE CARE

After an emergency Caesarean section many mothers are still in a 'state of shock' and disbelief over the suddenness of their surgery. Every effort should be made to provide an opportunity for her to discuss any concerns she may have. Emergency surgery is one of the moderate risk factors for deep vein thrombosis therefore TED stockings and the use of heparin is recommended.

SPECIFIC OBSTETRIC EMERGENCIES AND FETAL DISTRESS

CORD PROLAPSE

As neonatal prognosis is related to detection to delivery time, the decision as to whether the baby is viable or not needs to be made rapidly. Delivery by immediate Caesarean section is usually required, but manoeuvres to relieve cord compression should continue. In this situation, if the patient has an established epidural, then extension should be as quick as a general anaesthetic. If the patient is in the left lateral position and the fetal heart is reasonable, then subarachnoid injection may be attempted. In reality, the majority of cord prolapses require a general anaesthetic for fast delivery of the fetus, and as long as maternal safety is not unduly compromised it would seem an appropriate choice of anaesthetic.

MASSIVE OBSTETRIC HAEMORRHAGE

This is defined as blood loss of greater than 1500 ml. Antepartum haemorrhage is usually caused by bleeding from placental abruption, placenta previa or vasa previa. These situations are potentially life threatening to both mother and baby. Resuscitation of the mother must take priority over fetal well-being. Placental blood flow at term is about 500 ml/min, so the potential for massive blood loss is obvious. Evacuation of uterine contents is often essential to control blood loss. Maternal resuscitation may therefore require immediate Caesarean section, even if the fetus is not viable. In these situations, clotting abnormalities may develop rapidly and if the clotting status of the mother is unknown and anaesthesia is required, then it should be assumed to be abnormal until proven otherwise.

This means that regional techniques are not suitable in this situation, and general anaesthesia is the method of choice.

ABRUPTION OF THE PLACENTA

If this diagnosis has been made then delivery of the baby and placenta is required to prevent further blood loss. Continuing bleeding needs immediate delivery usually by Caesarean section, but treatment of maternal shock should be on-going. If, however, the mother is stable and the fetus has already died, then Caesarean section is seldom indicated. Monitoring of clotting status is important in this situation as DIC may rapidly occur.

PLACENTA PREVIA

Bleeding from a placenta previa or accreta (invasion of the myometrium by the placenta) will continue until the uterus is evacuated and may require Caesarean hysterectomy to control it in severe cases. In this situation, when maternal clotting status and extent of surgery is unknown, or the mother is already significantly hypovolaemic, then general anaesthesia is the method of choice.

VASA PREVIA

Bleeding from a vasa previa will rapidly lead to exsanguination of the mother unless the uterus is emptied. Again general anaesthesia is the method of choice.

UTERINE RUPTURE

If uterine rupture is suspected then immediate laparotomy is required. In cases where maternal shock occurs, resuscitation as for massive haemorrhage should be simultaneous with surgery. Extensive surgery may be essential to control bleeding and Caesarean hysterectomy is a distinct possibility. In this situation general anaesthesia is the best choice.

If uterine rupture is suspected but no signs of maternal shock are present, then extension of a pre-existing epidural may be possible. However, it is important to remember that signs of shock may be concealed until 20–30% of blood volume is lost and the use of regional anaesthesia can then unmask hypovolaemia, leading to profound hypotension. Single shot spinal anaesthesia is not appropriate in this situation, as this technique is not flexible enough if extended surgery time occurs.

THE MANAGEMENT OF MASSIVE OBSTETRIC HAEMORRHAGE

It is useful to have a designated 'haemorrhage trolley' so all the necessary fluids, cannula, giving-sets, forms and blood bottles can be rapidly accessed. A major haemorrhage 'fire drill' is useful to iron out any local problems with a major haemorrhage protocol and to make staff aware of the protocol.

GENERAL RULES

- A blood loss of around 1500 ml should activate the major haemorrhage protocol. If blood loss is estimated to be between 1000 and 1500 ml then at least some aspects of the protocol should be followed, e.g. post-delivery hourly urine output and haemoglobin estimate.
- It may be difficult to assess accurately blood loss, due to dilution of blood with amniotic fluid and very large amounts of blood may be hidden in the uterus and vagina.
- Patients tend to be otherwise young and fit. They compensate for hypovolaemia by increasing sympathetic activity with a tachycardia and vaso-constriction. Blood pressure will not fall until there is a blood loss of 30–50% of maternal blood volume. Hypotension is therefore a late and unreliable sign.
- Oliguria is an early sign.
- Hypotension is made worse by aorto-caval compression. Place the mother in full lateral position or in the supine position with lateral tilt if in theatre.
- Give the mother oxygen.

MAJOR HAEMORRHAGE PROTOCOL

An easily followed major haemorrhage protocol should cover the following points.

Activate staff

Dealing effectively with a major haemorrhage must involve a team approach. All members of the team must be aware of the protocol and must act promptly:

- Call senior midwife or designated team leader (to inform and liase with other team members, see below).
- Call senior obstetric help (low threshold for contacting obstetric consultant if possible).
- Call labour ward anaesthetist (low threshold for contacting consultant if possible).

- Call labour ward ODA and main theatre. The labour ward anaesthetic assistant should be rapidly available and may need additional assistance and equipment if the maternity unit is away from the main theatre site.
- Alert blood bank and haematology.
- Call for porters.

Initial resuscitation

The rapid initial resuscitation is usually given by the obstetric and anaesthetic team based on the delivery suite. Rapid assessment and simple initial manoeuvres can be life saving:

- Give oxygen face-mask. Give 8 l/min.
- Insert two 14G cannula.
- Take a blood sample for:
  – full blood count, urea and electrolytes.
  – clotting screen.
  – cross-match at least 8 units of blood.
- An arterial blood gas, to detect a metabolic acidosis which is a reliable and early method for evaluating the extent of hypovolaemic shock. A corrected base deficit of greater than minus five is significant.
- Keep the mother warm.

Monitoring

Basic non-invasive monitoring should be rapidly available. Insertion of CVP and arterial lines are less immediately important and can be considered if the mother needs to go to the operating theatre:

- All patients need ECG, NIBP and pulse oximetry.
- Urinary catheter for hourly urine output is a reliable early sign of hypovolaemia.
- CVP if blood loss is 1500 ml and continuing.
- Arterial line if haemodynamically unstable.

Fluids

Giving enough of the correct fluids, with the minimum of delay, is life saving. Delay in receiving blood can be very serious and it is important that haematology blood bank staff are told specifically of the situation:

- Crystalloids are needed at three times the estimated blood loss (EBL).
- Colloids (Gelofusin or Hespan) if hypotensive or EBL > 1500 ml.
- Blood if EBL > 1500 ml or earlier if there is pre-existing anaemia.
- O negative blood or group specific blood may be used whilst waiting for cross-matched blood. This must be clearly conveyed to the blood bank.
- Use active fluid warming devices.

Coagulation products

The optimum amount of blood products, to correct clotting deficits due to clotting factor dilution or DIC is controversial. Up-to-date coagulation studies are ideal, especially if a haematologist can interpret the results. In the clinical situation of severe and on going haemorrhage, waiting for clotting results before giving blood products can be detrimental:

- Coagulation results can lag behind the clinical situation. It is useful to be able to go on clinical grounds rather than wait for the laboratory results.
- Give blood products sooner rather than later.
- Give 6 units of FFP for every 10 units of blood for *ongoing* bleeding.
- Give 6 units of platelets for every 10 units of blood for *ongoing* bleeding.
- Keep platelet count $>50 \times 10^9$ and aim for 100.
- Give more FFP if PT or APPT > 3 s beyond control.
- Give cryoprecipitate if fibrinogen is very low or bleeding is severe, but FFP should be the mainstay of treatment. The only real value of cryoprecipitate is if volume over-load is a problem.
- If there are any coagulation abnormalities, discuss them with a haematologist if possible.
- Take blood for FBC, clotting and U&E for every 8 units of transfused blood given.

Drugs for uterine atonia

Drug therapy is an important part of the management of obstetric haemorrhage, particulary if related to uterine atonia. The anaesthetist is often asked to give these drugs:

- Syntocinon 5 unit bolus followed by a infusion at 10 units/h.
- Ergometrine 0.5 mg.
- Carboprost 250 μg at not more than every 15 min (contraindicated in asthmatics).

Anaesthesia

The choice of anaesthetic must be up to the individual anaesthetist and their experience in dealing with the situation. There are some general rules that can be followed:

- Choose general anaesthesia if haemorrhage is severe, hypovolaemia present or diagnosis uncertain.

- If there is a spinal or epidural block *in situ* then it may be used, as a general anaesthetic in addition to regional blockade may make haemodynamic instability worse in the presence of hypovolaemia.
- Indications for converting a regional to a general anaesthetic are
  - maternal unconsciousness due to hypotension,
  - maternal anxiety,
  - inadequate anaesthesia.

Continuing care

The mother who has had a major haemorrhage must be cared for in an appropriate environment and with great care. Maternal deaths have been attributed to substandard care in the post-partum period:

- Patients will need continuing observation once stable, in a high dependency area. This may be on the delivery suite or attached to an intensive care area.
- There must be close collaboration between obstetrician and anaesthetists and careful observations.
- Regular haemoglobin and coagulation studies will be needed if there has been a transfusion requirement of more than 8 units of blood.
- Continued bleeding, coagulopathy, hypothermia and anuria are indications for admission to an intensive care unit.

FURTHER READING

1. Davis AG. Anaesthesia for Caesarean section. The potential for regional block. *Anaesthesia* 1982; **37**: 748–753.
2. Morgan BM, Magni V, Goroszenuik T. Anaesthesia for emergency Caesarean section. *Br J Obstet Gynaecol* 1990; **97**: 420–424.
3. Marx GF, Luykx WM, Cohen S. Fetal-neonatal status following Caesarean section for fetal distress. *Br J Anaesth* 1984; **56**: 1009–1013.
4. Price ML, Reynolds F, Morgan BM. Extending epidural blockade for emergency Caesarean section. *Int J Obstet Anaesth* 1991; **1**: 13–18.
5. Department of Health. *Report on confidential enquires into maternal deaths in the United Kingdom 1991–1993*. Her Majesty's Stationary Office, London, 1996.
6. Chestnut D. Fetal monitoring and anaesthesia for fetal distress. *Can J Anaesth* 1993; **40**: R74–R77.

11

INTRAPARTUM FETAL MONITORING

Toby N. Fay & Bryony Strachen

INTRODUCTION

Patient monitoring is familiar to all anaesthetists during operative procedures and in intensive care units. Most women in labour go through a normal physiological process, which results in the expulsion of the fetus and placental products from the uterus. In the developed world this process usually occurs in the labour suite (>95%). A brief review of the history of midwifery and obstetrics reveals that early in the last century most efforts went in to tending to the mother and keeping her alive. The fetus was very much a secondary concern with intermittent auscultation as the mainstay of intrapartum fetal monitoring. The same could be said for current maternity strategies in many parts of the developing world. With advances in modern anaesthesia, obstetricians have the facility to intervene before or during labour and safely deliver the fetus earlier than previously would have been possible. Following the reduction in maternal morbidity and mortality, the focus has shifted towards a better outcome for the fetus. The stillbirth rate has halved in the last 30 years, the perinatal mortality has dropped to below eight deaths per 1000 maternities, and fetal death in labour is a rare event for babies over 1500 g, at a rate of 0.3 deaths per 1000 total births.[1] A part of this fall is due to the successful development of neonatal care, especially for the premature neonate. Obstetric interventions during pathological pregnancies and labours have also contributed to the improvement in perinatal survival.[2]

It is important for the anaesthetist to understand the major adverse patterns on the CTG and the results of interventions such as fetal blood sampling (FBS), to make communication easier with obstetricians and midwives. Appropriate anaesthetic intervention can more easily be made in good time, resulting in safer anaesthesia for mother and baby. Methods of fetal monitoring in the future may make obstetric decision making easier and the obstetric anaesthetist must be familiar with the techniques.

The fetus has proven to be a difficult and inaccessible patient to monitor during labour. It is true that many labours and babies require very little monitoring to ensure a successful outcome for both mother and baby. The danger of making unnecessary assessments and observations is that obstetricians intervene inappropriately, and consequently increase maternal morbidity with no real benefit to the fetus.[3] The widespread use of impreace nomenclature is a problem; terms like fetal distress, hypoxia and birth asphyxia should be avoided, as these terms are non-specific and inaccurate. The Greek translation of asphyxia is 'pulseless'. Reference should instead be made to objective, definable entities such as fetal bradycardia, umbilical artery pH values and hypoxic ischaemic encephalopathy.

FETAL PHYSIOLOGY

The fetus receives its nutrients from the placenta via the umbilical vein at a flow rate of approximately 100 ml/kg/min. The fetal circulation (Fig. 11.1) directs a blood flow preferentially to the fetal brain and heart. The fetal cardiac output varies with gestation and at 30 weeks is about 550 ml/min and is mainly controlled by heart rate rather than stroke volume. About 50% of the cardiac output is re-directed back to the umbilical circulation.

Vagal control of heart rate

The normal fetal heart rate is between 110 and 150 beats/min and is under cerebral control via the vagus nerve. Early heart rate decelerations are often seen in labour during contractions as a result of head or umbilical cord compression. The fetus also has a reflex compensatory mechanism whereby a re-distribution of blood-flow and a slowing in the fetal heart rate occurs during uterine diastole, which serves to improve oxygenation of the myocardium. These phenomena are referred to as variable or late fetal heart rate decelerations. In 50% of cases, variable or late decelerations are associated with fetal metabolic acidaemia (normal umbilical arterial pH: mean = 7.26, SD = 0.08), which

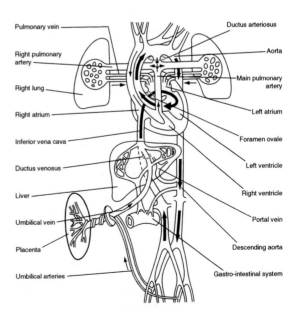

Figure 11.1 Fetal circulation.

represents a serious pathological decompensation. Fetal blood gas analysis is necessary to determine the difference between the physiological and pathological fetal heart rate responses (see later).

Hormonal control of heart rate

Probably the most important hormone responsible for these cardiovascular responses is arginine vasopressin (AVP). Experiments in fetal sheep have shown that AVP administration leads to transient bradycardia and hypertension, similar to that observed in acute hypoxia, and AVP levels increase in fetal plasma with induced acute hypoxia. Angiotensin II and catecholamine levels also seem to rise in acute hypoxia. Recent experiments suggest that these endocrine responses may be mediated via peripheral chemoreceptor signals relayed to the brain via vagal afferents.[4] However, at present, the knowledge and understanding of the relationship between human fetal heart rate patterns and fetal myocardial and cerebral oxygenation, is incomplete and more research is necessary.[5]

Sympathetic control of heart rate

The sympathetic nervous system, including adenomedullary catecholamine responses, can increase the fetal heart rate up to a maximum of about 220 beats/min in response to anaemia, hyperthermia, sepsis and hypoxia. In a healthy fetus, the heart rate would be expected to increase above the baseline, by more than 15 beats/min for more than 15 s, in response to fetal movements, tactile or auditory stimulation. This is known as fetal heart rate acceleration, and its presence indicates a healthy fetal brain and myocardium. The fetal heart rate is not constant but has an intrinsic degree of variability. This variability in fetal heart rate (5–25 beats/min) is another feature of a healthy fetus, although a brief (<20 min) loss of variability may merely represent fetal inactivity, or a fetal 'sleep' pattern.

OXYGEN TRANSFER

The transfer of oxygen and carbon dioxide occurs down pressure gradients shown in Table 11.1.

Although the fetal partial pressure of oxygen (P_aO_2) is lower than the adult, the total oxygen carrying capacity is higher in the fetus because:

- The fetus has a higher haemoglobin concentration (mean haemoglobin concentration = 18 g/dl).
- The haemoglobin in fetal red blood cells is composed mainly of fetal haemoglobin (HbF) which has a higher affinity for oxygen than haemoglobin A and A_2.

Table 11.1   Oxygen and carbon dioxide partial pressures in uterine and fetal circulation

Vessel	O_2 (kPa)	CO_2 (kPa)
Uterine artery	12.0	4.0
Umbilical vein	4.0	5.3
Umbilical artery	2.7	6.1
Uterine vein	5.3	4.8

- Fetal red cells have less 2,3-diphosphoglycerol and carbonic anhydrase activity and consequently the oxygen-dissociation curve is shifted to the left (the Bohr effect) and enables an arterial oxygen saturation (S_aO_2) of 80% at lower P_aO_2 (4.0 kPa). The fetal haemoglobin S_aO_2 is on the steep part of the oxygen-dissociation curve and thus fetal blood can easily surrender oxygen following a small drop in the P_aO_2 in peripheral tissues. Similarly, in the placenta, fetal haemoglobin can efficiently bind oxygen where there is a higher P_aO_2 from the maternal circulation. The Haldane effect is also observed with an increased transfer of CO_2 from the fetus to the mother at low P_aO_2.
- Fetal whole blood oxygen content of 19.0 ml/100 ml compared with 16.7 ml/100 ml in the adult.

Metabolism utilization in the healthy fetus

While oxygen is the essential substrate required by mitochondrial oxidative phosphorylation to produce high energy ATP in cellular, aerobic respiration, the main energy substrate for fetal cells, especially the myocardium and brain, is glucose. Glucose is absorbed from the maternal circulation by the placenta via a process of facilitated diffusion. Approximately 60% is utilized by the placenta itself. Under aerobic conditions intracellular glycolysis produces pyruvate which is converted into acetyl-CoA. This enters the Krebs Cycle and during oxidative phosphorylation, high energy ATP is produced for cellular metabolism and homeostasis. Other substrates can be utilised by the fetus, including amino acids and non-esterified free fatty acids. In a healthy intrauterine environment the fetus grows (mean growth rate = 13 g/day, range: 8–17 g/day) in anabolic metabolic conditions, laying down glycogen in the liver and white and brown fat in the peripheral tissues. This is largely mediated by the action of fetal insulin. Glycogen provides the substrate reserve for parturition and early neonatal life, while brown and white fat provide energy and insulation to help maintain body temperature post-partum.

Metabolism in the compromised fetus

Under pathological conditions, that results in intrauterine growth restriction such as placental insufficiency, the fetus may have been in a catabolic, rather than an anabolic state for some time prior to the onset of labour. Depleted hepatic glycogen reserves make it difficult for the fetus to cope with the energy demands that parturition imposes. If no glucose is available to maintain normal intracellular metabolic processes, cellular damage results in a metabolic acidosis. Where placental blood flow is impeded, as in pre-eclampsia or abruption, fetal blood oxygen falls and carbon dioxide accumulates. Following the consumption of the blood buffer reserves, the pH falls and a primary respiratory acidosis develops, with a normal base excess (mean umbilical arterial base excess = 6.7 mEq/l, SD = 3.6). This situation is not deleterious to the fetus as long there is sufficient oxygen for normal metabolism. If the fetus were to be delivered at this stage, the onset of normal neonatal respiration would 'blow off' the accumulated carbon dioxide and rapidly return the blood pH to normal.[6] If the placental blood flow is limited and fetal oxygenation further reduced, the peripheral fetal circulation is reduced to preserve blood flow to the fetal brain and myocardium. Under hypoxic conditions, intracellular anaerobic glycolysis would start to generate ATP; the Krebs Cycle and oxidative phosphorylation cannot produce ATP without oxygen. The resultant equation for the formation of ATP by anaerobic glycolysis is

$$\star \text{Glucose} + 2\text{ADP} + 2\text{P}_i \rightarrow 2\text{lactate} + 2\text{ATP}$$

$\star$(where P_i is the inorganic phosphate; ATP is adenosine triphosphate; ADP is adenosine diphosphate.) Lactic acid accumulates (normal umbilical arterial lactate = 2.41 mmol/l, SD = 1.21) leading to a metabolic acidosis with a large negative base excess (< -12 mEq/l), and possibly hypoxic ischaemic encephalopathy and its consequences. It has been shown in experimental animal studies that fetal neurological damage is related not to acidosis *per se*, but to the metabolic, rather than respiratory component of the acidosis.[7] Experiments with infant monkeys suggest that glucose infusions prior to a hypoxic insult appeared to enhance survival and prevent central nervous system injury.[8] The explanation for the observation that some fetuses can tolerate severe metabolic acidosis during labour (e.g. a well-grown healthy term infant) and some cannot, is dependent on the insults which occur during the development of the fetus in the antepartum period. At present it is not possible to identify all these 'at-risk' fetuses.

Most (90%) children born at term who develop cerebral palsy are likely to have had a pre-labour problem (genetic or developmental) or antenatal complication (e.g. antepartum haemorrhage, hypertension) rather than an intrapartum cause.[9]

Utero-placental/fetal circulation

The final physiological consideration relates to the utero-placental and fetal circulations. The uterine artery blood flow to the placenta (500–1000 ml/min) is severely diminished during uterine contractions so the fetus has to compensate during uterine diastole. Uterine hyperstimulation can seriously compromise fetal well-being, because of reduced time between contractions. This is a very common complication of the use of oxytocics for induction or augmentation of labour. The uterine artery is a low priority circulation in the maternal autonomic control of blood pressure and so if the maternal circulatory system is compromised by haemorrhage, postural supine hypotension or sympathetic blockade, during regional anaesthesia, the uterine arterial system will constrict and reduce maternal placental blood flow to the fetus. In the fetus with compromised placental function that results in catabolic metabolism or chronic lack of oxygen, there exists a sensitive and powerful autonomic control of blood flow to organs which, if activated, will preferentially supply the fetal brain, heart and placenta, at the expense of other vascular beds. With a reduction in renal blood flow, oliguria results in oligohydramnios, as fetal urine is the main constituent of amniotic fluid in the second half of pregnancy. As a result, oligohydramnios is an exceedingly important sign of the compromised fetus in both the antenatal and intrapartum periods. This preferential re-distribution of blood flow will ultimately contribute to the overall metabolic acidosis and explains the observation that a severely acidotic baby appears floppy, pale and shocked with poor peripheral circulation.

CURRENT PRACTICES IN INTRAPARTUM FETAL MONITORING

CARDIOTOCOGRAPHY

The introduction of continuous, routine, electronic fetal monitoring (EFM) in the clinical management of labour in the 1970s was based on sound scientific concepts and the initial results were promising.[10] Cardiotocography (CTG) was rapidly accepted as the modern method of monitoring the fetus, but without proper assessment of the test's performance in clinical practice (Fig. 11.2). Subsequently many randomized

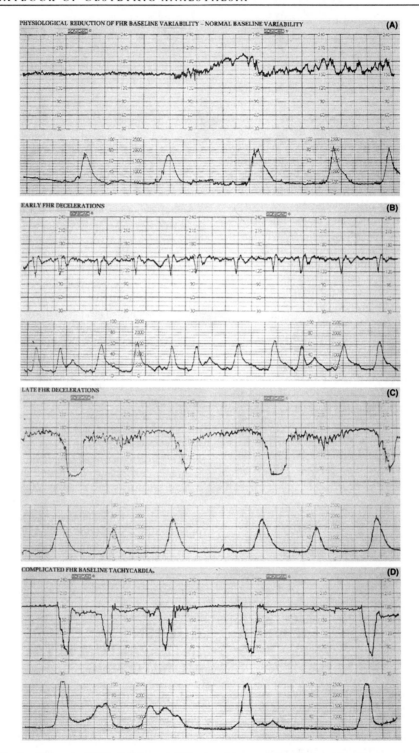

Figure 11.2   Cardiotocography (CTG): (A) Normal CTG: showing a period of reduced fetal heart rate variability followed by the normal pattern of fetal heart rate variability; (B) Early decelerations: slowing of the fetal heart begins at the start of uterine activity and recovers promptly as the uterus relaxes; (C) Late decelerations: the fetal heart rate slows and there is delayed recovery as the uterus relaxes; (D) Complicated tachycardia: the fetal heart rate is persistently elevated with decelerations during and after contractions.

Table 11.2 Prevalence of common neonatal outcomes as indicators requiring obstetric interventions for fetal distress not using EFM (except intrapartum deaths) adapted from Ref. 13

Neonatal outcome	Prevalence (%)
Apgar score <5 at 5 min	0.90
Umbilical artery pH < 7.0	0.65
Intubation at birth	0.50
Neonatal seizures	0.20
Perinatal mortality attributable to hypoxia	0.18
Hypoxic ischaemic encephalopathy	0.06
Intrapartum cerebral palsy	0.03
Intrapartum death >1500 g	0.03

trials failed to demonstrate significant benefits, although most were too small to assess adverse neonatal outcomes of low prevalence (Table 11.2), which were associated with high intervention rates for fetal distress: Caesarean section = 0.2–9.1%; instrumental delivery = 6.3–40%. A meta-analysis of these studies[11] and a large Dublin study,[12] have shown only a reduction in neonatal seizures (Grade II or III hypoxic ischaemic encephalopathy) when examining outcomes following complicated labours. This is an important benefit in itself but has been over-looked. In an erudite commentary on this complicated subject, Mongelli and colleagues[13] concluded ' … the flaws in much of the evidence has given special prominence to the negative aspects of EFM, whereas the possible benefits have been obscured by studies of insufficient numbers. This has provoked a drive to limit the use of EFM in labour before its potential is (has been) fully explored.'

In practical terms, the CTG as a test of fetal well-being has proven to be sensitive (about 98%) but not particularly specific (60–70%) for fetal acidosis, and there is considerable inter- and intra-observer variation in interpretation and classification.[14] In addition, the quality of recordings often confounds its interpretation.

As a test the CTG has four independent parameters:

- base rate,
- intrinsic variability,
- accelerations,
- decelerations.

Each of these parameters may have a different significance depending on the particular clinical situation. Some of the test parameters may be normal while others abnormal, which adds to the difficulties in interpretation. As the CTG is a test that has a high false positive rate (low specificity) it requires a second-line test to refute false positives, in order to reduce inappropriate interventions. FBS which, with a cut-off of pH = 7.20, enables the clinician to classify the CTG as a true or false positive and to act appropriately. This system requires a high standard of CTG interpretation otherwise too many FBS tests will be performed.

There are some CTG patterns that require immediate delivery of the fetus, for example prolonged fetal bradycardia, where time would be wasted performing an FBS. Also FBS may not be appropriate in the presence of fetal tachycardia associated with fetal infection. The fetus may respond to infection with a tachycardia, which can sometimes become complicated (with decelerations and/or loss of variability) and the development of fetal acidosis in these cases is a late and lethal complication of septicaemia and shock. Some would recommend that decisions concerning suspicious or abnormal CTGs should be made on the assessment of the FBS pH in conjunction with parameters such as the PCO_2 and base excess. This helps to differentiate between a metabolic acidosis, with immediate action required to deliver the baby, and the more conservative management of primary respiratory acidosis with correction of underlying causes such as uterine hyperstimulation, epidural complications and aorto-caval compression.[15] There is, however, only a weak relationship between fetal acidosis (pH < 7.11), condition at birth and longer term development.

CTG test should be applied to high-risk clinical situations but is not necessary for routine continuous use in all labours.[16] Continuous EFM during labours with an increased likelihood of fetal decompensation is accepted good practice (see Table 11.3).

What is not so clear-cut is the best method of monitoring the fetus in uncomplicated normal labour. As is often the case in obstetrics, too many assessments may lead to over-intervention. To make things more difficult, it is not always possible to identify pregnancies in which placental malfunction or insufficiency has occurred antenatally increasing the risk of intrapartum decompensation, acidosis and death. In a recent confidential enquiry into stillbirths and deaths in infancy, 9–10% of deaths reported occurred in the intrapartum period and hypoxia was thought to play a part, although half remained unexplained.[17] The enquiry also highlighted that abnormal CTGs went unrecognized with long delays to delivery after the onset of fetal compromise. This is not a defect of the monitoring tool but a reflection of poor education

Table 11.3 Conditions where continuous EFM should be employed during labour

Maternal
Hypertension and pre-eclampsia
Diabetes
Epilepsy
Rhesus disease
Heart disease
Respiratory conditions leading to hypoxia
Renal failure and transplants
Thyroid disease
Previous Caesarean section (uterine scar)
Inability to auscultate fetal heart (obesity)
Previous fetal loss

Fetal
Prolonged and/or augmented labour
Pre-term labour
Infection
Meconium stained liquor, oligohydramnios
Audible abnormal heart rate
Intrauterine growth restriction
Breech presentation
Multiple pregnancy
Antepartum or intrapartum haemorrhage

and response times. In the modern management of labour it is imperative to employ a system of assessments and recordings of the mother and baby that will help determine the correct level of fetal monitoring and intervention necessary for a satisfactory labour outcome.[18]

Admission testing to identify the high-risk fetus

Gibb and Arulkumaran[19] have proposed a set of assessments and recordings on admission to detect any at-risk fetuses that may have remained undetected throughout the antenatal period. Ingemarsson and colleagues[20] first described the admission test as a screening for fetal distress.

CTG

It consists of a CTG for 20–30 min immediately on admission in labour. If the CTG is classified as:

- reactive (about 88%), the chances of fetal acidosis is about 1%;
- suspicious or equivocal (8%), the fetal acidosis is about 10%;
- pathological (4%), the fetal acidosis rate is 50%.

Acidosis is defined as an FBS pH < 7.20 and a cord umbilical artery pH < 7.15, and/or an Apgar score of less than 7 at 1 min. If the admission CTG is satisfactory, intermittent auscultation every 15 min after contractions should be performed throughout the labour. There is evidence to suggest that the hand-held Doppler ultrasound monitor is more reliable than the Pinnard stethoscope in detecting fetal heart rate abnormalities and that its use is associated with a lower neonatal mortality and morbidity.[21]

The National Institute for clinical excellence has now issued guidlines on electoric fetal monitoring where routine admission CTGs are not required for low risk labours. A full list of the current guidlines can be found on www.nice.org.uk.

Fetal size

The second part of the assessment is an estimation of fetal size by a symphyseal-fundal height measurement in centimetres. If the measurement is 3 cm greater or less than the corresponding weeks of gestation, the fetus is monitored continuously and medical consultation is advised.

Amniotic fluid/meconium staining

Meconium stained liquor contains fetal faeces, which are sterile and contain bile acids, giving the characteristic green discolouration. Meconium is found in 15–20% of term labours, and is not always an indicator of fetal hypoxia. It may indicate either normal physiology or pathological processes such as fetal acidosis and fetal diarrhoea caused by infection, (especially *Listeria monocytogenes*), congenital thyrotoxicosis and some drugs. The grade or thickness of meconium staining is a function of the amount of liquor present at the time of fetal bowel action. The thicker the meconium the greater the risk of the meconium aspiration syndrome and associated intrapartum mortality. Attempts have been made to grade meconium, e.g. thin and stale green (Grade I), moderate (Grade II), thick and fresh green (Grade III) but this classification has not been found helpful in clinical practice. Amnioinfusion with warm isotonic saline in labour to dilute Grade III meconium in an attempt to reduce the risk of meconium aspiration syndrome has been described. This appeared successful, and perhaps should be considered as a possible therapeutic intervention in labour.[22]

Amniotic fluid/volume

Amniotic fluid volume measurements made during antenatal ultrasound scans correlate with perinatal

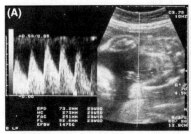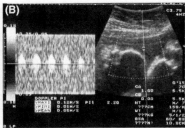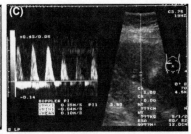

Figure 11.3   Doppler ultrasound of umbilical artery: (A) Normal Doppler wave forms showing flow in the artery during systole and diastole; (B) Absent end-diastolic flow; (C) Reversed end-diastolic flow.

mortality rates (PNMR):

- 1 cm pool, PNMR = 200/1000 births;
- 2 cm pool, PNMR = 50/1000 births;
- 3 cm pool, PNMR = 10/1000 births.

If little or no liquor is observed after spontaneous or artificial rupture of the fetal membranes or during labour, the pregnancy should be deemed to be complicated by oligohydramnios and monitored accordingly.

DOPPLER ULTRASOUND UMBILICAL ARTERY WAVEFORM ANALYSIS

This test is not used in intrapartum monitoring, but its antenatal use to determine need for early delivery has been found to halve the perinatal mortality rate when applied to high-risk pregnancies.[23] The absence of end diastolic flow or reverse diastolic flow in the cardiac cycle, represents increased upstream, (placental), resistance, associated with abnormal placental function and poor fetal and neonatal outcome. Absent end diastolic flow indicates a relative risk of fetal or neonatal death 30 times greater than if flow in diastole were to be observed, with a sensitivity of 67% and specificity of 98%. Doppler ultrasound umbilical artery waveform analysis often provides the clinician with evidence to justify intervention and delivery of the fetus. If the fetus is pre-term (<34 weeks gestation), this is whenever possible after the administration of corticosteroids to the mother, to enhance fetal lung surfactant production, and her transfer to a unit with appropriate neonatal facilities.

METHODS OF FETAL MONITORING UNDER INVESTIGATION

FETAL STIMULATION TESTS

Stimulation of the fetus by external stimuli provides useful information about fetal well-being and is usually applied in conjunction with continuous CTG monitoring. The fetal acoustic stimulation test consists of a burst of sound to which a healthy fetus will respond with an increase in heart rate. It appears to be a good discriminatory test with a sensitivity approaching 100% and a specificity of 70–80% and has been shown to reduce the need for an FBS by 50%.[24] Fetal scalp mechanical stimulation has also been described. In fact it is common to see an increase in the fetal heart rate during the performance of an FBS, (which is usually normal.) These tests are only applicable in term fetuses with no maternal narcotic analgesic administration and no fetal tachycardia.

FETAL PULSE OXIMETRY

While pulse oximetry has become an established tool for monitoring the anaesthetized patient, the transfer of the technology to the labour room has not been straightforward. For the last decade attempts have been made to adapt this technology to measure fetal oxygen saturation during labour, but problems of accessibility, reliability and whether the results are applicable, have been encountered.[25] Because of the lower range of oxygen saturation values in the fetus (mean value = 60–70%, range = 11–81%) the light wavelength range of adult probes (660 and 890 nm) must be replaced with wavelengths of 735 and 890 nm to improve accuracy. Fetal probes have been designed for reflectance oximetry in which both the light-emitting diode and the light receiving diode are integrated into one probe. There have been several prototypes developed to enable good surface contact between the presenting part of the fetus and the probe including a partial vacuum device[26] and a spiral electrode that secures the probe on to the fetal scalp.[27] The development of caput secundum on the fetal head in labour and the fetal scalp hair, have an adverse effect on the transmission signal.

A Probe has been designed to be placed over the fetal cheek. The balloon probe is passed around the presenting part and held in place by the inflation of a fluid-filled balloon. This probe also contains a contact ECG electrode and a transducer to provide a continuous measure of fetal heart rate and intra-uterine pressure.[28] There are problems with light transmission due to meconium and vernix caseosa and the signal is also subject to artefact from uterine contractions.

In practice, it appears that accurate values can be obtained in approximately 75% of labours in the first stage but success is less in the second stage. It has been suggested that the physiological re-distribution of blood flow in response to fetal compensation leads to a reduced flow in the peripheral circulation that in turn leads to insufficient pulsatility for detection by the pulse oximetry device.[29]

NEAR INFRA-RED SPECTROSCOPY

This technique was first described by Jobsis in 1977.[30] Light in the near infra-red spectrum (700–1000 nm) transmits up to a depth of 6 cm through fetal brain tissue.[31] Near infra-red spectroscopy (NIRS) has the potential to provide real-time continuous measurement of fetal cerebral oxygenation and haemodynamics during labour.[32] Absorption of light in this spectrum is mainly by two chromophores; haemoglobin and cytochrome aa3. By transillumination of the fetal brain by light of known wavelengths, changes in absorbance at these wavelengths can be converted into changes in concentrations of oxygenated haemoglobin, deoxygenated haemoglobin and cytochrome aa3. This technique differs from pulse oximetry in that total cerebral tissue oxygenation is measured as opposed to just arterial oxygenation. The pulse oximeter removes and ignores the effects of non-pulsatile light by measuring the ratio of change in light intensity during systole and diastole. Like pulse oximetry, a major problem with this technique is the development of a probe to attach to the fetal scalp. It is crucial that the pathway length along which the light is transmitted is constant. Unfortunately artefacts due to change in this length, caused by pressure effects during contractions, may occur. In two cases of known intrauterine death, mean cerebral oxygenated haemoglobin concentrations measurements were found to be the same as those taken from live fetuses during labour.[33] Therefore at present more research is necessary before NIRS can be used as a standard monitoring tool in labour.

FETAL ELECTROCARDIOGRAPHY

The idea behind the fetal electrocardiogram is that analysis may reveal fetal myocardial ischaemia before serious metabolic acidosis develops.[34] The main technical problem to overcome has been the acquisition of a decent and reliable signal. Initially the signal was obtained from electrodes placed on the maternal abdomen. The large signal from the maternal ECG and artefacts from maternal and fetal movements, meant that the fetal signal was of poor quality. Even with direct electrode placement through the cervix, the signal was small and prone to distortion and artefact. It is only with the aid of computer-assisted analysis and removal of distortion that an averaged ECG complex can be produced of sufficient quality for analysis.[35] There have been two main areas of interest: the morphologies of the T-wave and ST segment and time-interval analyses.

ST segment and T-wave analysis

Animal studies and observational studies in humans suggest that changes occur in this part of the ECG complex in the acidotic fetus. However these changes are not consistent and may be a late phenomenon. A major problem is that the vector of the ECG complex obtained by a direct fetal ECG electrode is largely unknown and may vary. Therefore the height of the ST segment is not reliable and T-wave inversion or an increase in T-wave height can occur.[36] In a prospective, randomized trial that compared conventional EFM with EFM plus ST waveform analysis, (both T/QRS ratio and ST morphology), in which 2434 women were recruited, results showed that there was a reduction in the number of deliveries for 'fetal distress' (61/1219 vs 111/1215), without an increase in the number of acidotic babies. The reduction in the operative delivery rate from 31% to 28% was not considered enough to justify the extra education, teaching and expense required to use the ST analyser.[37]

Time-interval analysis

Observational studies have demonstrated that there is normally a negative relationship between the PR interval and fetal heart rate (i.e. as the fetal heart slows the PR interval lengthens and vice versa). In the acidotic fetus this relationship is reversed (i.e. as the heart slows the PR interval shortens and vice versa).[38] This may be due to the different responses by the SA and AV nodes to hypoxaemia. The slow, oxygen-sensitive calcium channels within the SA node largely determine the threshold of the cardiac action potential and therefore the fetal heart rate. The PR interval is determined by the delay in propagation of the action potential by the AV node via both slow calcium and fast sodium channels. Fast sodium channels are resistant to changes in oxygen concentration. In the presence of hypoxaemia however, there is an increase in the threshold potential of the slow calcium channels at the SA node, and results in a slowing of the fetal heart rate. The threshold at the AV node is largely unchanged and therefore, as the fetal heart rate slows, the PR interval remains the same and may even shorten due to the effect of epinephrine.[39] There is, therefore, a positive relationship between the PR interval and the fetal heart rate under hypoxic conditions.[40] Measurements of this relationship over the short and long-term in labour have been made. A retrospective study carried out on over 250 women suggested that the addition of FECG time-interval analysis using such measurements could reduce the rate of unnecessary FBS or assisted delivery for presumed fetal distress. It also suggested that there could be a reduction in babies born with unsuspected acidosis at delivery.[41] A prospective trial has also been carried out. Although the initial study showed a significant reduction in the number of fetuses requiring FBS during labour, with a non-significant reduction in the number of acidotic infants delivered, these findings were not confirmed from an analysis of a further 1034 women. There were no differences in the Apgar scores, umbilical arterial pH or admission to the neonatal intensive care unit with the use of FECG time interval analysis. It may be that changes observed in the relationship between the PR interval and heart rate may vary between fetuses at differing levels of blood pH; so that in some fetuses the FECG changes may occur late, (at low pH) – not soon enough to allow intervention to prevent hypoxic ischaemic encephalopathy.[42]

CONTINUOUS FETAL MEASUREMENTS

Continuous fetal tissue pH and PCO_2 monitoring, show good correlation with both tissue pH and capillary blood pH, and avoids repeated FBS assessments. It has a high predictive value for poor neonatal outcome. In the past this technique has been expensive, technically difficult and required regular calibration of the glass electrodes, which are prone to damage.[43] More recently, fibreoptic pH electrodes have overcome some of these difficulties, but more data is awaited. Continuous fetal transcutaneous O_2 and CO_2 tension devices have been assessed but numerous factors may adversely influence recordings, including scalp blood flow, pressure effects and caput formation. At present neither of these techniques are ready for routine intrapartum use although the latter has been used in the management of unusual cases of fetal tachyarrhythmias.

FUTURE OF ELECTRONIC FETAL MONITORING

It is clear that at present and for the foreseeable future, the mainstay for fetal monitoring will continue to be the CTG. In order to reduce intrapartum mortality and hypoxic ischaemic encephalopathy there needs to be an improvement in the use and interpretation of cardiotocographs. Education, standard setting and audit are all required.[44] The whole process may be augmented and assisted by the computer-assisted learning programmes which are becoming available.[45]

COMPUTER SUPPORT

The interpretation of the CTG relies upon pattern recognition and understanding of the risks and variables of labour. Inter- and intra–observer errors continue to be a problem in interpretation. Replacing the observer with a computer may reduce these errors.[46] Data from each minute of the CTG is grouped into 16 epochs, the mean pulse interval is calculated and averaged. This enables the computation of short-term variation (STV). Results correlate with fetal outcome (STV $> 4\,ms$ = 0% metabolic acidosis or intrauterine death $< 2.5\,ms$ = 72% chance of metabolic acidosis or intrauterine death). Short-term variation cannot be deduced by naked-eye interpretation. Its application to intrapartum CTGs is soon to be available.[47]

There are several approaches to the design of such programmes: a decision-support system can be devised using the best expert knowledge. Software can be designed to analyse the fetal heart rate, and particularly decelerations on the CTG, in isolation from the clinical situation. The capacity for computerized analysis of the deceleration area after a contraction has been shown to be a reasonable predictor of a low arterial pH at delivery and FBS pH during labour.[48] Models using neural networks enable the computer to assign a risk to a combination of CTG parameters, e.g. tachycardia, low variability with late decelerations.[49] A further development is to combine the clinical features from the pregnancy and labour with the CTG analysis, to produce in a more sophisticated decision-support engine. Computerization of CTG interpretation may provide standardized decision-making in the future.

SUMMARY

Clinicians must decide which mothers require fetal monitoring and what type of monitoring is appropriate. Intermittent auscultation, if performed adequately, is acceptable in problem-free pregnancies, during low risk labours. A continuous programme of CTG education and audit for all birth attendants of locally-derived standards, definitions and actions is essential. Research into the basic pathophysiological responses of the human fetus during labour is required and, in combination with new rigorously tested technologies, may in the future help to more reliably identify labours which require intervention to prevent intrapartum-related morbidity and death.

REFERENCES

1. Spencer JAD. Deaths related to intrapartum asphyxia. *Br Med J* 1998; **316**: 640.

2. Yeh SY, Diaz F, Paul RN. Ten-year experience of intrapartum fetal monitoring in Los Angeles County/ University of Southern California Medical Centre. *Am J Obstet Gynecol* 1982; **143**: 496–500.

3. Prentice A, Lind T. Fetal heart rate monitoring during labour-too frequent intervention, too little benefit? *Lancet* 1987; **ii**: 1375–1377.

4. Stein PE, White SE, Homan J et al. Fetal endocrine responses to prolonged reduced uterine blood flow are altered following bilateral sectioning of the carotid sinus and vagus nerves. *J Endocrinol* 1998; **157**: 149–155.

5. Spencer JAD. Fetal response to labour. In: Spencer JAD, Ward RHT (eds) *Intrapartum fetal surveillance*. London: RCOG Press, 1993, pp 17–33.

6. Bruns PD, Bowes WA, Drose VE, Battaglia FC. Effect of respiratory acidosis on the rabbit fetus *in utero*. *Am J Obstet Gynecol* 1965; **87**: 1074–1080.

7. Myers RE. Two patterns of perinatal brain damage and conditions of occurrence. *Am J Obstet Gynecol* 1975; **112**: 246–276.

8. Johnson P, Sloper JJ, Powell TC. Glucose loading and cardiorespiratory and metabolic responses to hypoxia and outcomes in neonatal monkeys. *Early Hum Dev* 1988; **18**: 224–225.

9. Gaffney G, Sellers S, Flavell et al. Case–control study of intrapartum care, cerebral palsy, and perinatal death. *Br Med J* 1994; **308**: 743–750.

10. Shenker L, Post RC, Seiler JS. Routine electronic monitoring of the fetal heart rate and uterine activity during labour. *Obstet Gynecol* 1976; **46**: 185–189.

11. Neilson JP. EFM + scalp sampling vs intermittent auscultation in labour. In: Neilson JP, Crowther CA, Hodnett ED, Hofmeyer GJ, Keirse MJNC (eds) *The cochrane pregnancy and childbirth database,* Issue 1. Update Software, Oxford, 1995.

12. Macdonald D, Grant A, Sheridan-Pereira M et al. The Dublin randomised controlled trial of intrapartum fetal heart rate monitoring. *Am J Obstet Gynecol* 1985; **152**: 524–539.

13. Mongelli M, Chung TKH, Chang AMZ. Obstetric intervention and benefit in conditions of very low prevalence. *Br J Obstet Gynaecol* 1997; **104**: 771–774.

14. Lotgering FK, Wallenburg HCS, Schouten HJA. Interobserver and intraobserver variation in the assessment of antepartum cardiotocographs. *Am J Obstet Gynecol* 1982; **144**: 701–705.

15. Saling E, Langner K. Fetal acid base measurements in labour. In: Spencer JAD (ed) *Fetal Monitoring. Physiology and techniques of antenatal and intrapartum assessment*. Tunbridge Wells: Castle House Publication, 1989, pp 172–178.

16. Neilson JP. Cardiotocography during labour. *Br Med J* 1993; **306**: 347–348.

17. Maternal and Child Health Research Consortium. *Confidential enquiry into stillbirths and deaths in infancy (CESDI): 4th annual report*. Department of Health, London, 1997.

18. Fay TN. Modern management of labour. In: Bogod DG (ed) *Bailliere's clinical anaesthesiology – obstetric anaesthesia,* vol 9, Issue 4. London: Bailliere Tindall, 1995, pp 591–605.

19. Gibb D, Arulkumaran S. *Fetal monitoring in practice*. Oxford: Butterworth/Heinemann, 1992.

20. Ingemarsson I, Arulkumaran S, Ingemarsson E et al. Admission test – a screening test for fetal distress in labor. *Obstet Gynecol* 1986; **68**: 800–806.

21. Mahomed K, Nyoni R, Mulambo T, Kasule J, Jacobus E. Randomised controlled trial of intrapartum fetal heart rate monitoring. *Br J Med* 1994; **308**: 497–500.

22. Hofmeyer GJ. Amnioinfusion for meconium-stained liquor in labour. In: Neilson JP, Crowther CA, Hodnett ED, Hofmeyer GJ, Keirse MJNC, Renfrew MJ (eds) *Pregnancy and childbirth module, Cochrane database of systemic reviews*. Oxford: Update Software, 1996.

23. Alfirevic Z, Neilson JP. Doppler ultrasonography in high risk pregnancies: systematic review with meta-analysis. *Am J Obstet Gynecol* 1995; **172**: 1379–1387.

24. Ingemarsson I, Arulkumaran S, Paul RH et al. Fetal acoustic stimulation in early labour in patients screened with the admission test. *Am J Obstet Gynecol* 1988; **158**: 70–74.

25. Johnson N, Johnson VA, Fisher J et al. Fetal monitoring with pulse oximetry. *Br J Obstet Gynaecol* 1991; **98**: 36–41.

26. Konig V, Ullrich G, Huch A, Huch R. Reflectance pulse oximetry-experience in Zurich. In: Labfeber HN (ed) *Fetal and neonatal physiological measurements*. Amsterdam: Elsevier, 1991, pp 111–117.

27. Buschmann J, Knitza R, Rall G. Fetal oxygen saturation measurement by transmission pulse oximetry. *Lancet* 1992; **1**: 615.

28. Gardosi JO, Damianou D, Schram CMH. Artefacts in fetal pulse oximetry: sensor-to-skin contact. *Am J Obstet Gynecol* 1994; **170**: 1169–1173.

29. Dildy GA, Clarke SL, Loucks CS. Intrapartum pulse oximetry: past, present and future. *Am J Obstet Gynecol* 1996; **175**: 1–9.

30. Jobsis FF. Non-invasive infra-red monitoring of cerebral and myocardial oxygen sufficiency and circulatory parameters. *Science* 1977; **198**: 1265–1267.

31. Faris F, Rolfe P, Thorniley M et al. Non-invasive optical monitoring of cerebral blood oxygenation in the foetus and newborn: preliminary investigation. *J Biomed Eng* 1992; **14**: 303–306.

32. Peebles DM, Edwards AD, Wyatt JS et al. Changes in human fetal haemoglobin concentration and oxygenation during labour measured by near infrared spectroscopy. *Am J Obstet Gynecol* 1992; **166**: 1369–1373.

33. Hamilton RJ, O'Brien PMS, Wickramasinghe YABD, Rolfe P. Intrapartum fetal cerebral near infrared spectroscopy: apparent change in oxygenation demonstrated in a non-viable fetus. *Br J Obstet Gynaecol* 1995; **102**: 1004–1007.

34. Jenkins HML, Symonds EM, Kirk DL, Smith PR. Can fetal electrocardiography improve the prediction of intrapartum acidosis? *Br J Obstet Gynaecol* 1986; **93**: 6–12.

35. Marvell CJ, Kirk DL. A simple software routine for the reproducible processing of the electrocardiogram. *J Biomed Eng* 1980; **2**: 216–220.

36. MacLachlan NA, Spencer JAD, Harding K, Arulkumaran S. Fetal acidaemia, the cardiotocograph and the T/QRS ratio of the fetal ECG in labour. *Br J Obstet Gynaecol* 1992; **99**: 26–31.

37. Westgate J, Harris M, Curnow JSH, Greene KR. Plymouth randomised trial of CTG only versus ST waveform plus CTG for intrapartum monitoring in 2400 cases. *Am J Obstet Gynecol* 1995; **169**: 1151–1160.

38. Mohajer MP, Sahota DS, Reed NN et al. Cumulative changes in the fetal electrocardiogram and biochemical indices of fetal hypoxia. *Eur J Obstet Gynecol Reprod Biol* 1994; **55**: 63–70.

39. Reed NN, Mohajer MP, Sahota DS et al. The potential impact of PR interval analysis of the fetal electrocardiogram (FECG) on intrapartum fetal monitoring. *Eur J Obstet Gynecol Reprod Biol* 1996; **68**: 87–92.

40. Murray HG. The fetal electrocardiogram: current clinical developments in Nottingham. *J Perinat Med* 1996; **14**: 399–404.

41. Van Wijngaarden WJ, Sahota DS, James DK et al. Improved intrapartum surveillance with PR interval analysis of the fetal electrocardiogram. *Am J Obstet Gynecol* 1996; **174**: 1296–1299.

42. Strachan BK, Sahota DS, Chang AZM et al. Computerised intrapartum fetal heart rate and fetal electrocardiogram interpretation. *J Obstet Gynaecol* 1997; **17**(suppl 1): S18.

43. Weber T, Nickelsen C. Tissue pH/pCO₂ and continuous base excess monitoring in the human fetus. *J Perinat Med* 1988; **16**(suppl 1): 151–160.

44. Fay TN, Buckley ER (On behalf of the CTG Interpretation Group). Educating clinicians in CTG interpretation. *Br J Obstet Gynaecol* 1998; **105**(suppl 17). Abstract 219.

45. Beckley SL, Stenhouse E, Green KR. Evaluation of a computer-based teaching package for intrapartum fetal monitoring. *Book of abstracts, 4th international symposium on intrapartum surveillance*. Paris, 1997.

46. Pello LC, Rosevaer SK, Dawes GS et al. Computerized fetal heart rate analysis in labor. *Obstet Gynecol* 1991; **78**: 602–610.

47. Dawes G, Lobb M, Moulden M et al. Antenatal cardiotocogram quality and interpretation using computers. *Br J Obstet Gynaecol* 1992; **99**: 791–797.

48. Chung TK, Mohajer MP, Yang ZJ et al. The prediction of fetal acidosis at birth by computerised analysis of intrapartum cardiotocography. *Br J Obstet Gynaecol* 1995; **102**: 454–460.

49. Strachan BK, Sahota DS, Chang AZM et al. Validation of a computerised analysis of fetal heart rate decelerations. *Book of abstracts, 4th international symposium on intrapartum surveillance*. Paris, 1997.

SUGGESTED FURTHER READING

Gibb D, Arulkumaran S. *Fetal monitoring in practice*. Oxford: Butterworth/Heinemann, 1992.

Ingemarsson I, Ingemarsson E, Spencer JAD. *Fetal heart rate monitoring. A practical guide*. Oxford: Oxford University Press, 1993.

Spencer JAD. *Fetal monitoring. Physiology and techniques of antenatal and intrapartum assessment*. Tunbridge Wells: Castle House Publication, 1989.

Spencer JAD, Ward RHT. *Intrapartum fetal surveillance*. London: RCOG Press, 1993.

12

THE OBSTETRIC PATIENT WITH CARDIAC DISEASE

Sarah Hughes

INTRODUCTION

Although uncommon, cardiac disease in obstetric patients remains a significant cause of maternal mortality. The 1997–1999 maternal mortality report records 35 deaths associated with cardiac disease. 29% were due to congenital heart disease, 15% due to ischaemic heart disease, and the remainder due to other acquired cardiac conditions.[1]

Care was said to be substandard in a significant proportion of cases. Although in a few, failure of the mother to take medical advice was the cause, failure to seek early, senior and specialist assistance, and poor co-operation between specialities were mentioned frequently. The report emphasizes the need to follow-up all signs and symptoms of cardiac disease, particularly in Asian immigrants when communication may be difficult and relevant medical history, (such as rheumatic fever, now rarely seen in the UK), difficult to obtain.

Information about how patients with cardiac disease should best be managed is hard to acquire because of the relatively small number of cases and lack of any controlled trials. Most information is acquired from ad hoc case reports and retrospective studies. The setting up of regional and national databases to store details of patients treated should aid the dissemination of information in the future.

The likelihood of a favourable outcome to a pregnancy is dependent in part on the functional state of the patient before pregnancy. Those who are functionally New York Heart Association (NYHA) class I or II (Box 12.1) have a good chance of a favourable outcome. Those who are class III or IV have a 25–30% risk of maternal mortality[2] and are generally advised against pregnancy. In addition, certain conditions carry a particularly high risk of maternal mortality and morbidity; these include Eisenmenger's syndrome, pulmonary hypertension, Marfan's syndrome with aortic root involvement, and tight aortic or mitral stenosis.[1]

GENERAL CONSIDERATIONS

The mother with significant cardiac disease should be managed in a hospital with a well-defined multi-disciplinary approach to her ante-natal follow-up, delivery and post-delivery care. The anaesthetist should be aware of the potential problems early in the pregnancy, and be involved in decision making with obstetricians and cardiologists. The plans for labour management or Caesarean delivery must be practical for any time of the day or night. All senior members of the on-call teams must be equally familiar with the

- Class I   Asymptomatic with activity
- Class II   Some functional limitation
- Class III   Limitation of most activity
- Class IV   Symptomatic at rest

Box 12.1   NYHA classification.

case and happy to manage the situation. A specialist cardiologist who can be rapidly available at any time is an invaluable resource.

Vaginal delivery has traditionally been favoured for patients with cardiac disease. Induction of labour under these circumstances facilitates the co-ordination of all the specialists involved in the care of a patient and permits reversal of anticoagulation, if necessary. It does, however, expose the patient to the potentially harmful cardiovascular side effects of the drugs used to induce labour. Labour and vaginal delivery are also associated with profound haemodynamic changes (see below) which may be undesirable in patients with cardiac disease. Shortening the second stage by assisted delivery may be appropriate in some patients, to avoid pushing and the associated valsalva effect.

Good analgesia minimizes the cardiovascular changes, which accompany labour, but in the case of regional analgesia consideration must be given to the effects of sympathetic blockade on the cardiovascular system in the presence of a given cardiac lesion. The widespread use of dilute local anaesthetic solutions and epidural opioids for labour analgesia has increased the number of patients with cardiac disease for whom regional analgesia is appropriate.

Caesarean section is associated with a greater blood loss than vaginal delivery, but avoids exposing the patient to the cardiovascular changes of labour, and minimizes the risk to the fetus. In addition, Caesarean section may be appropriate because the condition of the mother or fetus necessitates delivery at a time when induction of labour is not appropriate.

Full-dose spinal anaesthesia is rarely, if ever, appropriate for patients with cardiac disease. However, the use of carefully controlled epidural or incremental combined spinal-epidural anaesthesia for Caesarean section, in the presence of conditions in which general anaesthesia was formerly thought mandatory, is being described more frequently in the literature.

General anaesthesia remains necessary for some patients because regional anaesthesia is contraindicated, or because the urgency of the situation does not allow the institution of regional anaesthesia. Many patients with cardiac disease will not tolerate the vasodilatation and myocardial depression associated with a standard rapid sequence induction. A 'cardiac' type induction, using high dose opioids may be more appropriate. It should, however, be borne in mind that this method of induction increases the risk to the patient of aspiration of gastric contents. H_2 antagonists, prokinetic agents and antacids should be used to optimize the volume and pH of gastric contents prior to induction of anaesthesia. If high dose intravenous opioids are given prior to delivery, the attending paediatrician should also be alerted.

MONITORING DURING LABOUR OR CAESAREAN SECTION

The extent to which patients should be monitored depends on each individual case. The location of the delivery should also be considered. In a hospital where maternity services are on a remote site it may be more appropriate for delivery to be carried out closer to the intensive care or high dependency unit, if appropriate monitoring is not available within the delivery suite (Box 12.2).

For all patients with cardiac disease, a certain minimum level of monitoring is essential. This includes cardiotocography, continuous ECG monitoring, preferably leads II and V5, non-invasive blood pressure and pulse oximetry. An arterial cannula is helpful if tight control of blood pressure is important as in Marfan's syndrome. A central venous line may provide helpful information about filling pressures and permits the administration of vasoactive drugs. Most controversial

is the use of pulmonary artery catheters, as their use is complicated by the most serious side effects. They are however useful if left ventricular pre-load needs to be maintained within a narrow range as in severe mitral or aortic stenosis, or if there is significant ventricular dysfunction, ischaemia or cardiomyopathy.

Full monitoring should be continued in an appropriate high dependency area for at least 24 h postpartum as patients are at high risk of fluid overload and other complications during this time.

CHANGES IN CARDIOVASCULAR PHYSIOLOGY DURING PREGNANCY AND DELIVERY

Cardiac output increases during the first and second trimester and reaches 60% above pre-pregnant levels by 28 weeks. This is achieved by a combination of increased heart rate (15%) and increased stroke volume (30%). Plasma volume increases by 50% during pregnancy due to salt and water retention. Red cell mass increases by 20%, stimulated by erythropoietin.

During the latter half of pregnancy, the mass of the uterus compresses the vena cava when the patient is supine, reducing venous return. Prevention of vena cava compression is an important consideration in all pregnant patients, but especially so for the mother with cardiac disease.

During the first stage of labour, cardiac output rises by a further 10% above pregnant levels. During uterine contractions blood from the placental bed enters the circulation, an effect equivalent to the transfusion of approximately 500 ml of blood. During the second stage of labour, cardiac output may reach 50% above pregnant levels, and immediately after delivery, the relief of vena cava compression and the autotransfusion of blood from the placental bed result in a cardiac output, which may reach 80% above the pregnant level.

CARDIOVASCULAR DRUG THERAPY IN PREGNANCY

Whenever possible, medication should be avoided during pregnancy. Many patients with cardiac disease, however, will need to continue to take drugs during pregnancy, and may need additional or different medication at this time. A number of factors must be considered when prescribing for the pregnant patient:

• the effect of the drugs on the fetus and its development;

For all patients:
• Large bore venous cannula and continuous oxygen
• ECG leads II and V5
• Non-invasive blood pressure
• Pulse oximetry
• CTG

For selected patients:
• Invasive blood pressure
• Central venous line
• Pulmonary artery catheter

Box 12.2   Monitoring patients with cardiac disease.

- the effect of the drugs on uteroplacental blood flow;
- the effect of the drugs on uterine contractility.

There are few controlled studies of the effects of drugs during pregnancy, and many older agents remain in use because they have been found, with prolonged use and through anecdotal evidence, not to have deleterious effects in the pregnant patient.

In addition to the above considerations, the absorption, distribution, metabolism and elimination of many drugs will be altered during pregnancy. Where it is available, close monitoring of plasma drug levels is advisable during pregnancy.

ANTICOAGULANTS

Pregnant patients may need to take anticoagulant medication for prophylaxis or treatment of thromboembolic disease, or because of the presence of a diseased or mechanical heart valve.

Heparin is a large, highly polarized molecule, which does not cross the placenta, and does not appear to have any adverse effects on intrauterine fetal development. Prolonged use, however, is related to maternal thrombocytopenia and osteoporosis. Its use is generally restricted to the first trimester when organogenesis is taking place, and to late pregnancy when it is desirable to be able to reverse anticoagulation rapidly before delivery. For full anticoagulation heparin must be given as an intravenous infusion.

Low molecular weight heparin (LMWH) has replaced much of the unfractionated heparin that was previously used. It has gained ground in the treatment of thromboembolic disease but has not been widely used in cases of high-risk mechanical valves.

Warfarin has the advantage that it can be taken orally. It is a smaller molecule, which readily crosses the placenta and has been associated with the fetal warfarin syndrome. This is a diverse collection of developmental abnormalities including hydrocephalus, microcephaly, growth retardation, and ophthalmic abnormalities.[3] The incidence of these abnormalities is related to the dose of warfarin rather than the INR. Warfarin is thus particularly unsuitable for those mothers who need to take a large dose, either because of drug resistance or because of the need to have a high INR. Warfarin is not used in the first trimester when the risks are highest, but may be used in the second and third, before heparin is restarted near term.

ANTIDYSRHYTHMIC DRUGS

Treatment of dysrhythmias in the pregnant patient does not differ significantly from that in non-pregnant patients. The effects of any drugs used on the fetus must however be considered.

Digoxin crosses the placenta readily. At term fetal levels are similar to maternal levels.[4] There are no reports of teratogenicity or untoward fetal effects associated with the prolonged use of digoxin during pregnancy, but fetal deaths have been reported in association with maternal digoxin toxicity.[5] Monitoring of maternal serum digoxin concentrations is important for this reason. In addition, the renal clearance of digoxin may be increased due to the increase in renal blood flow.

Amiodarone has not been widely used during pregnancy, but there are reports of its use with no adverse fetal effects.[6,7] However, because of limited experience and its general toxicity, it is generally reserved for dangerous dysrhythmias which are refractory to treatment with other agents.

Adenosine is a newer agent with a very short half life, which is widely used to treat supraventricular tachydysrhythmias. There are reports of its use in pregnant patients[8,9] without adverse fetal effects, and it can be used to terminate SVT in labour.

β BLOCKERS

Propranolol has been widely used during pregnancy in the treatment of hypertension, thyrotoxicosis and obstructive cardiomyopathy. There are no reports of fetal abnormalities associated with its use, but it has been associated with fetal hypoglycaemia, bradycardia and apnoea.[10,11] It may be given orally or, at much lower doses, intravenously.

Labetolol has both α and β blocking activity. It has been used for many years in the treatment of hypertension during pregnancy, and is not associated with any adverse fetal effects.[12] It may be given as intravenous boluses. An infusion may be used to gain rapid control of blood pressure.

VASODILATORS

Hydralazine has been used for many years to treat hypertension during pregnancy, and appears to have no adverse effect on uterine blood flow or fetal development. It may be given orally, or intravenously in the treatment of severe hypertension.[13]

Nifedipine is not licensed for use during pregnancy, but has been extensively used for the treatment of hypertension and premature labour, and appears to be safe.[14] It may be given sub-lingually in patients who are unable to take oral medication.

ANGIOTENSIN CONVERTING ENZYME (ACE) INHIBITORS AND DIURETICS

There is little experience in the use of ACE inhibitors during pregnancy. Because of reports of an increase in intrauterine deaths and stillbirths in animals treated with captopril they are avoided if possible.[15,16]

Diuretics in the large part can be used safely to control heart failure and fluid over-load in pregnancy.

VASOPRESSORS

Epidural and spinal blockade can produce maternal systemic hypotension, which if profound or prolonged, may have a detrimental effect on fetal well-being.[17] Vasopressors are widely used to provide a rapid restoration of blood pressure.

Ephedrine, a mixed α and β adrenergic agonist, is widely used in obstetric practice because of animal studies that suggest it maintains uterine perfusion better than other agents.[18] In the presence of cardiovascular disease however, the inotropic and chronotropic actions of ephedrine may be undesirable for the mother.

Phenylephrine and methoxamine are both α adrenergic agonists and have been used in small doses (boluses of 100 μg and 2 mg respectively) to correct maternal hypotension without deleterious effects on the fetus.[19,20]

ANTIBIOTIC PROPHYLAXIS

Antibiotic cover is required for all procedures which are likely to cause a bacteraemia in women with prosthetic or rheumatic valves, congenital cardiac lesions and surgically produced shunts. The recommendations of a working party are:[21] i.v. amoxycillin 1 g and gentamicin 120 mg, followed by amoxycillin 500 mg given orally 6 h later. For patients who are allergic to penicillin, vancomycin 500 mg should be given in place of amoxycillin.

OBSTETRIC DRUG THERAPY IN THE PRESENCE OF CARDIAC DISEASE

Oxytocic agents are widely used in obstetric practice for the induction of labour and prevention or treatment of postpartum haemorrhage, but their use may be associated with cardiovascular side effects, which are undesirable in the presence of cardiac disease:

- Oxytocin in bolus doses of 5–10 IU causes vasodilatation and may cause significant hypotension.
- Ergometrine causes vasoconstriction and may precipitate pulmonary oedema in the presence of cardiac disease.
- Prostaglandin F2α has been shown to increase pulmonary arterial pressure and pulmonary capillary wedge pressure.

Infusion of dilute solutions of oxytocin appears to be associated with minimal cardiovascular changes and is the agent of choice in the treatment of uterine atony.[22,23] Five units of syntocinon diluted to 10 ml and given slowly, followed by a further 5 units given as a slow infusion as necessary is recommended.

VALVULAR HEART DISEASE

MITRAL STENOSIS

Mitral stenosis is a common isolated valve lesion seen in pregnant patients and is generally rheumatic in origin, with symptoms developing 10–15 years after the initial illness (Box 12.3).[24]

The primary physiological abnormality in mitral stenosis is obstruction to the flow of blood from the left atrium to the left ventricle. Blood flow across the valve depends on the area of the valve, the atrio-ventricular pressure gradient, and the time available for blood flow. The normal valve area is 4–$6\,cm^2$. Typically symptoms of mitral stenosis occur when this is reduced to $2\,cm^2$. A valve area of less than $1\,cm^2$ represents severe mitral stenosis and requires an AV pressure gradient of 20 mmHg to maintain the cardiac output at rest.[25]

In overcoming the obstruction, left atrial pressure and volume increase. This is followed by a rise in pulmonary venous pressure and pulmonary capillary pressure. Long-standing pulmonary hypertension results in

---

- Avoid increases in heart rate. Treat dysrhythmias aggressively
- Monitor and maintain pre-load within a narrow optimal range
- Avoid sudden and severe decreases in systemic vascular resistance
- Avoid increases in pulmonary vascular resistance (e.g. hypoxia, hypercarbia, PEEP)

Box 12.3   Mitral stenosis and pregnancy.

pulmonary artery medial thickening and an irreversible rise in pulmonary vascular resistance. Right ventricular hypertrophy, dilatation and failure ensue, with tricuspid regurgitation, hepatic and peripheral congestion.

Any increase in heart rate results in a disproportionate reduction in the length of diastole, the time available for blood flow across the valve. Tachycardia therefore increases the pressure gradient across the valve and further elevates the left atrial pressure.

Left atrial enlargement predisposes to the development of supraventricular dysrhythmias. The sudden onset of atrial fibrillation may precipitate acute pulmonary oedema and cardiac decompensation. Long-standing atrial fibrillation predisposes to the formation of left atrial thrombi and systemic emboli. Such patients require long-term anticoagulation with warfarin, which should be changed to heparin during early pregnancy.

Clinical findings

The main symptom of mitral stenosis is dyspnoea due to reduced pulmonary compliance; initially on exertion only, later occurring at rest. Orthopnoea and paroxysmal nocturnal dyspnoea also occur later in the course of the disease as a result of increased pulmonary pressures. Symptoms may become apparent for the first time during pregnancy, because of the increase in blood volume, heart rate, and cardiac output, all of which contribute to a rise in left atrial pressure.[25] Presentation with decompensated heart failure usually occurs in the mid-trimester.

Examination reveals a mid-diastolic murmur with presystolic accentuation, loudest with the patient lying on her right side, and an opening snap following the second heart sound. The duration, but not intensity of the murmur is related to the severity of valve stenosis. If right ventricular hypertrophy is present, a right ventricular heave will be palpable. The jugular venous pressure may be normal or increased in the presence of pulmonary hypertension and a raised right ventricular end diastolic pressure.

Left atrial enlargement is shown by the presence of P mitrale on the ECG, there may also be evidence of right ventricular hypertrophy. Atrial fibrillation is a common finding in patients with mitral stenosis. The chest X-ray may be normal in mild mitral stenosis. As the disease progresses the enlarged left atrium appears as a double shadow on the right border of the heart, with a bump on the left border. Right ventricular enlargement may also be seen. On echocardiography, the valve is seen to open less and close more slowly than normal. Doppler echocardiography combined with conventional techniques, permits estimation of the cross-sectional area of the valve and the blood flow across it.

Patients with severe mitral stenosis and intractable cardiac failure may require surgical intervention during pregnancy. Closed mitral valvotomy has been performed successfully during pregnancy with good maternal and fetal survival.[26]

Anaesthesia

Patients with mitral stenosis, who are asymptomatic, generally tolerate pregnancy and delivery well, and do not require invasive monitoring. Patients with severe or symptomatic mitral stenosis may benefit from the use of arterial and pulmonary artery catheters to aid fluid management.[27] The time of greatest risk during labour is delivery and the early postpartum period, when the most marked haemodynamic changes occur.

Pre-load must be preserved to maintain cardiac output. Decreases in right atrial filling, which may occur with aorto-caval compression, anaesthesia or blood loss, can precipitate a fall in cardiac output. Rises such as those that may occur with autotransfusion from the uteroplacental bed, are also poorly tolerated and may result in pulmonary oedema. The pulmonary capillary wedge pressure will tend to overestimate the left ventricular filling pressure, but the trend is a reliable guide to changes in pre-load and can be used to maintain the pre-load within the narrow optimal range.

Increases in heart rate reduce the time available for ventricular filling and increase the pressure gradient across the valve. Steps should therefore be taken to avoid increases, which can occur with pain, stress, light general anaesthesia, and in response to tracheal intubation. Dysrhythmias such as atrial fibrillation compromise ventricular filling and should be treated aggressively with drugs or cardioversion.

In severe mitral stenosis, the stroke volume is fixed and cannot be increased to compensate for decreases in systemic vascular resistance. Cardiac output can only be increased by increasing heart rate, which may in itself have a deleterious effect on cardiac function.

Factors which increase the pulmonary vascular resistance should be avoided. These include hypoxia, hypercarbia, acidosis, and lung hyperinflation. Prostaglandins used in the treatment of uterine atony increase pulmonary vascular resistance and can precipitate right ventricular failure.

Regional anaesthesia

In the absence of adverse obstetric factors, vaginal delivery is preferred in patients with mild to moderate mitral stenosis. Pain and stress cause tachycardia, and can be avoided through the use of regional analgesia. Regional blockade should be instituted slowly with low concentrations of local anaesthetic. The addition of opioids is helpful in reducing the local anaesthetic requirement. Hypotension should be treated with intravenous fluid if the wedge pressure suggests that this is appropriate, or small increments of a vasoconstrictor. Ephedrine is best avoided because of its effect on heart rate, as are epinephrine containing local anaesthetic solutions. Assisted delivery using forceps of vacuum extraction may be useful to prevent the valsalva effect produced by expulsive efforts.

General anaesthesia

Regional anaesthesia can also be used for Caesarean section, but for patients who are NYHA functional class III or IV, most reviews favour general anaesthesia. It may also be necessary in patients who are anticoagulated. The rise in heart rate, which accompanies intubation may be prevented by the use of opioids or β blockers. Patients with severe mitral stenosis may not tolerate the reduction in systemic vascular resistance, which occurs with the use of thiopentone and volatile agents. In such cases, the use of a high dose opioid anaesthetic technique is appropriate.

Post-delivery care

High dependency care is advisable for at least 48 h postpartum, as this is a period when there is a high risk of pulmonary oedema. The increase in pre-load associated with the withdrawal of sympathetic blockade is accompanied by an increase in circulating blood volume as the uterus contracts and there is relief of vena cava compression. Treatment with a diuretic may be necessary. Adequate pain control is important to prevent tachycardia. This can be achieved through the use of parenteral or epidural opioids.

AORTIC STENOSIS

Aortic stenosis is usually congenital in origin and is more common in males than females. When severe, it is associated with significant maternal and fetal mortality.[28,29]

The primary physiological abnormality in aortic stenosis is obstruction to left ventricular outflow. The chronic pressure overload produces a hypertrophied left ventricle, which is susceptible to ischaemia even in the presence of normal coronary arteries.

The symptoms of aortic stenosis are dyspnoea on exertion, syncope and angina. Unlike mitral stenosis, symptoms occur relatively late in the course of the disease, the absence of symptoms therefore does not necessarily imply mild disease. Because of the late on-set of symptoms, a pre-pregnancy exercise test will help to identify those women with the reserve to tolerate pregnancy.

Examination reveals a pulse which is slow rising and plateau in character; the pulse pressure may be reduced in tight aortic stenosis. An ejection systolic murmur can be heard in the aortic area; as the stenosis becomes more severe the murmur lengthens. Eventually left ventricular exceeds right ventricular ejection time and the aortic component of the second heart sound is heard after the pulmonary component (reverse splitting).

The ECG in significant aortic stenosis shows left ventricular hypertrophy and strain. Left ventricular enlargement may also be evident on the chest X-ray. Doppler echocardiography can be used to measure the gradient across the valve. A gradient of greater than 50 mmHg is considered to represent significant aortic stenosis. Echocardiography can also be used to determine the area of the valve. Since the pressure gradient across the valve is flow dependent, the gradient and valve area should be used together to determine disease severity. This is especially relevant in pregnancy because of the increased cardiac output. A gradient measured across the valve is virtually meaningless unless it is a pre-pregnancy value with valvular area. A cross-sectional valvular area of less than $1 \, cm^2$ represents significant aortic stenosis and less than $0.7 \, cm^2$ severe aortic stenosis (normal $2.5–3.6 \, cm^2$).

Anaesthesia

Pre-load

The hypertrophied, non-compliant left ventricle is sensitive to changes in pre-load: A small change in fluid loading can produce a significant change in left ventricular end diastolic pressure. Haemorrhage and aorto-caval compression can have severe effects. Decreases in left ventricular filling will reduce stroke volume and cardiac output, but increases can cause pulmonary oedema. The range of appropriate fluid loading is therefore narrow. In a normal heart, atrial systole accounts for approximately 20% of ventricular filling. In the presence of aortic stenosis, its contribution may be as much as 40%.[30] Dysrhythmias therefore have an adverse effect on cardiac output.

After-load

In the presence of aortic stenosis, cardiac output is relatively fixed and cannot be increased to compensate for reductions in systemic vascular resistance which can result in severe hypotension. The only mechanism by which the cardiac output can be increased is by an increase in heart rate, therefore drugs which produce bradycardia are poorly tolerated. Heart rates above 140 bpm however are also undesirable because the time available for ventricular filling and coronary perfusion is reduced, increasing the risk of ischaemia.

Patients with significant aortic stenosis may benefit from invasive monitoring. An arterial line is essential and in the most difficult cases a pulmonary artery catheter allows accurate monitoring of left ventricular pre-load, which needs to be maintained within narrow limits. The most serious risk associated with its use is the precipitation of dysrhythmias, which can adversely affect ventricular filling.[31]

Regional analgesia and anaesthesia

The tachycardia associated with pain and stress during labour is undesirable. Epidural analgesia, although traditionally considered to be contraindicated in the presence of aortic stenosis, has been performed successfully using dilute local anaesthetic solutions and opioids, to minimize the haemodynamic changes associated with labour and delivery.[32] Pre-load should be closely monitored during regional analgesia and fluids given as needed to avoid hypotension and fluid overload. Epinephrine containing local anaesthetic solutions are best avoided because of their potential for producing tachycardia. Similarly if a vasopressor is needed, ephedrine should be avoided because of its effect on heart rate, especially if her heart rate is towards the upper range of normal. Phenylephrine is a suitable alternative.

The haemodynamic aims in the presence of aortic stenosis are well established (Box 12.4), but how they may best be achieved in the obstetric patient remains controversial.[33,34]

- Avoid decreases in systemic vascular resistance
- Monitor and maintain left ventricular pre-load
- Avoid bradycardia
- Avoid tachycardia
- Treat dysrhythmias aggressively
- Avoid myocardial depression

Box 12.4   Aortic stenosis and pregnancy.

Historically, regional anaesthesia was considered contraindicated in the presence of aortic stenosis, because of the reduction in after-load associated with sympathetic blockade. There are, however, a growing number of reports in the literature of successful Caesarean section under both epidural anaesthesia[31,32] and, more recently, spinal anaesthesia employing a subarachnoid catheter[35] or incremental combined spinal-epidural, to allow careful titration of local anaesthetic dose to level of block.

General anaesthesia

If general anaesthesia is employed, the standard obstetric 'rapid sequence' induction may produce a catastrophic fall in cardiac output and systemic vascular resistance, and the response to intubation, an undesirable tachycardia. A high dose opioid, 'cardiac' anaesthetic technique minimizes the haemodynamic response to intubation, and the need for volatile agents with their undesirable effects on systemic vascular resistance and myocardial contractility.

Bolus injections of oxytocin can cause a decrease in systemic vascular resistance and should be avoided; infusions of dilute solutions have been used without adverse consequences.[31,33]

Post-delivery care

High dependency care with full haemodynamic monitoring are advisable for 24–48 h postpartum, in patients with aortic stenosis. Post-operative analgesia is important to prevent tachycardia due to pain, which will have an undesirable effect on myocardial oxygen supply and ventricular filling. The combination of the withdrawal of the vasodilator action of anaesthetic agents and autotransfusion from the uterine bed may result in fluid overload and require treatment with a diuretic.

MITRAL REGURGITATION

Mitral regurgitation is usually rheumatic in origin and often occurs in association with mitral stenosis (Box 12.5).[36] Non-rheumatic causes include mitral valve prolapse, connective tissue disorders, papillary muscle or chordae tendinae dysfunction.

Failure of the mitral valve to close completely during ventricular systole results in the regurgitant flow of blood into the left atrium. The degree of regurgitant flow depends on the size of the orifice through which flow occurs, the ventriculo-atrial pressure gradient, and the time available for flow. The retrograde flow

- Maintain adequate left ventricular pre-load
- Avoid bradycardia
- Avoid vasoconstriction
- Treat dysrhythmias aggressively

Box 12.5 Mitral regurgitation and pregnancy.

of blood increases left atrial volume and eventually pressure, and producing pulmonary congestion and oedema. The volume load of the left ventricle from the dilated left atrium is also increased. An increase in left ventricular compliance maintains the left ventricular end diastolic pressure within normal limits until late in the course of the disease. An increased stroke volume maintains the forward flow of blood in the early stages of the disease, until a deterioration of left ventricular function due to chronic volume overload, causes a reduction in forward flow and the symptoms of fatigue and weakness follow.

Late sequelae of mitral regurgitation include pulmonary hypertension, right ventricular hypertrophy and biventricular failure.[37] Complications of the condition include supraventricular dysrhythmias, systemic emboli and bacterial endocarditis.

Clinical findings

The main symptoms of mitral regurgitation are those of left ventricular failure and the main sign is a pan-systolic murmur, which is transmitted to the left axilla. In severe mitral regurgitation, a third heart sound may also be heard. The ECG is normal except in the presence of severe mitral regurgitation when P mitrale and evidence of left ventricular hypertrophy may be seen. The chest X-ray shows left ventricular hypertrophy and a double right heart border indicating left atrial enlargement. Pulmonary oedema may also be evident in late disease.

Anaesthesia

The decreased systemic vascular resistance and tachycardia of pregnancy are beneficial in mitral regurgitation. The increase in blood volume is generally accommodated by the compliant left ventricle, but may cause pulmonary congestion in patients with symptomatic mitral regurgitation. Patients with moderate to severe symptomatic disease benefit from haemodynamic monitoring with arterial and pulmonary artery catheters during labour and delivery or Caesarean section.[38]

Regional anaesthesia

Epidural blockade is appropriate for both vaginal delivery and Caesarean section, as the decrease in systemic vascular resistance favours the forward flow of blood. Volume loading is helpful to prevent a fall in pre-load, in severe mitral regurgitation invasive monitoring of the left ventricular pre-load may be helpful. Blood loss must be treated aggressively to prevent a fall in pre-load and cardiac output. Ephedrine is a suitable agent to treat the hypotension associated with sympathetic block as a slight tachycardia is helpful. Atrial dysrhythmias and left atrial enlargement are relatively common in mitral regurgitation and patients may therefore be anticoagulated, which will limit the use of regional techniques, unless reversed.

General anaesthesia

If general anaesthesia is necessary, steps should be taken to prevent the pressor response to intubation. Light anaesthesia causes vasoconstriction and should be avoided. A rapid sequence induction followed by maintenance with isoflurane and narcotics following delivery, achieves vasodilatation and a mild tachycardia. Supraventricular dysrhythmias may cause left ventricular decompensation and require immediate treatment with pharmacological or DC cardioversion.

MITRAL VALVE PROLAPSE

Mitral valve prolapse is the most common congenital heart lesion affecting 5–10% of the population.[39] In most patients it has a benign course, and causes no symptoms. A small proportion of patients have significant mitral regurgitation. The characteristic sign of mitral valve prolapse is a mid to late systolic click, which is sometimes followed by a late systolic murmur. The timing and duration of the murmur reflect the severity of mitral regurgitation.

Conditions which decrease left ventricular volume cause earlier prolapsing of the valve and exacerbate mitral regurgitation. These factors include a decrease in pre-load, an increase in airway pressure, increased contractility and tachycardia.[40]

In patients who are asymptomatic, pregnancy and delivery generally cause no problems, provided account is taken of the above factors. Ephedrine is best avoided in the management of hypotension because of its effect on heart rate and contractility. Phenylephrine and methoxamine are suitable alternatives. Patients with significant mitral regurgitation should be managed as outlined above.

AORTIC REGURGITATION

Aortic regurgitation is uncommon in pregnant women. It is usually due to rheumatic fever, but may also be seen in association with aortic stenosis after valvotomy, connective tissue disorders such as systemic lupus erythematosus, or Marfan's syndrome.

In aortic regurgitation, the retrograde flow of blood across the aortic valve imposes a chronic volume overload on the left ventricle. This results in left ventricular distension, but an increase in left ventricular compliance means that the left ventricular end diastolic pressure remains normal until late in the course of the disease. The degree of regurgitation depends on the area of the regurgitant orifice, the aortic-left ventricular pressure gradient and the duration of diastole.

The increase in circulatory volume associated with pregnancy is generally well tolerated by patients with aortic regurgitation, and the increase in heart rate encourages forward flow.

Clinical findings

The usual symptoms of aortic regurgitation are those of congestive cardiac failure. Angina and syncope occur less commonly. The pulse pressure is wide with bounding peripheral pulses and a low diastolic pressure. An early diastolic murmur is audible at the left sternal edge. Left ventricular hypertrophy is evident on the ECG and chest X-ray. Pulmonary congestion may also be seen on the chest X-ray.

Anaesthesia

The anaesthetic considerations in aortic regurgitation are similar to those in mitral regurgitation, with most authors considering regional blockade to be appropriate for vaginal delivery and Caesarean section.[38] There is however a report of cardiovascular collapse following epidural anaesthesia in a patient with aortic regurgitation. The cause was thought to be myocardial ischaemia due to hypotension. The case underlines the importance of aggressive treatment of hypotension, with vasopressors and positioning the mother to avoid aorto-caval compression, in order to maintain diastolic pressure and myocardial perfusion.[41]

Unlike patients with aortic stenosis, those with aortic regurgitation tolerate a wide range of left ventricular pre-loads, and the use of a pulmonary artery catheter is rarely necessary.

ISCHAEMIC HEART DISEASE

Myocardial infarction is unusual in pregnancy, with an estimated incidence of 1 in 10 000 pregnancies.[42] It is a major cause of death in UK, and coupled with a trend towards later childbearing, it may become a more common complication of pregnancy in the future. During the period 1997–1999, 5 deaths were reported in which ischaemic heart disease was the cause.[1]

In addition to coronary artery disease, there are other aetiological factors that may be relevant in the pregnant patient; the hypercoagulable state, which is associated with pregnancy, may predispose to the formation of coronary thrombus, and coronary artery spasm may be related to renin release from the placenta, which contains 160 times more renin than human plasma.[43] The hormonal changes which accompany pregnancy may contribute to the relatively high incidence of coronary artery dissection noted in pregnant patients after myocardial infarction.[44]

Mortality depends on the timing of the infarction, being highest in the puerperium. The overall mortality is estimated to be 28%. Most deaths occur at the time of infarction, or within 2 weeks. Delivery during this time is associated with a particularly high mortality (50%).[45]

MANAGEMENT OF ACUTE MYOCARDIAL INFARCTION IN PREGNANCY

Diagnosis of acute myocardial infarction is usually based on a characteristic history, ECG changes, and a rise in cardiac enzyme levels in blood. The situation in pregnancy is complicated by the frequent occurrence during pregnancy of non-cardiac chest pain related to gastro-oesophageal reflux, and the non-specific ECG changes which accompany pregnancy.[46]

The management of an acute myocardial infarction during pregnancy is similar to that in a non-pregnant patient and includes admission to a coronary care unit, supplementary oxygen, analgesia, intravenous nitrates, and bed rest. In addition, care must be taken to avoid vena cava compression by maintaining a left lateral tilt. Thrombolytic therapy with streptokinase is now routine therapy after myocardial infarction to limit infarct size and reduce mortality. In pregnancy, streptokinase has been associated with maternal bleeding, premature labour and dysfunctional uterine contraction, and is therefore not used routinely.[47] Some authors, however, recommend its use in potentially life threatening situations such as a large anterior myocardial infarction, provided that there are no other contraindications.[48] The successful use of tissue plasminogen activator following a myocardial infarction in a pregnant patient has been described.[49]

If angina persists after a myocardial infarction, angiography should be considered, and if necessary, angioplasty or bypass surgery performed. Both are reported to have been carried out successfully during pregnancy,[50–52] although by-pass surgery carries a high mortality to the fetus, which if viable, should be delivered.

MANAGEMENT OF DELIVERY AFTER MYOCARDIAL INFARCTION

Patients who have had a myocardial infarction during pregnancy, may have to undergo delivery within 3 months of that infarct, when they are most at risk of further adverse cardiac events. Whenever possible, delivery should be delayed until at least 2 weeks after a myocardial infarction, because of the particularly high mortality associated with delivery within this period.[45] No consensus exists on the best mode of delivery in these patients. Elective Caesarean section allows the time of delivery to be planned and all necessary medical personnel to be available, but exposes the patient to the stress of surgery and the risk of increased blood loss. Vaginal delivery removes the stress of surgery, but labour itself may be prolonged and stressful, and is associated with rises in cardiac output which may reach 80% above pregnant levels immediately postpartum.[44,53,54]

Regional anaesthesia

Most authors conclude that in the absence of obstetric indications for Caesarean section, or significant myocardial dysfunction,[55] vaginal delivery with regional analgesia is the preferred method of delivery. The use of forceps or ventouse extraction to shorten the second stage may be appropriate.[55] A low dose local anaesthetic and an opioid epidural will provide good analgesia and prevent breakthrough pain and the need for large boluses of local anaesthetic. Epinephrine containing local anaesthetics should be avoided, since the tachycardia produced may have an adverse effect on the balance of myocardial oxygen supply and demand.

Epidural anaesthesia is also appropriate for Caesarean section. The level of anaesthesia should be controlled with careful infusion of fluid to maintain pre-load and blood pressure. High dose spinal anaesthesia carries the risk of rapid onset of block with severe hypotension and tachycardia and should be avoided, although an incremental combined spinal-epidural can be used.

General anaesthesia

If general anaesthesia is employed for Caesarean section, steps should be taken to minimize the pressor response that occurs in response to intubation. Opioids, β blockers and lidocaine have been used for this purpose. If opioids are given to the mother before delivery the paediatrician should be advised of this and the baby given naloxone if necessary. Parenteral nitrates have been used in parturients with ischaemic heart disease, but care must be taken if they are used in combination with epidural anaesthesia, as the combination may produce marked hypotension and reduce myocardial oxygen supply.

The extent to which a patient needs to be monitored should be assessed on an individual basis. Non-invasive monitoring of blood pressure, ECG, and pulse oximetry is advisable in all patients with ischaemic heart disease. Invasive monitoring with a pulmonary artery catheter is useful in the management of patients with significant myocardial dysfunction; the pulmonary capillary wedge pressure (PCWP) provides a guide to fluid therapy. A rapid rise may reflect deteriorating left ventricular function and the need for intervention.

Post-delivery care

Continuous monitoring and care in a high dependency area are necessary for at least 24 h postpartum, as the risk of adverse cardiac events remains high at this time. Analgesia in the postpartum period can be provided with epidural local anaesthetic and opioid infusions, or a parenteral opioid infusion. Pre-load may increase as anaesthesia subsides and intravascular volume increases after delivery and may require treatment with a diuretic or nitrate.

CARDIAC ARREST

Cardiac arrest during pregnancy is unusual, occurring approximately once in every 30 000 pregnancies.[56,60]

Basic life support should be instituted as soon as possible after cardiac arrest. Because of the physiological changes, which occur during pregnancy, certain modifications are necessary to resuscitation protocols for the non-pregnant patient (Box 12.6).[61]

Aorto-caval compression must be relieved by tilting the patient to the left. This can be achieved using a

- Relieve vena cava compression
- Early endotracheal intubation. Cricoid pressure during facemask ventilation
- Altered drug therapy after epidural local anaesthetic
- Early Caesarean section

Box 12.6   Cardiopulmonary resuscitation in pregnancy.

'Cardiff' wedge[57] or human wedge.[58] If the patient cannot be tilted, the gravid uterus should be displaced manually by an assistant.

Standard protocols for the treatment of dysrhythmias and asystole apply during pregnancy. The exception is the patient who has received epidural local anaesthetics;[62] in this situation lidocaine should be avoided because of the risk of precipitating local anaesthetic toxicity. Bretylium tosylate is a suitable alternative agent for the treatment of refractory VF.[59]

CONGENITAL HEART DISEASE

The frequency with which congenital heart disease is encountered during pregnancy is increasing, as improved medical and surgical management results in growing numbers of women with congenital heart disease reaching childbearing age. At the same time rheumatic heart disease is declining, producing a reversal in the ratio of congenital to rheumatic heart disease seen during pregnancy.[38]

Many patients with congenital heart disease will have undergone cardiac surgery which may have been corrective or palliative, and may have taken place many years previously. Details of the procedure performed and its results may be difficult to obtain. It is helpful if such patients are seen, assessed, and if necessary, investigated with echocardiography or cardiac catheterization before pregnancy is considered, in order that the effects of pregnancy and of anaesthetic interventions can be more accurately predicted. Unfortunately this may not be the case and the mother presents once pregnant, when a full assessment is not possible.

Congenital heart disease falls into four broad categories:

- left to right shunts (ASD, VSD, PDA);
- right to left shunts (Fallot's, Eisenmenger's syndrome);
- vascular lesions (coarctation of the aorta);
- valvular lesions.

Generally, for patients with acyanotic heart disease who are functionally New York Heart Association class I or II the risk of pregnancy is small. For patients with cyanotic heart disease, who are NYHA class III or IV or have pulmonary hypertension, the maternal and fetal mortality is significant, and many consider pregnancy contraindicated in such patients. Surgical correction of cyanotic lesions improves the outcome of subsequent pregnancies.[63]

All patients with structural cardiac lesions are at risk of developing bacterial endocarditis, and need cover with appropriate antibiotics in the peripartum period. Guidelines are given above. Patients with right-to-left shunts are also at risk from emboli of blood clot, air, or bacteria, which can enter the systemic circulation across the defect, bypassing the filtering action of the lungs. Strict asepsis is necessary when establishing any form of vascular access, and care must be taken to remove all air from giving sets and lines before they are connected to the patient. The use of saline, not air, to identify the epidural space is recommended as there is a report of air embolism from the epidural veins.[64]

ATRIAL SEPTAL DEFECT

Atrial septal defects rarely produce symptoms until the fourth and fifth decades, and provided there is no evidence of right ventricular failure or pulmonary hypertension, pregnancy is usually straightforward.

Most patients with atrial septal defects are asymptomatic and the lesion is discovered on routine examination. An ejection systolic murmur can be heard at the left sternal edge. This is due to increased flow across the pulmonary valve; blood flowing across the lesion itself cannot be heard. In addition there is fixed splitting of the second heart sound. In the presence of a significant left to right shunt, a rumbling diastolic tricuspid flow murmur may be heard. The ECG may show right axis deviation or right bundle branch block. The chest X-ray is often normal, but may show right atrial enlargement and plethoric lung fields.

Patients with atrial septal defects are prone to supraventricular dysrhythmias, which tend to be poorly tolerated in pregnancy, and should be treated aggressively with DC cardioversion, β blockers or digoxin. Increases in systemic vascular resistance occurring, for example in response to blood loss, may increase the shunt across the defect and are poorly tolerated.

Regional blockade is ideal for either vaginal delivery or Caesarean section as it prevents pain and stress thus minimizing rises in systemic vascular resistance. If general anaesthesia is necessary, care is needed to avoid rises in systemic vascular resistance, which may occur in response to endotracheal intubation or light anaesthesia.

VENTRICULAR SEPTAL DEFECTS

Ventricular septal defects are more common than atrial septal defects. Most close spontaneously in childhood or are surgically corrected. Small shunts, which persist into adulthood are generally well tolerated in pregnancy and require no particular intervention other than the general precautions for patients with structural heart defects. The presence of a large shunt or pulmonary hypertension is an indication for invasive monitoring with arterial and central venous catheters during labour or Caesarean section.

Most patients with ventricular septal defects are asymptomatic. A pansystolic murmur can be heard at the left sternal edge, in the presence of a large shunt, a mid-diastolic mitral flow murmur may also be audible. The ECG and chest X-ray may show evidence of right ventricular enlargement.

Patients with uncomplicated ventricular septal defects should be allowed to deliver vaginally unless there are obstetric indications for Caesarean section. Changes in systemic vascular resistance are poorly tolerated. Increases, which may occur with pain or in response to endotracheal intubation, increase the left-to-right shunt precipitating right ventricular, and eventually biventricular, failure with pulmonary oedema and a low cardiac output. A fall in systemic vascular resistance or rise in pulmonary vascular resistance may reverse the flow through the defect, producing a right-to-left shunt with an increased left ventricular output. Cyanosis may result from either of these mechanisms. If it is accompanied by evidence of a low cardiac output, with cool peripheries and an elevated central venous pressure, the former mechanism should be suspected and treatment with inotropes and vasodilators instituted. Cyanosis in the presence of an elevated cardiac output suggests reversal of the flow through the defect, and should be treated with 100% oxygen and small doses of a vasopressor. Increases in heart rate also increase flow through the shunt and can cause pulmonary hypertension and right ventricular failure.

For vaginal delivery, epidural analgesia prevents the rise in systemic vascular resistance associated with pain and anxiety. The valsalva manoeuvre has an undesirable effect on cardiac output and pushing should, therefore, be minimized; assisted delivery may be necessary. Epidural anaesthesia is also suitable for Caesarean section. High dose spinal anaesthesia is not recommended because of the rapid associated haemodynamic changes. If general anaesthesia is necessary, increases in systemic vascular resistance due to endotracheal intubation or light anaesthesia should be avoided with an appropriate anaesthetic technique.

PATENT DUCTUS ARTERIOSUS

Patent ductus arteriosus is rarely seen in women of childbearing age, as most are corrected surgically in childhood. Small shunts, which produce no symptoms, are well tolerated and do not usually cause problems during pregnancy or delivery. Larger shunts (greater than 1 cm diameter) produce a significant increase in pulmonary blood flow, which can eventually cause pulmonary hypertension, biventricular failure, and shunt reversal.

Anaesthetic considerations are similar to that outlined above for patients with ventricular septal defects. The use of pulse oximeters on both the right hand (to which blood flow is pre-ductal) and the right foot allows detection of right-to-left shunting.

FALLOT'S TETRALOGY

Fallot's tetralogy is the most common cause of cyanotic heart disease.[65] The primary cardiac defects are:

- right ventricular outflow obstruction: this may be a fixed valvular stenosis, or dynamic infundibular obstruction;
- overriding aorta;
- ventricular septal defect;
- right ventricular hypertrophy.

Pulmonary blood flow is reduced, with right-to-left shunting of blood through the VSD. The reduction in systemic vascular resistance associated with pregnancy may increase the right to left shunt and worsen cyanosis. Uncorrected, Fallot's Tetralogy is associated with significant maternal and fetal mortality. A haematocrit of greater than 60%, arterial oxygen saturation of less than 80%, and the presence of syncopal episodes are considered to be very poor prognostic indicators.[66] Surgical correction improves maternal and fetal outcome,[63,65] but there may be residual right ventricular dysfunction.

Anaesthesia

Patients with uncorrected or partially corrected Fallot's tetralogy need invasive monitoring with radial arterial and central venous lines for anaesthetic intervention.

Reductions in systemic vascular resistance increase the right-to-left shunt and worsen cyanosis. Regional anaesthesia is therefore inadvisable in these patients and Caesarean section under general anaesthesia is generally the preferred mode of delivery. Intravascular volume must be maintained, blood loss replaced promptly with strict avoidance of aorto-caval compression, as decreases in venous return reduce the ability of the right ventricle to perfuse the lungs.

In patients with dynamic right ventricular outflow obstruction, increases in contractility and heart rate will worsen the obstruction and cyanosis. Treatment consists of deepening anaesthesia, increasing venous return and decreasing myocardial contractility. In patients in whom the obstruction is fixed, worsening cyanosis is usually due to a decrease in systemic vascular resistance and should be treated by the administration of oxygen, and reducing depth of anaesthesia.

EISENMENGER'S SYNDROME

Eisenmenger's syndrome was first described by Victor Eisenmenger in 1897, and later redefined by Wood in the 1950s as pulmonary hypertension with a right-to-left or bidirectional shunt and peripheral cyanosis.[67] The shunt may be atrial, ventricular, or aorto-pulmonary. The syndrome represents the end stage in the pathophysiology of atrial septal defect, ventricular septal defect, or patent ductus arteriosus. It is seen less commonly as more congenital defects are corrected in childhood. Once it occurs it is not amenable to surgical correction, except by heart–lung transplantation, because the high pulmonary vascular resistance is fixed and cannot be reversed. Maternal mortality in patients with Eisenmenger's has been estimated at 30–70%, with most deaths occurring at the time of delivery, and in the first postpartum week, when the additional cardiovascular stresses are at their greatest.[68] Most authors agree that patients with the syndrome should be advised against becoming pregnant.[69]

Anaesthesia

The reduction in systemic vascular resistance, which occurs during pregnancy, is not matched, in patients with Eisenmenger's syndrome, by a fall in pulmonary vascular resistance, because of the hypertrophic changes that have occurred in the pulmonary arteries; pregnancy, therefore, increases the right-to-left shunt. Further increases in pulmonary vascular resistance may be precipitated by hypoxia, hypercarbia, or acidosis, and will increase the shunt further. Reductions in intravascular volume or pre-load to the right heart are not tolerated by the poorly compliant right ventricle, but increases may result in right ventricular failure and an increase in right-to-left shunt.

The ideal mode of delivery in patients with Eisenmenger's syndrome is highly controversial. Those who advocate Caesarean section cite the avoidance of the pain and fatigue of labour, the valsalva manoeuvre associated with the second stage, and the greater ease of coordinating the multidisciplinary team involved as arguments in favour of this mode of delivery.[70] Against this is the greater, and less predictable, blood loss associated with Caesarean section, and the need for general or regional anaesthesia.[71] Since the haemodynamic changes which accompany labour can be minimized by careful, controlled regional analgesia and the use of dilute local anaesthetic solutions, in the absence of adverse obstetric factors, vaginal delivery with careful regional anaesthesia, and an assisted second stage, may be an appropriate method of delivery for some patients with Eisenmenger's syndrome. In a mother who has such severe cardiac problems it is unusual to carry the pregnancy to term, because of her deteriorating medical condition. She will therefore most likely have a Caesarean section early in the third trimester.

Regional anaesthesia

Epidural blockade has been described for both vaginal delivery and Caesarean section in the presence of Eisenmenger's syndrome.[68,70] Strict aseptic conditions are essential and the use of saline, not air, for loss of resistance is recommended because of the risk of systemic embolization of air or bacteria from the epidural veins, in the absence of the filtering effect of the lungs. Many patients with congenital heart disease will have been anticoagulated as prophylaxis against thromboembolic events. This needs to be stopped or reversed, and the clotting times checked to permit the use of epidural anaesthesia. Epinephrine should not be used in local anaesthetic mixtures, as the resultant tachycardia may impair right ventricular filling and function. Epidural opioids are useful for labour, Caesarean section and in the postpartum period, allowing lower doses of local anaesthetic to be used, and thus minimizing the degree of sympathetic blockade. Phenylephrine in small increments is an appropriate agent to correct hypotension secondary to vasodilatation.

General anaesthesia

If general anaesthesia is employed, the same principles apply and the anaesthetic technique should minimize any decreases in systemic vascular resistance and venous return. High dose opioids are appropriate to minimize the use of induction agents and volatile agents. Factors such as hypoxia and hypercarbia which increase pulmonary vascular resistance should be avoided. Induction and emergence from anaesthesia are equally times of high risk.

Monitoring

Patients with Eisenmenger's syndrome require full non-invasive cardiovascular monitoring. Most authors also agree on the value of direct arterial pressure and central venous pressure monitoring. More controversial is the use of a pulmonary artery catheter:

- In the presence of a structural cardiac defect, insertion of a pulmonary artery catheter may be difficult, and the catheter may traverse the lesion.
- Placement of the catheter may cause dysrhythmias, emboli to the systemic circulation, or pulmonary artery rupture.
- In the presence of pulmonary vascular disease, the pulmonary artery wedge pressure will not accurately reflect either the left ventricular end diastolic pressure or volume.
- In Eisenmenger's syndrome, it is the right, not left ventricle, which is at highest risk of dysfunction, and measurement of the right atrial pressure should allow assessment of the intravascular volume.
- Estimates of cardiac output using thermodilution techniques will be inaccurate in the presence of an intracardiac shunt.[72,73]
- A pulmonary artery catheter will, however allow estimation of the pulmonary vascular resistance, and observation of the effect of therapeutic manoeuvres on the pulmonary vascular resistance.

The risks of the procedure need to be weighed against the value of any information which may be obtained and a decision made based on the circumstances of each individual case.[74]

Post-delivery

Many of the deaths of patients with Eisenmenger's syndrome occur in the first week postpartum.[75] After delivery, patients need to be monitored in an Intensive Care Unit for several days. The onset of pain and increase in sympathetic tone that occur when the epidural block recedes, and the increase in the intravascular volume in the early postpartum period can precipitate right ventricular overload and failure. Analgesia should be provided with either epidural or systemic opioids. Oxygen is given to help reduce

pulmonary vascular resistance and therefore should be provided throughout the peripartum period.

PRIMARY PULMONARY HYPERTENSION

Pulmonary hypertension is defined as a systolic pulmonary artery pressure of greater than 30/15 mmHg or mean pulmonary artery pressure of greater than 25 mmHg. Most cases are secondary to cardiac or pulmonary disease such as mitral stenosis, left ventricular failure, or pulmonary emboli. Primary pulmonary hypertension exists in the absence of any underlying disease and represents a disorder of the pulmonary vasculature. It is a condition which affects mainly young women.[76] Periods of high cardiac output, such as pregnancy, can precipitate vascular changes. The onset of problems can therefore occur in pregnancy, and worsen during subsequent pregnancies. It results in progressive right ventricular hypertrophy and failure, and unless treated by heart–lung transplantation, most patients die within 5 years.[77] Patients with primary pulmonary hypertension do not tolerate pregnancy well. The associated mortality is in excess of 50%[78] and avoidance or termination of pregnancy is therefore recommended for patients with pulmonary hypertension.[79] In patients who decide to continue with pregnancy or who present too late for termination to be considered, the mode of delivery should be determined by obstetric indications, the aim being vaginal delivery.

Anaesthesia

The principles of management of parturients with pulmonary hypertension are well established (Box 12.7). Less clear is how these objectives should be achieved in practice. Factors, which increase pulmonary vascular resistance should be avoided. These include hypoxaemia, hypercarbia, acidosis, extremes of lung volume, positive end expiratory pressure (PEEP), α agonists,

---

- Avoid increases in pulmonary vascular resistance (hypoxia, hypercarbia, acidosis)
- Maintain venous return and intravascular volume
- Maintain systemic vascular resistance
- Avoid myocardial depression

Box 12.7   Primary pulmonary hypertension.

and endogenous catecholamines. Falls in venous return due to vasodilatation, aorto-caval compression and blood loss are not tolerated by the hypertrophied, poorly compliant right ventricle; cardiac output falls further and cardiovascular collapse may follow. Falls in systemic vascular resistance may also result in profound hypotension, since the output of the right ventricle is fixed and cannot be increased to compensate for changes in resistance. Agents which depress myocardial contractility are poorly tolerated by the failing right ventricle.[38]

Early cardiovascular assessment of patients with primary pulmonary hypertension is important to assess the degree of pulmonary hypertension, the state of the right ventricle, its response to fluid challenges and the responsiveness of the pulmonary vasculature to vasodilators such as prostacyclin, diltiazem, nifedipine, isoprenaline, and oxygen. Nitric oxide may in future be useful in the management of patients with primary pulmonary hypertension, but its place is yet to be fully established.

Regional anaesthesia

Pain, anxiety and stress during labour and delivery increase pulmonary vascular resistance. Good analgesia is therefore essential. Because of concerns about the effects of epidural anaesthesia on venous return and systemic vascular resistance, inhalational analgesia, systemic or high dose intrathecal opioids, paracervical and pudendal nerve blocks have been recommended.[38,80] The analgesia produced by these techniques however is unreliable and a growing number of reports in the literature suggest that a carefully titrated epidural using dilute solutions of local anaesthetic and opioids can be employed successfully in labouring patients with primary pulmonary hypertension.[81–83]

Caesarean section may be necessary because continuation of pregnancy to term would endanger the life of mother, or because of obstetric factors. Traditionally, general anaesthesia has been considered the technique of choice, there are, however, several reports in the literature of the successful use of epidural anaesthesia for Caesarean section in patients with primary pulmonary hypertension.[84–86]

General anaesthesia

If general anaesthesia is employed, the principles outlined above apply. Laryngoscopy and intubation raise pulmonary artery pressure and steps should be taken to minimize this effect. A high dose narcotic technique has been advocated,[87] but this increases the risks of aspiration of gastric contents at the time of induction. Hyperinflation of the lungs when positive pressure ventilation is employed, will raise pulmonary vascular resistance and should be avoided.

There is little data available on the effects of anaesthetic agents on pulmonary vascular resistance. Barbiturates reduce pulmonary vascular resistance and pulmonary artery pressure, but only at high doses.[88] Narcotics have no direct effect on pulmonary artery pressure, but in spontaneously breathing patients may have an effect secondary to their respiratory depressant action and the resultant hypercarbia. Nitrous oxide may increase pulmonary vascular resistance, particularly in the presence of pre-existing pulmonary hypertension.[89] The omission of its use, however, from an anaesthetic will necessitate the use of higher concentrations of volatile agents with their attendant undesirable effects on myocardial contractility and systemic vascular resistance. There is some data available to suggest that isoflurane has a beneficial action on pulmonary vascular resistance and right ventricular output.[88]

In the early postpartum period, the large amounts of fluid which have accumulated in the interstitial tissues shift into the maternal circulation, increasing venous return and aggravating pulmonary hypertension. This may account for the fact that many of the deaths of patients with pulmonary hypertension occur during the first postpartum week. High dependency care and monitoring should therefore be continued for several days postpartum.

The use of pulmonary artery catheters in primary pulmonary hypertension is controversial. The arguments against their use are similar to those outlined above for patients with Eisenmenger's syndrome, and while their use may aid decision making in the management of such patients, this has not been reflected in improved outcome.[87] If a pulmonary artery catheter is used, the balloon should be inflated as infrequently as possible because of the increased risk of pulmonary artery rupture.

MARFAN'S SYNDROME

Marfan's syndrome is a hereditary disorder of connective tissue, which is inherited in an autosomal dominant fashion (Box 12.8). It has an incidence of approximately six cases per 100 000 births.[90] Diagnosis is based on a positive family history and involvement of two systems, or no family history and the involvement of three systems.[91] The characteristic histopathological lesion is cystic medial necrosis of the walls of blood vessels. This results in weakening of the aortic wall and predisposes to aneurysm formation and dissection.[92]

- Most problems occur in patients with pre-existing cardiovascular involvement and in the third trimester
- An arterial cannula is useful during vaginal delivery or Caesarean section, central venous cannulation is only indicated if a valve lesion is significant
- Patients may be at increased risk of postpartum haemorrhage

Box 12.8   Marfan's syndrome in pregnancy.

Features of importance to the anaesthetist include mitral and aortic regurgitation, kyphoscoliosis, difficulties in airway management and spontaneous pneumothorax. Life expectancy in patients with the syndrome is reduced, mainly because of the associated cardiovascular complications (aortic dilatation, dissection, and rupture).

Pregnancy in patients with the syndrome poses a significant risk to both mother and fetus. Aortic dissection and rupture occur with increased frequency during pregnancy, compared with the non-pregnant state. Among the possible reasons for this are the hyperdynamic, hypervolaemic state of the circulation during pregnancy, and the effect of increased oestrogen and progesterone on collagen deposition in the aorta.[93]

The incidence of complications in pregnant patients with Marfan's syndrome is not known, and uncomplicated pregnancies are probably under reported, but it would seem that aortic dissection and rupture occur most frequently in patients with pre-existing cardiovascular abnormalities and in the third trimester.[94] An aortic root diameter of greater than 40 mm is associated with a high risk of dissection during pregnancy and it is recommended that such patients are counselled against becoming pregnant.[91] A straightforward pregnancy, however, cannot be guaranteed for any patient with the syndrome, even in the presence of a normal cardiovascular system. Pregnancy is associated with an increase in cardiac output which may be as high as 60–80% above pre-pregnant levels immediately after delivery.[95] This increase in cardiac output increases the shear force (dP/dt) of the blood within the aorta, making dissection and rupture more likely.

Transoesophageal echocardiography is the investigation of choice and superior to transthoracic echocardiography for the assessment of the aortic root, and detection of aortic dilatation.[96] Serial examinations should be carried out throughout pregnancy to allow early detection of changes in the aortic root. If significant dilatation is detected either before or during pregnancy or the aortic root diameter reaches 55 mm, surgery should be considered. This can be carried out after a therapeutic abortion, during pregnancy, or with a concomitant Caesarean section if fetal maturity permits.

Prophylactic medical therapy

β blockers appear to have a beneficial effect on the rate of progression of aortic dilatation in children and adolescents.[97,98] Their use in the pregnant patient has not been extensively investigated, but in the light of available information the use of prophylactic β blockers would seem reasonable, despite their potential side effects (reduced fetal growth, fetal bradycardia, hyperbilirubinaemia, hypoglycaemia, and apnoea).[99,100] Most studies have looked at the non-selective β blocker propranolol, but in pregnancy, a more cardioselective agent such as atenolol may be preferable to limit the effects on uterine activity.

Anaesthesia

The aim of anaesthetic management in patients with Marfan's syndrome is to minimize sudden changes in blood pressure and increases in contractility, which increase the shear force within the aorta. An arterial cannula is useful for labour, delivery and for all anaesthetic interventions, regional or general. Central venous cannulation is only of value if there is significant valvular involvement. Any existing drug therapy such as β blockers should be continued and antibiotic prophylaxis against bacterial endocarditis given.

Regional anaesthesia

Vaginal delivery is safe in patients with no significant cardiovascular involvement.[101,102] Regional analgesia is beneficial as it reduces pain and anxiety thereby reducing endogenous catecholamine release. There may however be technical difficulties siting an epidural in the presence of significant kyphoscoliosis. The use of forceps or ventouse in the second stage to avoid pushing, seems prudent.

Increases in blood pressure during contractions should be anticipated, and controlled with a β blocker or hydralazine. Decreases in blood pressure during epidural anaesthesia should be treated with intravenous fluids, atropine if the hypotension is due to bradycardia, or small doses of a vasoconstrictor such as phenylephrine. Ephedrine because of its effects on contractility may increase the shear forces within the aorta and should only be used with caution.

Caesarean section may be necessary because of cardio-vascular involvement, or for obstetric indications. Regional anaesthesia with an epidural is a suitable technique. A high dose spinal technique should be avoided because of the rapid haemodynamic changes which can occur.

General anaesthesia

If general anaesthesia is necessary, steps should be taken to prevent the cardiovascular responses to endotracheal intubation. Opioids or β blockers to control the blood pressure should be readily available. Total intra-venous anaesthesia using propofol has been used successfully to provide anaesthesia for Caesarean section in a patient with Marfan's syndrome.[103]

Post-delivery

Monitoring should extend into the postpartum period when cardiac output remains elevated, and the patient should remain in an intensive care unit for at least 24 h after delivery. Patients with Marfan's syndrome appear to be at increased risk of postpartum haemorrhage, possibly because of involvement of the uterine arteries in the pathological process.[104] Adequate post-operative analgesia is important and can be provided by either epidural or intravenous opioids.

PERIPARTUM CARDIOMYOPATHY

DEFINITION

Cardiac failure in the postpartum period was described in the 19th century,[105] but has only been described as a separate disease entity since the 1930s.[106] In 1971 Demakis et al established diagnostic criteria for peri-partum cardiomyopathy[107] which include:

- The development of cardiac failure during the last month of pregnancy, or the first 5 months post-partum.
- Absence of any obvious precipitating cause of cardiac failure.
- Absence of previous cardiac disease.

Some authors also include echocardiographically demonstrable impairment of ventricular function as a criterion for the diagnosis of peripartum cardiomy-opathy.[108]

INCIDENCE AND RISK

The incidence of peripartum cardiomyopathy is estimated to be between 1 in 3000 and 1 in 15 000

pregnancies.[108] It is more common in patients over the age of 30, multiparous women,[109] those with twin pregnancies,[110] and in the presence of pregnancy induced hypertension. It is also more common among women of African descent.

Nutritional, hormonal, inflammatory and immuno-logical mechanisms have been proposed as possible aetiological factors in peripartum cardiomyopathy, but at present no study has identified a distinct cause of the disorder.[108]

CLINICAL PRESENTATION

Peripartum cardiomyopathy presents commonly in the first or second month postpartum, with the symptoms and signs of left or right ventricular failure. Fatigue, dyspnoea, and oedema are frequently encountered. Evidence of pulmonary or systemic emboli may be the presenting feature of the disorder. It can, however present at any stage during pregnancy.

Examination may demonstrate elevated or decreased blood pressure, cardiomegally, gallop rhythm, a mitral regurgitant murmur, pulmonary crepitations and peripheral oedema. Many of these signs and symptoms are present in late pregnancy in normal patients, which may make diagnosis difficult. The ECG may be normal, or may show non-specific ST, or T-wave changes, or evidence of left ventricular hypertrophy. Atrial or ventricular dysrhythmias or conduction defects are sometimes seen. The chest X-ray usually shows cardiomegaly, pulmonary congestion, and sometimes pleural effusions. Echocardiography reveals a dilated heart with a global reduction in ventricular performance, and haemodynamic studies demonstrate reduced cardiac output in the presence of high left and right sided filling pressures.

TREATMENT

Medical therapy for peripartum cardiomyopathy is similar to that for other forms of congestive cardiac failure. The mainstays of treatment are digoxin, diuretics, sodium restriction and after-load reduction. Digoxin is generally considered to be safe in pregnancy, but levels must be monitored closely because this group of patients appears to be extremely sensitive to it. Angiotensin-converting-enzyme (ACE) inhibitors are well established in the treatment of cardiac failure in non-pregnant patients, but there are reports of neonatal renal failure and death in neonates whose mothers had taken captopril, and it is now considered to be contraindicated in pregnancy.[15,16] Diuretics may be used.

Because if the high frequency of thromboembolic events, both pulmonary and systemic, in these patients, prophylactic anticoagulation is recommended in those considered to be at highest risk. This includes patients with significant haemodynamic compromise, or ventricular thrombus seen on echocardiography.

ANAESTHESIA

If peripartum cardiomyopathy presents before delivery, vaginal delivery is preferred to Caesarean section. Anticoagulants should be stopped or reversed and the coagulation status of the patient checked prior to delivery by either method. Stress and pain increase myocardial oxygen consumption, and should be prevented by regional analgesia using low concentrations of local anaesthetics and epidural opioids.

Caesarean section may be necessary for obstetric reasons, or because the increasing cardiovascular stress make continuation of the pregnancy dangerous for the mother. Both regional and general anaesthesia have been described in this situation. If general anaesthesia is employed, the increases in systemic vascular resistance, which occur with endotracheal intubation or light anaesthesia may precipitate ventricular failure. The myocardial depressant effects of induction agents and volatile agents are also undesirable and a 'cardiac anaesthetic' with high dose opioids is the technique of choice, although this does not include a rapid sequence induction and increases the risk of aspiration of gastric contents.

Patients with significant impairment of ventricular function may require invasive cardiovascular monitoring with arterial and pulmonary artery catheters during delivery and need high dependency care for several days postpartum. Sometimes a period of ventilatory or inotropic support is necessary. Ventricular assist devices have been employed in patients with severe left ventricular failure.

The mortality from peripartum cardiomyopathy is 30–60%, and the risk of recurrence in subsequent pregnancies is approximately 50%. The prognosis is dependent on the duration of the cardiomyopathy, with those who have not recovered after 6 months having a poor outlook. For those whose condition cannot be stabilized, or who have a persistent dilated cardiomyopathy, cardiac transplantation has been reported.

CARDIAC SURGERY DURING PREGNANCY

Cardiac surgery was first performed during pregnancy in 1952. Cardiopulmonary bypass during pregnancy has been described since 1959.[111] A review of reports of cardiac surgery with cardiopulmonary bypass performed during pregnancy up to 1990 recorded 115 cases.[112] The overall maternal mortality was 2%. This did not differ from that which would be expected in a non-pregnant population, and was related to the procedure performed and the maternal cardiovascular status. The risk to the fetus however was considerable with fetal mortality estimated to be 15–20% after cardiac surgery with cardiopulmonary bypass (Box 12.9).

The optimal time for the performance of cardiac surgery during pregnancy is the second trimester. This coincides with the time when cardiac output is highest and the mother's condition has decompensated. Surgery during this period avoids organogenesis of the first trimester when the risk of congenital malformations is greatest, or the third trimester when the risk of premature labour is high. If the fetus is considered viable, Caesarean section immediately prior to cardiopulmonary bypass may be considered to avoid exposure of the fetus to the hazards of cardiopulmonary bypass.

Cardiopulmonary bypass has a number of effects which may be detrimental to uteroplacental perfusion, including non-pulsatile blood flow, haemodilution, the release of vasoactive substances, the risk of air or particulate embolism, hypotension and hypothermia. Most authors recommend the use of high flow ($2.5 l/min/m^2$), high pressure (MAP 70 mmHg), normothermic cardiopulmonary bypass during pregnancy.[111,113]

Anaesthesia

As with all pregnant patients, aorto-caval compression must be avoided, and a left lateral tilt maintained. The standard rapid sequence induction normally employed during pregnancy is not appropriate for patients with cardiac disease. Generally a high dose narcotic technique is preferred, however, it increases the risk of

---

- When possible perform surgery during the second trimester
- Avoid aorto-caval compression and aspiration of gastric contents
- High flow, high pressure cardiopulmonary bypass
- Monitor fetal heart rate and uterine contractility
- Facilities for simultaneous Caesarean section if the fetus is viable

Box 12.9   Cardiac surgery during pregnancy.

aspiration of gastric contents. H_2 receptor antagonists, prokinetic agents and antacids should be employed to optimize gastric pH and volume preoperatively. Uterine blood flow is pressure dependent; fluids and vasopressors should therefore be used as necessary to maintain maternal blood pressure. Maternal hyperventilation and hypocarbia have undesirable effects on uterine blood flow and should be avoided. Inotropic and chronotropic agents should be employed as indicated according to maternal cardiovascular status.

In addition to the invasive cardiovascular monitoring normally employed during cardiac surgery, continuous fetal monitoring should be used. In the majority of cases reported, fetal bradycardias during cardiopulmonary bypass have responded to increases in bypass flow rates. Uterine contractility should also be monitored as there is a risk of premature labour particularly during rewarming and tocolysis using inhalational agents or $\beta 2$ agonists may be necessary.[114] In the presence of a viable fetus, facilities should be available to perform a simultaneous Caesarean section for fetal distress, or premature labour unresponsive to treatment.[115] Fetal and uterine monitoring should be continued for several days post-operatively, while the risk of premature labour persists.

PREGNANCY FOLLOWING CARDIAC TRANSPLANTATION

The improved survival of patients following cardiac transplantation has resulted in an increasing number of these patients becoming pregnant. A recent review documented thirty such patients.[116] Chronic hypertension, pre-eclampsia and preterm delivery were common problems, but there were no adverse fetal effects or congenital abnormalities related to the use of long-term immunosuppressive drugs.[116]

A non-rejecting cardiac allograft usually shows good ventricular function, but has no autonomic innervation. Patients with a transplanted heart have a baseline tachycardia because of the absence of vagal tone, and the absence of autonomic innervation means that high regional anaesthesia (T4) will not result in bradycardia. The ventricular performance of a transplanted heart is dependent on the Starling mechanism. It is essential therefore that vena cava compression is avoided, and it is advisable to increase the pre-load before undertaking anaesthetic manoeuvres such as administration of intravenous induction agents, or the institution of regional anaesthesia.

In the absence of obstetric indications for Caesarean section, vaginal delivery is preferred in patients following heart transplantation. Epidural anaesthesia has been described for both vaginal delivery[117,118] and Caesarean section following cardiac transplantation[119] and is preferred to spinal anaesthesia. Gradual volume loading is used to compensate for the fall in systemic vascular resistance. The dennervated, transplanted heart is extremely sensitive to β agonists because of 'up-regulation' of β receptors in the myocardium[120] and it has been suggested that local anaesthetic solutions which contain epinephrine are best avoided in this situation.

If general anaesthesia is necessary for a patient with a transplanted heart, a cardiac type anaesthetic will be better tolerated than a conventional rapid sequence induction by a patient whose cardiac output is dependent on pre-load.

As infection is a major cause of morbidity and mortality in immuno-compromised patients, strict asepsis is essential for all invasive procedures, including intubation. The benefit to be gained from the use of invasive monitoring lines in the presence of good ventricular function should be weighed against the potential morbidity from line sepsis.

REFERENCES

1. *Why mothers die 1997–1999.* The confidential enquiries into maternal deaths in the UK. RCOG Press, 2001.

2. Gianopoulous JG. Cardiac disease in pregnancy. *Med Clin N Am* 1989; **73**: 639–651.

DRUG THERAPY

3. Stevenson RE, Burton M, Ferlanto GJ et al. Hazards of oral anticoagulants during pregnancy. *JAMA* 1980; **243**: 1549–1551.

4. Rogers MC, Willerson JT, Goldblat A et al. Serum digoxin concentrations in the human fetus, neonate and infant. *New Engl J Med* 1972; **287**: 1010–1013.

5. Sherman JL, Locke RV. Transplacental neonatal digitalis intoxication. *Am J Cardiol* 1960; **6**: 834–837.

6. McKenna WJ, Harris L, Rowland E et al. Amiodarone therapy during pregnancy. *Am J Cardiol* 1983; **51**: 1231–233.

7. Robson DJ, Raj MVJ, Storey GCA et al. Use of amiodarone during pregnancy. *Postgrad Med J* 1985; **61**: 75–77.

8. Harrison JK, Greenfield RA, Wharton JM. Acute termination of supraventricular tachycardia by adenosine during pregnancy. *Am Heart J* 1992; **123**: 1386–1388.

9. Podolsky SM, Varon J. Adenosine use during pregnancy. *Ann Emerg Med* 1991; **20**: 1027–1028.

10. O' Connor PC, Jick H, Hunter JR, Stergachis A, Madsen S. Propranolol and pregnancy outcome (letter). *Lancet* 1981; **21**: 1168.

11. Tunstall ME. The effect of propranolol in the onset of breathing at birth. *Br J Anaesth* 1969; **41**: 792.

12. Michael CA. The evaluation of labetolol in the treatment of hypertension complicating pregnancy. *Br J Clin Pharmacol* 1982; **13**(suppl 1): 127–131.

13. Lunell NO, Lewander R, Nylund L et al. Acute effect of dihydralazine on uteroplacental blood flow in hypertension during pregnancy. *Gynecol Obstet Invest* 1983; **16**: 274–282.

14. Constantine G, Beevers DG, Reynolds AL et al. Nifedipine as a second line antihypertensive drug in pregnancy. *Br J Obstet Gynaecol* 1987; **94**: 1136–1142.

15. Broughton Pipkin F, Synonds EM, Turner SR. The effect of captopril on mother and fetus in the chronically cannulated ewe and in the pregnant rabbit. *J Physiol* 1982; **323**: 415–422.

16. Anon (Editorial). Are ACE inhibitors safe in pregnancy? *Lancet* 1989; **2**: 482.

17. Antoine C, Young BK. Fetal lactic acidosis with epidural anaesthesia. *Am J Obstet Gynecol* 1982; **142**: 55–59.

18. Ralston DH, Schneider SM, Delorimer AA. Effects of equipotent ephedrine, mephenteramine and methoxamine on uterine blood flow in the pregnant ewe. *Anaesthesiology* 1974; **40**: 354–369.

19. Ramanathan S, Grant GJ. Vasopressor therapy for hypotension due to epidural anaesthesia for Caesarean section. *Acta Anaesth Scand* 1988; **32**: 559–565.

20. Wright PMC, Ifhikhar M, Fitzpatrick KT et al. Vasopressor therapy for hypotension during epidural anaesthesia for Caesarean section. Effects on maternal and fetal flow velocity ratios. *Anaesth Analg* 1992; **75**: 56–63.

21. Working Party of the British Society for Antimicrobial Chemotherapy. Antibiotic prophylaxis and infective endocarditis. *Lancet* 1992; **I**: 1292–1293.

22. Secher NJ, Arnsbo P, Wallin L. *Acta Scand Obstet* 1978; **57**: 97–103.

23. Weis FR, Markello R, Mo B et al. Cardiovascular effects of oxytocin. *Obstet Gynecol* 1975; **46**: 211–214.

24. Szekly P, Turner R, Snaith L. Pregnancy and the changing pattern of rheumatic heart disease. *Br Heart J* 1973; **35**: 1293–1303.

25. Brady K, Duff P. Rheumatic heart disease and pregnancy. *Clin Obstet Gynecol* 1989; **31**: 21–40.

26. Becker RM. Intracardiac surgery in pregnant women. *Ann Thor Surg* 1983; **36**: 453–458.

27. Clark SL, Phelan JP, Greenspoon J et al. Labour and delivery in the presence of mitral stenosis: central haemodynamic observations. *Am J Obstet Gynecol* 1985; **152**: 984–988.

28. Sullivan JM, Ramanathan KB. Current concepts. Management of medical problems in pregnancy –

29. Arias F, Pineda J. aortic stenosis and pregnancy. *J Reprod Med* 1978; **20**(4): 229–232.

30. Stott DK, Marpole DG, Bristow JD, Kloster FE, Griswold HE. The role of left atrial transport in aortic and mitral stenosis. *Circulation* 1970; **41**: 1031–1041.

31. Brian JE, Seifen AB, Clark RB, Robertson DM, Quirk JG. Aortic stenosis, Caesarean delivery and epidural anaesthesia. *J Clin Anaesth* 1993; **5**: 154–157.

32. Easterling TR, Chadwick HS, Otto CM, Benedetti TJ. Aortic stenosis in pregnancy. *Obstet Gynecol* 1988; **72**: 113–117.

33. Brighouse D. Anaesthesia for Caesarean section in patients with aortic stenosis: the case for regional anaesthesia. *Anaesthesia* 1998; **53**: 107–119.

34. Whitfield A, Holdcroft A. Anaesthesia for Caesarean section in patients with aortic stenosis: the case for general anaesthesia. *Anaesthesia* 1998; **53**: 109–112.

35. Pittard A, Vucevic M. Regional anaesthesia with a subarachnoid microcatheter for Caesarean section in a patient with aortic stenosis. *Anaesthesia* 1998; **53**: 169–173.

36. Stoelting RK, Dierdorf SF, McCamnon RL. Valvular heart disease. In: *Anaesthesia and co-existing disease*. New York: Churchill Livingstone.

37. Szekely P, Snaith L. *Heart disease and pregnancy*. London: Churchill Livingstone, 1994.

38. Mangano DT. Anaesthesia for the pregnant cardiac patient. In: Shnider SM, Levinson G (ed) *Anaesthesia for obstetrics*, 3rd edn. Baltimore: Williams and Wilkins, 1993.

39. Barlow JB, Polock WA. The problem of nonejection systolic clicks and associated mitral valve murmurs: emphasis on the billowing mitral valve leaflet syndrome. *Am Heart J* 1976; **90**: 636–655.

40. Alcantara LG, Marx GF. Caesarean section under epidural analgesia in a parturient with mitral valve prolapse. *Anaesth Analg* 1987; **66**: 902–903.

41. Alderson JD. Cardiovascular collapse following epidural anaesthesia for Caesarean section in a patient with aortic incompetence. *Anaesthesia* 1987; **42**: 643–645.

ISCHAEMIC HEART DISEASE

42. Ginz B. Myocardial infarction in pregnancy. *J Obstet Gynaecol Br Commonw* 1970; **77**: 610–615.

43. Skinner SL, Lumbers ER, Symonds EM. Renin concentration in human fetal and maternal tissues. *Am J Obstet Gynecol* 1968; **101**: 529–533.

44. Aglio LS, Johnson MD. Anaesthetic management of myocardial infarction in a parturient. *Br J Anaesth* 1996; **55**: 258–261.

45. Hankins GDV, Wendel GD, Leveno KJ, Stoneham J. Myocardial infarction during pregnancy – a review. *Obstet Gynecol* 1985; **65**: 139–146.

46. Caruth JE, Mivis SB, Brogan DR et al. The ECG in pregnancy. *Am Heart J* 1981; **102**: 1075–1078.

47. Pfeifer GW. The use of thrombolytic therapy in obstetrics and gynecology. *Aust Ann Med* 1970; **19**: 28.

48. Oakley CM. Coronary artery disease. In: *Heart disease in pregnancy*. BMJ Publishing Group, 1997.

49. Schumacher B, Belfort MA, Card RJ. Successful treatment of acute myocardial infarction during pregnancy with tissue plasminogen activator. *Am J Obstet Gynecol* 1997; **176**: 716–719.

50. Cowan NC, deBelder MA, Rothman MT. Coronary angioplasty in pregnancy. *Br Heart J* 1988; **59**: 588–592.

51. Saxena R, Nolan TE, von Dohlen T, Houghton JL. Postpartum myocardial infarction treated by balloon coronary angioplasty. *Obstet Gynecol* 1992; **79**: 810–812.

52. Majdan JF, Walinsky P, Cowchock SF, Wapner RJ, Plzak L. Coronary artery bypass surgery during pregnancy. *Am J Cardiol* 1983; **52**: 1145–1146.

53. Adams JQ, Alexander AM. Alterations in cardiovascular physiology during labour. *Obstet Gynecol* 1958; **13**: 542–547.

54. Walters WAW, MacGregor WG, Hills M. Cardiac output at rest, during pregnancy, and in the puerperium. *Clin Sci* 1966; **30**: 1–11.

55. Soderlein MK, Purhonen S, Haring P et al. Myocardial infarction in a parturient. A case report with emphasis on medication and management. *Anaesthesia* 1994; **49**: 870–872.

CARDIAC ARREST

56. Turnbull AC, Tindall VR, Robson G et al. *Report on confidential enquiries into maternal deaths in England and Wales 1982–1984*. London: HMSO, 1989.

57. Rees GAD, Willis BA. Resuscitation in late pregnancy. *Anaesthesia* 1988; **43**: 347–349.

58. Goodwin APL, Pearce AJ. The human wedge – a measure to relieve aortocaval compression in late pregnancy. *Anaesthesia* 1992; **47**: 433–434.

59. Handley AJ, Swain A. *Advanced life support manual,* 2nd edn. Resuscitation Council, 1996.

60. Lindsay SL, Hanson GC. Cardiac arrest in near term pregnancy. *Anaesthesia* 1987; **42**: 1074–1077.

61. O Connor RL, Sevarino FB. Cardiopulmonary arrest in the pregnant patient. A report of a successful resuscitation. *J Clin Anaesth* 1996; **6**: 66–68.

62. Hawthorne L, Lyons G. Cardiac arrest complicating spinal anaesthesia for Caesarean section. *Int J Obstet Anaesth* 1997; **6**: 126–129.

CONGENITAL HEART DISEASE

63. Weiss BM, Atanassoff PG. Cyanotic congenital heart disease and pregnancy: natural selection, pulmonary hypertension and anaesthesia. *J Clin Anaesth* 1993; **5**: 332–341.

64. Naulty JS, Ostheimer GLJ, Datta S et al. Incidence of venous air embolism during epidural catheter insertion. *Anaesthesiology* 1982; **57**: 410–412.

65. Singh H, Bolton PJ, Oakley CM. Pregnancy after surgical correction of tetralogy of Fallot. *Br Med J* 1982; **285**: 168–170.

66. Vaclavinova V, Machado L. Delivery in a multipara with unoperated Fallot's tetralogy. *Int J Gynecol Obstet* 1994; **44**: 165–171.

67. Wood P. Pulmonary Hypertension. *Br Med Bull* 1952; **8**: 348–353.

68. Atanassoff P, Alon E, Schmid ER et al. Epidural anaesthesia for Caesarean section in a patient with severe pulmonary hypertension. *Acta Anaesth Scand* 1989; **33**: 75–77.

69. Cardiac disease in pregnancy. *Am Coll Obstet Gynecol Tech Bull* 1992; **168**: 1–8.

70. Spinnato JA, Kraynack BJ, Cooper MW. Eisenmengers syndrome in pregnancy: epidural anaesthesia for elective Caesarean sedtion. *New Engl J Med* 1981; **304**: 1215–1217.

71. Gleicher N, Midwall J, Hochberger D et al. Eisenmengers syndrome and pregnancy. *Obstet Gynecol Surv* 1979; **34**: 721–741.

72. Schwalbe SS, Desmulch S, Marx GF. Use of pulmonary artery catheterisation in patients with Eisenmengers syndrome. *Anaes Analg* 1990; **71**: 442–443.

73. Robinson S. pulmonary artery catheters in Eisenmengers syndrome: many risks, few benefits. *Anaesthesiology* 1983; **58**: 588–589.

74. Weiss BM, Atanassoff PG. Cyanotic congenital heart disease and pregnancy: natural selection, pulmonary hypertension and anasthesia. *J Clin Anaesth* 1993; **5**: 332–341.

75. Elkayam W, Gleicher N. Congenital heart disease in pregnancy. *Heart Failure* 1993; **9**: 46–51.

PRIMARY PULMONARY HYPERTENSION

76. Weiss BM, Atanassoff PG. Cyanotic congenital heart disease and pregnancy: natural selection, pulmonary hypertension and anaesthesia. *J Clin Anaesth* 1993; **5**: 332–341.

77. Fuster V, Steele PM, Edwards WD, Gersh BJ, McGoon MD, Frye RL. Primary pulmonary hypertensin: natural history and the importance of thrombosis. *Circulation* 1984; **70**: 580–587.

78. Roberts NV, Keast PJ. Pulmonary hypertension and pregnancy – a lethal combination. *Anaesth Intens Care* 1990; **18**: 366–374.

79. Slomka F, Salmeron S, Zetlaowi P, Cohen H, Simonneau G, Samii K. Primary pulmonary hypertension and pregnancy: anaesthetic management for delivery. *Anaesthesiology* 1988; **69**: 959–961.

80. Abboud TK, Raya J, Noweihed R, Daniel J. Intrathecal morphine for the relief of labour pain in

a parturient with severe pulmonary hypertension. *Anaesthesiology* 1983; **59**: 477–479.

81. Smedstad KG, Cramb R, Morison DH. Pulmonary hypertension and pregnancy. A series of eight cases. *Can J Anaesth* 1994; **41**: 502–512.

82. Robinson DE, Leicht CH. Epidural anaesthesia with low dose bupivacaine for labour and delivery in a parturient with severe pulmonary hypertension. *Anaesthesiology* 1988; **68**: 285–288.

83. Power KJ, Avery AF. Extradural anaesthesia in the intrapartum management of a patient with pulmonary hypertension. *Br J Anaesth* 1989; **63**: 116–120.

84. Kiss H, Egarter C, Asseryanis E, Putz D, Kneussl M. Primary pulmonary hypertension in pregnancy – a case report. *Am J Obstet Gynecol* 1995; **172**: 1052–1054.

85. Breen TW, Janzen JA. Pulmonary hypertension and cardiomyopathy: anaesthetic management for Caesarean section. *Can J Anaesth* 1991; **38**: 895–899.

86. Khan MJ, Bhatt SB, Krye JJ. Anaesthetic considerations for parturients with primary pulmonary hypertension: a review of the literature and clinical presentation. *Int J Obstet Anaesth* 1996; **5**: 36–42.

87. Weeks SK, Smith JB. Obstetric anaesthesia in patients with primary pulmonary hypertension. *Can J Anaesth* 1991; **38**: 814–816.

88. Cheng DCH, Edelist G. Isoflurane and primary pulmonary hypertension. *Anaesthesia* 1988; **43**: 22–24.

89. Schulte-Sasse U, Hess W, Tarnow J. Pulmonary vascular responses to nitrous oxide in patients with normal and high pulmonary vascular resistance. *Anaesthesiology* 1982; **57**: 9–13.

MARFAN'S SYNDROME

90. Pyeritz RE, McKusick VA. The Marfan syndrome: diagnosis and management. *New Engl J Med* 1979; **300**: 772–777.

91. Pyeritz RE. Maternal and fetal complications of pregnancy in the Marfan syndrome. *Am J Med* 1981; **71**: 784–790.

92. Baer RW, Taussig HB, Oppenheimer EH. Congenital aneurysmal dilatation of the aorta associated with arachnodactyl. *Bull Johns Hopkins Hosp* 1943; **72**: 309–331.

93. Elkayam U, Ostrzega E, Shotan A, Mehra A. Cardiovascular problems in patients with the Marfan syndrome. *Ann Int Med* 1995; **123**: 117–122.

94. Hussebye KO, Wolff JH, Friedman LL. Aortic dissection in pregnancy: a case of Marfan syndrome. *Am Heart J* 1958; **55**: 662–676.

95. Gordon CF, Johnson MD. Anaesthetic management of the pregnant patient with Marfan syndrome. *J Clin Anaesth* 1993; **5**: 248–251.

96. Simpson IA, deBelder MA, Treasure T, Camm AJ, Pumphry CW. Cardiac manifestations of Marfan's syndrome: improved evaluation by transoesophageal echocardiography. *Br Heart J* 1993; **69**: 104–108.

97. Zahka KG, Hensley C, Glesby M, Pyeritz RE. The impact of medical and surgical therapy on the cardiovascular prognosis of the Marfan syndrome in early childhood (abstract). *J Am Coll Cardiol* 1989; **13**: 119A.

98. Shores J, Berger KR, Murphy EA, Pyeritz RE. Progression of aortic dilatation and the benefit of long term β adrenergic blockade in Marfan's syndrome. *New Engl J Med* 1994; **330**: 1335–1341.

99. O Connor PC, Jick H, Hunter JR, Stergachis A, Madsen S. Propranolol and pregnancy outcome [letter]. *Lancet* 1981; **2**: 1168.

100. Tunstall ME. The effect of propranolol on the onset of breathing at birth. *Br J Anaesth* 1969; **41**: 792.

101. Donaldson LB, DeAlverez RP. The Marfan syndrome and pregnancy. *Am J Obstet Gynaecol* 1965; **92**: 629–641.

102. Elias S, Berkowitz RL. The Marfan syndrome and pregnancy. *Obstet Gynecol* 1976; **47**: 358–361.

103. Llopis JE, Garcia-Aguado R, Sifre C, Tommasi Rosso M, Vivo M, Martin-Jurado J, Grau F. Total intravenous anaesthesia for Caesarean section in a patient with Marfan's syndrome. *Int J Obstet Anaesth* 1997; **6**: 59–62.

104. Irons DW, Pollard KP. Post partum haemorrhage secondary to Marfan's disease of the uterine vasculature. *Br J Obstet Gynaecol* 1993; **100**: 279–281.

PERIPARTUM CARDIOMYOPATHY

105. Richie C. Clinical contribution to the pathology, diagnosis and treatment of certain chronic conditions of the heart. *Edinb Med Surg J* 1849; **2**: 333.

106. Hull E, Hafkesbring E. Toxic post partal heart disease. *New Orleans Med Surg J* 1937; **89**: 550–557.

107. Demakis JG, Rahimtoola SH, Sutton GC, Meadows R, Szanto PB, Tobin JR, Gunnar RM. Natural course of peripartum cardiomyopathy. *Circulation* 1971; **44**: 1053–1061.

108. Lampert MB, Lang RM. Peripartum cardiomyopathy. *Am Heart J* 1995; **130**: 860–870.

109. Veille JC. Peripartum cardiomyopathies: a review. *Am J Obstet Gynecol* 1984; 805–818.

110. Fillmore SJ, Parry EO. The evolution of peripartal heart failure in Zaria. *Circulation* 1977; **56**: 1058–1061.

CARDIAC SURGERY

111. Chambers CE, Clark SL. Cardiac surgery during pregnancy. *Clin Obstet Gynaecol* 1994; **37**: 316–323.

112. Westaby S, Parry AJ, Forfar JC. Reoperation for prosthetic valve endocarditis in the third trimester of pregnancy. *Ann Thorac Surg* 1992; **53**: 263–265.

113. Bernal JM, Miralles PJ. Cardiac surgery with cardiopulmonary bypass during pregnancy. *Obstet Gynecol Surv* 1986; **41**: 1–6.

114. Pomini F, Mercogliano D, Cavalletti C, Caruso A, Pomini P. Cardiopulmonary bypass in pregnancy. *Ann Thorac Surg* 1996; **61**: 259–268.

115. Martin MC, Pernoll ML, Boruszak AN, Jones JW, Lo Cicero J. Caesarean section while on cardiopulmonary bypass: a report of a case. *Obstet Gynecol* 1981; **57**(suppl): 41S–45S.

CARDIAC TRANSPLANTS

116. Scott JR, Wagoner LE, Olsen SL, Taylor DO, Renlund DG. Pregnancy in heart transplant recipients: management and outcome. *Obstet Gynecol* 1993; **82**: 324–327.

117. Camann WR, Jarcho JA, Mintz KJ et al. Uncomplicated vaginal delivery 14 months after cardiac transplantation. *Am Heart J* 1991; **121**: 939–941.

118. Kirk EP. Organ transplantation and pregnancy. *Am J Obstet Gynecol* 1991; **164**: 1629–1634.

119. Camann WR, Goldman GA, Johnson MD, Moore J, Greene M. Caesarean delivery in a patient with a transplanted heart. *Anaesthesiology* 1989; **71**: 618–620.

120. Yusef S, Theodoropoulos S, Mathias CJ et al. Increased sensitivity of the dennervated transplanted heart to isoprenaline both before and after β adrenergic blockade. *Circulation* 1987; **75**: 696–704.

13

THE OBSTETRIC PATIENT WITH RESPIRATORY, NEUROLOGICAL AND ENDOCRINE DISEASE

Sarah Hughes

ASTHMA

Asthma is a respiratory disorder that is characterized by

- airway obstruction, reversible either spontaneously or with treatment;
- airway inflammation;
- hyper-reactivity of the airway in response to a variety of stimuli.

It is common, occurring in approximately 5% of the adult population, and has a prevalence of approximately 1% among pregnant patients.[1,2] Despite the availability of effective and safe therapy, the tendency is for asthma to be underdiagnosed and undertreated.

THE EFFECT OF PREGNANCY ON ASTHMA

Hyperventilation begins in the first trimester, and is achieved by a small increase in respiratory rate, and an increase of approximately 50% in tidal volume. These changes result in a fall in alveolar and arterial pCO_2. Arterial pH is maintained within normal limits, by an increase in the renal excretion of bicarbonate; arterial blood gases therefore show a picture of a compensated respiratory alkalosis. This reduction in normal arterial pCO_2 must be borne in mind when interpreting the results of arterial blood gas estimation in pregnant women. Whilst these changes are well tolerated by patients with normal respiratory function, patients with pre-existing lung disease and limited respiratory reserve will need careful monitoring and management to prevent maternal and fetal complications.

Studies reveal no clear changes in the severity of asthma during pregnancy. Most of the published studies report approximately a quarter of patients whose asthma improves during pregnancy, a quarter in whom it deteriorates, and approximately half who experience no change.[3] Increased levels of endogenous steroids may account for the improvement in asthma during pregnancy.[4] One possible explanation for a worsening of asthma during pregnancy is a reluctance, on the part of the patient, to take medication, fearing an adverse effect on the fetus.[1] The hyperventilation and subjective dyspnoea associated with pregnancy may cause anxiety and also precipitate bronchospasm.

The pattern of asthma in a pregnant individual appears to be predictable, in that asthma tends to return to its pre-pregnant severity within 3 months post-partum, and the pattern of change tends to recur in subsequent pregnancies.[5]

THE EFFECT OF ASTHMA ON PREGNANCY

Asthma potentially has a number of adverse effects on the fetus:

- Maternal hypoxaemia due to chronic or acute asthma will reduce oxygen delivery to the fetus.
- Maternal hypocarbia during an acute asthma attack causes umbilical artery vasoconstriction, and a shift to the left in the maternal oxy-haemoglobin dissociation curve. Both these factors will reduce oxygen delivery to the fetus.
- A rise in intrathoracic pressure, which may occur with expiration during an acute attack, will reduce venous return and cardiac output, hence reducing oxygen delivery to the fetus.[6]

Studies of asthma in pregnancy have reported numerous and sometimes conflicting effects on the fetus. Consistent findings appear to be an increase in preterm labour, low birthweight,[1] increased perinatal mortality, hyperemesis gravidarum,[3] pre-eclampsia[7] and complicated labour. There is apparently no increase in the incidence of congenital malformations. It is unclear whether these effects are due to exposure of the fetus to drugs or to episodes of hypoxia, but good control of asthma tends to be associated with a better outcome of the pregnancy.

MANAGEMENT OF ASTHMA

The management of asthma in the pregnant patient does not differ significantly from that in the non-pregnant patient. The aim of treatment is to avoid maternal and fetal hypoxaemia by the prevention of acute attacks of bronchospasm whilst minimizing fetal exposure to potentially harmful drugs.[8]

Asthma is an underdiagnosed condition, it is therefore helpful to ask at the antenatal booking clinic not only about a history of asthma, but also about any symptoms, which may be due to undiagnosed asthma such as wheezing, waking at night with noisy breathing or coughing. Asthmatic mothers already on medication should be assessed to ensure that their asthma control is optimal and their medication should be continued or adjusted if necessary. Those with symptoms of asthma who are not on medication should be referred to a specialist chest physician for assessment, treatment and advice.

It is recognized that subjective reporting of symptoms is a poor guide to the severity of asthma. The advent of readily available home peak flow meters has aided the monitoring of asthma. Mothers with anything but mild asthma should be taught to measure, record and interpret peak flow readings. They should be given a self-management plan involving a change in dose of inhaled medication or the introduction of oral steroids, to use in the event of a deterioration. Several factors may precipitate an attack of asthma and mothers should be advised to avoid them. They include drugs such as non-steroidal anti-inflammatory agents and β blockers, allergens such as dust, cold weather, and cigarette smoke.

β2 agonists used to be the mainstay of treatment of asthma, and remain so for mild forms of the condition. There are however concerns that their frequent use may actually worsen asthma. Salbutamol is the most commonly used agent. It may be used by metered inhaler, nebulized or given intravenously in the management of severe, acute bronchospasm. There is no evidence for any teratogenic effect, nor has it been demonstrated to delay the onset or slow the progress of labour when given in the inhaled form, despite the fact that intravenous β2 agonists are used to delay labour. Inhaled or nebulized salbutamol should not be withheld if needed.[1]

The long acting β agonist salmeterol is not used for the acute treatment of asthma, but has been increasingly used in the long-term control of symptoms. It has been used in pregnancy and may reduce the rate of acute exacibations.

Corticosteroids may be given by inhalation or orally. They have no direct bronchodilator action, but are anti-inflammatory and reduce airway reactivity. Synergism exists between the actions of β agonists and steroids. Regular inhaled steroids are the mainstay of treatment in moderate or severe asthma. Beclomethasone is the drug of choice in pregnancy because of its widespread and long-standing use during pregnancy, without evidence of fetal harm.[9] Mothers should be given instructions to increase the dose of their inhaled steroid in the event of a deterioration in peak flow readings to a predetermined value.

Systemic absorption of inhaled steroids is minimal. Mothers with more severe asthma may require short courses of high dose oral steroids, or chronic use of smaller oral doses. Those with particularly severe asthma may be given a course of oral steroid and instructions to take them if peak flow readings drop below a given value. This is an attempt to prevent further deterioration in pulmonary function. When steroids are used in acute asthma, it should be borne in mind that the onset of action takes 4–6 h, and that they should be given early in the management of a mother with an acute asthma attack. Mothers who have received oral steroids within the previous

12 months will require intravenous steroids during labour and delivery, or Caesarean section, because of the risk of adrenal suppression.

Steroids given by either route do not increase the risk of congenital malformations, nor do they appear to cause significant neonatal adrenal suppression, probably because they are transported across the placenta slowly.[3] Chronic use of steroids may be associated with impaired glucose tolerance in pregnant patients.

Methylxanthines act by inhibiting phosphodiesterase, and thus increase levels of intracellular c-AMP. They have a weak bronchodilator action, but are also anti-inflammatory. Theophylline is the oral preparation and is sometimes used in the long-term control of asthma. Aminophylline is the only drug available for intravenous use in the management of acute asthma.

The pharmacokinetics of these agents are altered in pregnancy, with studies showing both increased and decreased levels.[10,11] Blood levels should be checked regularly and the dosage adjusted to maintain therapeutic levels. There is no evidence of a teratogenic effect, but fetal levels tend to be similar to maternal levels with the risk of fetal toxicity if levels are not carefully monitored.

Ipratropium bromide is an anticholinergic agent used occasionally in the management of chronic obstructive pulmonary disease. It is rarely used in the prevention of asthma, but may be used in the nebulized form in the management of acute asthma, which is not responding to nebulized salbutamol. There are no reports of fetal malformations associated with its use.[12]

Sodium cromoglycate may be used by inhaler in the management of asthma. It acts by inhibiting mast cell degranulation, and hence has an anti-inflammatory action. There is no evidence that it causes fetal harm.[13]

It is clear that there is a wide range of drugs that have been used during pregnancy for many years in the management of asthma, without hazard to the fetus. It is important to emphasise to patients that the risk to the fetus from uncontrolled asthma is far greater than that from the medication used to control it.

MANAGEMENT OF ACUTE ASTHMA

An acute asthma attack may be life threatening and should be treated as a medical emergency. The symptoms are breathlessness, wheezing and cough. The inability to speak in sentences is an indication of extreme

- Prevent aorta-cava compression
- Give oxygen in high concentrations
- Establish venous access and give fluids
- Give nebulized salbutamol, consider adding ipratropium bromide
- Give intravenous steroids
- Give intravenous aminophylline if condition does not improve
- Investigations: FBC, theophylline level, artrial blood gases CXR and PEFR
- Obtain senior help and establish fetal monitoring
- Consider ITU admission

Box 13.1   The management of acute asthma.

severity. Examination usually reveals widespread expiratory wheezing; a silent chest with little air entry is an ominous sign. Objective signs of severe asthma are a respiratory rate of greater than 30 breaths/min, a forced expiratory volume (FEV1) of less than 1L, a heart rate of greater than 120 beats/min and a pulsus paradox of greater than 15 mmHg. Blood gases that show a normal P_aCO_2 may indicate decompensating asthma because of the normal hyperventilation seen in pregnancy. Management of an acute attack is not significantly different from that in a non-pregnant patient (Box 13.1):

- Oxygen via a facemask should be given immediately, in the highest concentration available, in an attempt to prevent maternal and fetal hypoxaemia. There is no place for 24% or 28% oxygen in the management of acute asthma.
- Steps should be taken to prevent aorto-caval compression, particularly since placental blood flow may already be compromised by maternal hypocarbia.
- The administration of intravenous fluids will help to prevent dehydration, which can compound the problem of thick bronchial secretions. Intravenous fluids will also improve placental perfusion.
- Nebulized β2 agonists such as salbutamol 5 mg should be given and repeated until bronchospasm begins to subside. Care is needed if terbutaline is used in late pregnancy because of the risk that it may precipitate pulmonary oedema.[14] If the response to β2 agonists is poor, nebulized ipatroprium bromide can be added, alternating with nebulized salbutamol.
- If the response to salbutamol is poor, intravenous aminophylline may be added. If the patient is not already taking oral aminophylline, a loading dose of 5 mg/kg should be given over 20–30 min followed by a maintenance infusion of 0.5 mg/kg. For patients already taking aminophylline, the loading dose is omitted. Plasma levels should be monitored frequently to ensure therapeutic levels are achieved and toxicity avoided in the presence of altered pharmacokinetics.
- Intravenous steroids take around 6 h to be effective and should therefore be given early in the management of severe asthma. They should then be given 4 hourly in the first instance.
- Investigations required include a full blood count, theophylline levels if necessary, arterial blood gases, and a chest X-ray to exclude pneumothorax.
- Any obvious precipitating cause such as infection should be treated appropriately.
- Peak expiratory flow rate (PEFR) should be measured and recorded frequently to monitor the response to therapy.

Senior help from obstetricians, anaesthetists and physicians should be sought early in the course of the illness and fetal monitoring commenced as soon as possible. Occasionally patients with severe asthma require admission to an intensive care unit for monitoring of their condition or mechanical ventilation, if arterial gases continue to deteriorate or exhaustion occurs.

MANAGEMENT OF LABOUR AND DELIVERY

Several basic principles apply to the management of all asthmatic mothers during labour. An early assessment should be made of respiratory function, and help sought from a respiratory physician if necessary. Any medication the patient is currently taking should be continued, and additional medication given if bronchospasm is present. Intravenous steroids should be given to those at risk of adrenal suppression. Intravenous fluids will prevent dehydration and help to maintain placental blood flow. Supplementary oxygen is beneficial to patients with all but mild asthma.

The pain of labour is associated with a rise in oxygen consumption and minute ventilation. This is well tolerated by most mothers, but in those with asthma, pain may precipitate an acute attack. Regional anaesthesia helps to obtund these changes[15] and should be considered early in labour in patients with all but mild asthma. Careful monitoring of the level of anaesthesia should prevent any significant effect on maternal respiratory function.

Prostaglandins should be avoided whenever possible. PGF2α has vasoconstrictor and bronchoconstrictor actions. PGE2, generally has vasodilator and bronchodilator actions and should be used instead of PGF2α in the presence of severe, life threatening post-partum haemorrhage, but it has occasionally been reported to cause bronchospasm.[7] Oxytocin is the agent of choice for augmentation of labour and in the management of post-partum haemorrhage, as it does not have an adverse effect on respiratory function.

ANAESTHESIA FOR CAESAREAN SECTION

All forms of anaesthesia have been used successfully in mothers with asthma. Regional techniques have the advantage of avoiding airway instrumentation, which carries the risk of precipitating bronchospasm. Regional anaesthesia also permits verbal contact with the patient and early recognition of respiratory symptoms.

Regional anaesthesia

Research has suggested the level of motor block in epidural anaesthesia is approximately four segments below the level of sensory block, in spinal anaesthesia the difference is 1–2 segments.[16] The significance of these findings in clinical practice is, however, unclear. Blockade of the intercostal nerves interferes with the ability to cough and clear secretions, epidural anaesthesia therefore offers the advantages over spinal anaesthesia of a more controllable level of block and theoretically less motor involvement. There is one report in the literature of severe bronchospasm following spinal anaesthesia for Caesarean section,[17] this is attributed to a decreased level of circulating catecholamines following sympathetic blockade, but it does not appear to be a common problem. The motor block associated with spinal anaesthesia may not be as predictable, but does not last as long when compared with epidural anaesthesia. This is also a theoretical advantage.

General anaesthesia

General anaesthesia may be occasionally necessary for emergency surgery or when regional anaesthesia is contraindicated. A rapid sequence induction is necessary because of the risk of aspiration of gastric contents, but intubation under these circumstances may provoke bronchospasm. The use of a short acting narcotic at induction will reduce the risk. In the presence of severe bronchospasm, ketamine may be an appropriate induction agent, because of its bronchodilator properties. All the volatile agents used in the maintenance of anaesthesia are bronchodilators, but in the presence of aminophylline, halothane is best avoided because of the risk of precipitating ventricular dysrhythmias.[18] Vecuronium is preferable to atracurium as it does not cause histamine release.

If bronchospasm occurs perioperatively it should be treated by deepening anaesthesia in the first instance and if necessary giving bronchodilators, either via the breathing system or intravenously. The differential diagnosis of perioperative wheezing includes a blocked or kinked endotracheal tube, an anaphylactic reaction to an intravenous or oral drug, amniotic fluid embolism or pneumothorax. These should be excluded or treated if present.

At the end of surgery, the endotracheal tube should remain in place until the mother is awake and able to protect her airway. This technique however may precipitate bronchospasm. Small doses of an opioid or intravenous lidocaine will help to smooth extubation and minimize the risk of bronchospasm.

Post-delivery care

Post-operative management should include humidified oxygen, intravenous fluids, inhaled bronchodilators and regular monitoring of respiratory function. Good analgesia is very important to enable active physiotherapy. Morphine potentially releases histamine so pethidine or fentanyl are alternatives. Maintaining epidural analgesia for the first 24 h may be beneficial, especially as many post-operative regimes are not as effective without the use of a non-steroidal anti-inflammatory, which may be contraindicated in the asthmatic.

CYSTIC FIBROSIS

Cystic fibrosis is an autosomal recessive disorder that affects approximately 1 in 2000 live births. The main features of the disease are

- chronic obstructive pulmonary disease;
- pancreatic exocrine insufficiency;
- increased concentrations of electrolytes in sweat; these arise because of an underlying defect in c-AMP mediated chloride transport across cell membranes.

Pulmonary involvement is characterized by acute on chronic episodes of pulmonary infection, airway obstruction due to mucus plugging, fibrosis and bronchiectasis. Progressive pulmonary impairment is the major cause of morbidity and mortality in cystic fibrosis[19] and haemoptysis, pneumothorax and respiratory failure are common complications. Patients with severe pulmonary disease are at risk of developing pulmonary hypertension and cor pulmonale. This is indicated by the presence of right ventricular hypertrophy on the ECG, a P_aO_2 of less than 7 kPa, a vital capacity of less than 60% of the predicted value, clinical evidence of CCF and increased pulmonary artery or cardiac size on the chest X-ray.[20] The mortality associated with pulmonary hypertension and pregnancy has been reported as 30–50%. Most authors consider pregnancy contraindicated in this situation.[20]

Pancreatic involvement in cystic fibrosis results in a reduction in pancreatic digestive enzymes and pancreatic duct obstruction. Eventually pancreatic fibrosis may encroach on endocrine secretory cells causing diabetes mellitus. The clinical consequences of pancreatic involvement are maldigestion, malabsorbtion, and malnutrition.

Due to improvements in nutrition and respiratory care, the median age of survival in cystic fibrosis is now 29 years.[19,21] Despite reduced fertility, possibly due to the abnormal electrolyte content of cervical mucus,[22] increasing numbers of patients with cystic fibrosis are becoming pregnant. The first report of pregnancy in a patient with cystic fibrosis was in 1960,[23] since then there have been many more reported in the literature. Pregnancy imposes additional cardiovascular, respiratory and nutritional stresses on patients with limited reserves. Despite this, studies suggest that mothers with good nutritional status, near normal chest X-rays and mild obstructive pulmonary disease tolerate pregnancy well.[24]

Pregnant patients with cystic fibrosis require management by a specialized multidisciplinary team. Exacerbations of their chronic respiratory problems need to be treated promptly with physiotherapy and antibiotics. The pharmacokinetics of some antibiotics such as the β-lactams are altered during pregnancy and doses will need to be altered accordingly.[25,26] Other antibiotics such as tetracyclines must not be used during pregnancy, as they are taken up into the developing bones and teeth of the fetus. The nutritional state of patients with cystic fibrosis also requires careful monitoring. Dietary supplements or additional nasogastric feeding may be necessary. Supplementary parenteral nutrition has also been described during pregnancy (Box 13.2).[27,28]

ANAESTHETIC MANAGEMENT

Unless there are obstetric indications for operative delivery, vaginal delivery should be the aim for patients with cystic fibrosis. Many patients with cystic

---

- Patients have limited respiratory reserves to deal with the increased demand of pregnancy. Patients with severe respiratory disease may have pulmonary hypertension and cor pulmonale
- Dietary supplements or additional nasogastric or parenteral feeding may be necessary to provide adequate nutrition during pregnancy
- Anaesthetic management should provide good analgesia with minimal respiratory depression due to opioids, or high motor block

Box 13.2   Cystic fibrosis and pregnancy.

---

fibrosis will however require delivery by Caesarean section before induction of labour is feasible, because of deteriorating maternal respiratory function.

Regional analgesia and anaesthesia

During labour, maternal hydration requires careful monitoring. Dehydration will exacerbate the problem of mucus plugging, but patients with impaired right ventricular function are at risk of fluid overload. Supplementary humidified oxygen will reverse the hypoxic component of pulmonary vasoconstriction and should be administered during labour. Oxygenation should be monitored by continuous pulse oximetry.

As in all patients with respiratory disease, adequate analgesia during labour is important, but drugs with a respiratory depressant action should be avoided whenever possible. Regional blockade provides excellent analgesia for labour. Local anaesthetic agents may be used alone or in combination with small doses of epidural opioids. The level of the block requires close monitoring, as a high thoracic block will impair the ability to cough and clear secretions.

Regional anaesthesia is appropriate for Caesarean section, but may cause technical difficulties for the surgeon in mothers who are unable to lie flat. Epidural anaesthesia may be preferable to spinal anaesthesia because greater control over the height of the block and possibly less motor involvement may minimize the respiratory effects of the technique. An incremental combined spinal–epidural is a useful alternative.

General anaesthesia

General anaesthesia with endotracheal intubation offers the opportunity for tracheobronchial toilet, but in the presence of significant respiratory involvement, weaning from mechanical ventilation may be problematic. If general anaesthesia is undertaken, it should be remembered that uptake of volatile agents will be delayed by ventilation-perfusion inequalities. Because there is a risk that the thick bronchial secretions may block the endotracheal tube, all inspired gases should be humidified. Ventilator settings should provide adequate time for expiration in order to prevent gas trapping. Anticholinergic agents will exacerbate the problem of mucus plugging and should be avoided if possible.

Post-delivery care

In the post-operative period supplementary oxygen should be provided and adequate hydration maintained. Good analgesia will permit chest physiotherapy and clearing of secretions.

DIABETES MELLITUS

Diabetes is a chronic metabolic disorder caused either by a failure of insulin production or resistance to the actions of insulin. The results is an abnormal metabolism of glucose, lipids and protein.

The incidence of diabetes mellitus in pregnancy is 2–3 per 1000 pregnancies. The majority, (approximately 95%), of these are patients with pre-existing, type I, insulin dependent diabetes. In addition, some women develop impaired glucose tolerance and diabetes mellitus during pregnancy; gestational diabetes. This condition affects approximately 2% of pregnancies.[29] The majority of patients with gestational diabetes do not require insulin and can be managed using diet alone, although insulin and dextrose may be required around delivery.

EFFECTS OF DIABETES ON THE PREGNANT PATIENT

Diabetic mothers are at increased risk from the systemic consequences of the disease and the disease process can accelerate during the pregnancy (Box 13.3). In addition the incidence of obstetric complications such as pre-eclampsia, polyhydramnios and preterm labour is higher in diabetic mothers.[30]

EFFECTS OF PREGNANCY ON DIABETES

During the first half of pregnancy, increased levels of oestrogen increase pancreatic secretion of insulin and peripheral utilization of glucose. This results in the

- *Cardiovascular*: Increased incidence of ischaemic heart disease, cerebrovascular disease and peripheral vascular disease
- *Renal*: Microvascular damage causing proteinuria and impaired renal function
- *Neurological*: Sensory and autonomic neuropathy, causing urinary retention and cardiovascular instability
- *Diminished resistance to infection*: Diabetic control may be difficult while infection is present
- *Ophthalmic*: Retinopathy and cataracts

Box 13.3   Systemic consequences of diabetes.

reduction in fasting plasma glucose and improved glucose tolerance. In diabetic patients, insulin requirements often fall at this time.[31]

In the latter half of pregnancy, insulin resistance and decreased tissue sensitivity results from the actions of human placental lactogen, prolactin, cortisol and progesterone. Insulin requirements may increase at this time.[32] Failure to increase insulin secretion to compensate for relative peripheral insulin resistance results in the development of gestational diabetes and may make control of the diabetic already on insulin worse.

Following delivery, insulin requirements fall rapidly and close monitoring of blood glucose levels is essential to prevent hypoglycaemia at this time.

PLACENTAL AND FETAL EFFECTS

Studies have demonstrated that uteroplacental perfusion is impaired in diabetic patients. This may be due either to a reduction in placental blood flow or an alteration in placental structure with enlarged villi and a reduced area available for gas exchange.[33,34] Haemoglobin A_{1c}, which is increased in patients with poor glycaemic control and used as a laboratory index of that control, may also impair oxygen delivery to the fetus.[35]

Despite reductions in perinatal mortality in diabetic mothers, it remains approximately five times higher than the general population.[36] The incidence of congenital abnormalities is also estimated to be between 4 and 10 times higher than in the general population.[36,37] Poor control of diabetes at the time of conception and in early pregnancy may be a contributing factor, and careful control of blood sugar at this time lowers the incidence.[38,39] Commonly encountered abnormalities in

- Uteroplacental perfusion may be impaired
- Increased risk of fetal death, stillbirth and perinatal mortality
- Increased incidence of macrosomia and congenital malformations
- Increased risk of infant respiratory distress syndrome
- Neonatal hypoglycaemia, hypocalcaemia, polycythaemia and hyperbilirubinaemia

Box 13.4   Fetal effects of diabetes in pregnancy.

the infants of diabetic mothers include spina bifida, hydrocephalus, cardiac abnormalities such as atrial and ventricular septal defects and transposition of the great vessels, renal agenesis, and polycystic kidney disease.

Glucose readily crosses the placenta and maternal hyperglycaemia causes fetal hyperglycaemia and insulin secretion. This results in increased skeletal growth and fat deposition in the fetus. A large fetus is at increased risk of nerve injury and shoulder dystocia during delivery. At the time of delivery the source of glucose from the mother ceases, but high insulin levels in the fetus may persist for longer, resulting in neonatal hypoglycaemia in the offspring of mothers with poorly controlled diabetes (Box 13.4).

There is some evidence that the fetal hyperglycaemia and hyperinsulinaemia, which results from poor diabetic control, is associated with impaired surfactant production and lung maturation, increasing the incidence of respiratory distress syndrome in infants of diabetic mothers. Estimations of the lecithin:sphingomyelin ratio can be used to assess lung maturity and guide the timing of delivery.

MANAGEMENT OF LABOUR

The aim of management of diabetic patients in labour is the maintenance of a normal plasma glucose. This is achieved by infusions of dextrose and insulin, either separately or together as in the Alberti regime.[39] This has the advantage that dextrose and insulin are infused together and one cannot be given in error without the other, but it may involve several changes of infusion if insulin concentrations need alteration. In addition, because the Alberti regime requires the infusion of 100 ml/h of dextrose, it is probably best reserved for short-term use only because of the risk of precipitating hyponatraemia.

Analgesia may be provided by any of the usual methods; intramuscular opioids or entonox may be sufficient for some mothers. Lumbar epidural analgesia reduces circulating catecholamine levels, which may be beneficial to glycaemic control and placental perfusion. Mothers with juvenile onset diabetes appear to have lower epidural local anaesthetic requirements than non-diabetic mothers of a similar age,[40] care is therefore needed when using epidural infusions or giving top ups.

After delivery insulin requirements fall rapidly, often to less than pre-pregnant levels. Close monitoring of blood glucose is essential with a reduction in the rate of insulin infusion if necessary. Continuing care in the delivery suite or HDU is essential for the first 24 h.

ANAESTHESIA FOR CAESAREAN SECTION

The perioperative management of diabetic patients undergoing elective Caesarean section should be determined by local policy drawn up in consultation with a diabetic physician. Whenever possible, diabetic patients should be scheduled first on a morning operating list. It is usual to give insulin as normal the evening before surgery and omit the dose on the morning of surgery. Insulin and dextrose can then be given during the perioperative period as for mothers in labour. Diet controlled diabetics can usually be managed by avoiding intravenous solutions which contain dextrose and lactate, with regular monitoring of blood glucose.

Spinal, epidural and general anaesthesia can all be employed in diabetic mothers with the usual precautions to avoid aspiration of gastric contents and aortocaval compression. Fetal monitoring, prevention of hypotension and maintenance of placental perfusion are particularly important in diabetic patients because the fetus is at greater risk of hypoxia. The paediatrician attending the delivery should be alerted to the fact that the mother is diabetic, and monitor the baby's blood sugar regularly.

DIABETIC KETOACIDOSIS

Diabetic ketoacidosis is a serious and potentially fatal complication of diabetes. Maternal mortality is similar to that in the general population; approximately 5%. Fetal mortality however may be as high as 50%.[41]

The most common cause of ketoacidosis is infection. Other factors, which may be relevant in the pregnant patient are the use of sympathomimetic agents to delay premature labour and the use of maternal steroids to promote fetal lung maturation.

- Avoid aorto-caval compression
- Treat dehydration; use 0.9% NaCl. Up to 6l may be needed
- Treat hyperglycaemia: use insulin by intravenous infusion, guided by regular blood glucose estimation
- Replace potassium – give 20–40mmol in each litre of NaCl. Check plasma potassium level regularly
- Consider giving bicarbonate only if pH <7.1.
- Monitor fluid input and output. Insert central venous line and urinary catheter
- Insert a nasogastric tube to minimize the risk of aspiration in the presence of gastric stasis
- Look for and treat the underlying cause, e.g. infection
- Involve senior medical and obstetric staff as soon as possible. Consider admission to intensive care

Box 13.5 The management of diabetic ketoacidosis.

	Normal	Hyperthyroid
Total T3	↑	↑
Total T4	↑	↑
Free T3	→	↑
Free T4	→	↑
TSH	→	↓

Box 13.6 Thyroid function tests in pregnancy.

Symptoms of ketoacidosis are usually nausea, vomiting, polydipsia, polyuria, drowsiness and occasionally unconsciousness. Investigations will reveal an elevated plasma glucose (>20 mmol/l), low plasma bicarbonate (<15 mmol/l), and a metabolic acidosis (pH < 7.30).

The treatment aims to replace the fluid deficit, which may be as high as 5–8l, with normal saline and correct the hyperglycaemia with a loading dose of 10 units of insulin, followed by an infusion of 5–10 units/h. Potassium will be required as the plasma glucose is corrected. Bicarbonate is rarely necessary to correct the acidosis, and should not be used unless the pH is <7.10 as it may worsen the intracellular acidosis. Urine output, central venous and arterial cannulation may also be helpful in monitoring fluid replacement. Blood for glucose, potassium and bicarbonate measurement should be taken regularly. Mothers will need to be treated in an intensive or high dependency unit, and the fetus monitored for evidence of fetal distress. In the severest cases a Caesarean should be considered if ketoacidosis persists, because of the increased metabolic demands of the pregnancy (Box 13.5).

THYROTOXICOSIS

Hyperthyroidism affects approximately 0.2% of pregnancies. 85% of cases are due to Grave's disease,

which is an autoimmune condition associated with the production of thyroid stimulating antibodies. Grave's disease may present for the first time or relapse during pregnancy or the puerperium.[42]

In women who remain untreated, or who do not respond to medical treatment, there is an increased incidence of pre-eclampsia and congestive cardiac failure during pregnancy. Rates of preterm labour, preterm delivery, stillbirth, and perinatal mortality are also increased.[43–45]

DIAGNOSIS

The heat intolerance and hyperdynamic state of the cardiovascular system during pregnancy can make hyperthyroidism difficult to diagnose. Weight loss, pretibial myxoedema, eye signs such as exophthalmos or lid lag, and the presence of a thyroid bruit or goitre suggest a diagnosis of hyperthyroidism.

High oestrogen levels during pregnancy cause an increase in thyroid binding globulin (TBG). Total serum T3 and T4 are therefore elevated during normal pregnancy. Elevated free T3 and T4 and reduced serum levels of thyroid stimulating hormone (TSH) are the most accurate indicators of hyperthyroidism (Box 13.6).

MANAGEMENT

The treatment of hyperthyroidism aims to block the production of further T3 and T4 with drugs such as propylthiouracil (PTU) or carbimazole, and to control the peripheral manifestations of the condition with β blocking agents. Propranolol is the β blocker most commonly used.

PTU and carbimazole both cross the placenta and can cause fetal hypothyroidism and goitre. Treatment therefore should aim to achieve euthyroidism with the lowest possible dose of either agent. There is no evidence that either drug is teratogenic and both are now considered safe in breastfeeding.[44,46] Carbimazole occasionally causes agranulocytosis. It is important therefore to check a full blood count regularly, and advise mothers to report any symptoms such as sore throat.

The action of a β blocker is not dependant on preventing the synthesis of further thyroid hormone and its onset of action is therefore more rapid. β blockers do not reduce the increased metabolic rate associated with hyperthyroidism and must not be used as the sole medical therapy for the condition.[47-49]

The use of radioactive iodine to treat hyperthyroidism is contraindicated during pregnancy and surgery should be reserved for patients in whom control cannot be achieved using medical therapy.

THYROID STORM

Thyroid storm is a medical emergency and is associated with significant maternal and fetal mortality. It typically occurs in an undiagnosed or untreated patient, precipitated by infection or stress, such as labour or Caesarean section. The clinical features of thyroid storm are fever, tachycardia and high output cardiac failure. Central nervous system manifestations such as restlessness, confusion or seizures and gastrointestinal symptoms may also be present.

If a diagnosis of thyroid storm is suspected, T3, T4 and TSH should be urgently measured. Treatment cannot wait for the results of such tests to be available, and should be commenced as soon as possible. The drug treatment of thyroid storm involves the use of high dose carbimazole (20 mg qds) or PTU (600–800 mg stat, then 200 mg qds) to suppress the production of further thyroid hormone, and β blockers (propranolol 5 mg i.v. or 20 mg p.o.) to control the symptoms. Lugol's iodine (0.2 ml qds) should be commenced after the PTU or carbimazole has been given; this achieves a transient inhibition of thyroid hormone formation. Glucocorticoids reduce the peripheral conversion of T4–T3 and therefore hydrocortisone 100 mg qds should be included in the treatment of thyroid storm (Box 13.7).

In addition to drug therapy, supportive care is required in a unit where continuous, invasive cardiac monitoring is available. Intravenous fluids and electrolytes are needed to replace increased gastrointestinal and insensible losses. Nutrition should be provided enterally if possible and parenterally if the patient is unable to eat. Supplementary thiamine and vitamins B and C are also required as levels may be depleted.[47] Supplementary oxygen is necessary to meet the increase in consumption associated with

- PTU 200 mg qds or carbimazole 20 mg qds
- Lugol's iodine 0.2 ml qds after PTU or carbimazole
- Hydrocortisone 100 mg qds
- Propranolol 20–80 mg p.o. or 5 mg i.v. 4 hourly
- Intravenous fluids and electrolytes
- Supplementary oxygen
- Cooling
- Enteral or parenteral nutrition and supplementary vitamins

Box 13.7   Management of thyroid storm.

hyperthyroidism. Body temperature should be monitored and reduced if necessary using paracetamol, cooling blankets and cold intravenous fluid.

ANAESTHESIA

Most patients with hyperthyroidism are well controlled and tolerate pregnancy and delivery without complications. Whenever possible, patients with hyperthyroidism should be rendered euthyroid prior to delivery or Caesarean section. For patients in whom hyperthyroidism is uncontrolled at the time of delivery, β blockers and antithyroid drugs should be commenced as soon as possible to control maternal heart rate. Lugol's iodine and hydrocortisone should also be given.

If general anaesthesia is considered, the airway should be carefully assessed for evidence of distortion or compression by a goitre. Drugs which increase the heart rate (e.g. ketamine, pancuronium) should be avoided. Care is needed to avoid injury to the eyes in the presence of exophthalmos. In addition to standard monitoring, temperature monitoring is advisable.

Regional anaesthesia has been performed safely in hyperthyroid patients.[43,50] Epidural is preferable to spinal anaesthesia because the changes in blood pressure occur less rapidly. Epinephrine containing local anaesthetic solutions are best avoided, as is ephedrine because of their undesirable effect on heart rate. Alternative vasopressors are discussed in the chapter on cardiac disease.

Patients with hyperthyroidism remain at risk from thyroid storm post-partum. High dependency care and invasive monitoring may therefore be appropriate at this time. Close monitoring of fluid and electrolyte balance, nutrition and thyroid status is essential. The baby may also develop a thyroid storm if the mother is undertreated.

EPILEPSY

Epilepsy is one of the most commonly encountered neurological disorders during pregnancy, affecting approximately 0.5% of the pregnant population.[51] Seizures may be generalized or partial, and in a pregnant patient, may be related to the pregnancy itself for example pre-eclampsia. It may be due to a pre-existing condition, e.g. metabolic disorders and intracranial vascular disorders. Seizures may be idiopathic or related to trauma.

THE EFFECT OF PREGNANCY ON EPILEPSY

Studies have shown an unpredictable effect of pregnancy on epilepsy, with approximately 30% of patients reporting an increase in seizure frequency, the remainder remaining unchanged or reporting a decrease in frequency.[52,53] Several factors may account for these changes:

- Many of the physiological changes associated with pregnancy, e.g. hormonal changes, hyperventilation and respiratory alkalosis, sodium and water retention, may exacerbate seizure disorders.
- The pharmacokinetics of anticonvulsant drugs may be altered. Absorption may be reduced as a result of reduced gastric motility, protein binding, volume of distribution, clearance and elimination of half life may all be altered in pregnant patients.[54] For this reason monitoring of plasma drug concentrations to maintain therapeutic levels is essential.
- Compliance with drug therapy may be altered, with some patients becoming more compliant because of fears about the effect of seizures on the fetus, and others stopping drug therapy because of fears about drug effects on the fetus.

THE EFFECTS OF EPILEPSY ON PREGNANCY

The prevention of seizures during pregnancy is of paramount importance during pregnancy because of the potentially serious consequences for both mother and fetus. The apnoea and increased maternal oxygen consumption, which occur during seizures, can cause fetal hypoxia and prolonged or frequent seizures can result in fetal death.

The incidence of congenital malformations are increased in the offspring of mothers with epilepsy, both treated and untreated. Congenital malformations are also increased in the offspring of epileptic fathers.[53] All the commonly used anticonvulsant agents have been implicated in teratogenesis, particularly facial, cardiac, neural tube and limb abnormalities. No agent can be considered entirely safe during pregnancy.[55] The aim of management should be to control seizures using the lowest possible dose of anticonvulsant drugs.

MANAGEMENT OF LABOUR AND VAGINAL DELIVERY

Adequate analgesia during labour is of benefit to mothers with epilepsy because it will prevent hyperventilation and respiratory alkalosis that may precipitate a seizure. For some mothers, pethidine or entonox is adequate, but epidural analgesia can be used safely and does not appear to increase seizure frequency. For instrumental delivery in patients without an epidural *in situ*, spinal anaesthesia is a suitable alternative.[56]

ANAESTHESIA FOR CAESAREAN SECTION

The choice of anaesthetic technique for Caesarean section in mothers with epilepsy should be based on the usual considerations, and takes into account maternal preference, urgency and any specific contraindications. Both spinal and epidural anaesthesia has been widely used and appears safe in epileptic patients. If general anaesthesia is employed, account should be taken of the interaction between anaesthetic and anticonvulsant drugs, and the effect of anaesthetic agents on epilepsy. Phenytion and carbamazepine may antagonise non-depolarizing muscle relaxants[57,58] and monitoring of neuromuscular blockade is important. Phenobarbitone is an enzyme inducing agent and will alter the metabolism of a wide range of drugs. Anaesthetic agents that lower the seizure threshold, notably enflurane and ketamine should be avoided.

In the post-partum period, anticonvulsant drug requirements may fall by up to 50%. Regular monitoring of drug levels should be continued.

MANAGEMENT OF SEIZURES AND STATUS EPILEPTICUS

There is an important differential diagnosis to be made when seizures occur in the latter half of pregnancy. The presence of hypertension, proteinuria, deranged clotting, deranged liver enzymes or elevated plasma urate suggest a diagnosis of eclampsia, in which case magnesium sulphate is the anticonvulsant

- The patient should be placed in a wedged position to avoid vena cava compression
- The airway should be cleared and oxygen administered in the highest possible concentration by facemask
- If the fit continues drug therapy should be instituted using diazepam 5–10 mg i.v. or pr or phenytoin 10 mg i.v. slowly
- If fits are prolonged with no return on consciousness between convulsions, endotracheal intubation may be necessary, and the patient admitted to the intensive care unit. The help of senior anaesthetic and obstetric staff should be sought
- Fetal monitoring should be instituted as soon as possible

Box 13.8   The management of non-eclamptic seizures during pregnancy.

of choice, though if this is not readily available, any other parenteral anticonvulsant may be used. The immediate management of a seizure is the same however, irrespective of the cause. Later management will depend on the underlying condition; patients with eclamptic fits require urgent delivery of the fetus whilst those with an exacerbation of an underlying seizure disorder may not (Box 13.8).

MULTIPLE SCLEROSIS

Multiple sclerosis is a chronic demyelinating disease of unknown aetiology, which is seen most commonly in young adults. It is characterized by intermittent relapses, separated by remission of symptoms, but in the later stages it may become chronically progressive. Factors that have been implicated in relapses include stress, exhaustion, a rise in body temperature, and infection. Symptoms are variable but most commonly include ataxia, spasticity, diplopia, and sphincter dysfunction. Patients with respiratory muscle involvement are at risk of pulmonary complications. Those with bladder involvement are at risk of recurrent urinary tract infections and renal impairment.

The effect of pregnancy on the course of multiple sclerosis is difficult to study. In the small number of mothers involved it would appear that the relapse rate during pregnancy is the same as would be expected in the non-pregnant population. The relapse rate during the first 3 months post-partum is however approximately twice the expected rate. Stress and

exhaustion may contribute although breast feeding does not appear to be a cause. Multiple sclerosis does not appear to have an adverse effect on the course or outcome of pregnancy.[59–61]

ANALGESIA FOR LABOUR AND DELIVERY

The issue of regional analgesia for labour and delivery or anaesthesia for Caesarean section is complex because of fears that relapses may be blamed on the anaesthetic technique. There is a risk therefore that mothers with multiple sclerosis will be denied the benefits of regional anaesthesia. It is important that all mothers are seen antenatally by an anaesthetist in order that the issues of anaesthesia and analgesia may be discussed fully. Mothers should be made aware of the risk of relapse in the post-partum period, regardless of the anaesthetic technique employed. In the antenatal clinic a full record should be made of any pre-existing neurological deficit, and an assessment made of the effect of the disease on respiratory and renal function.

The effect of regional blockade on mothers with multiple sclerosis is difficult to study because numbers are small. It would appear that the number of relapses following epidural blockade is no higher than would be expected if mothers had not received regional blockade.[61] In addition regional analgesia may be of benefit to mothers with multiple sclerosis by reducing stress and anxiety during labour. Where relapses have been linked with regional techniques, the use of high concentrations of local anaesthetic may be significant and local anaesthetic dose should be kept to a minimum.[61] Epidural opioids such as fentanyl may reduce the local anaesthetic requirement, but the effect of epidural opioids on the course of multiple sclerosis has not been studied.

ANAESTHESIA FOR CAESAREAN SECTION

Whilst it is now generally acknowledged that the use of epidural anaesthesia is safe in multiple sclerosis, the issue of spinal anaesthesia is more controversial.[62,63] There have been reports of relapses following spinal anaesthesia. The higher CSF concentrations of local anaesthetic, which are associated with spinal anaesthesia may be responsible for this observation.[60] It is very important to discuss the pros and cons of the various techniques well before delivery.

If general anaesthesia is necessary, conventional techniques are appropriate. The exception to this is the mother in whom significant muscle wasting is present and in this situation suxamethonium should be avoided because of the potential for hyperkalaemia. Intubation should be achieved either awake or using a non-depolarizing muscle relaxant. Care should be taken to maintain a normal body temperature with warming devices but overheating should be avoided as this may contribute to a relapse.

SPINAL CORD INJURY

In women of childbearing age, the most common cause of spinal cord injury is trauma, although infection and neoplasm do occur. Following the acute phase which lasts for up to 72 h, patients with spinal cord injuries develop a picture of paralysis below the level of the injury, muscle spasticity and disuse atrophy. Associated problems include: osteoporosis, pressure sores, impaired thermoregulation, impaired pulmonary function, renal impairment secondary to chronic urinary tract infections, and autonomic hyperreflexia. In addition, anatomical abnormalities may make procedures such as venepuncture or regional anaesthesia technically difficult or impossible. Mothers with a spinal cord lesion should receive an anaesthetic assessment in the antenatal clinic. Depending on the level of the lesion, pulmonary function tests, arterial blood gas measurement, and an assessment of the anatomy of the spine may be helpful particularly in those above T8. A neurological examination should also be documented as early as possible. Involvement of specialists from other disciplines such as neurology, rehabilitation medicine, respiratory medicine, and urology may be helpful.

AUTONOMIC HYPERREFLEXIA

Autonomic hyperreflexia was first described in 1917 by Head and Riddoch.[64] It is a syndrome that consists of sweating, mydriasis, flushing, paroxysmal hypertension, which may be sufficient to cause convulsions or intracerebreal haemorrhage, and cardiac dysrhythmias. It occurs in response to contraction or distension of a hollow viscus below the level of the spinal injury. Subsequent sympathetic discharge is not inhibited or modified by higher centres and results in intense vasoconstriction below the level of injury leading to hypertension. Hypertension is accompanied by a fall in heart rate and vasodilatation above the level of the lesion mediated by the aortic and carotid baroreceptors. Phentolamine, sodium nitroprusside, trimetaphan and labetolol have been used to achieve control of hypertension[65–67] in this situation. The syndrome of autonomic hyperreflexia may occur in 85% of patients with cord injuries above T6.[68] In the pregnant patient the most important differential diagnosis is with pre-eclampsia. Failure to recognize and treat the syndrome appropriately may have disastrous consequences for the mother.[69]

ANALGESIA FOR LABOUR

Mothers with complete cord transection above the level of T10 will not experience pain in labour. They are however at risk of autonomic hyperreflexia in response to uterine contractions. The symptoms and signs of flushing, palpitations, headache and visual disturbance may be the only indicators of the onset of labour. Epidural analgesia with local anaesthetic agents abolishes this response by blocking sensory stimuli from the uterus and should be considered for patients with lesions above T6. Care is needed when instituting epidural anaesthesia because a test dose may not identify accidental intrathecal injection in the presence of a high spinal cord lesion and monitoring the level of the block is only possible by testing segmental spinal reflexes. Regional anaesthesia may be technically difficult in mothers with spinal deformity.[70] Epidural pethidine,[71] but not fentanyl[72] appears to be effective in preventing autonomic hyperreflexia, this may be because of the local anaesthetic properties of pethidine.

Mothers with spinal cord lesions should have additional cardiovascular monitoring, which should include a continuous ECG for detection of dysrhythmias, non-invasive or invasive arterial blood pressure and pulse oximetry.

ANAESTHESIA FOR CAESAREAN SECTION

Caesarean section in patients with spinal injuries is reserved for obstetric indications such as pelvic deformity. Regional anaesthesia is the technique of choice. Spinal anaesthesia carries the risk of profound hypotension and unpredictable spread in the presence of abnormal spinal anatomy so epidural anaesthesia is preferred. If general anaesthesia is necessary, suxamethonium should be avoided for a period of 48 h to 1 year following the injury because of the risk of

---

- Pulmonary function may be impaired
- Increased risk of urinary tract infection and renal impairment secondary to recurrent infections
- Risk of autonomic hyperreflexia during labour
- Increased risk of pressure sores and venous thrombosis in the peripartum period
- Technical difficulties with venous access, anaesthetic and surgical procedures

Box 13.9   Spinal cord injury and pregnancy.

hyperkalaemia. A non-depolarizing muscle relaxant should be used to aid endotracheal intubation but the same precautions for any mother requiring a general anaesthetic applies, and awake fiberoptic intubation is probably safer.

Patients with severe respiratory impairment may need a period of mechanical ventilation post-operatively. Careful monitoring of renal function, prophylaxis against deep vein thrombosis and prevention of pressure sores are important considerations in the post-operative period (Box 13.9).

REFERENCES

ASTHMA

1. Moore Gillon J. Asthma and pregnancy. *Br J Obstet Gynaecol* 1994; **101**: 658–660.

2. Huff RW. Asthma in pregnancy. *Med Clin N Am* 1989; **73**: 653–660.

3. Turner ES, Greenberger PA, Patterson R. Management of the pregnant asthmatic patient. *Ann Intern Med* 1980; **93**: 905–918.

4. Gee JBL, Pacher BS, Miller JE, Robin ED. Pulmonary mechanics during pregnancy. *J Clin Invest* 1967; **46**: 945–952.

5. Schatz M, Harden K, Forsythe A et al. The course of asthma during pregnancy, postpartum and with successive pregnancies: a prospective analysis. *J Allergy Clin Immunol* 1988; **81**: 509–517.

6. Schatz M. Asthma during pregnancy: interrelationships and management. *Ann Allergy* 1992; **68**: 123–133.

7. Lehrer S, Stone J, Lockwood CJ et al. Association between pregnancy induced hypertension and asthma during pregnancy. *Am J Obstet Gynecol* 1993; **168**: 1463–1466.

8. Greenberg PA, Patterson R. Management of asthma during pregnancy. *New Engl J Med* 1985; **312**: 897–902.

9. Mabie WC. Asthma in pregnancy. *Clin Obstet Gynecol* 1996; **39**: 56–89.

10. Carter BL, Driscoll CF, Smith GD. Theophylline clearance during pregnancy. *Obstet Gynecol* 1986; **68**: 555–559.

11. Frederikson MC, Ruo TL, Chow MJ et al. Theophylline pharmacokinetics in pregnancy. *Clin Pharmacol Ther* 1986; **40**: 321–328.

12. Gross NJ, Skorodin MS. Anticholinergic, antimuscarinic bronchodilators. *Am Rev Respir Dis* 1984; **129**: 856–870.

13. Wilson J. Use of chromoglycate during pregnancy. *J Pharmacol Med* 1982; **8**: 45.

14. Benedetti TJ. Maternal complications of parenteral β sympathomimetic therapy for premature labour. *Am J Obstet Gynecol* 1983; **145**: 1–6.

15. Hagerdal M, Morgan CW, Sumner AE, Gutsche BB. Minute ventilation and oxygen consumption during labour with epidural anaesthesia. *Anaesthesiology* 1983; **59**: 425–427.

16. Freund FG, Bonica JJ, Ward RJ, Akamatsu TJ, Kennedy WF. Ventilatory reserve and level of motor block during high spinal and epidural anaesthesia. *Anaesthesiology* 1967; **28**: 834–837.

17. Mallampati SR. Bronchospasm during spinal anaesthesia. *Anaesth Analg* 1981; **60**: 839.

18. Roizen MF, Stevens WC. Multiform ventricular tachycardia due to the interaction of aminophylline and halothane. *Anesth Analg* 1978; **57**: 738–741.

CYSTIC FIBROSIS

19. Hilman BC, Aitken ML, Constantinescu M. Pregnancy in patients with cystic fibrosis. *Clin Obstet Gynecol* 1996; **39**: 70–86.

20. Norris MC, Chan L. Respiratory disease. In: *Anaesthetic and obstetric management of high risk pregnancy*. St Louis: Mosby Year Book, 1991.

21. Kotkoff RM, Fitzsimmons SC, Fiel SB. Fertility and pregnancy in patients with cystic fibrosis. *Clin Chest Med* 1992; **13**: 623.

22. Kopito LE, Kosasky HJ, Schwachman H. Water and electrolytes in cervical mucus from patients with cystic fibrosis. *Fertil Steril* 1973; **24**: 512–516.

23. Siegel B, Siegel S. Pregnancy and delivery in a patient with cystic fibrosis of the pancreas. Report of a case. *Obstet Gynecol* 1960; **16**: 439–440.

24. Palmer J, Dillon Baker C, Tecklin JS et al. Pregnancy in patients with cystic fibrosis. *Ann Intern Med* 1983; **99**: 596–600.

25. Heilcka A, Erkkola R. Review of β lactam antibiotics in pregnancy – the need for adjustment of dose schedules. *Clin Pharmacokinet* 1994; **27**: 49–62.

26. Hedstrom S, Martens MG. Antibiotics in pregnancy. *Clin Obstet Gynecol* 1993; **36**: 886–892.

27. Cole BN, Seltzer MN, Kassabrau J et al. Parenteral nutrition in a pregnant cystic fibrosis patient. *J Parent Nutri* 1987; **11**: 205–207.

28. Bose D, Yentis SM, Fauvel NJ. Caesarean section in a parturient with respiratory failure caused by cystic fibrosis. *Anaesthesia* 1997; **52**: 576–582.

DIABETES MELLITUS

29. Gillmer MD. Management of pre-existing disorders in pregnancy: diabetes mellitus. *Prescribers J* 1996; **36**: 159–164.

30. Roberts AB, Pattison NS. Pregnancy in women with diabetes mellitus; 20 years experience. *New Zed Med J* 1990; **103**: 211–213.

31. Barss VA. Diabetes and pregnancy. *Med Clin N Am* 1989; **73**: 685–700.

32. Landon MB, Gabbe SG. Diabetes and pregnancy. *Med Clin N Am* 1988; **72**: 1493–1511.

33. Nylund L, Lunell NO, Lewander R et al. Uteroplacental blood flow in diabetic pregnancy – measurements with indium 113 m and a computer linked gamma camera. *Am J Obstet Gynecol* 1982; **144**: 298–302.

34. Bjork O, Persson B. Placental changes in relation to the degree of metabolic control in diabetes mellitus. *Placenta* 1982; **3**: 267.

35. Madsen H, Ditzel J. Changes in red blood cell oxygen transport in diabetic pregnancy. *Am J Obstet Gynecol* 1982; **143**: 421–424.

36. Hawthorne G, Robson S, Ryall EA et al. Prospective population based survey of outcome of pregnancy in diabetic women: results of the Northern Diabetic Pregnancy Audit 1994. *Br Med J* 1997; **315**: 279–281.

37. Casson IF, Clarke CA, Howard CV et al. Outcomes of pregnancy in insulin dependant diabetic women: results of a five year population cohort study. *Br Med J* 1997; **315**: 275–278.

38. Fuhrmann K, Reiher H, Semmler K et al. The effect of intensified conventional insulin therapy before and during pregnancy on the malformation rate in the offspring of diabetic mothers. *Exp Clin Endocrinol* 1984; **83**: 173–179.

39. Alberti KGMM, Thomal BJB. The management of diabetes during surgery. *Br J Anaesth* 1979; **51**: 693–710.

40. Bromage PR. Physiology and pharmacology of epidural analgesia. *Anaesthesiology* 1967; **28**: 592–622.

41. Datta S, Greene MF. The diabetic parturient. In: Datta S (ed) *Anaesthetic and obstetric management of high risk pregnancy*. St Louis: Mosby Year Book, 1991.

THYROTOXICOSIS

42. Mestman JH. Hyperthyroidism in pregnancy. *Clin Obstet Gynecol* 1997; **40**: 45–64.

43. Van der Spuy ZM, Jacobs HS. Management of endocrine disorders in pregnancy. Part I. Thyroid and parathyroid disease. *Postgrad Med J* 1984; **60**: 245–252.

44. Davies LE, Lucas MJ, Hankins GDV et al. Thyrotoxicosis complicating pregnancy. *Am J Obstet Gynecol* 1989; **160**: 63–70.

45. Clark SL, Phelan JP, Montcro, Mestman. Transient ventricular dysfunction associated with Caesarean section in a patient with hyperthyroidism. *Am J Obstet Gynecol* 1985; **151**: 384–386.

46. Momotani N, Noh J, Oyanagi H, Ishikawa N, Ito K. Antithyroid drug therapy for Graves' disease during pregnancy. Optimal regimen for fetal thyroid status. *New Engl J Med* 1986; **315**: 24–28.

47. Molitch ME. Endocrine emergencies in pregnancy. *Balliere Clin Endocrinol Metabol* 1992; **6**(1): 167–191.

48. Tunstall ME. The effect of propranolol on the onset of breathing at birth. *Br J Anaesth* 1969; **41**: 792.

49. Burrow GN. Current concepts: the management of thyrotoxicosis in pregnancy. *New Engl J Med* 1985; **313**: 562–566.

50. Mayer DC, Thorp J, Baucom D et al. Hyperthyroidism and seizures during pregnancy. *Am J Perinatol* 1995; **12**: 192–194.

EPILEPSY

51. Dalessio DJ. Current concepts: seizure disorders and pregnancy. *New Engl J Med* 1985; **312**: 559–563.

52. Schmidt D, Canger R, Avanzini G et al. Change of seizure frequency in pregnant women. *J Neurol Neurosurg Psych* 1983; **46**: 751–755.

53. Patterson RM. Seizure disorders in pregnancy. *Med Clin N Am* 1989; **73**: 661–665.

54. Lander CM, Edwards VE, Eadie MJ, Tyrer JH. Plasma anticonvulsant concentrations during pregnancy. *Neurology* 1977; **27**: 128–131.

55. Kelly TE. Teratogenicity of anticonvulsant drugs 1: review of the literature. *Am J Med Genet* 1984; **19**: 413–434.

56. Aravapelli R, Abouleish E, Aldrete JA. Anaesthetic implications in the parturient epileptic patient. *Anaesth Analg* 1988; **67**: S266.

57. Ornstein E, Matteo RS, Young WL, Diaz J. Resistance to metocurine induced neuromuscular block in patients receiving phenytoin. *Anaesthesiology* 1985; **63**: 294–298.

58. Roth S, Ebrahim ZY. Resistance to pancuronium in patients receiving carbamazepine. *Anaesthesiology* 1987; **66**: 691–693.

MULTIPLE SCLEROSIS

59. Birk K, Smeltzer S, Rudick R. Pregnancy and multiple sclerosis. *Semin Neurol* 1988; **8**: 205–213

60. Sweeney W. Pregnancy and multiple sclerosis. *Am J Obstet Gynecol* 1953; **66**: 124–130.

61. McArthur JC, Young F. Multiple sclerosis in pregnancy. In: Goldstein PJ (ed) *Neurological disorders of pregnancy*, 1986.

62. Bader AM, Hunt CO, Datta S et al. Anaesthesia for the pregnant patient with multiple sclerosis. *J Clin Anaesth* 1988; **1**: 21–24.

63. Bamford C, Sibley W, Laguna J. Anaesthesia in multiple sclerosis. *Can J Neurol Sci* 1978; **5**: 41–44.

SPINAL CORD INJURY

64. Head H, Riddoch G. The automatic bladder, excessive sweating and some other reflex conditions in gross injuries of the spinal cord. *Brain* 1917; **40**: 188–263.

65. Erickson R. Autonomic hyperreflexia, pathophysiology and medical management. *Arch Phys Med Rehabil* 1980; **61**: 431–440.

66. Ravindran RC, Cummings DF, Smith IE. Experience with the use of nitroprusside and subsequent epidural anaesthesia in the pregnant quadriplegic patient. *Anaesth Analg* 1981; **60**: 61–63.

67. Stirt JA, Marco A, Conkin KA. Obstetric anaesthesia for a quadriplegic patient with autonomic hyperreflexia. *Anaesthesiology* 1979; **51**: 560–562.

68. Kurnick NB. Autonomic hyperreflexia and its control in patient with spinal cord lesions. *Ann Intern Med* 1956; **44**: 678–686.

69. Abouleish E. Hypertension in a paraplegic parturient. *Anaesthesiology (Letter)* 1980; **53**: 948–949.

70. Ahmed AB, Bogod DG. Anaesthetic management of a quadriplegic patient with severe respiratory insufficiency undergoing Caesarean section. *Anaesthesia* 1996; **51**: 1043–1045.

71. Baraka A. Epidural meperidine for control of autonomic hyperreflexia in a paraplegic parturient. *Anaesthesiology* 1985; **62**: 688–690.

72. Abouleish E, Hanley ES, Palmer SM. Can epidural fentanyl control autonomic hyperreflexia in a quadriplegic parturient. *Anaesth Analg* 1989; **68**: 523–526.

Andrew H. Shennan

INTRODUCTION

Pre-eclampsia is a condition peculiar to pregnancy characterized by raised blood pressure and proteinuria. It can be associated with seizures, (eclampsia) and multi-organ failure in the mother. The fetus is susceptible to growth restriction and other complications such as abruption of the placenta. The pre-eclamptic woman commonly presents to the obstetric anaesthetist, and the underlying pathophysiology can result in challenging management issues. This chapter will outline what those problems are likely to be and how they can be overcome. In addition some insight into the magnitude of the problem in modern antenatal care, the definition and classification of the syndrome, and the current theories as to the possible causes of pre-eclampsia will be discussed. It will also describe the characteristic cardiovascular changes that occur with this disease and whether pre-eclampsia can be predicted or prevented. Risk factors will be discussed. Some of the latest developments in the management of both the maternal and fetal disease associated with the condition will be considered.

PREVALENCE AND IMPORTANCE

The prevalence of pre-eclampsia varies and is dependant on the characteristics of the population studied, as well as the definitions of pre-eclampsia used. It occurs in less than 5% of most antenatal populations. Recent prospective studies have shown the incidence to be low at 2.2%, even in a primigravid population in which the condition is known to occur more frequently.[1] Gestational hypertension (hypertension without proteinuria) is approximately three times as common, but carries far less perinatal risk. Most clinicians who deal with pregnancy will have to deal with pre-eclampsia on a regular basis.

The consequences of pre-eclampsia are well defined. There is increased morbidity and mortality to the mother and fetus, and in the developed world pre-eclampsia and eclampsia are leading causes of maternal death. Of particular concern is the fact that most of these deaths in the UK are associated with suboptimal care, particularly by intrapartum carers.[2] In the UK less than 10 women will die each year but once a women suffers an eclamptic seizure, the mortality increases to 2%.[3] Throughout the world, pre-eclampsia is believed to account for more than 100 000 maternal deaths per year. Up to a quarter of antenatal admissions are directly related to the need for managing women with hypertension. Antenatal care is structured towards identifying women with hypertension and proteinuria.

The association between pre-eclampsia, placental abruption and increased perinatal mortality may be explained by the pathological changes within the placenta.[4] Proteinuria is associated with increased fetal risk.[5] Pre-eclampsia is associated with intrauterine growth restriction except when it presents late in gestation. Women may need to be delivered early; currently delivery is the only known cure for the disease. The resulting iatrogenic prematurity accounts for 15% of all premature births[6] but also a disproportionate number of very low birth weight infants with their associated long-term complications.[7] Severe maternal disease is not always associated with fetal problems; babies of women who have eclampsia at term have normal birth weight.[3]

IDENTIFYING THE AT-RISK WOMAN

Diagnosing the disease by the presence of hypertension and proteinuria is imprecise. These two clinical findings are not fundamental to the aetiology, but represent end organ damage. These clinical findings are used as they are easy to measure with high sensitivity but have low specificity. An isolated finding of hypertension (or proteinuria) is unlikely to be significant. There is however a clear relationship between persistently raised blood pressure and morbidity and mortality; still-birth rates are higher at *any* gestation when the maternal diastolic pressure is equal to or greater than 95 mmHg.[8] The term 'pre-eclampsia' is used to represent the syndrome characterized by hypertension, proteinuria associated with increased perinatal risk. 'Pregnancy induced hypertension' identifies hypertension in isolation, and is not associated with increased perinatal risk, as long as pre-eclampsia does not materialize. The International Society for the Study of Hypertension in Pregnancy (ISSHP) has adopted the recommendation of Davey and MacGillivray[9] which uses the term 'gestational hypertension' to cover all hypertensive women whether proteinuric or not, as long as they had been previously normotensive and not proteinuric. Once proteinuria has developed this is assumed to be pre-eclampsia (Table 14.1).

DEFINITIONS

Hypertension in pregnancy:
A. Diastolic BP $\geq$ 110 mmHg on any one occasion or

Table 14.1   A summary of the ISSHP classification

A. Gestational hypertension and/or proteinuria developing during pregnancy, labour or the puerperium in a previously normotensive non-proteinuric woman
   1. Gestational hypertension (without proteinuria)
   2. Gestational proteinuria (without hypertension)
   3. Gestational proteinuric hypertension (pre-eclampsia)
B. Chronic hypertension (before the 20th week of pregnancy) and chronic renal disease (proteinuria before the 20th week of pregnancy)
   1. Chronic hypertension (without proteinuria)
   2. Chronic renal disease (proteinuria with or without hypertension)
   3. Chronic hypertension with superimposed pre-eclampsia (new onset proteinuria)
C. Unclassified hypertension and/or proteinuria
D. Eclampsia

B. Diastolic BP $\geq$ 90 mmHg on two or more consecutive occasions $\geq$ 4 h apart.

Proteinuria in pregnancy:
A. One 24 h collection with total protein excretion $\geq$ 300 mg/24 h or
B. Two 'clean-catch – midstream' or catheter specimens of urine collected $\geq$ 4 h apart with $\geq$ 2+ on reagent strip.

There is very little agreement in published papers as to how to define pre-eclampsia.[10] A high index of suspicion is required when any organ system, known to be affected in pre-eclampsia, is involved. Hypertension and proteinuria cannot be the only findings used to diagnose the woman at risk. These signs must remain hallmarks for classifying pre-eclampsia for pragmatic reasons, but liver, kidney, blood and placental involvement should always be looked for if the condition is suspected (see below).

UNDERLYING PATHOPHYSIOLOGY

Pre-eclampsia is associated with abnormal implantation of the placenta and shallow invasion of the trophoblast[11] associated with reduced perfusion of the placenta. The maternal spiral arteries do not undergo their normal physiological vasodilatation and may become obstructed through acute atherotic change. Only the most superficial decidual portion of the spiral artery is invaded by the trophoblast. However, inadequate trophoblast invasion is also seen in pregnancies complicated by fetal growth restriction in women without pre-eclampsia. This suggests that the maternal syndrome of pre-eclampsia must also be

related to additional factors. The pathology results in increased resistance in the utero-placental circulation and an impaired intervillous blood flow. Ischaemia and hypoxia is found in the second half of pregnancy.[12] There is an associated production of reactive oxygen species and oxidative stress in the placenta.[13] The widespread manifestations of the disease can be explained by endothelial cell activation as vascular endothelium supplies all organ systems involved; markers of endothelial damage are in fact raised in women with pre-eclampsia. There is also a two-fold increase in triglyceride and free fatty acid concentrations,[14] possibly related to the pathology associated with acute atherosis. Increased lipid peroxidation, occurring both in the placenta and systemically, in pre-eclamptic women causes further oxidative stress. Oxidative stress is the imbalance between free radical synthesis and antioxidant defence, resulting in lipid peroxidation, which can damage the endothelium, leading to the manifestations of pre-eclampsia. A better understanding of the pathophysiology has led to more targeted prophylactic treatment such as the use of the antioxidants vitamins C and E to prevent pre-eclampsia (see later).

CARDIOVASCULAR CHANGES

A range of haemodynamic states has been demonstrated in hypertensive pregnant women, ranging from high output–low resistance to low output–high resistance states. The best studies suggest a reduced pre-load and cardiac output in association with a markedly increased after load in pre-eclamptic women. These observations are be consistent with the reduced plasma volume found in pre-eclampsia (volumes similar to those found in non-pregnant women). As blood pressure is a function of peripheral vascular resistance and cardiac output, these findings suggest that pre-eclampsia is associated with a huge increase in peripheral vascular resistance. These findings are particularly important when managing the sick pre-eclamptic (see later); the circulation is particularly sensitive to vasodilatation and fluid shifts.

WHO IS AT RISK?

A knowledge of who is at risk is essential: the majority of *eclamptic* women present either intra- or post-partum (18% and 44% respectively).[3] Diagnosis of pre-eclampsia at this time is confounded by the difficulties of blood pressure and protein assessment in labour or following delivery. Once diagnosed with pre-eclampsia, women should be closely monitored as inpatients. Delivery is the only cure.

RISK FACTORS

There are many risk factors for pre-eclampsia; a careful history will allow the clinician to assess the risk. There is a well-established genetic influence in the aetiology of pre-eclampsia; a family history in either mother or sister increases the risk four- to eight-fold. A woman has twice the risk of pre-eclampsia if pregnant by a partner who had previously fathered an affected pregnancy:[15] exposure to the paternal antigen, either from the fetus or partner influences the risk of pre-eclampsia, suggesting an immunological element. Pre-eclampsia is ten times more likely to occur in first pregnancies; even miscarriages and terminations of pregnancy provide some reduction in risk in subsequent pregnancies.[16] A new partner returns a woman's risk to that of a primigravidae.[17]

Risk is *reduced* with non-barrier methods of contraception,[18] increased duration of sexual cohabitation[19] and with the practice of oral sex[20] (i.e. it appears to be decreased by increased exposure to the foreign antigens found in the partner's semen). Lack of exposure to these antigens may explain why teenage girls[21] and pregnancies conceived by donor insemination[22] have increased risk of pre-eclampsia.

Underlying medical disorders can be strongly associated with the risk of pre-eclampsia in particular vascular disease, which highlights the importance of maternal susceptibility as well as the placental aetiology in the disease process. About 20% of women with chronic hypertension develop pre-eclampsia[23], and chronic hypertension without other evidence of pre-eclampsia is also associated with growth restriction.[24] Women with previous pre-eclampsia with severe complications or requiring delivery before 37 weeks, have about a 20% chance of developing pre-eclampsia again. Glucose intolerance, including gestational diabetes, is associated with an increased risk of pre-eclampsia.[25] Obesity predisposes to pre-eclampsia;[26] a BMI of greater than 29 increases the risk approximately four-fold.[27] Women with underlying thrombotic tendency, particularly antiphospholipid syndrome, are at increased risk of pre-eclampsia.[28] Multiple pregnancies have more than double the risk,[27] possibly due to increased size of the placenta. Molar pregnancies have been associated with pre-eclampsia, as well as hydrops fetalis (Mirror syndrome) and trisomy chromosomal complement, all of which are associated with large placentas.

BIOPHYSICAL TESTS

Various forms of blood pressure assessment in association with isometric exercise or rolling over have been used to identify women likely to become pre-eclamptic. If a woman tends to have higher blood pressures in pregnancy her risk of pre-eclampsia increases.

Doppler assessment of the utero-placental circulation has predictive powers, which are as good as any other test, whilst being relatively quick, inexpensive and non-invasive. Poor placental perfusion appears to be a characteristic feature of pregnancies destined to develop pre-eclampsia, and this can be evaluated with Doppler ultrasound to identify abnormal flow velocity waveforms in the uterine artery. There is a persistence of a relatively high resistant circulation with a notch as the pregnancy advances (Fig. 14.1). At 20 weeks gestation in a low-risk population, approximately one in five women will develop pre-eclampsia if they have an abnormal waveform.[29] If the test is repeated at 24 weeks, the prediction values are even greater.

BIOCHEMICAL TESTS

A large number of biochemical tests have also been investigated as potential predictors or risk accessors of pre-eclampsia. The angiotensin 2 sensitivity test is no better than Doppler[30] and is also invasive, time-consuming and costly. The simpler measurements of plasma volume, haemoglobin concentration and haematocrit have a weak association with the development and severity of pre-eclampsia. Measurements

Abnormal (High resistance and notch)

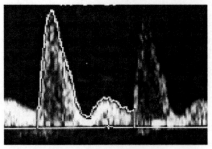

Normal (Low resistance)

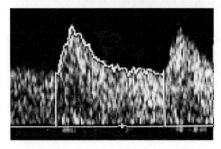

Figure 14.1   A comparison of normal and abnormal fetal velocity waveforms.

of uric acid and platelets can be used in women with chronic hypertension to predict superimposed pre-eclampsia, but all have poor sensitivity and specificity both as predictors or markers of severity. Increased maternal levels of second trimester human chorionic gonadotrophin and maternal serum alpha feto-protein are associated with a two-fold increase in pre-eclampsia. This reflects the disease process that occurs at the utero-placental interface. Markers of endothelial activation are often increased in pre-eclampsia and some will rise before the clinical manifestations of the disease; there is always cross-over between the women who are subsequently normal and those who develop pre-eclampsia, again limiting the clinical usefulness of such markers. Urinary excretion of a number of substances has a weak relationship with pre-eclampsia, but again are not clinically useful.

PREVENTATIVE THERAPIES

Some women who present to the obstetric anaethetist will be on preventative therapies for pre-eclampsia, and therefore an understanding of the rationale and the effects of this treatment is important. Work has principally focussed on aspirin, calcium and fish oils, although other substances such as magnesium, zinc

and even rhubarb[31] have been investigated. Aspirin acts as an endothelial cyclo-oxygenase inhibitor, reversing the imbalance between thromboxane and the more favourable prostacyclin, found to occur in pre-eclampsia. There are currently 42 randomized trials reported by the Cochrane Collaboration[32] demonstrating a 15% relative reduction in the risk of pre-eclampsia associated with the use of aspirin or other antiplatelet agents. There is also a significant reduction in the risk of preterm delivery and risk of death to the baby. Low dose aspirin is therefore often given to high-risk women. There is no reason to continue it to delivery, unless there is an additional risk of thromboembolism, and it can be stopped at 36 weeks. These trials have demonstrated that the use of low-dose aspirin is likely to be safe. There is no increased risk to the mother who receives regional block.

There are currently 10 trials in women that are investigating the role of calcium as prophylaxis for pre-eclampsia. Benefit seems to be restricted to women with poor nutritional status, and this the subject of a large WHO trial at present. Fish oils that contain n-3 fatty acids are thought to inhibit platelets thromboxane A2. However, the four trials that have investigated their use have not shown any reduction in the incidence of pre-eclampsia.

As oxidative stress may play a role in the aetiology of the maternal syndrome of pre-eclampsia, we have investigated the role of vitamins C and E supplementation from the second trimester of pregnancy. In 283 women identified as high risk of pre-eclampsia (principally because of an abnormal uterine artery Doppler), vitamins C and E supplementation reduced the likelihood of developing pre-eclampsia by more than 75%. Even those women who withdrew from treatment after 1 month (because of normalization of their Doppler), this single month of treatment was associated with a 50% reduction; 1000 mg of vitamin C and 400 IU of vitamin E were used and had a synergistic effect. A trial to see if this benefit can relate to other high risk populations and also to the low-risk primigravid population, where a large proportion of pre-eclamptic women originate, is planned.[33]

DIAGNOSIS

ESTABLISHING A DIAGNOSIS

As many as one in five women will be hypertensive in pregnancy, whereas less than 10% of these will get serious disease. A very important risk factor for adverse perinatal events is the gestation at which women present with hypertension. Late onset hypertension (after 37 weeks), rarely results in serious morbidity to mother or baby, but hypertension that presents early results in the majority of women developing the classical syndrome of pre-eclampsia.

PROBLEMS WITH BLOOD PRESSURE MEASUREMENT

Care with blood pressure measurement technique is essential as there is ample evidence to suggest that this is poorly performed and impacts on practice. Digit preference in antenatal care, (rounding the final digit of the blood pressure to 0), occurs in more than 80% of blood pressure measurements; in effect, an imprecise measurement is being made worse. In the UK, the antenatal population has one of the highest rates of obesity in Europe. The standard bladder used in sphygmomanometer cuffs (23 × 12 cm) is too small for approximately 25% of the antenatal population, resulting in the over-diagnosis of hypertension. This type of 'undercuffing' results in greater than a 10 mmHg over-read in blood pressure whereas over-cuffing has the opposite effect, but to a much smaller degree (less than 5 mmHg).

Keeping the rate of deflation during measurement to 2–3 mm/s will prevent over-diagnosis of diastolic hypertension. Korotkoff 4 is no longer recommended as it is not reproducible[34] and randomized controlled clinical trials have demonstrated it is both appropriate and safe to use Korotkoff 5.[35] By using Korotkoff 5, there will be less over-diagnosis of hypertension.

Automated blood pressure devices usually under-record the blood pressure in pre-eclampsia. Table 14.2 demonstrates those machines that have been evaluated in pregnancy and pre-eclampsia (both intra-arterially and against mercury sphygmomanometry), showing that most are under-recording by significant amounts. Even the ubiquitous DINAMAP under-records by an average of 15 mmHg for systolic blood pressure. Care must be taken when interpreting these readings from oscillometric devices.

There are similar problems with the interpretation of proteinuria; both false positives and false negatives are commonplace with dipstick urinalysis. Twenty-four hour collections of urine are required to confirm the diagnosis; women with more than 300 mg in 24 h should be considered at risk. In the near future newer automated devices that can be used by the bedside, which relate the proteinuria to creatinine are almost as good as 24 h collections and are likely to aid clinical practice.

The clinician cannot rely on blood pressure and proteinuria alone; the syndrome of pre-eclampsia is multi-system and these two findings are used mainly because they are easy to measure. Only just over half of women who present with eclampsia have had prior hypertension and proteinuria identified.[3] Other organ involvement must be sought. The diagnosis must be considered in women with fetal involvement or other signs such as epigastric tenderness. For pragmatic reasons, other signs have not been used to define the disease, but are equally important.

ANTENATAL MANAGEMENT

A common problem with early onset pre-eclampsia is placental insufficiency. This can result in intrauterine growth restriction, abruption of the placenta or fetal

---

Table 14.2   Mean and standard deviation (mmHg) of differences in BP measurements between standard and device (standard minus device) in pregnancy and pre-eclampsia

	Pregnancy		Pre-eclampsia	
	Systolic	Diastolic	Systolic	Diastolic
SpaceLabs 90207	3(4)	4(4)	19(8)*	0.6(3)
QuietTrak	0.34(9)	1.6(8)	25(16)*	18(8)
Omron Hem 705 CP	0.9(10)	1.5(10)	2(10)	8(8)
Dinamap XL 301			15(9)*	11(7)
SpaceLabs Scout			18(10)*	4(10)
Welsh Allyn Lifesign	2(7)	3(6)	8(6)*	6(5)*

Acceptable standard 5(8) mmHg (Association for the Advancement of Medical Instrumentation).
*Denotes comparison with intra-arterial measurement.

death. A cardiotocogram (CTG) and symphyseal fundal height should be carefully measured in all women who present with pre-eclampsia and it is usual to confirm fetal growth with ultrasound at early gestations, along with amniotic fluid index and umbilical artery Doppler analysis. Deterioration of the fetal condition is a frequent cause for delivery, and the obstetrician may consider Caesarean section for these reasons.

Equally the maternal condition must also be carefully monitored in women who present with hypertension and proteinuria, particularly the involvement of other organ systems. Endothelial dysfunction results in platelet dysfunction. If the platelet count is greater than $50 \times 10^9/l$, there is likely to be normal haemostasis, but delivery is often considered if the platelet count falls to less than 100. Haemoglobin is often higher than normal due to the hypovolaemia of pre-eclampsia, which results in an increased haematocrit. As pre-eclampsia can cause disseminated intravascular coagulation, if delivery is likely to be imminent, it is also sensible to screen clotting parameters, particularly if a regional block is to be considered.

Uric acid or urate levels are used to assess the severity of the disease and its progression, although severe disease can occur in the presence of normal uric acid concentrations. Extremely raised uric acid levels should alert the clinician to the possibility of acute fatty liver of pregnancy, which is associated with high maternal mortality. Raised plasma urea and creatinine concentrations are generally associated with late renal involvement and serious disease, and are not useful as an early indicators of disease severity, but should be sought longitudinally to assess renal disease progression. Pre-eclampsia can cause sub-capsular haematoma of the liver, liver rupture and hepatic infarction. The syndrome of haemolysis, elevated liver enzymes and low platelets, (HELLP syndrome), is a severe variant of pre-eclampsia, often with mild hypertension or proteinuria in its early phase. Pre-eclampsia is the commonest cause of nephrotic syndrome in young women and high levels of proteinuria may result in hypoalbuminaemia, increasing the risk of pulmonary oedema. Raised levels of aspartate aminotransferase (AST) and other transaminases indicate hepatocellular damage and may signal the need for early delivery. Haemolysis is associated with increased lactate dehydrogenase levels and to a lesser degree with increases in AST.

ANTIHYPERTENSIVE THERAPY AND STEROIDS

Blood pressure control without the decision to deliver is controversial as there is some evidence that treating moderate levels of hypertension may be detrimental to fetal growth,[36] although most clinicians agree that severe hypertension should be avoided. Blood pressures of greater than 170/110 mmHg are likely to require urgent therapy. The obstetrician may consider loading with a centrally acting drug such as methyldopa to make subsequent management of severe hypertension easier. Other drugs such as labetalol and nifedipine are commonly used, although their safety profile is not as well established; in particular there is a paucity of follow-up studies in children. Beta-blockers may have a detrimental effect on fetal growth. ACE inhibitors should be avoided as they cause fetal renal toxicity and diuretics should only rarely be used, and usually only to treat fluid over-load or pulmonary oedema.

The Royal College of Obstetricians and Gynaecologists (1996) recommend that corticosteroids should be given to enhance fetal lung maturity and should be given between 24 and 36 weeks gestation. Steroids may assist in the recovery from HELLP syndrome and have been used in the postpartum period. It is not unusual to see a slight improvement in biochemical parameters associated with corticosteroid use.

THE DECISION TO DELIVER

Most obstetricians will consider delivery once fetal maturity is unlikely to be a concern. Beyond 36 weeks women with severe pre-eclampsia should be delivered. Onset of pre-eclampsia at early gestations can often be managed conservatively with significant fetal benefit regarding maturity, without significantly increasing maternal morbidity.

In the mother, inability to control the blood pressure, deteriorating liver or renal function, progressive fall in platelets or neurological complications usually indicate delivery is necessary. In the fetus a non-reactive CTG with decelerations to the fetal heart rate or a fetal condition that is clearly deteriorating also warrants delivery.

MANAGEMENT IN LABOUR

Many units have now developed a severe pre-eclampsia protocol. Cases which require protocol determined management are defined as those with severe hypertension, (greater than 170/110 mmHg), or hypertension with an additional complication such as headache, visual disturbance, epigastric pain, clonus, (more than three beats), or a platelet count less than 100 or AST more than 50 IU/l.

Table 14.3 Maternal mortality 1985–1999: immediate hypertensive deaths

Intracerebral haemorrhage	36 (33%)
ARDS	33 (30%)
Other	41 (37%)
Total	110

Data from the confidential enquiry into maternal deaths suggests there are two main reasons why women die: cerebral haemorrhage and adult or acute respiratory distress syndrome (Table 14.3).

Severe hypertension and excess fluid intake are the most important preventable factors in the aetiology of mortality. Management therefore involves control of blood pressure and fluid balance.

BLOOD PRESSURE CONTROL PERIPARTUM (FIG. 14.2)

Blood pressure should be measured frequently, (every 15 min), and to facilitate this, automated sphygmomanometers are used. As already mentioned there is evidence that these oscillometric devices under-read the blood pressure in pre-eclampsia.[37] Significant changes in blood pressure should be confirmed with a mercury sphygmomanometer that does not have this error. Protocols frequently use mean arterial pressure, (MAP), to guide management; at MAPs over 150 mmHg there is serious risk that cerebral autoregulation is overwhelmed, resulting in intracerebral haemorrhage. At MAPs about 140 mmHg, urgent treatment is required if sustained over 15 min. Pressures between 125 and 140 mmHg, that are sustained over 45 min, also require treatment. Intravenous hydralazine (5 mg) has proved to be a very good first line therapy for severe hypertension in labour. If the baby is still undelivered at the time of treatment, then colloid should be infused prior to treatment to protect the utero-placental circulation and prevent hypotension and fetal distress. Should the blood pressure remain high after repeated doses, labetalol may be added or used as an alternative if hydralazine results in significant tachycardia.

Figure 14.2 shows the blood pressure protocol adopted by Guy's and St. Thomas' NHS Trust to manage blood pressure in the severe pre-eclamptic.

FLUID MANAGEMENT

Pre-eclampsia is associated with a reduced intravascular volume, leaky capillary membranes and low albumen concentrations all of which increase the risk of pulmonary oedema, particularly if there is over-zealous administration of intravenous fluid given in response to oliguria. A urine output of 100 ml/4 h should be sufficient. Most protocols will now limit fluid in the form of intravenous crystalloid to 85 ml/h (Fig. 14.3). A Foley catheter should be inserted and strict fluid balance maintained and recorded.

Careful monitoring is mandatory with a low threshold for central venous pressure, (CVP), assessment. Fluid above maintenance levels should only be given when oliguria is associated with a low CVP. Persistent oliguria associated with a high CVP (>8 mmHg), may indicate the need for dopamine by infusion, (1 μg/kg/min). Should the creatinine or potassium rise, haemodialysis or haemofiltration may be necessary. If there are signs of pulmonary oedema then frusemide 40 mg can be given and repeated.

ANTICONVULSANT THERAPY

As less than 1% of women with severe pre-eclampsia will have an eclamptic fit, uncertainly whether prophylactic anticonvulsants are justified. This was the subject of the 'Magpie Trial', which evaluated the use of magnesium sulphate versus placebo as prophylaxis in women with pre-eclampsia. Early results suggest that magnesium prophylaxis may be benefit in severe pre-eclampsia. It is now clear that if a woman does have an eclamptic fit, magnesium sulphate is the drug of choice, as shown by the Eclampsia Trial. There are additional benefits to be gained from the use of magnesium sulphate in preference to both diazepam and phenytoin: as well as preventing further fits more effectively, magnesium was associated with a significantly lower need for maternal ventilation, less pneumonia and fewer intensive care admissions. Magnesium sulphate acts as a membrane stabilizer and vasodilator and reduces intracerebral ischaemia. It is given as a 2 g intravenous loading dose (20 ml) and a maintenance infusion at 1–2 g/h. Magnesium sulphate can be used up to a dose of 8 g to abort a fit although diazepam is a more familiar drug to most clinicians and is a very effective anticonvulsant. Most fits are self-limiting and prolonged fitting probably requires a brain scan to rule out other pathology such as an intracerebral bleed.

When oliguria is present, care must be taken, as excretion of magnesium sulphate is predominately renal. Toxicity can be detected by absence of the patella reflexes (but not after regional blockade) and ultimately respiratory arrest and muscle paralysis can occur, as well as cardiac arrest.

In the event of an eclamptic fit, it is crucial that the mother is stabilized before delivery. A general

Antihypertensive therapy

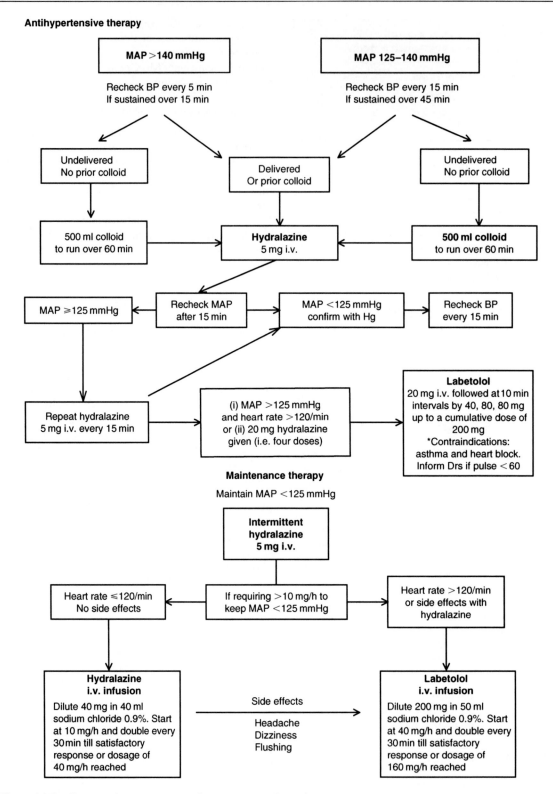

Figure 14.2 Hypertensive management for severe pre-eclampsia.

Fluid regime

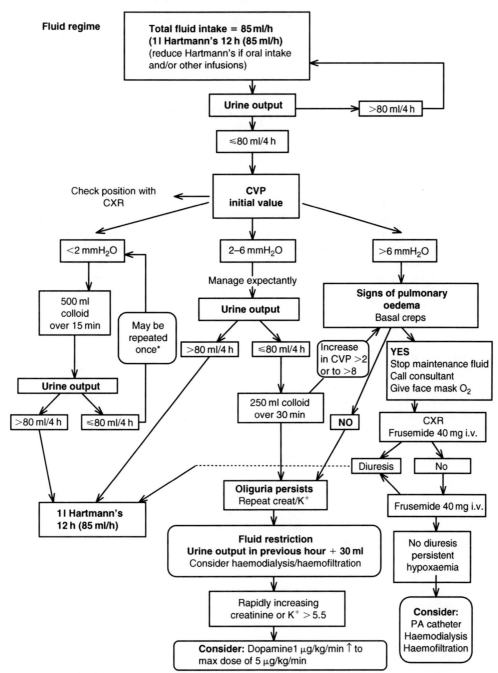

Figure 14.3   Fluid management for severe pre-eclampsia.

*Do not forget

Patients with marked **hypovolaemia** due to haemorrhage (>500 ml), underestimated blood loss at APH/CS, intravascular haemolysis or DIC are obvious exceptions. They will often be thirsty.

They need: **CVP monitoring**
             Blood ± blood products

anaesthetic can be dangerous as intubation can cause severe hypertension.

EFFECTS OF INTUBATION ON BLOOD PRESSURE

As intracranial haemorrhage is a common cause of death in the pre-eclamptic woman, stable systemic arterial and intracranial pressures are desirable. Large fluctuations in systemic and pulmonary arterial pressure can occur in association with endotracheal intubation, and are exaggerated in the pre-eclamptic state. A number of therapeutic measures have been described to ameliorate this response including opioids, vasodilators, anaesthetic agents and beta adrenoreceptor antagonists. However magnesium itself is effective at reducing the pressor response to intubation, without causing profound hypotension or harming the fetus.[38] However, where possible regional blockade should be used in preference to general anaesthesia.

ANAESTHETIC ISSUES

Regional blockade is the recommended method of analgesia for labour and anaesthesia for operative deliveries, as long as coagulopathy has been ruled out. If the platelet count is above 100 and the levels have been stable, most obstetric anaesthetists would insert a regional block. If the platelet count is below 100 a coagulation screen is necessary senior obstetric anaesthetic and haematological advice should be sought under these circumstances. Care must be taken to avoid arterial hypotension in view of the vasoconstriction and reduced intravascular volume. Hypotension following postpartum haemorrhage is relatively common and may be very severe. In view of the reduced intravascular volume, great care must be taken in managing haemorrhage in pre-eclamptic woman. A very low threshold for central invasive monitoring is wise in the sick pre-eclamptic woman who requires a Caesarean section.

Following delivery, intensive monitoring is required for up to 48 h, as a third of eclamptic fits occur during this time.[4] Although eclampsia is reported beyond this time, it is not likely to be associated with serious morbidity. Blood pressure is frequently at its highest 3–4 days after delivery and therefore it is usual to continue antihypertensive therapy until checked by the GP at 6 weeks.

If methyldopa has been used antenatally, it should be changed to a less depressive drug when there are no longer fetal considerations. Of the women who die from eclampsia, the vast majority are preterm and death is approximately 10 times more likely to occur in a multiparous woman. Multiparas are more likely to have an underlying cause for the disease process.

CONCLUSION

Pre-eclampsia remains a major cause of maternal and fetal morbidity and mortality throughout the world. Careful management, with a good understanding of the disease process is crucial in preventing serious morbidity. An improved understanding of the aetiology and pathophysiology is likely to lead to the development of therapeutic options that reduce the impact of this disease in the future. Delivery is currently the only definitive treatment but the careful management of the blood pressure and fluid balance are essential to maintain maternal well-being.

REFERENCES

1. Higgins JR, Walshe JJ, Halligan A, O'Brien E, Conroy R, Darling MR. Can 24-hour ambulatory blood pressure measurement predict the development of hypertension in primigravidae? *Br J Obstet Gynaecol* 1997; **104**: 356–362.

2. CEMD: Department of Health. *Why mothers die? Report on confidential enquiries into maternal deaths in the United Kingdom 1997–1999.* London: 2001.

3. Douglas KA, Redman CWG. Eclampsia in the United Kingdom. *Br Med J* 1994; **309**: 1395–1400.

4. Kaunitz AM, Hughes JM, Grimes DA, Smith JC, Rochat RW, Kafrissen ME. Causes of maternity mortality in the United States. *Obstet Gynecol* 1985; **65**: 605–612.

5. Chua S, Redman CW. Prognosis of pre-eclampsia complicated by 5 g or more of proteinuria in 24 hours. *Eur J Obstet Gynaecol Reprod Biol* 1992; **43**: 9–12.

6. Ales KL, Frayer W, Hawks G, Auld PM, Druzin ML. Development and validation of a multivariate predictor of mortality in very low birth weight. *J Clin Epidemiol* 1988; **41**: 1095–1103.

7. Whitfield MF, Grunau RVE, Holsti L. Extremely premature (<or=to 800 g) schoolchildren: multiple areas of hidden disability. *Arch Dis Child Fetal Neonat* 1997; **77**: 85F–90F.

8. Freidman EA, Neff RK. Pregnancy outcome is related to hypertension, oedema and proteinuria. In: Churchill D, Beevers DG (eds) *Hypertension in pregnancy.* London: BMJ Books, 1996.

9. Davey DA, MacGillivray I. The classification and definition of the hypertensive disorders of pregnancy. *Am J Obstet Gynecol* 1988; **158**: 892–898.

10. Chappell LC, Poulton L, Halligan A, Shennan AH. Lack of consistency in research papers over the definition of pre-eclampsia. *Br J Obstet Gynaecol* 1999; **106**: 983–985.

11. Pijnenborg R. Trophoblast invasion. *Reprod Med Rev* 1994; **3**: 53–73.

12. Graham CH, Postovit LM, Park H, Canning MT, Fitzpatrick TE. Adriana and Luisa Castellucci award lecture 1999: role of oxygen in the regulation of trophoblast gene expression and invasion. *Placenta* 2000; **21**: 443–450.

13. Hubel CA. Oxidative stress in the pathogenesis of pre-eclampsia. *Proc Soc Exp Biol Med* 1999; **222**: 222–235.

14. Hubel CA, McLaughlin MK, Evans RW, Hauth BA, Sims CJ, Roberts JM. Fasting serum triglycerides, free fatty acids, and malondialdehyde are increased in pre-eclampsia, are positively correlated, and decrease within 48 hours post partum. *Am J Obstet Gynecol* 1996; **174**: 975–982.

15. Lie RT, Rasmussen S, Brunborg H, Gjessing HK, Lie-Nielsen E, Irgens LM. Fetal and maternal contributions to risk of pre-eclampsia: population based study. *Br Med J* 1998; **316**: 1343–1347.

16. Strickland DM, Guzick DS, Cox K, Gant NF, Rosenfeld CR. The relationship between abortion in the first pregnancy and development of pregnancy-induced hypertension in the subsequent pregnancy. *Am J Obstet Gynecol* 1986; **154**: 146–148.

17. Robillard PY, Dekker GA, Hulsey TC. Revisiting the epidemiological standard of pre-eclampsia: primigravidity or primipaternity? *Eur J Obstet Gynecol Reprod Biol* 1999; **84**: 37–41.

18. Klonoff-Cohen HS, Savitz DA, Cefalo RC, McCann MF. An epidemiologic study of contraception and pre-eclampsia. *JAMA* 1989; **262**: 3141–3147.

19. Robillard PY, Hulsey TC, Perianin J, Janky E, Miri EH, Papiernik E. Association of pregnancy-induced hypertension with duration of sexual cohabitation before conception. *Lancet* 1994; **344**: 973–975.

20. Koelman CA, Coumans AB, Nijman HW, Doxiadis II, Dekker GA, Claas FH. Correlation between oral sex and a low incidence of pre-eclampsia: a role for soluble HLA in seminal fluid? *J Reprod Immunol* 2000; **46**: 155–166.

21. Sellmann AH. Blood pressure, edema and proteinuria in pregnancy. Edema-plus-proteinuria relationships. *Prog Clin Biol Res* 1976; **7**: 193–214.

22. Need JA, Bell B, Meffin E, Jones WR. Pre-eclampsia in pregnancies from donor insemination. *J Reprod Immunol* 1983; **5**: 329–338.

23. Rey E, Couturier A. The prognosis of pregnancy in women with chronic hypertension. *Am J Obstet Gynecol* 1994; **171**: 410–416.

24. McCowan LM, Buist RG, North RA, Gamble G. Perinatal morbidity in chronic hypertension. *Br J Obstet Gynaecol* 1996; **103**: 123–129.

25. Sibai BM. Risk factors, pregnancy complications, and prevention of hypertensive disorders in women with pregravid diabetes mellitus. *J Mat Fetal Med* 2000; **9**: 62–65.

26. Stone JL, Lockwood CJ, Berkowitz GS, Alvarez M, Lapinski R, Berkowitz RL. Risk factors for severe pre-eclampsia. *Obstet Gynecol* 1994; **83**: 357–361.

27. Conde-Agudelo A, Belizan JM. Risk factors for pre-eclampsia in a large cohort of Latin American and Caribbean women. *Br J Obstet Gynaecol* 2000; **107**: 75–83.

28. Lockshin MD. Pregnancy loss in the antiphospholipid syndrome. *Thromb Haem* 1999; **82**: 641–648.

29. Mires GJ, Williams FL, Leslie J, Howie PW. Assessment of uterine arterial notching as a screening test for adverse pregnancy outcome. *Am J Obstet Gynecol* 1998; **179**: 1317–1323.

30. Kyle PM, Buckley D, Kissane J, de Swiet M, Redman CW. The angiotensin sensitivity test and low-dose aspirin are ineffective methods to predict and prevent hypertensive disorders in nulliparous pregnancy. *Am J Obstet Gynecol* 1995; **173**: 865–872.

31. Zhang ZJ, Cheng WW, Yang YM. Low-dose of processed rhubarb in preventing pregnancy induced hypertension. *Zhonghua Fu Chan Ke Za Zhi* 1994; **29**: 463–464.

32. Duley L, Henderson-Smart D, Knight M, King J. Antiplatelet drugs for prevention of pre-eclampsia and its consequences: systematic review. *Br Med J* 2001; **322**: 329–333.

33. Chappell LC, Seed PT, Briley AL, Kelly FJ, Lee R, Hunt BJ, Parmar K, Bewley SJ, Shennan AH, Steer PJ, Poston L. Prevention of pre-eclampsia by antioxidants: a randomized trial of vitamins C and E in women at increased risk of pre-eclampsia. *Lancet* 1999; **354**: 810–816.

34. Shennan A, Gupta M, Halligan A, Taylor DJ, de Swiet M. Lack of reproducibility in pregnancy of Korotkoff phase IV as measured by mercury sphygmomanometry. *Lancet* 1996; **347**: 139–142.

35. Brown MA, Buddle ML, Farrell T, Davis G, Jones M. Randomised trial of management of hypertensive pregnancies by Korotkoff phase IV or phase V. *Lancet* 1998; **352**: 777–781.

36. Von Dadelszen P, Ornstein MP, Bull SB, Logan AG, Koren G, Magee LA. Fall in mean arterial pressure and fetal growth restriction in pregnancy hypertension: a meta-analysis. *Lancet* 2000; **355**: 87–92.

37. Penny JA, Shennan AH, Halligan AW, Taylor DJ, de Swiet M, Anthony J. Blood pressure measurement in severe pre-eclampsia. *Lancet* 1997; **349**: 1518.

38. Allen RW, James MF, Uys PC et al. Attenuation of the pressor response to tracheal intubation in hypertensive proteinuric pregnant patients by lignocaine, alfentanil and magnesium sulphate. *Br J Anaesth* 1991; **66**: 216–223.

15

INTENSIVE AND HIGH DEPENDENCY CARE OF THE OBSTETRIC PATIENT

Girish R. Dhond & Saxon A. Ridley

INTRODUCTION

The majority of women of child-bearing age are healthy and pregnancy is a natural physiological process that proceeds without complication. Occasionally, the pregnant patient may develop critical illness as a result of either her pregnancy or a coincidental medical or surgical problem, which may be aggravated by the physiological changes of pregnancy. Thus the critically ill pregnant patient presents a unique challenge to the intensivist in terms of altered maternal physiology, diseases specific to pregnancy and the presence of a fetus.

Whilst the general principles of diagnoses and management are similar to those for other seriously ill patients, there are epidemiological, physiological and therapeutic issues to be addressed in the pregnant patient. This chapter initially considers the epidemiology of obstetric admissions to intensive care. There follows a discussion on the general principles of intensive care monitoring and management with reference to the pregnant patient. In the remainder of the chapter, a number of the circulatory and respiratory disorders that most commonly require intensive care are reviewed.

OBSTETRIC MORTALITY AND MORBIDITY

The 1997–1999 Confidential Enquiries into Maternal Deaths shows a stabilization in maternal mortality overall but an increase in deaths associated with indirect causes.[1] The major causes of death remain thrombosis and thromboembolism, hypertensive disorders of pregnancy and haemorrhage. One of the report's concerns relate to the level of care provided to the obstetric patient when clinical problems arose; care was judged to have been substandard in 60% of the deaths and this was commonest in hypertensive disorders (80%) and massive haemorrhage (71%). Two of the three anaesthetic deaths occurred due to problems on the intensive care unit and the report also drew attention to deficiencies in the provision of intensive care facilities for obstetric patients with delayed admission to intensive care contributing to maternal death in some cases.

While maternal death is a vital index in the assessment of obstetric care, it does not address the issue of maternal morbidity. A rational approach would be to consider rates of admission of obstetric patients to intensive care, indications for admission, severity of illness at time of admission and outcome, with particular reference to residual disability. Intensive care

unit (ICU) admission may become necessary for managing obstetric complications in approximately 0.1–0.9% of all pregnancies.[2–4] The major indications for admission include hypertensive disorders of pregnancy, acute respiratory failure and sepsis (Table 15.1).[5] Although the overall maternal mortality rate is stable, the age adjusted mortality rate for obstetric patients admitted to ICU remains high at 4.5–20%.[5–7] A number of recent studies have characterized obstetric admissions in terms of ICU utilization rates, management and outcome.[3–8] In terms of outcome prediction, the APACHE scoring system is a commonly used measure of severity of illness in the ICU, but has not been validated for use in the obstetric population. In pregnant patients, the normal values for some of the measured physiological variables are altered (e.g. heart rate, respiratory rate and haematocrit). Furthermore, certain variables likely to be of predictive value in the pregnant patient are not included in the APACHE score (e.g. platelet count and liver function tests). The reliability of APACHE scores as a predictor of illness severity in pregnancy remains controversial and lower than predicted, higher than predicted and appropriate mortality rates have all been reported.[8,9]

Failure to provide optimum care has repeatedly been shown to be associated with increased mortality and morbidity in obstetric patients.[10] The requirement for or availability of ICU beds worldwide has been variously reported as between 1 and 9 beds per 1000 deliveries.[6] It is clear that intensive care facilities must be readily available for obstetric patients in the same hospital as the maternity unit and, in the opinion of the authors, such patients should be managed on

Table 15.1	Main indications for obstetric admission to ICU
Condition	Percent of total
Hypertensive disorders	32
Massive haemorrhage	7.3
Medical problems	
Cardiac	30.3
Pulmonary	6.6
Renal	4.9
Sepsis	4.2
Gastrointestinal	3.1
Endocrine	2.8
Central nervous system	2.4
Other	3.8

Source: Mabie et al[5] with permission.

a general ICU following the same basic tenets of supportive care as for other critically ill patients.

There is emerging evidence that early provision of intensive care for the obstetric patient can minimize progression to multiple organ failure and reduce mortality and morbidity.[10] It behoves all the relevant specialists to liaise effectively so that an optimum level of care is achieved for these patients when clinical problems arise.

FETAL CONSIDERATIONS

The management of the critically ill mother requires an understanding of the normal mechanisms controlling fetal oxygenation. Oxygen delivery to the placenta and fetus is dependent on maternal arterial oxygen content and uterine blood flow. The anaemia of pregnancy, which reduces arterial oxygen content by 20–25%, renders the mother more dependent on cardiac output to maintain fetal oxygen delivery. Under normal circumstances the uterine vasculature may be maximally dilated and therefore poorly able to adapt to a fall in maternal cardiac output. This may be particularly dangerous for the fetus if superimposed upon maternal hypoxaemia.

Effects of ICU management on fetal well-being should be considered in any critically ill obstetric patient. Depending on gestational age, delivery of the baby may be the most appropriate solution. Failing this, uteroplacental oxygen delivery must be maximized. Simple manoeuvres such as supplemental oxygen and tilting the patient to the left lateral position should not be overlooked. Increasing maternal oxygen carrying capacity by transfusion, enhancing cardiac output and oxygenation can often serve to improve fetal oxygen delivery.

GENERAL PRINCIPLES OF ICU MANAGEMENT

Pregnancy may not always be obvious when a critically ill woman presents to the ICU and, for optimal management, it is incumbent on the intensivist to be vigilant and to confirm or exclude this diagnosis when suspected. The following section will consider the general principles of respiratory support, haemodynamic monitoring, drug therapy, nutrition and cardiopulmonary resuscitation as they apply to the pregnant patient receiving intensive care.

RESPIRATORY SUPPORT

The management of the pregnant patient with respiratory failure is similar to that of the non-pregnant patient with certain additional considerations. For example, in addition to maternal indications for oxygen, a hypoxic fetus may benefit from maternal oxygen administration in the presence of normal maternal cardiorespiratory status. Indeed maternal oxygen administration has been demonstrated to improve some of the indices of fetal well-being.[13]

Indications for intubation and ventilation in pregnancy are essentially the same as for the non-pregnant patient, namely airway protection, pulmonary toilet, management of severe hypoxia or ventilatory failure as manifest by significant non-compensated respiratory acidosis. Mucosal hyperaemia of the upper respiratory tract results in narrowed and friable airways so rendering intubation more hazardous. Nasotracheal intubation is best avoided and endotracheal intubation should be undertaken carefully, possibly using a smaller endotracheal tube than in the non-pregnant patient. The increased oxygen consumption and decreased FRC in pregnancy predisposes the patient to rapid arterial desaturation during periods of apnoea;[11,12] preoxygenation with 100% oxygen is mandatory.

Data concerning mechanical ventilation in pregnancy are derived principally from experience with anaesthetic ventilation for operative delivery and there is little information concerning prolonged ventilation of the pregnant patient. In the absence of metabolic dysfunction, it is appropriate to aim for P_aCO_2 of 4 kPa to mimic the mild respiratory alkalosis of pregnancy. Greater hyperventilation causing hypocapnia and alkalosis may decrease uteroplacental blood flow and fetal oxygenation. In the absence of pulmonary pathology, mild hypocapnia may be achieved with tidal volumes in the range of 10 ml/kg and respiratory rates of 15–18 breaths/min.

The current trends in mechanical ventilation of avoiding high ventilatory pressures (and hence alveolar over-distention) by controlled hypoventilation and permissive hypercapnia have not yet been fully evaluated in pregnancy and are probably best avoided if possible. In terms of the degree of permissible hypercapnia, a maternal P_aCO_2 of up to 8 kPa with adequate supplemental inspired oxygen does not appear to adversely affect the fetus and may actually improve fetal oxygenation.[14] In the event of a diffuse lung pathology, sufficient positive end-expiratory pressure (PEEP) should be added to correct hypoxaemia with inspired oxygen fractions initially of less than 0.5.

Little data exists concerning the use of non-invasive ventilation in acute respiratory failure during pregnancy. However, potential hazards include exacerbation of the upper airway oedema and the risk of oesophageal reflux and aspiration. Obstetric patients, like all young previously fit patients, tend to compensate until there is severe physiological derangement; at this stage, conventional ventilation is the preferred initial course of therapy. The use of a variety of unconventional modes of respiratory support in pregnant patients including extracorporeal membrane oxygenation,[15] extracorporeal carbon dioxide removal,[16] high-frequency jet ventilation and the use of an intracaval oxygenator[17] have been described in case reports but clinical experience is limited.

HAEMODYNAMIC MONITORING

Pregnancy does not represent a contraindication to invasive monitoring and, in general, the indications are similar to those in the non-obstetric patient. Most of the data on invasive monitoring in obstetric patients is derived from preeclamptic women; it is of value in a number of conditions including cardiac disease, sepsis, acute lung injury and amniotic fluid embolism. Invasive monitoring is particularly valuable during labour and delivery when marked fluctuations in haemodynamics occur. Despite the normally elevated cardiac output and reduced systemic vascular resistance during pregnancy, filling pressures are usually unchanged from non-pregnant values and left ventricular function is well preserved even in the presence of significant pre-eclampsia. Although guidelines have been suggested for the use of pulmonary artery catheters in obstetrics (Table 15.2), controversy exists as to whether clinical outcome is improved. When used judiciously, invasive monitoring provides additional information in the management of complex

---

Table 15.2   Indications for pulmonary artery catheterization

Pre-eclampsia
   Congestive heart failure
   Oliguria despite adequate central
     venous pressure
   Postpartum cardiac failure
   Hypertension unresponsive to
     conventional therapy
Amniotic fluid embolism
Cardiac disease
   Congenital
   Valvular
   Ischaemia/infarction
   Postpartum cardiomyopathy
Sepsis
Tocolytic-induced pulmonary oedema

---

haemodynamic disturbances. However, no study in pregnant patients has demonstrated a significant outcome benefit of invasive monitoring and therefore recommendations for its use must remain qualified.

DRUG THERAPY

The pregnant woman represents two potential targets for drug therapy and consideration must be given to the pharmacological and teratogenic effects on the fetus. The major risk period for teratogenesis is in the first 10 weeks of gestation. During the second and third trimesters drugs may affect the growth and functional development of the fetus or have toxic effects on fetal tissues.

Drugs given shortly before term or during labour may have adverse effects on labour or on the neonate after delivery. Risk status may be assigned to a drug based on the level of risk it poses to the fetus. The British National Formulary contains a list of drugs to be avoided or used with caution in pregnancy,[18] although absence of a drug from the list does not imply safety. In the United States, drugs may be classified according to safe use in pregnancy and receive 'use-in-pregnancy' ratings. The following section discusses some of the commonly used drugs in ICU.

Inotropes

Vasoactive drugs are frequently employed in the treatment of maternal hypotension but have a potentially hazardous effect on the uteroplacental circulation. The commonly used catecholamines, including dobutamine, norepinephrine and epinephrine, have been shown to adversely affect uterine blood flow in animal studies despite favourable maternal haemodynamic responses.[19,20] Conflicting results concerning dopamine usage have been reported.[21,22] Ephedrine is routinely used to prevent or treat maternal hypotension following spinal anaesthesia; use of this agent has been shown to increase maternal blood pressure while preserving uterine blood flow and is associated with an improvement in fetal hypoxia and acidosis.[23] Recently both ephedrine and phenylephrine have been shown to be safe and effective in treating maternal hypotension following spinal anaesthesia without adversely affecting neonatal outcome.[24] In animal studies, the phosphodiesterase III inhibitor, amrinone, did not significantly alter uterine blood flow while acting as an ino-dilator.[21]

Antihypertensive drugs

Vasodilator agents, used in the treatment of pregnancy-induced hypertension, may produce excessive hypotension compromising uteroplacental perfusion. Hydralazine is the most widely used agent and has a good record of safety and efficacy in pregnancy.[25] Labetalol, a valuable alternative, combines alpha- and beta-adrenoreceptor blocking activity and has been shown to effectively control maternal blood pressure without adversely affecting uterine blood flow.[26] Methyldopa has a long history of effective use for the treatment of essential hypertension in pregnancy and a good record with respect to fetal and neonatal safety.[27]

The use of nifedipine, a calcium-channel blocking agent, during pregnancy remains controversial. Animal studies demonstrate that the hypotensive effect of nifedipine may result in a decrease in uterine blood flow with fetal hypoxaemia and acidosis.[28] Experience with nifedipine in human pregnancy is limited; however, severe adverse reactions have been reported when nifedipine was used in combination with intravenous magnesium sulphate resulting in severe hypotension and neuromuscular blockade due to the synergistic actions of these two agents.[29,30] Sodium nitroprusside is effective in acute hypertensive crises in pregnancy, but risks of fetal cyanide toxicity imposes a relative contraindication and restricts its use to short term peripartum management of severe hypertensive episodes.[31] Angiotensin-converting enzyme inhibitors are contraindicated in pregnancy due to risk of fetal renal dysfunction. There are now more than 30 cases reported of perinatal renal failure, many of which have been fatal, following *in utero* exposure to captopril or enalapril.[32]

Antiarrhythmic agents

Pregnancy is associated with an increased incidence of both supraventricular and ventricular arrhythmias, which though well tolerated under normal circumstances, may be life-threatening in the setting of critical illness.

The use of intravenous adenosine for the treatment of supraventricular arrhythmias during pregnancy has been reported.[33] Because of its mode of action; slowing conduction through the AV node, heart block or transient asystole may occur. It is likely that adenosine crosses the placenta, but no adverse fetal effects have been identified.[33] Verapamil, a calcium-channel blocking agent, terminates paroxysmal supraventricular tachycardia and may be used in pregnancy. It crosses the placenta and has been used for control of fetal arrhythmias.[34]

Ventricular tachyarrhythmias in pregnancy are often responsive to beta-adrenoceptor blockade or to type I antiarrhythmic drugs. Nevertheless cardioversion or synchronous defibrillation should not be withheld during pregnancy if clinically indicated. Quinidine, a type I antiarrhythmic agent, controls both supraventricular and ventricular arrhythmias. However transplacental passage of quinidine has been shown and it may cause fetal thrombocytopaenia and damage to the developing eighth cranial nerve.[35] Procainamide appears to be a relatively safe antiarrhythmic agent for use in pregnancy as no adverse fetal effects have been reported to date.[36] Disopyramide, whilst better tolerated than quinidine, has a proarrhythmic activity and has been reported to increase uterine contractions.[37] Lidocaine, an agent administered intravenously to terminate ventricular arrhythmias, has been found to be safe and effective in the pregnant patient. It does cross the placenta and high maternal plasma levels may be associated with neonatal depression.[35] Amiodarone has been used during pregnancy for maternal and fetal arrhythmias[38] and the drug appears to be well tolerated by both mother and fetus. Its major metabolite, desethylamiodarone, crosses the placenta and raises the potential risk of neonatal hypothyroidism which should be excluded in all new-borns exposed to amiodarone *in utero*.

Drugs for analgesia, sedation and neuromuscular blockade

There is relatively little data on the adverse fetal effects of these groups of drugs; assessment of their effects is complicated by numerous other circumstances that may commonly occur on the ICU. Benzodiazepines cross the placenta, 'midazolam to a lesser extent than diazepam', and may increase the risk of cleft palate when used early in pregnancy. No significant risk of congenital malformation has been associated with opiate analgesics such as morphine, pethidine and fentanyl. Most non-depolarizing neuromuscular blocking agents cross the placenta to a small degree but short term use is not associated with adverse effects on the fetus. The use of any sedative agents near delivery should signal the need for neonatal ventilatory support.

NUTRITION

Nutritional support is vital to the critically ill patient, even more so if they are pregnant. During starvation, maternal body stores are preserved at the expense of the fetus. This may result in intrauterine growth retardation and neurological impairment if the starvation occurs before 26 weeks gestation. Pregnancy increases calorie requirements by approximately 300 kcal/day to 40 kcal/kg/day. In the event of coincidental critical illness, current information suggests that optimal nutritional support may be provided by supplying approximately 80% of estimated energy requirements with approximately 20% of the calories administered as lipids.[39] Protein intake should be augmented by 20–50% to 1.5 g/kg/day in order to meet the demand for maternal and fetal protein synthesis; all protein or amino acid preparations should include glutamine.[40] Due to concerns over macrosomia and other adverse effects of hyperglycaemia, good control of maternal blood glucose levels is important. Most vitamins and trace elements need only modest supplementation but there is an increased need for vitamins (especially A, C and E) and minerals including iron, zinc and magnesium. Serum calcium, phosphate and magnesium levels should be monitored, as these tend to fall in critical illness.

Enteral nutrition is the method of choice and, due to reduced lower oesophageal sphincter tone in pregnancy, nasoduodenal feeding is the preferred route of delivery. However, feeding tube placement may prove difficult as there is no guarantee that the tube will remain in the small bowel. Total parenteral nutrition has been successfully administered to pregnant patients for several months in a variety of disorders including inflammatory bowel disease, oesophageal stricture and malignancy; its use in obstetric patients on the intensive care unit is less well described. Theoretical concerns over the use of lipid emulsions leading to fatty infiltration of the placenta and premature labour have not been supported by clinical studies.

RADIOLOGICAL CONSIDERATIONS

Despite the risk of exposing the fetus to ionizing radiation, radiological procedures are often necessary for the diagnosis and management of the critically ill obstetric patient. A chest radiograph exposes the maternal lungs to approximately 0.5 cGy; techniques such as shielding the abdomen with lead and using a well collimated X-ray beam can reduce fetal exposure to about 0.001 cGy. Significantly more fetal exposure occurs with abdominal and pelvic investigations such as computed tomography, which can deliver between 5 and 10 cGy to the fetus. The potential adverse effects of radiation exposure to the fetus include teratogenicity and oncogenicity; low dose (under 5 cGy) exposure is associated with a slightly increased risk of childhood cancer but does not predispose to congenital developmental abnormalities. It is likely that the risk to the fetus increases with the dose of radiation and therefore every effort should be made to limit this, particularly in the first trimester.

CARDIOPULMONARY RESUSCITATION

Standard ATLS or ACLS protocols for the management of cardiac arrest may require minor modification in the pregnant patient. Fetal monitoring should be removed prior to cardioversion or defibrillation to prevent arcing. Perimortem Caesarean section may be indicated when there is no response to standard resuscitative measures in a pregnancy of greater than 24–26 weeks gestation. In such cases, the likelihood of infant survival without neurological sequelae is greatest when Caesarean section is initiated within 4 min of the cardiac arrest.[40,41] See Chapter 16.

CIRCULATORY DISORDERS OF PREGNANCY

HYPERTENSIVE DISORDERS OF PREGNANCY (see Chapter 14)

Hypertensive disorders of pregnancy are common, affecting more than 10% of pregnant women. In the 1997–1999 UK Confidential Enquiry into Maternal Deaths, hypertensive disorders were the second most common cause of death, accounting for many of those transferred to ICU.[1] Pre-eclampsia is a pregnancy-induced disorder characterized by hypertension, proteinuria and generalized oedema, occurring primarily in primigravidas after the 20 weeks of gestation. Pre-eclampsia is responsible for 20–60% of obstetric admissions to the ICU; the main admission indications for ICU in pre-eclampsia are listed in Table 15.3.

From a critical care perspective, it is an unpredictable disease that can progress rapidly producing life-threatening complications such as DIC, seizures, pulmonary oedema, acute renal failure and liver dysfunction. The initial examination of the pre-eclamptic patient should assess the severity of the disease and the presence of complications with particular emphasis

Table 15.3	Indications for ICU admission in preeclampsia

Invasive haemodynamic monitoring
    Hypertensive crisis
Mechanical ventilation
    Acute respiratory distress syndrome
    Pulmonary oedema
    Aspiration
Airway protection
    Seizures
    Upper airway oedema
Disseminated intravascular coagulation
HELLP syndrome
Acute renal failure

on the cardiorespiratory status, neurological disturbances and laboratory evidence of organ dysfunction (coagulation, renal and hepatic indices). Seizures are the most common neurological complication and herald the syndrome of eclampsia. Cerebral oedema is an uncommon sequelae of pre-eclampsia and is thought to occur secondary to hypoxia or severe hypertension; it may be exacerbated by aggressive fluid administration and is an important cause of mortality in preeclamptic patients.

The definitive treatment of pre-eclampsia is delivery of the baby where feasible and this should be expedited if severe pre-eclampsia develops. However, during early pregnancy or when unstable, preeclamptic patients pose greater difficulties. Treatment is essentially supportive, including control of blood pressure and seizures, fluid management and epidural anaesthesia.

Eclampsia

Eclampsia occurs in around 1 in 2000 deliveries in developed countries and as frequently as 1 in 700 in developing countries. The cause of eclamptic seizures is multifactorial and related to elements of cerebral vasospasm, ischaemia and oedema. Management includes anticonvulsants for control of the seizures, treatment of the underlying preeclamptic condition and prompt delivery of the baby. Magnesium sulphate is the agent of choice, being more effective, in preventing the recurrence of seizures in eclampsia than either diazepam or phenytoin. Magnesium therapy was associated with fewer ICU admissions and a lower incidence of pneumonia.[42] Magnesium sulphate is usually given as an intravenous loading dose of 2–4 g over 10–20 min followed by an infusion of 1 g/h. The infusion is usually continued for 12–24 h postpartum. Respiratory depression due to respiratory muscle weakness and cardiac conduction defects are recognized complications and may be preceded by loss of patellar reflexes. Thus, use of magnesium sulphate should be accompanied by appropriate monitoring of respiratory function and reflexes particularly in cases of renal dysfunction.

Pulmonary oedema

Pulmonary oedema is a rare complication occurring in 2.9% of severely preeclamptic patients. It presents most commonly in the postpartum period and may be associated with aggressive fluid administration in relatively hypovolaemic patients. Such patients may also have a decreased colloid osmotic pressure, which promotes egress of fluid into the alveoli. Management

is supportive involving fluid restriction, oxygen and diuretic therapy and may be guided by invasive haemodynamic monitoring such as pulmonary artery catheterization. There is a subgroup of chronically hypertensive, obese women who readily develop pulmonary oedema associated with pre-eclampsia. They exhibit evidence of left ventricular dysfunction with elevated filling pressures; acute pulmonary oedema is most frequently precipitated by the volume overload of pregnancy and the haemodynamic stress of labour.[43]

Renal dysfunction

Intravascular volume depletion and generalized arterial vasospasm is universal in pre-eclampsia and commonly results in oliguria; fortunately it only rarely proceeds to frank renal failure. Fluid status may be difficult to assess accurately in preeclamptic patients who may have generalized oedema and expansion of the interstitial space in the face of a constricted intravascular compartment. This paradox is, in part, due to an increase in vascular permeability and a fall in plasma colloid osmotic pressure. Patients with oliguria unresponsive to a 500 ml intravenous crystalloid challenge or a central venous pressure that does not appear to correlate to degree of hypovolaemia may benefit from pulmonary artery catheterization to guide fluid and drug therapy. Fortunately, the acute renal dysfunction associated with pre-eclampsia only rarely results in residual impairment of function.

HELLP syndrome

Between 4% and 20% of patients with severe pre-eclampsia may develop the HELLP syndrome characterized by microangiopathic haemolytic anaemia, elevated liver enzymes and low platelets. The syndrome is associated with a poor outcome. Maternal and perinatal mortality rates of 24% and 33% respectively have been reported.[44] Approximately 30% of cases of HELLP syndrome present in the postpartum period.

The definitive management of the HELLP syndrome is primarily obstetric with prompt delivery of the fetus, which may require blood product support. Regional anaesthesia is contraindicated in the presence of thrombocytopaenia. Supportive ICU management of HELLP syndrome alone is associated with a poor outcome despite a number of novel strategies including antiplatelet agents, thromboxane synthetase inhibition, steroids and plasmapheresis.

The maternal complications of HELLP syndrome include acute renal failure, acute respiratory distress syndrome and haemorrhage. Profound hypoglycaemia has been reported and blood glucose should be closely monitored. Hepatic haemorrhage occurs in 2% of cases and may progress to catastrophic hepatic rupture. Thus all patients with HELLP should have their abdomen assessed clinically and, if necessary, by ultrasound.

OBSTETRIC HAEMORRHAGE

Obstetric haemorrhage can be massive and devastating and is a leading cause of maternal mortality despite modern improvements in obstetric practice and transfusion services. Failure to appreciate severity of bleeding in cases where haemorrhage is concealed may be a contributory factor; in cases of placental abruption leading to fetal death, blood loss averages 2–3 l but can exceed 5 l and yet still remained concealed within the uterus.

The most common causes of haemorrhagic shock in pregnancy are listed in Table 15.4. Most significant antepartum haemorrhage is due to either placental abruption (premature separation of a normally implanted placenta) or placenta praevia (disruption of an abnormally sited placenta). Placental abruption occurs in 1/77 to 1/250 pregnancies, is usually associated with hypertension and multiparity and often presents with uterine irritability and pain. Placenta praevia occurs in 1/200 pregnancies with an increased incidence in multiparous, older patients. It is frequently associated with massive haemorrhage either during labour as the cervix dilates, or postpartum, due to ineffective contraction of the lower uterine segment. Most obstetric haemorrhage occurs postpartum and is usually due to uterine atony following placental separation, retention of placental fragments and operative delivery. Maternal mortality, usually from the haemorrhage itself, may be up to 5%, while fetal mortality is even higher. Maternal complications include DIC and acute renal failure.

Management of severe obstetric haemorrhage comprises both initial resuscitative measures and specific obstetric interventions to ameliorate the cause. Establishing good venous access, rapid volume replacement, supplemental oxygen and left lateral positioning are essential prerequisites to control of bleeding. Obstetric haemorrhage is one setting in which initial resuscitation may require the use of unmatched type-specific blood until more complete crossmatching has been achieved. Pre-existing consumptive coagulopathy should be excluded and a dilutional coagulopathy anticipated and so managed with appropriate blood product support (e.g. fresh frozen plasma, cryoprecipitate, and platelet concentrates). In addition to monitoring vital signs, central venous pressure monitoring may be valuable but should not delay initial resuscitation. The antecubital site may be preferred in the presence of significant coagulopathy as iatrogenic haemorrhage may be more easily controlled.

TRAUMA

Death from road traffic accidents is a leading cause of non-obstetric maternal mortality.[45,46] While trauma during pregnancy does not carry a higher mortality rate than in the non-pregnant woman,[46] there may be a significant impact on the outcome of the pregnancy, particularly if there is disruption of the maternal pelvis. Fetal demise is related to severity of maternal injury and haemodynamic compromise as well as to direct fetoplacental injury.[47] The gravid uterus renders the pregnant woman susceptible to unique injuries including amniotic membrane rupture, uterine rupture, premature labour and direct fetal trauma. As pregnancy progresses the uterus becomes increasingly vulnerable to trauma and the patient is at particular risk of haemorrhage as blood flow to the pelvis is increased. A series reported placental abruption and uterine rupture as the most serious sequelae of blunt abdominal trauma in late pregnancy.[48] Cephalad displacement of abdominal contents by the uterus increases the risk of visceral injury following penetrating trauma of the abdomen. The bladder becomes a target for injury after the 12th week of gestation due to its intra-abdominal position.

The physiological changes of pregnancy may make accurate assessment of the patient more difficult; the increased blood volume of pregnancy tends to delay signs of hypovolaemia until blood loss is very severe. Lesser degrees of hypovolaemia may induce vasoconstriction that maintains perfusion to maternal vital organ at the expense of uteroplacental blood flow. Signs of fetal distress are a sinister, if late, marker of significant maternal haemodynamic compromise and often herald impending catastrophe. Passive

Table 15.4 Main causes of massive haemorrhage in pregnancy	
Early	Late (third trimester)
Trauma	Trauma
Ectopic pregnancy	Placenta praevia
Abortion	Placental abruption
Disseminated intravascular coagulation	Disseminated intravascular coagulation
Hydatidiform mole	Uterine rupture

stretching of the peritoneum can decrease peritoneal sensitivity so diminishing signs of tenderness and guarding.

Initial management follows the established protocols of airway management, oxygenation and volume replacement. If necessary, emergency intubation should be performed by a skilled operator because of the increased risk of aspiration during later pregnancy. Once cervical spine injury has been excluded, the woman should be nursed in the left lateral tilt position. The diagnosis of pelvic or abdominal injuries may be aided by ultrasound, computed tomography, (bearing in mind fetal radiation exposure), and peritoneal lavage; the latter procedure may be safely and effectively performed under direct vision via mini-laparatomy to avoid the uterus.

Obstetric opinion should be sought early and, in addition to formal examination of uterus and vagina, fetal monitoring should also be instituted. Cardiotocography may predict placental abruption when used in trauma patients beyond 20 weeks gestation. Fetomaternal haemorrhage may be identified by the Kleihauer–Betke test. This involves mixing a sample of maternal blood with a specific elutant which selectively causes lysis of the maternal red blood cells so that an accurate assessment of fetal transfusion to the mother can be made. Anti-D immune globulin must be administered to the Rhesus-negative woman in a dose that depends on gestational age and degree of fetomaternal haemorrhage. Close obstetric follow-up is essential and Caesarean section should be considered in situations of fetal distress and in states of refractory maternal shock.

SEPTIC SHOCK

Infection is an important cause of maternal mortality, accounting for approximately 15% of maternal deaths.[49] Pregnant patients may have a decreased cell-mediated immunity and a susceptibility to the systemic effects of endotoxaemia has been reported in animal studies.[50] Septic shock occurs most commonly peripartum and following abortions. It often follows chorioamnionitis, postpartum endometritis, septic abortion and urinary tract infection. There is an association with operative delivery, prolonged rupture of membranes, retained products of conception and prior instrumentation of the genito-urinary tract. Although Gram-negative coliforms are the most frequent causative organisms, aerobic and anaerobic streptococci, bacteroides and clostridia have been implicated.

The physiological changes of pregnancy may confound the presentation and alter the course of septic shock. The management of sepsis in the obstetric setting follows the general principles of care of the septic patient. Prompt volume expansion to optimize cardiac output and tissue oxygen delivery in conjunction with invasive haemodynamic monitoring to guide inotropic therapy is indicated. Empirical antibiotic regimes should provide broad Gram negative, Gram positive and anaerobic cover for what is typically a polymicrobial infection. Commonly used combinations include ampicillin, gentamicin and clindamycin; ampicillin-sulbactam; or cefoxitin. A microbiological diagnosis should be sought in guiding therapy and surgical drainage of infected collections is usually indicated. Although high dose steroids have not proven useful in septic shock, novel immunotherapeutic agents such as antilipopolysaccharide immunoglobulin are currently undergoing clinical evaluation and are likely to play a role in the treatment of septic shock in the future.[51]

RESPIRATORY DISORDERS OF PREGNANCY

ACUTE LUNG INJURY

Acute respiratory failure is rarely encountered in association with pregnancy, but with the decline in other causes of maternal death, it is becoming an increasingly important cause of maternal mortality and morbidity. Acute lung injury is frequently the prelude to development of multiorgan failure. The pregnant patient is at risk of acute lung injury from both uniquely obstetric causes and other coincidental pulmonary insults (Table 15.5).[52] The leading obstetric causes include pre-eclampsia, obstetric haemorrhage, amnionitis or endometritis and amniotic fluid embolism.[53]

The management of acute lung injury in pregnancy includes diagnosis, maternal stabilization, investigation and treatment of underlying causes, fetal monitoring and evaluation for delivery. The diagnosis is established, as for non-pregnant individuals, on clinical and radiological grounds. Maternal stabilization and the general principles of respiratory support have been discussed earlier; careful attention must be paid to oxygenation, maintenance of an adequate cardiac output, preservation of coagulation and renal function and optimal nutritional support. Management strategies must consider the cardiorespiratory alterations of pregnancy and the well-being of the fetus.

The dependence of the fetus on maternal cardiac output places important limitations on therapy for acute lung injury during pregnancy. Both diuresis and

Table 15.5   Causes of acute respiratory failure in pregnancy

Specific to pregnancy
  Amniotic fluid embolism
  Pulmonary oedema due to pre-eclampsia
  Pulmonary oedema due to tocolytic therapy
  Peripartum cardiomyopathy
  Acute lung injury due obstetric sepsis
Increased risk during pregnancy
  Venous thromboembolism
  Pulmonary oedema due to pre-existing
    cardiac disease
  Acute lung injury due to massive transfusion
  Aspiration pneumonitis
  Pneumonia due to varicella, listeria
    monocytogenes, coccidioidomycosis
  Venous air embolism
Coincidental
  Trauma
  Drugs and toxins
  Pneumonia

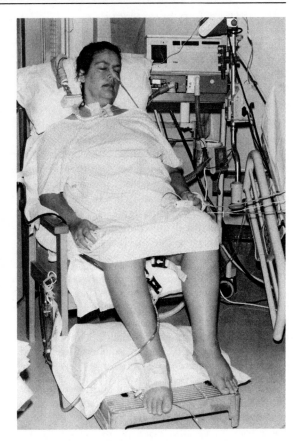

Figure 15.1   Management of acute lung injury may include tracheostomy if the patient requires respiratory support for more than 1–2 weeks. Sitting upright puts the diaphragm at a mechanical advantage, increases the thoracic wall compliance and so decreases the work of breathing. Critical illness and operative intervention frequently lead to long lastinggastrointestinal dysfunction as testifiedby the bile stained nasogastric aspirate. Expansion of the extracellular spaceand peripheral oedema is almost universal in these patients.

PEEP may diminish cardiac output and vasopressor agents may adversely affect uteroplacental perfusion (vide supra). Furthermore, prostaglandin E_1, which has been used in the treatment of acute lung injury,[54] is contraindicated because of its tendency to induce uterine contractions. Non-steroidal anti-inflammatory agents, potentially beneficial early in the course of acute lung injury, must be used with caution in pregnancy because they precipitate premature closure of the fetal ductus arteriosus and decrease fetal urine output.[55] Prolonged or high dose use of non-steroidal anti-inflammatory agents has been reported to reduce fetal survival and predispose to intraventricular haemorrhage in premature neonates.[56]

Efforts must be directed at determining the underlying cause of the acute lung injury and early treatment of surgically remediable causes of infection has been recommended.[57,58] In any pregnant patient with unexplained acute lung injury, amnionitis must be considered and diagnostic amniocentesis for Gram's stain and culture of organisms undertaken.

Finally, delivery of the baby should be considered as a therapeutic option if the maternal condition continues to deteriorate. This is likely to be advantageous for three reasons. Firstly, the fetus is unlikely to prosper in an increasingly hostile environment and abrupt fetal deterioration may accompany progression of acute lung injury in the mother.[59] Secondly, delivery *per se* has been reported to have a positive impact on the maternal condition in this setting,[60] and lastly, delivery of the baby increases the range of treatment options available for the mother in the postpartum period.

Currently it is not possible to reliably predict which patients with acute lung injury during pregnancy will survive; however, it is evident that prolonged ventilation does not necessarily imply excessive maternal mortality[53] (Fig. 15.1). The outcome of acute lung injury during pregnancy appears to be marginally better than in the general population probably reflecting the young age of the group, their proven ability to tolerate pregnancy and the reversibility of many of the predisposing conditions.[61]

AMNIOTIC FLUID EMBOLISM

The reported mortality rate has fallen from over 80% in the 1970s to approximately 60% more recently,[62] although only 15% of survivors are free of significant neurological damage and there is a high rate of fetal demise.

The mechanisms of respiratory and circulatory failure in amniotic fluid embolism remain unclear but appear to involve amniotic fluid entering the circulation through endocervical veins or uterine tears. Although elevation in right sided pressures suggests that acute right ventricular strain is the principal cause of circulatory failure, there is evidence that acute left ventricular dysfunction and an anaphylactic reaction may play a role in pathogenesis of this condition.[63]

The diagnosis of amniotic fluid embolism is frequently a presumptive one; confirmation with the presence of fetal squames in the buffy coat of maternal pulmonary arterial blood does not appear to be reliable.[64] More recent diagnostic approaches include a monoclonal antibody to fetal mucin[65] and measurement of elevated maternal serum zinc coproporphyrin.[66]

Management of amniotic fluid embolism is supportive with resuscitation aimed at ensuring adequate oxygenation, stable circulation and control of bleeding. Pulmonary artery catheterization aids diagnosis and may be used to guide efforts to achieve haemodynamic stability. (See Chapter 17.)

VENOUS THROMBOEMBOLISM

Thromboembolic disease is a complication of 0.3–1.3% of pregnancies. Following massive pulmonary embolism, some patients collapse and die; however, increasing numbers of patients survive long enough to be transferred to ICU.

The pregnant woman is at considerably increased risk of thromboembolism due to a number of factors including the hypercoagulable state in pregnancy, hormonally-mediated venous stasis and local pressure effects of the uterus on the venous system. Although some thromboembolic deaths occur without warning, symptoms of dyspnoea or chest pain may precede the catastrophic event and should not be overlooked. A high index of suspicion should alert the physician to such sentinel symptoms in this at-risk population. Diagnostic techniques include Duplex ultrasound, ventilation-perfusion scanning and pulmonary angiography. Venous doppler assessment is prone to false-positive results due to venous obstruction by the gravid uterus. Ventilation-perfusion scans and angiography

via the brachial route may be performed with minimal fetal radiation exposure.

With respect to anticoagulant therapy, warfarin is usually avoided during pregnancy as it is associated with congenital defects following exposure during the first trimester and central nervous system abnormalities following later in pregnancy. Heparin is the agent of choice in pregnancy. It does not cross the placenta, is readily reversed and has no adverse effects on the fetus. Although pregnancy is a relative contraindication to thrombolytic therapy, this form of treatment has been used successfully, even in late pregnancy.[67] When clinically indicated, a transvenous filter may be sited in the inferior vena cava during pregnancy but there is a risk of dislodgement during labour.[68]

VENOUS AIR EMBOLISM

Venous air embolism, an uncommon complication of pregnancy, may account for 1% of all maternal deaths and is associated with placenta praevia, normal labour, Caesarean delivery and criminal abortion using air. Air is thought to enter the subplacental venous sinuses and pass through the right ventricle to produce obstruction of pulmonary blood flow. Furthermore, leucocyte activation and formation of fibrin microemboli at the air-blood interface may contribute to the clinical picture, which is characterized by sudden profound hypotension followed by respiratory failure. Patients who survive the initial cardiovascular collapse may go on to develop acute respiratory distress syndrome.

Management is essentially supportive and includes measures such as flooding of the surgical site with saline, fluid resuscitation and oxygen administration. Embolus size may be reduced by aspiration of air directly from the right ventricle if a central venous line is in place and, where available, by hyperbaric oxygen therapy.

ASPIRATION OF GASTRIC CONTENTS

Aspiration of gastric contents is a well recognized complication of the peripartum period. Predisposing factors include the increased intra-abdominal pressure, relaxation of lower oesophageal sphincter and delay in gastric emptying during labour. The early injury results from a chemical pneumonitis, the extent of which is related to the acidity and volume of the aspirated material. Diffuse lung injury with development of adult respiratory distress syndrome may develop 24–72 h after the aspiration and may be complicated by a polymicrobial bacterial pneumonia. Prevention of aspiration should be the primary goal.

RESPIRATORY INFECTIONS

Although the spectrum of causative organisms that result in bacterial pneumonia is similar to that in the non-pregnant population, pregnancy is associated with a change in cell-mediated immunity, which may increase susceptibility to a number of infections including varicella, herpes simplex, listeria monocytogenes and coccidioidomycosis. HIV infection may precipitate acute lung injury during pregnancy and an association between pyelonephritis and acute lung injury has been described in pregnancy.[69] One review of pneumonia in pregnancy reported maternal and fetal mortality rates of 4% and 12% respectively.[69] One fifth of the patients required mechanical ventilation and 44% went into premature labour.

Choice of antibiotic therapy should reflect both microbiological diagnosis and concern for fetal toxicity. Although penicillins and cephalosporins are considered safe, tetracycline is contraindicated and sulpha-containing agents should be avoided near term. The early use of acyclovir decreases the otherwise high mortality of disseminated herpes or varicella infection without adverse fetal effects. Amphotericin B has been used successfully in the treatment of coccidioidomycosis in pregnancy.

PULMONARY OEDEMA

There are a number of conditions that may cause pulmonary oedema during pregnancy including pre-eclampsia (*vide supra*), tocolytic therapy and cardiac dysfunction.

Tocolytic-induced pulmonary oedema

Acute pulmonary oedema is a recognized complication of beta-adrenergic agonists, such as ritodrine and terbutaline, which are used to delay onset of labour. The incidence of tocolytic-induced pulmonary oedema is quoted at between 0.3% and 9% of pregnancies. Typically it presents with acute respiratory distress, substernal chest pain in 25% of cases and signs of pulmonary oedema during or within 12 h of discontinuing tocolytic therapy. The pathophysiological mechanisms remain unclear but may involve a combination of catecholamine-induced myocardial dysfunction, fluid overload, increased capillary permeability and the reduced colloid osmotic pressure in pregnancy. The concomitant use of steroids to enhance fetal lung maturation may contribute by promoting fluid retention.

Recognition of the cause, discontinuation of the tocolytic agents and supportive measures such as oxygen supplementation and diuretic therapy are often all that is called for; invasive monitoring is seldom warranted. Failure of pulmonary oedema to resolve within 12–24 h should alert the physician to alternative pathologies.

Cardiogenic pulmonary oedema

The increased cardiovascular demands of pregnancy place the woman with pre-existing cardiac disease, particularly stenotic lesions, at considerable risk of decompensation. Cardiogenic pulmonary oedema is an important differential diagnosis of acute respiratory failure in pregnancy. The prevalence of heart disease in pregnancy ranges from 0.4% to 4%, with a maternal mortality rate of 25–30% in patients classified in class III or IV heart failure (New York Heart Association).[71] Cardiac failure may also occur as a result of hypertensive disease in pregnancy or peripartum cardiomyopathy.

The haemodynamic stress of labour and delivery make this an especially hazardous time for women with cardiac dysfunction. Invasive monitoring may be helpful in following fluid shifts and to optimize haemodynamic parameters. The vasodilatory effects of epidural anaesthesia may be of benefit in these patients; however, caution needs to be exercised as a precipitous fall in afterload may lead to acute decompensation in patients with aortic stenosis, hypertrophic cardiomyopathy or pulmonary hypertension.[71]

CONCLUSION

The critically ill obstetric patient poses a number of problems to the intensive care physician, the successful management of which requires an awareness of the normal cardiorespiratory changes of pregnancy, familiarity with pregnancy-specific diseases that may cause critical illness and a consideration for the well-being of both mother and fetus. Of equal importance in delivering the optimal standard of care to the critically ill pregnant patient, is the need for greater co-operation between the relevant specialities to ensure a prompt, integrated and multidisciplinary approach when clinical problems first arise. Recognition of the severity of the patient's condition followed by rapid referral to an ICU is vital in reducing maternal mortality and morbidity in pregnancy related critical illness.

REFERENCES

1. *Why Mothers Die 1997–1999.* The confidential enquiries into maternal deaths in the UK. RCOG Press, 2001.

2. Wheatley E, Farkas A, Watson D. Obstetric admissions to an intensive therapy unit. *Int J Obstet Anaesth* 1996; **5**: 221–224.

3. Graham SG, Luxton MC. The requirement for intensive care support for the pregnant population. *Anaesthesia* 1989; **44**: 581–584.

4. Stephens ID. ICU admissions from the obstetrical hospital. *Can J Anaesth* 1991; **38**: 677–681.

5. Mabie WC, Sibai BM. Treatment in an obstetric intensive care unit. *Am J Obstet Gynecol* 1990; **162**: 1–4.

6. Kilpatrick SJ, Matthay MA. Obstetric patients requiring critical care: a five-year review. *Chest* 1992; **101**: 1407–1412.

7. Collop NA, Sahn SA. Critical illness in pregnancy: an analysis of 20 patients admitted to a medical intensive care unit. *Chest* 1993; **103**: 1548–1552.

8. Lewinsohn G, Herman A, Leonov Y, Klinowski E. Critically ill obstetrical patients: outcome and predictability. *Crit Care Med* 1994; **22**: 1412–1414.

9. El-Solh AA, Grant BJB. A comparison of severity of illness scoring systems for critically ill obstetrical patients. *Am J Resp Crit Care Med* 1996; **153**: A362.

10. Department of Health. *Report on confidential enquiries into maternal deaths in the United Kingdom 1988–1990.* London: Her Majesty's Stationary Office, 1994.

11. Hollinsworth HM, Pratter MR, Irwin RS. Acute respiratory failure in pregnancy. *J Intens Care Med* 1989; **4**: 11.

12. Bernard F, Louvard V, Cressy ML, Tanguy M, Malledant Y. Preoxygenation before induction for caesarean section. *Annals de Francais Anesthesie Reanimation* 1994; **13**: 2–5.

13. Bartnicki J, Saling E. The influence of maternal oxygen administration on the fetus. *Int J Gynecol Obstet* 1994; **45**: 87–95.

14. Ivankovic AD, Elam JO, Huffman J. Effect of maternal hypercarbia on the new-born infant. *Am J Obstet Gynecol* 1970; **107**: 939–946.

15. Clark GP, Dobson PM, Thickett A, Turner NM. Chickenpox pneumonia, its complications and management: a report of three cases, including the use of extracorporeal membrane oxygenation. *Anaesthesia* 1991; **46**: 376–380.

16. Abrams JH, Gilmour IJ, Kriett JM, Bitterman PB, Irmiter RJ, McComb RC, Cerra FB. Low-frequency positive-pressure ventilation with extracorporeal carbon dioxide removal. *Crit Care Med* 1990; **18**: 212–220.

17. Conrad SA, Eggerstedt JM, Morris VM, Romero MD. Prolonged intracorporeal support of gas exchange with an intracaval oxygenator. *Chest* 1993; **103**: 158–161.

18. British Medical Association and Royal Pharmaceutical Society of Great Britain, London. British National Formulary 1997; **33**: 585–594.

19. Fishburne JI, Meis RB, Urban RB, Greiss FC, Wheeler AS, James FM, Swain MF, Rhyne AL. Vascular and uterine responses to dobutamine and dopamine in the gravid ewe. *Am J Obstet Gynecol* 1980; **137**: 944–952.

20. Rosenfeld CR, Barton MD, Meschia G. Effects of epinephrine on distribution of blood flow in the pregnant ewe. *Am J Obstet Gynecol* 1976; **124**: 156–163.

21. Fishburne JI, Dormer KJ, Payne GG. Effects of amrinone and dopamine on uterine blood flow and vascular responses in the gravid baboon. *Am J Obstet Gynecol* 1988; **158**: 829–837.

22. Clark RB, Brunner JA. Dopamine for the treatment of spinal hypotension during caesarean section. *Anesthesiology* 1980; **53**: 514–517.

23. Shnider SM, De Lormier AA, Holl JW, Chapler FK, Morishima HO. Vasopressors in obstetrics: correction of fetal acidosis with ephedrine during spinal hypotension. *Am J Obstet Gynecol* 1968; **102**: 911–919.

24. LaPorta RF, Arthur GR, Datta S. Phenylephrine in treating maternal hypotension due to spinal anaesthesia for caesarean delivery: effects on neonatal catecholamine concentrations, acid base status and Apgar scores. *Acta Anaesth Scand* 1995; **39**: 901–905.

25. Mabie WC, Gonzalez AR, Sibai BM, Amon E. A comparative trial of labetalol and hydrallazine in the acute management of severe hypertension complicating pregnancy. *Obstet Gynecol* 1987; **70**: 328–333.

26. Riley AJ. Clinical pharmacology of labetalol in pregnancy. *J Cardiovas Pharmacol* 1981; **3**: 53–59.

27. Redman CWG, Beilin LJ, Bonnar J. Fetal outcome in trial of antihypertensive treatment in pregnancy. *Lancet* 1976; **1**: 753–756.

28. Harake B, Gilbert RD, Ashwal S, Power GG. Nifedipine: effects on foetal and maternal haemodynamics in pregnant sheep. *Am J Obstet Gynecol* 1987; **157**: 1003–1008.

29. Synder SW, Cardwell MS. Neuromuscular blockade with magnesium sulphate and nifedipine. *Am J Obstet Gynecol* 1989; **161**: 35–36.

30. Waisman GD, Mayorga LM, Camera MI, Vignolo CA, Martinotti A. Magnesium plus nifedipine: potentiation of hypotensive effect in pre-eclampsia? *Am J Obstet Gynecol* 1988; **159**: 308–309.

31. Shoemaker CT, Meyers M. Sodium nitroprusside for control of severe hypertensive disease in pregnancy: a case report and discussion of potential toxicity. *Am J Obstet Gynecol* 1984; **149**: 171–173.

32. Shotan A, Widerhorn J, Hurst A, Elkayam U. Risks of angiotensin-converting enzyme inhibition during pregnancy: experimental and clinical evidence, potential mechanisms, and recommendations for use. *Am J Med* 1994; **96**: 451–456.

33. Afridi I, Moise KJ, Rokey R. Termination of supraventricular tachycardia with intravenous adenosine in a pregnant woman with Wolff–Parkinson–White syndrome. *Obstet Gynecol* 1992; **80**: 481–483.

34. Byerly WG, Hartmann A, Foster DE. Verapamil in the treatment of maternal paroxysmal supraventricular tachycardia. *Ann Emer Med* 1991; **20**: 552–554.

35. Berkowitz RL, Coustan DR, Mochizuki TK. *Handbook for prescribing medications during pregnancy.* Boston, Little: Brown, 1986.

36. Rotmensch HH, Elkayam U, Frishman W. Antiarrhythmic drug therapy during pregnancy. *Ann Int Med* 1983; **98**: 487–497.

37. Tadmor OP, Keren A, Rosenak D. The effect of disopyramide on uterine contractions during pregnancy. *Am J Obstet Gynecol* 1990; **162**: 482–486.

38. Mckenna W, Harris L, Rowland E. Amiodarone therapy during pregnancy. *Am J Cardiol* 1983; **51**: 1231–1233.

39. DeBiasse MA, Wilmore DW. What is optimal nutritional support? *New Horizons* 1994; **2**: 122–130.

40. Strong TH, Lowe RA. Perimortem cesarean section. *Am J Emer Med* 1989; **7**: 489–494.

41. Katz VL, Dotters DJ, Droegemueller W. Perimortem cesarean delivery. *Obstet Gynecol* 1986; **68**: 571–576.

42. The Eclampsia Trial Collaborative Group. Which anticonvulsant for women with eclampsia? Evidence from the collaborative eclampsia trial. *Lancet* 1995; **345**: 1455–1463.

43. Mabie WC, Ratts TE, Ramanathan KB, Sibai BM. Circulatory congestion in obese hypertensive women: a subset of pulmonary oedema in pregnancy. *Obstet Gynecol* 1988; **72**: 553–558.

44. Sibai BM, Taslimi MM, El-Nazer A, Amon E, Mabie BC, Ryan GM. Maternal-perinatal outcome associated with the syndrome of hemolysis, elevated liver enzymes and low platelets in severe pre-eclampsia-eclampsia. *Am J Obstet Gynecol* 1986; **155**: 501–509.

45. Rothenberger D, Quattlebaum FW, Perry JF, Zabel J, Fischer RP. Blunt maternal trauma: a review of 103 cases. *J Traum* 1978; **18**: 173–179.

46. Drost TF, Rosemurgy AS, Sherman HF, Scott LM, Williams JK. Major trauma in pregnant women: maternal/fetal outcome. *J Traum* 1990; **30**: 574–578.

47. Kissinger DP, Rozycki GS, Morris JA, Knudson M, Copes WS, Bass SM, Yates HK, Champion HR. Trauma in pregnancy: predicting pregnancy outcome. *Arch Surg* 1991; **126**: 1079–1086.

48. Williams JK, McClain L. Evaluation of blunt abdominal trauma in the third trimester of pregnancy: maternal and fetal considerations. *Obstet Gynecol* 1990; **75**: 33–35.

49. Gibbs RS. Severe infections in pregnancy. *Med Clin N Am* 1989; **73**: 713–725.

50. O'Brian WF, Golden SM, Davis SE. Endotoxemia in the neonatal lamb. *Am J Obstet Gynecol* 1985; **151**: 651–653.

51. Lackman E, Pitsoe SB, Gaffin SL. Anti-lipopolysaccharide immunotherapy in management of septic shock of obstetric and gynaecological origin. *Lancet* 1984; **1**: 981–984.

52. Lapinsky SE. Respiratory care of the critically ill pregnant patient. *Curr Opin Crit Care* 1996; **3**: 1–5.

53. Catanzarite VA, Willms D. Adult respiratory distress syndrome in pregnancy: report of three cases and review of the literature. *Obstet Gynecol Surv* 1997; **52**: 381–392.

54. Shoemaker WC, Appel PI. Effects of prostaglandin E₁ in adult respiratory distress syndrome. *Surgery* 1986; **99**: 275–282.

55. Major CA, Lewis DF, Harding JA. Tocolysis with indomethacin increases the incidence of necrotising enterocolitis in the low-birth weight neonate. *Am J Obstet Gynecol* 1994; **170**: 192–196.

56. Norton ME, Merrill J, Cooper BAB. Neonatal complications after the administration of indomethacin for preterm labour. *New Engl J Med* 1993; **329**: 1602–1607.

57. Smith JL, Thomas F, Orme JF. Adult respiratory distress syndrome during pregnancy and immediately postpartum. *Western J Med* 1990; **153**: 508–510.

58. Lee W, Clark SL, Cotton DB. Septic shock during pregnancy. *Am J Obstet Gynecol* 1988; **159**: 410–416.

59. Richey SD, Roberts SW, Ramin KD. Pneumonia complicating pregnancy. *Obstet Gynecol* 1994; **84**: 525–528.

60. Daily WH, Katz AR, Tonnesen A. Beneficial effect of delivery in a patient with adult respiratory distress syndrome. *Anesthesiology* 1990; **72**: 383–386.

61. Mabie WC, Barton JR, Sibai BM. Adult respiratory distress syndrome in pregnancy. *Am J Obstet Gynecol* 1992; **167**: 950–957.

62. Clark SL, Hankins GD, Dudley DA, Dildy GA, Porter TF. Amniotic fluid embolism: analysis of the national registry. *Am J Obstet Gynecol* 1995; **172**: 1158–1167.

63. Clark SL, Montz FJ, Phelan JP. Hemodynamic alterations associated with amniotic fluid embolism: a reappraisal. *Am J Obstet Gynecol* 1985; **151**: 617.

64. Clark SL, Pavlova Z, Greenspoon J. Squamous cells in the maternal pulmonary circulation. *Am J Obstet Gynecol* 1986; **154**: 104–106.

65. Kobayashi H, Ohi H, Terao T. A simple noninvasive, sensitive method for diagnosis of amniotic fluid embolism by monoclonal antibody TKH-2 that recognises NeuAca2-6GaINAc. *Am J Obstet Gynecol* 1993; **168**: 848–853.

66. Kanayama M, Yamazaki T, Naruse H, Sumimoto K, Horiuchi K, Terao T. Determining zinc coproporphyrin in maternal plasma – a new method for diagnosing amniotic fluid embolism. *Clin Chem* 1992; **38**: 526–529.

67. Turrentine MA, Braems G, Ramirez MM. Use of thrombolytics for the treatment of thromboembolic

disease during pregnancy. *Obstet Gynecol Surv* 1995; **50**: 534–541.

68. Narayan H, Cullimore J, Krarup K, Macvicar J, Bolia A. Experience with the cardial inferior vena cava filter as prophylaxis against pulmonary embolism in pregnant women with extensive deep venous thrombosis. *Br J Obstet Gynaecol* 1992; **99**: 637–640.

69. Cunningham FG, Leveno KJ, Hankins GDV. Respiratory insufficiency associated with antepartum pyelonephritis. *Obstet Gynecol* 1984; **63**: 121–125.

70. Madinger NE, Greenspoon JS, Ellrodt AG. Pneumonia during pregnancy: has modern technology improved maternal and fetal outcome? *Am J Obstet Gynecol* 1989; **161**: 657.

71. Sullivan JM, Ramanathan KB. Management of medical problems in pregnancy – severe cardiac disease. *New Engl J Med* 1985; **313**: 304.

CARDIOPULMONARY RESUSCITATION IN PREGNANCY

Nigel W. Penfold

INTRODUCTION

Fortunately, cardiac arrest of the mother in pregnancy is an uncommon event;[1,2] the incidence has been estimated to be one in 30 000 pregnancies.[1] The survival rate of mothers sustaining a cardiac arrest in the third trimester is unknown[3] due to the small number of case reports.[3–11] However, it may be that the incidence of cardiac arrest in pregnancy is increasing as a result of social trends and medical progress. More mothers with pre-existing medical conditions progress to term, and there are more medical procedures available to the gravid woman. In the 1997–1999 report into maternal deaths in the United Kingdom[12] the baseline mortality rate had increased from 9.8 in the 1991–93 report to 11.4 per 100 000 maternities, with 106 direct causes of death attributable to pregnancy. This overall rise may be explained in part by increased reporting. It has also been stated that approximately 50% maternal deaths are due to acute potentially treatable causes.[13] Indeed, maternal cardiopulmonary resuscitation (CPR) in pregnancy requires particular emphasis in educational programmes since success results in saving two 'hearts and brains too good to die'.[13]

The aetiology of cardiac arrest in pregnancy is the same as that of the general population, such as congenital

---

Table 16.1 Causes of cardiac arrest in the obstetric patient

General population
Congenital and aquired heart disease
  (increased risk in pregnancy)
Dysrrhythmias
Pulmonary embolus (increased risk
  in pregnancy)
Trauma (increased risk of blunt trauma)
Anaphylaxis

Specific to pregnancy
Peripartum haemorrhage
Pregnancy induced hypertension
Laryngeal oedema
Amniotic fluid embolus
Peripartum cardiomyopathy
Anaesthetic related problems
  General anaesthesia
    Airway management problems
    Anaphylaxis
  Regional anaesthesia
    Intravascular drug toxicity
    Accidental total spinal anaesthesia

---

and acquired heart disease, dysrrhythmias, pulmonary embolism, trauma, anaphylaxis and myocardial infarction, the latter having a reported incidence of one in 10 000 deliveries.[14] Causes specifically related to the state of being pregnant include amniotic fluid embolism,[15] peripartum haemorrhage, pregnancy induced hypertension, laryngeal angioedema, aortic dissection, peripartum cardiomyopathy (which may first present at the induction of anaesthesia[16]), bupivacaine toxicity from regional analgesia, and subarachnoid opioid-induced respiratory depression.[11] To this may be added the complications of tocolytic therapy, (arrhythmias and pulmonary oedema), and hypermagnaesaemia from the treatment of pre-eclampsia and eclampsia (Table 16.1).

The dramatic changes in maternal physiology that occur in pregnancy mean that resuscitation in this group of patients has many unique characteristics but, regretfully, since there is a paucity of research into cardiac arrest and CPR in pregnancy[13] many recommendations are based on studies in the non-pregnant situation and from assumptions made from our current understanding of the dynamic alterations in maternal physiology.

PHYSIOLOGICAL CHANGES OF PREGNANCY INFLUENCING CPR

CARDIOVASCULAR SYSTEM

As yet there are no systematic studies of the haemodynamic effects of cardiopulmonary resuscitation in pregnant humans.[13] Therefore, much of what is known clinically relies on studies of the normal changes of physiology during pregnancy. (See Table 16.2.)

The gravid uterus may significantly affect the maternal cardiovascular system by virtue of its size and weight causing mechanical obstruction particularly to the inferior vena cava. This compression leads to a reduction in cardiac output of between 10% and 25% when the mother is supine with a spontaneous cardiac output, and further compromises the already poor venous return that exists during cardiopulmonary resuscitation.[4] Abdominal aortic arterial flow distal to the obstruction from the gravid uterus is reduced and further compromises uteroplacental blood flow. Either manually displacing the uterus in a left and cephalad direction, or placing the supine gravida in a left lateral position is essential to minimize aorto-caval compression.[1,17]

Table 16.2   The significance of the physiological changes of pregnancy to CPR

Organ system	Significance to maternal CPR
Cardiovascular system	
Increased blood volume, with relative haemodilution and increased heart rate. Decreased blood pressure, systemic vascular resistance, pulmonary vascular resistance and wedge pressure	Minimal impact during resuscitation but needs to be considered post-resuscitation
Increased cardiac output with uteroplacental redistribution	Require high cardiac output during CPR
Aortocaval compression decreasing venous return and reducing cardiac output	Effect on maternal cardiac output and blood flow unknown. Uteroplacental flow improved with left lateral decubitus position
Increased sensitivity of uteroplacental bed to adrenergic vasopressors during maternal hypoxia and hypovolaemia	Dilemma as uteroplacental flow dependent maternal output, which is improved with high dose epinephrine
Respiratory system	
Decreased total lung compliance	Increased difficulty of external chest compression and positive pressure ventilation
Decreased FRC	More susceptible to hypoxia
Increased oxygen consumption and basal metabolic rate	More susceptible to hypoxia
Respiratory alkalosis	Decreased buffering capacity
More vascular, oedematous airway	Possibly need smaller endotracheal tube. Intubation may be more difficult
Gastrointestinal system	
Reduction in motility, and relaxation of lower oesophageal sphincter	Increased risk of aspiration requiring prompt intubation

RESPIRATORY SYSTEM

The respiratory system, like the cardiovascular, undergoes significant changes which enhance fetal oxygenation during pregnancy[18,19] but unfortunately, make the mother less able to tolerate the insults of a cardiac arrest. The overall effect of the changes is to render the parturient more susceptible to hypoxia when apnoeic, and to render the thorax less compressible to external pressure and so complicating any resuscitative measures.

The hyperventilation of pregnancy leads to a partially renal compensated respiratory alkalosis, with lowered serum bicarbonate levels. Thus the mother's buffering capacity during periods of hypotension or cardiac arrest is reduced. The airway becomes more vascular and oedematous and the rise in progesterone leads to a decrease in gastro-intestinal motility and a reduction in

lower gastro-oesophageal tone. These changes combine to increase the risk of pulmonary aspiration of gastric contents and render intubation more difficult. Hence prompt definitive airway control with a cuffed endotracheal tube assumes even greater importance during a cardiac arrest in pregnancy.

FETAL PHYSIOLOGY AND MATERNAL CPR

It can be of no surprise that the altered physiology during a maternal cardiac arrest significantly influences fetal outcome. Experience with perimortem Caesarean section shows that fetal survival and neurological outcome are improved if delivery occurs within 5 min of maternal arrest.[20] However, primate experiments and occasional case reports show that intact survivors may be delivered after 20 min of maternal CPR.[6,20] This variation may relate to the difficulty in timing the onset of true maternal arrest.

The fetus has, however, several adaptive physiological responses to hypoxia.[4,21] Although the supply to vital organs can be preserved for a limited period of time with central redistribution, if asphyxia persists, such physiological compensations become overwhelmed and neurological deficit and fetal death result. It is in the interest of both the mother and fetus that time to delivery is as short as possible, and certainly within 5 min of maternal arrest.[2]

CARDIOPULMONARY RESUSCITATION IN PREGNANCY

While there is a paucity of research relating to cardiopulmonary resuscitation in pregnancy,[13] it is generally accepted that standard resuscitation protocols should be followed for basic and advanced life support, albeit with some modifications for the pregnant patient.[2] The reader is advised to consult the European Resuscitation Council guidelines[22,23] or find them on the Resuscitation Council (UK) web site on www.resus.org.uk.

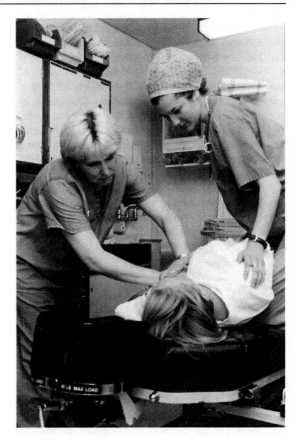

Figure 16.1   Human wedge technique.

BASIC LIFE SUPPORT

Basic life support refers to maintaining airway patency and supporting breathing and the circulation without recourse to specialized equipment, other than a protective face shield.[24] Conventional basic life protocols should be followed,[22] with important consideration being made to minimize the adverse cardiovascular effects of aorto-caval compression by displacing the uterus cephalad and leftwards. The anatomical changes in advanced pregnancy including flared ribs, breast hypertrophy, raised diaphragm and frequently obesity may make chest compression technically more difficult to perform. Minimizing the effect of aorto-caval compression may be achieved, with only a small reduction in applied chest compression force, by utilizing a tilting device such as the Cardiff resuscitation wedge.[1] If such a wedge is not immediately available then judicious use of pillows or foam wedges may be used, or preferably the human wedge technique,[17] in which the patient is tilted onto one of the rescuer's knees (Fig. 16.1). Whatever technique is employed, the important principle is to relieve the aorto-caval compression while allowing adequate chest compression to be performed. However, even optimal chest compression in the

supine non-pregnant victim produces at best only 30% of normal cardiac output, 30–50% cerebral of blood flow, and only 5–20% of coronary blood flow,[25] and it is not known if the output from chest compressions with the pregnant patient in the lateral position is sufficient for the maternal or uteroplacental circulation.[13] It remains to be seen whether the use of active compression–decompression devises, for example, the Ambu Cardiopump, will be advocated in pregnancy. In non-pregnant subjects the use of these devises improves the haemodynamic performance of cardiopulmonary resuscitation[26] but studies to date have not confirmed benefit in relation to survival or neurological outcome.[25] Furthermore since early Caesarean section is recommended in such resuscitation situations, open-cardiac compression has been advocated since the simple equipment required is at hand.

As in all cases of cardiopulmonary resuscitation, it is imperative that a clear airway is established immediately. In the absence of adequate respiration, intermittent positive pressure ventilation should commence by either mouth-to-mouth, mouth-to-nose, or mouth-to-airway adjunct (e.g. Laerdal pocket mask), until a means of giving high concentration oxygen is available. The recommendations advocate using breaths of 400–600 ml, delivered over 1.5–2 s, at a ratio of one ventilation to five chest compressions when two rescuers are present, the compression rate being at 100 compressions per minute with a pause for ventilation.[22] A single rescuer is recommended to perform two ventilations to 15 compressions. Maternal basic life support has fundamentally no different recommendations to that of the non-pregnant victim. Due to the previously stated physiological changes there is a high risk of pulmonary soiling during resuscitation in pregnancy and consideration should be given to applying cricoid pressure until the airway is secured by a cuffed endotracheal tube.[27]

ADVANCED LIFE SUPPORT

As is the case with basic life support, the European Resuscitation Council guidelines should be followed (Fig. 16.2).[23]

INTUBATION

In all arrest situations adequate ventilation assumes the utmost importance. In view of the changes in the respiratory system outlined above, secure control of the airway with an endotracheal tube should occur as soon as facilities and skill allow. Obviously ventilation during basic life support should have been initiated if required. The mother may have a short obese neck and full breasts making insertion of the laryngoscope blade difficult, in which case a short blade or angled blade laryngoscope may be needed. Visualization of the larynx can also be difficult due to laryngeal oedema. Confirmation of correct tube positioning in the trachea ideally would include using capnography to measure end-tidal expired carbon dioxide levels, but reliance on clinical methods may be necessary depending on the location of the arrest and available equipment.

DEFIBRILLATION

If the patient is discovered during the arrest to be in a shockable rhythm (i.e. ventricular fibrillation or pulseless ventricular tachycardia) then direct current defibrillation using the current guidelines should be implemented immediately. There are no contradictions to external defibrillation during pregnancy and case reports have shown that shocks of 300 J have not led to adverse effects on the fetus.[4,28,29] Elective cardioversion of mothers with supraventricular tachycardias

suggests that the fetal heart is not compromised by the external shock applied to the mother's chest.[30]

PHARMACOLOGICAL INTERVENTIONS

Drug delivery

Venous administration remains the optimal method of drug delivery during cardiopulmonary resuscitation, with central venous injection being the preferred option. If such a line is not in place then the risks associated with the technique, which in themselves may be life-threatening, mean that in an individual case the decision as to peripheral or central drug administration relates to the skills of the operator and availability of equipment. When peripheral cannulation is used this should be into as proximal a vein as possible (e.g. antecubital fossa), and drugs should be flushed in with 20 ml saline.[23]

The administration of drugs by the trans-tracheal route remains very much a second line approach due to erratic absorption and unpredictable pharmokinetics. It is limited to epinephrine, atropine and lidocaine, requires doses 2–3 times the intravenous dose, and drug need to be diluted to at least 10 ml with saline. Absorption is enhanced by applying five ventilations to increase dispersion to the distal bronchial tree.[23]

Intravenous fluids

The requirement for intravenous fluids in terms of the volume, speed of administration and the nature of the solutions, whether crystalloid or colloid, is dependent on the clinical assessment of the patient and presumed aetiology of the arrest. In general, acute collapse from hypovolaemia would require rapid infusion of plasma expanders (e.g. gelofusin or starch solutions), and blood replacement when available. Crystalloid replacement is also often employed to maintain line potency and for flushing in drugs. Care must be used to avoid maternal hyperglycaemia as this is associated with a poorer neurological outcome in survivors from cerebral hypoxia.

Pharmacological agents

Although some of the drugs used in advanced CPR would be classified as unsuitable for use in pregnancy by the licencing board in the United States (the Food and Drug Administration), the consensus view allows their utilization in this context.[2,31] This situation holds in the United Kingdom. Standard pharmacological therapy should therefore be utilized without

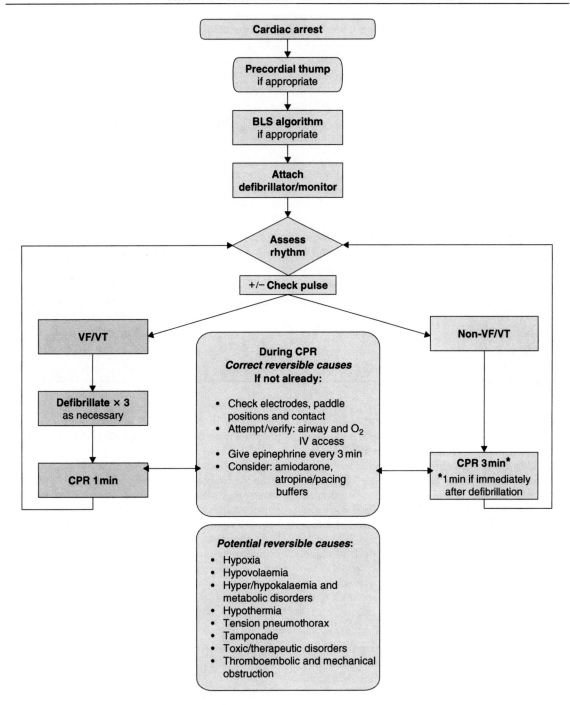

Figure 16.2   Algorithm for adult advanced life support.

modification in pregnancy, as the primary goal is maternal resuscitation.[32] The vasopressors, in particular epinephrine, which induce uteroplacental vasoconstriction, especially in the presence of maternal hypotension and hypoxia, should not be withheld if clinically indicated and should be used in accordance with the current resuscitation protocols (see Fig. 16.2). Indeed studies exist to suggest that the success of cardiac arrest in adults is enhanced by higher doses of epinephrine,[25] although other vasopressors, for example, vasopressin are being evaluated.[33] As resuscitation protocols have been re-evaluated over the years,

Table 16.3   Drugs used in CPR: considerations in pregnancy

Drug	Indication	
Atropine	Bradycardia	Crosses placenta. Not teratogenic, but may cause fetal tachycardia
Bretylium	Resistant ventricular fibrillation. Local anaesthetic induced arrhythmias	Safety not established in pregnancy. Use only if clinically necessary
Calcium gluconate	Antidote to Mg induced respiratory arrest	Crosses placenta, but not teratogenic
Dopamine/dobutamine	Inotropic support post-arrest	Non-teratogenic in animal studies. Effects in human pregnancy unknown
Epinephrine	Enhancing cerebral and cardiac blood flow during CPR	May induce uteroplacental vasoconstriction. Non-teratogenic in animal studies
Lidocaine	Reduction of ventricular tachyarrhythmia post-arrest	Crosses placenta but non-teratogenic; mild transient neurobehavioural depression
Sodium bicarbonate	Controversial	Paradoxical fetal acidosis
Amiodarone	Reduce ventricular tachyarrhthmia post-arrest. Now first line treatment	Considered safe in pregnancy

intravenous calcium and sodium bicarbonate have fallen from favour. However, calcium gluconate may be indicated in the treatment of magnesium toxicity in the management of severe pre-eclampsia leading to respiratory depression or arrest. The use of sodium bicarbonate in the gravida is more controversial, despite not being recommended in general resuscitation situations. The maternal administration of bicarbonate will lead to fetal hypercarbia and acidosis.[13] However, since maternal metabolic acidosis increases the reactivity of the uteroplacental vasculature to α-adrenergic agents, bicarbonate may be considered to correct acidosis if the maternal PO_2 and PCO_2 are normal.[18]

In general, drugs other than epinephrine and atropine have little place in the early stages of a resuscitation attempt in pregnancy and are very much second line therapy after measures detailed in the algorithm, coupled with rapid surgical delivery of the fetus. Table 16.3 outlines the major points relating to drugs used in resuscitation and the implications specific to the parturient.

Magnesium therapy

The use of magnesium sulphate in the treatment of some cases of pre-eclampsia and eclampsia is now established in the United Kingdom. One of the potential side effects, however, is drug induced respiratory depression, and this should be considered in the possible aetiology of a cardiac arrest in such a patient receiving magnesium.[34] Strict adherence to unit policies using volumetric infusion pumps and regular serum analysis should prevent inadvertent overdosage, but such cases leading to cardiopulmonary arrest have been reported.[10,16] Should such a situation arise then management is directed to supportive measures, cessation of the magnesium infusion, slow intravenous infusion of calcium gluconate or chloride (initially 10 ml of a 10% solution)[2] and consideration of the need for Caesarean section.

THORACOTOMY AND OPEN CARDIAC MASSAGE

The performance of a thoracotomy and open cardiac massage is infrequent during resuscitation attempts despite this technique permitting an adequate cardiac output to be established. Indeed this may lead to a reduced need for the administration of epinephrine and its associated uteroplacental vasoconstriction.[4,18] However since, particularly when the fetus is viable from 24 weeks, urgent Caesarean delivery is an essential part of maternal resuscitation, open cardiac compression should be considered if a spontaneous maternal circulation is not established soon after Caesarean delivery.

CAESAREAN SECTION

While the majority of the techniques of modern cardiopulmonary resuscitation have been described in recent years, this cannot be said for the role of peri-mortem Caesarean delivery, which was established in Roman Law in the eighth century BC, and was practised in Egyptian, Persian, Hindu, Finnish and North American Indian culture amongst others.[20] Even Shakespeare[35] in *Macbeth* refers to this practice when Macduff during his duel with Macbeth states 'Despair thy charm; and let the angel whom thou has serv'd tell thee, Macduff was from his mother's womb untimely ripp'd'.

Perimortem Caesarean delivery is a rare procedure and the decision to perform one may be difficult. Perinatal outcome is determined by many factors, the most per-tinent being the gestational age of the fetus, the time from maternal arrest to delivery, the nature of the maternal insult, pre-arrest morbidity, and perhaps the availability of neonatal intensive care resources.

Infant survival decreases and neurological damage increases with the time taken to deliver. When Cae-sarean section is performed within 5 min of maternal arrest the outcome is generally good, from 10 to 15 min fair, and longer than this the chances of good infant survival is poor, although not unknown.[20,36] It has been suggested that fetal prognosis is better after the sudden death of a previously healthy mother rather than from a mother who had been suffering from a prolonged or debilitating illness.[20,37]

Once the decision has been made to perform a peri-mortem Caesarean section, cardiopulmonary resuscita-tion should be continued as described on the mother from the time of arrest until post-delivery. While a few seconds of sterile abdominal preparation are suggested, delivery should occur rapidly, and the use of a vertical incision has been recommended.[37] In this situation while it is ideal that consent for the operation is obtained, no delay should occur in obtaining it.[20,37]

COMPLICATIONS OF CPR IN PREGNANCY

It is evident that the techniques used in cardiopul-monary resuscitation can lead to post-arrest compli-cations. The obstetric patient is particularly at risk from laceration of her internal organs, most likely

being the liver, (especially with the spontaneous intra-hepatic haemorrhage associated with pre-eclampsia), uterus and spleen, in addition to the general risks of fractured ribs and sternum, haemopneumothorax and haemopericardium.[18]

Potential fetal risks range from cardiac arrhythmias from defibrillation or drug therapy, central nervous toxicity from medication, altered uterine activity or reduced or absent placental perfusion from maternal hypoxia, hypovolaemia, acidosis or vasoconstriction, to fetal non-survival. As stated previously fetal sur-vival is enhanced if delivery occurs within 5 min of maternal circulatory arrest.[20]

To ensure survival of the mother and fetus each indi-vidual needs to be admitted to the appropriate inten-sive care facility for further investigation and treatment.

SUMMARY

Due to the infrequency of resuscitation in preg-nancy and the difficulty of accurately reproducing the cardiopulmonary effects of human pregnancy in an animal model, accurate research of CPR in the gravid woman is significantly absent. The absolute degree to which the decreased cardiac output due to aorto-caval compression compromises blood flow during CPR, or the effect of open cardiac compression and early abdominal decompression by Caesarean deliv-ery on blood flow to the maternal cardiac and cere-bral circulations requires clarification.

CPR in early pregnancy differs marginally from that of the non-pregnant, but recommendations can only be supported by case reports, a knowledge of the physio-logical changes in pregnancy, and research into CPR in non-human pregnant models, with assumption then being made. As pregnancy advances, changes in mater-nal physiology and anatomy require modifications to a more aggressive airway management policy, and meas-ures to cause left displacement of the enlarging uterus. Recognition of the aetiology of the cardiac arrest may lead to specifically aimed therapy, but in essence, guide-lines for defibrillation and drug treatment are unchanged. In the second and especially the third trimester urgent perimortem Caesarean section should be seriously considered in all cases in an attempt to save the infant and improve the maternal haemodynamics such that maternal survival is possible.

REFERENCES

1. Rees GAD, Willis BA. Resuscitation in late pregnancy. *Anaesthesia* 1988; **43**: 347–349.

2. International Liaison Committee on Resuscitation. Special resuscitation situations. *Resuscitation* 1997; **34**: 129–149.

3. Parker J, Balis N, Chester S, Adey D. Cardiopulmonary arrest in pregnancy: successful resuscitation of mother and infant following immediate Caesarean section on labour ward. *Aust NZ J Obstet Gynaecol* 1996; **36**(2): 207–210.

4. Seldon BS, Burke TJ. Complete maternal and fetal recovery after prolonged cardiac arrest. *Ann Emerg Med* 1988; **17**: 346–348.

5. O'Connor RL, Sevarino FB. Cardiopulmonary arrest in the pregnant patient: a report of a successful resuscitation. *J Clin Anesth* 1994; **6**: 66–68.

6. Lanoix R, Akkapeddi V, Goldfeder B. Perimortem Caesarean section: case reports and recommendations. *Acad Emerg Med* 1995; **2**: 1063–1067.

7. Oates S, Williams GL, Rees GAD. Cardiopulmonary resuscitation in late pregnancy. *Br Med J* 1988; **297**: 404–405.

8. Linsay SL, Hansen GC. Cardiac arrest in near-term pregnancy. *Anaesthesia* 1987; **42**: 1074–1077.

9. DePace NL, Betesh JS, Kotler MN. Post mortem Caesarean section with recovery of both mother and off-spring. *J Am Med Assoc* 1982; **248**: 971–973.

10. McCubbin JH, Sibai BM, Abdella TN, Anderson GD. Cardiopulmonary arrest due to acute maternal hypermagnaesaemia. *Lancet* 1981; **1**: 1058.

11. Myint Y, Bailey PW, Milne BR. Cardiorespiratory arrest following combined spinal and epidural anaesthesia for Caesarean section. *Anaesthesia* 1993; **48**: 684–686.

12. *Why Mothers Die 1997–1999*. The confidential enquiries into maternal deaths in the UK. RCOG Press, 2001.

13. Ornato JP, Paradis N, Bircher N, Brown C et al. Future directions for resuscitation research. III. External cardiopulmonary resuscitation advanced life support. *Resuscitation* 1996; **32**: 139–158.

14. Ginz B. Myocardial infarction in pregnancy. *J Obstet Gynaecol* 1970; **77**: 610–615.

15. Morgan M. Amniotic fluid embolism. *Anaesthesia* 1979; **34**: 20–34.

16. McIndoe AK, Hammond EJ, Babington PC. Peripeartum cardiomyopathy presenting as a cardiac arrest at induction of anaesthesia for emergency Caesarean section. *Br J Anaesth* 1995; **75**: 97–101.

17. Goodwin APL, Pearce AJ. *Anaesthesia* 1992; **47**: 433–434.

18. Lee W, Cotton DB. Cardiorespiratory changes during pregnancy. In: Clarke SL, Cotton DB, Hankins GD, Phelan JP (eds) *Critical care obstetrics*, 2nd edn. Boston: Blackwell Scientific Publications, 1991, p 2.

19. Sherman HF, Scott LM, Rosemurgy AS. Changes affecting the initial evaluation and care of the pregnant trauma victim. *J Emerg Med* 1990; **8**: 575.

20. Katz VL, Dotters DJ, Droegemuller W. Perimortem Cesarean delivery. *Obstet Gynaecol* 1986; **68**: 571–576.

21. Thorp JM, Cefalo RC. Maternal-fetal physiological interactions in the critically ill pregnant patient. In: Clark SL, Cotton DB, Hankins GDV, Phelan JP (eds) *Critical care obstetrics*. Boston: Blackwell Scientific Publications, 1991, p 102.

22. Basic Life Support Working Group of the European Resuscitation Council. The 1998 European Resuscitation Council guidelines for adult single rescuer basic life support. *Br Med J* 1998; **316**: 1870–1876.

23. Advanced Life Support Working Group of the European Resuscitation Council. The 1998 European Resuscitation Council guidelines for adult advanced life support. *Br Med J* 1998; **316**: 1863–1868.

24. Chamberlain DC, Cummins RO. Task force. Recommended guidelines for uniform reporting of data from out-of-hospital cardiac arrest: the 'Utstein style'. *Resuscitation* 1991; **22**: 1–26.

25. Lindner KH. Cardiopulmonary resuscitation. *Curr Opin Anaesth* 1997; **10**: 114–118.

26. Lurie KG. Active compression-decompression CPR: a progress report. *Resuscitation* 1994; **28**: 115–122.

27. Rees GAD, Willis BA. Resuscitation in pregnancy. In: Colquhoun MC, Handley AJ, Evans TR (eds) *ABC of resuscitation*, 3rd edn. BMJ Publishing Group, 1995, p 32.

28. Curry JJ, Quintana FJ. Myocardial infarction with ventricular fibrillation during pregnancy treated by direct current defibrillation with fetal survival. *Chest* 1970; **58**: 82.

29. Stokes IM, Evans J, Stone M. Myocardial infarction and cardiac arrest in the second trimester followed by assisted vaginal delivery under epidural analgesia at 38 weeks gestation: case report. *Br J Obstet Gynaecol* 1984; **91**: 197.

30. Cullhed I. Cardioversion during pregnancy. A case report. *Acta Med Scand* 1983; **214**: 169–172.

31. Special resuscitation situations. *J Am Med Assoc* 1992; **268**: 2242.

32. Dildy GA, Clark SL. Cardiac arrest during pregnancy. *Obstet Gynaecol Clin N Am* 1995; **22**(2): 303–314.

33. Lindler KH, Prengel AW, Brinkmann A, Strohmenger HU et al. Vasopressin administration in refractory cardiac arrest. *Ann Int Med* 1996; **124**: 1061–1064.

34. Wax JR, Segna JA, Vandersloot JA. Magnesium toxicity and resuscitation – an unusual case of postcaesarian evisceration. *Int J Gynaecol Obstet* 1995; **48**: 213–214.

35. Shakespeare W. *Macbeth*. Act V, Scene viii. William Sheakespeare: The Complete Works. Hamlyn Publishing Group Ltd., 1968.

36. Lopez-Zeno JA, Carlo WA, O'Grady JP. Infant survival following delayed post-mortem Cesarean delivery. *Obstet Gynaecol* 1990; **76**: 991.

37. Strong TH, Lowe RA. Perimortem Cesarean section. *Am J Emerg Med* 1989; **7**: 489–494.

OTHER USEFUL REFERENCES

Albright GA. Cardiac arrest following regional anaesthesia with etidocaine or bupivacaine. *Anaesthesiology* 1979; **51**: 285–287.

Archer GW, Marx G. *Br J Anaesth* 1974; **46**: 358–360.

Caplan et al. Unexpected cardiac arrest under spinal anaesthesia. *Anaesthesiology* 1988; **68**: 5–11.

Clark SL, Cotton DB, Lee W. Central hemodynamic assessment of normal term pregnancy. *Am J Obstet Gynaecol* 1989; **161**: 1439.

Clarkson CW, Houdegham LM. *Anaesthesiology* 1985; **62**: 396–405.

Davis MG, Harrison JC. Amniotic fluid embolism: maternal mortality revisited. *Br J Hosp Med* 1992; **47**: 775.

Kouwenhoven WB et al. *J Am Med Assoc* 1960; **173**: 1064–1067.

Lee RV, Rodgers BD, White LM, Harvey RC. Cardiopulmonary resuscitation of pregnant women. *Am J Med* 1986; **81**: 311–318.

Marx GF. CPR of late pregnancy. *Anaesthesiology* 1982; **56**: 156.

Riley DP, Burgess RW. External abdominal aortic compression: a study of a resuscitation manoeuvre for postpartum haemorrage. *Anaesth Intens Care* 1994; **22**: 571–575.

Werner JA, Green et al. *Circulation* 1981; **63**: 1417–1421.

17

AMNIOTIC FLUID EMBOLISM

Paul Howell

INTRODUCTION

Since its first appearance in the English language literature in 1941,[1] amniotic fluid embolism (AFE) has probably become the single most feared diagnosis in pregnancy. A major review in 1979 by Morgan confirmed the dramatic nature of the condition.[2] However, in the past decade, evolution in our understanding of this potentially devastating condition has lead to a re-evaluation of many long-held beliefs. Several of the traditional concepts in AFE were based on early experiments in lower animal models with inappropriate extrapolation to humans. It is apparent that the clinical and pathophysiological profile of AFE is much more complex and variable than previously believed. It would now appear likely that the classic, sudden, largely fatal, collapse represents the lethal extremity of a continuum, which includes less dramatic presentations of AFE, and possibly even a sub-clinical, asymptomatic state.

There is currently considerable debate (i.e. confusion) about what exactly should be considered in the diagnosis of AFE, the validity of histological evidence, the natural pathophysiological course of AFE, and the opportunities for therapeutic intervention. Much of the credit for advancing our understanding of AFE must be given to Steven Clark, who has written extensively on the subject and who was instrumental in establishing the US national registry for AFE.[3–10]

This voluntary registry was set up in 1988 to collect and review cases of suspected AFE occurring since 1983 according to strict, and somewhat classical, diagnostic criteria (Table 17.1).[10] Initial data on 46 patients were published in 1995, although several other patients who were considered to have an AFE-like syndrome but did not meet the strict entry criteria were excluded.

Despite being a condition associated almost invariably with death, the English language literature currently contains details of over 130 survivors from AFE.[11–100] As our awareness of the complexities and inconsistencies in our understanding of AFE grows, so our perspective of this condition must evolve. In 1990, Clark wrote *'That the syndrome of AFE exists is irrefutable; the exact relationship of this syndrome to amniotic fluid, however, remains somewhat more obscure'*.[7] Unfortunately, it appears that the US AFE Registry is no longer collecting data, although a similar register has recently been established in the UK.[101]

INCIDENCE

AFE is an uncommon condition, and the classic presentation of sudden collapse and death is indeed

---

Table 17.1   US National AFE Registry: entry criteria

1. Acute hypotension or cardiac arrest
2. Acute hypoxia, defined as dyspnoea, cyanosis or respiratory arrest
3. Coagulopathy, defined as laboratory evidence of intravascular consumption or fibrinolysis or severe clinical haemorrhage in the absence of other explanations
   [NB: *patients meeting all other criteria including abrupt cardiorespiratory arrest who died before coagulopathy could be assessed are included in the primary analysis*]
4. Onset of the above during labour, Caesarean section, or dilation and evacuation, or within 30 min postpartum
5. Absence of any other significant confounding or potential explanation or the signs and symptoms observed
6. Occurrence within 5 years of registry opening (i.e. not before 1983)

From Ref. 10.

---

markedly rare, but there now is growing evidence that other less dramatic, less lethal, presentations may also occur. The incidence is widely reported to lie between 1:80 000 and 1:8000 births, but the true figure is almost impossible to ascertain. One of the most significant problems is that clinical and laboratory diagnostic criteria vary greatly. However, cases with an AFE component probably occur more frequently than is generally realized.

On the one hand there has probably been significant under-reporting of AFE since fatal outcome has previously been considered almost essential for the diagnosis to be made, and hence many of the less severe, non-lethal, non-typical cases would have been missed. In addition, survival is reported less reliably than mortality. On the other hand it is likely that AFE has been diagnosed in a number of cases of sudden, unexpected death which were due to other causes (e.g. massive abruption, pulmonary embolism). Over-reporting may also occur in litigious societies since the low expectation of survival following a diagnosis of AFE may reduce the likelihood of medico-legal action against the medical teams involved.[102,103]

OUTCOME

MORTALITY

Whilst AFE may be a rare condition, it is the commonest cause of peripartum death in the UK and associated with a very high mortality rate, often quoted as being in excess of 80%.[2] A more recent review from the USA of severe 'classic' cases (i.e. those fulfilling strict diagnostic entry criteria) reported lower mortality (61%), although there was significant morbidity in the survivors – only 15% of women made full recoveries.[10] Mortality reports from the UK, however, show little improvement in the number of deaths due to AFE over the past 20 years, and in 1994–96 it was the fourth most common direct cause of maternal death.[101]

World-wide, as deaths due to other causes fall (e.g. sepsis, haemorrhage, hypertensive disorders), AFE becomes relatively more important. Published statistics most commonly suggest AFE cause between 4% and 8% of maternal deaths (Table 17.2). Isolated reports quote much higher figures, and one extraordinary report from Miami, USA, details six cases of AFE occurring amongst nine maternal deaths that occurred in 1970.[104] The cause of these surprisingly high incidence rates is unclear, but may reflect some of the diagnostic difficulties of this condition.

Of the various mortality figures shown in Table 17.2, data from the UK is probably the most reliable, due to

the vigorous and comprehensive nature of the triennial 'Report on confidential enquiries into maternal deaths in the United Kingdom'. Data during 1985–93 suggests that AFE causes 7.3% of direct maternal deaths and that the incidence of lethal AFE is approximately 4 per 1 000 000 maternities, although the (1994–96) report suggests a higher death rate (5.6 per million maternities).[101,105]

Death is frequently rapid, with 25% mortality at 1 h reported by Morgan,[2] and 24% mortality and 39% mortality reported at 2 and 5 h respectively.[10] Mortality data from the UK suggests two groups of patients; those that die within a few hours of collapse (of haemorrhage or failed resuscitation), and those in whom resuscitation is successful enough to allow transfer to an intensive care facility, where they die several days later.[101]

At the time of Morgan's extensive review in 1979 there had been few published reports of survival following AFE.[2] However, the number of published reports of survivors confirms that AFE need not be lethal under certain conditions.[11–100] Several factors are probably involved. Some of the cases reported appear to be of a less severe nature than that seen in 'classic' AFE, and the diagnostic criteria are evolving and being broadened, possibly including patients that would not, previously, have been labelled 'AFE'. However, the lower mortality rate (61%) reported in patients entered into the US AFE registry has occurred in a group of patients with the most severe, 'classic' forms.[10]

Table 17.2 World-wide maternal mortality from AFE

Country	Period	Number of AFE deaths	(Direct)* maternal deaths (%)	Reference number
Australia	1964–84	54	4.5	76
Australia	1970–90	34	7.5	197
Ireland	1989–91	2**	40**	198
Israel	1955–66	13	4.4	133
Japan	1964–80	15	4.9	199
Malaysia	1991	15	7.4	200
Sweden	1971–80	8	16.5	44
Sweden	1973–79	6	30	201
UK	1985–93	30	7.3	105
USA	1974–78	189	7.6	202
USA (New York)	1981–83	11	16.6	203
USA (Pennsylvania)	1959–73	6	19.4	204
USA (S Carolina)	1970–84	13	7.7	102

*Direct maternal deaths specified.
**NB: small numbers (2/5 direct maternal deaths due to AFE).

In other cases, therefore, the fall in mortality may have resulted from a more aggressive clinical response to the suspected diagnosis of AFE, with rapidly instituted haemodynamic monitoring, and efficient clinical and haematological back-up available. Clark reported survival of four women with AFE in whom early pulmonary artery catheterization guided appropriate haemodynamic manipulation.[6] It is interesting to note from the 1991–93 UK data that, whilst there was no change in mortality, more patients survived long enough to be transferred to an ITU facility than previously.[105] Hopefully, this reflects improved immediate management of maternal collapse (although there is little evidence to suggest that this has led to improved outcome).

MORBIDITY FOLLOWING SURVIVAL

Whilst there is some evidence that maternal mortality from AFE may have fallen slightly in recent decades, it is disappointing that long-term morbidity in survivors may be significant.[10] Clark reported that approximately 85% of cases of 'classic' AFE die or survive with permanent neurological damage, particularly in the presence of meconium or a dead baby.[10] This represents a 15% 'intact' survival rate, which is similar to previous outcome reports.[2] However, contrary to these findings, another review of survivors of AFE suggests that most patients appear to make a full recovery. Overall, persistent neurological deficit, (the commonest persistent problem), was reported in only 15% of survivors. The paucity of reports of acute renal failure and the requirement for short- or long-term haemodialysis or haemofiltration in survivors is perhaps surprising, although renal support has been described in isolated cases. Chronic pulmonary impairment has also been reported. The vast majority of survivors may therefore make a good recovery from AFE, and in fact a few have been able to overcome the physical and emotional scars of AFE and have subsequently undergone pregnancy with successful outcomes.[9,20,56,106,107]

FETAL OUTCOME

When AFE occurs prior to delivery, fetal outcome is poor, and although US registry data shows only 21% perinatal mortality, half the surviving neonates had permanent neurological injury (i.e. 39% intact survival).[10] In survivors, fetal survival has been reported at 88%, although few reports comment on subsequent morbidity. Fetal bradycardia is commonly reported and may be an inevitable consequence of AFE, but may also precede maternal collapse.[10,29,108] In the event of maternal cardiac arrest with a live fetus

in utero, intact neonatal survival appears inversely related to the cardiac arrest-to-delivery time interval (Table 17.3).[10,109] Hence immediate delivery is indicated for both maternal and neonatal survival.

CLINICAL PRESENTATION

'CLASSIC' AFE COLLAPSE

In their landmark article of 1941, Steiner and Lushbaugh presented a series of eight maternal deaths in which similar, characteristic clinical and histological features were present.[1] Since then, there have been a large number of similar cases reported in the literature. It is clear that (whatever the cause) there is a rare, but highly lethal, condition in pregnancy, which presents, usually during labour or the immediate postpartum period, with the clinical features of the 'classic' AFE collapse (Box 17.1).

Table 17.3 Cardiac arrest-to-delivery interval and neonatal outcome in AFE

Interval (min)	Survival no.	Intact survival no. (%)
<5	3/3	2/3 (67)
5–15	3/3	2/3 (67)
16–25	2/5	2/5 (40)
26–35	3/4	1/4 (25)
36–54	0/1	0/1 (0)

From Ref. 10.

- Cyanosis
- Respiratory distress
- Cardiovascular collapse
- Cardiac arrest
- Pulmonary oedema
- Agitation/confusion/delirium
- Coma
- Convulsions
- Fetal distress
- Uterine atony
- Haemorrhage
- Coagulopathy
- Death

Box 17.1 Clinical features of 'classic' AFE collapse.

VARIANTS

Morgan considered cardiorespiratory collapse to be invariable in his large review of cases in 1979,[2] and these features were also included in the diagnostic entry criteria for the US Registry.[10] Whilst hypotension is the predominant occurrence, in a few patients this is preceded by a short period of hypertension,[10,36] a feature also noted in animal models.[110] However, a number of cases with less dramatic presentations have been described where haemodynamic instability is less severe, many of whom have survived. In two reported cases, the clinical picture was of acute allergic reaction, but the timing (onset at membrane rupture or delivery) was highly suggestive of AFE aetiology.[45,58]

In addition, a 'forme fruste' variant of AFE has been proposed where isolated (but potentially lethal) coagulopathy develops in the relative absence of hypotension, hypoxia or other characteristic AFE problems.[25,47,52,71] The mortality risk associated with 'forme fruste' is unclear: despite several isolated reports of survival,[24,25,47,52,53] data from eight cases submitted to the US National Registry showed 75% mortality, implying that this may not be a 'mild' form of AFE.[71]

Whilst the diagnosis of AFE may be questioned in a few of these 'variant' cases, it is now apparent that there is a broad spectrum of clinical presentation and severity of this condition which can allow survival with full recovery (Box 17.2)(Chart 17.1).

Coagulopathy is very common (78%)

Less severe haemodynamic disturbance
   50% suffer 'classic' collapse
   35% develop pulmonary oedema
   25% develop cardiac arrest
   11% show minimal CVS depression
    6% show only coagulopathy ('forme fruste')

Persistent neurological damage is rare (15%)

Box 17.2   Features of reported survivors.

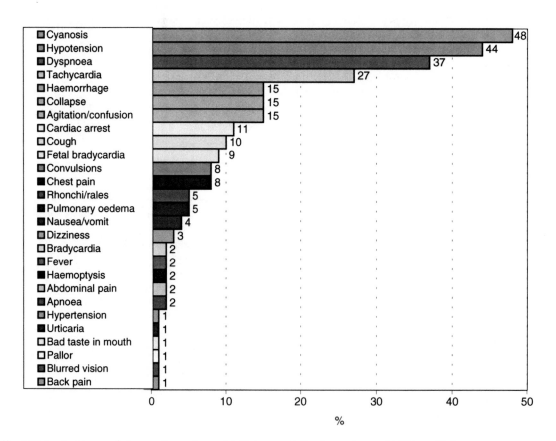

Chart 17.1   Incidence of signs and symptoms at initial presentation in survivors of AFE (n = 130).

INITIAL PRESENTATION

Steiner and Lushbaugh's original report of AFE described rapid onset of cardiovascular collapse ('shock') and cyanosis in association with air hunger or tachypnoea.[1] Many other authors since have reported similar early respiratory symptoms followed by sudden and dramatic collapse. Morgan's review from 1979 of 272 cases showed that the most common presenting complaint was of respiratory difficulty with cyanosis (51%). Less common initial presentations included cardiovascular collapse (27%), haemorrhage (12%) and convulsions (10%).[2] Quance reported an isolated fall in oxygen saturation following delivery by Caesarean section under epidural anaesthesia, which was followed over 1 h later by other characteristic (and fatal) features of AFE.[111] As a result of this experience the author recommended the routine use of pulse oximetry at all deliveries.

More recent data from the US Registry suggests that in women presenting before delivery seizures, or seizure-like activity, are as common as respiratory symptoms (30% each).[10] Although cardiovascular symptoms were the presenting complaint in only 13% of patients, cardiac arrest occurred in 83% patients within 1 h of AFE symptom onset, and in over one-third of these patients, the arrest occurred within 5 min. Fetal bradycardia was the presenting condition in 17% cases, preceding maternal haemodynamic decompensation, a feature that has been noted by others.[29]

Cardiovascular:	Myocardial infarction
	Primary arrhythmia
	Haemorrhage (especially placental abruption)
	Aortocaval compression
Respiratory:	Pulmonary embolism
	Air embolism
	Aspiration pneumonitis
Central nervous system:	Eclampsia
	Intra-cranial pathology
Regional anaesthesia:	Total spinal/high block
	Local anaesthetic toxicity
Anaphylactoid reaction	
Septic shock	
Substance abuse	

Box 17.3 Differential diagnosis of AFE collapse.

It is interesting to compare these figures (from reviews with 86% and 61% mortality respectively) with those of patients who have survived AFE, many of whom did not appear to suffer the severe 'classic' AFE syndrome (Chart 17.1, Table 17.4). Review of the published case reports of 135 survivors of AFE reveals a remarkably similar picture at presentation: cyanosis, hypotension and shortness of breath (or other respiratory complaint) and tachycardia were most common (occurring in between 25% and 50% of survivors). Other dramatic presentations include sudden collapse (15%), cardiac arrest (10%) and convulsions (8%), although convulsions appear much less commonly in survivors compared to Clark's data.[10]

Some patients may present with rather subtle complaints, including restlessness, confusion or altered level of consciousness, chest pain or tightness, tachycardia or bradycardia. AFE may also present with unexplained haemorrhage or fetal distress (particularly fetal bradycardia) which may precede maternal signs and symptoms. In a number of women who survived the 'forme fruste' variant haemorrhage (coagulopathy) was the main clinical feature.[24,25,47,52,53,71]

It would appear, therefore, that the signs and symptoms seen at presentation of AFE are not predictive of survival except, possibly, convulsions. AFE should be suspected, (if only to be excluded), in any pregnant patient who complains of respiratory difficulty, or sudden onset of chest pain, confusion or cough, or who develops unexplained cyanosis, hypotension, tachycardia or bradycardia, or haemorrhage in the peripartum period. Convulsions should be remembered in the differential diagnosis, along with eclampsia, epilepsy, intra-cranial pathology and substance abuse. AFE is, of course, not the only cause of collapse in pregnant women, and other diagnoses must be considered (Box 17.3).

CLINICAL COURSE

Whilst the signs and symptoms of AFE at presentation in survivors appear indistinguishable from those in fatal cases, the clinical course may show some differences. Compared to data from Morgan[2] and, particularly, Clark,[10] survivors appear to suffer less severe effects from AFE, with a lower incidence of convulsions (12% vs. 48%), severe cardiovascular collapse (70% vs. 100%), cardiac arrest (25% vs. 87%), pulmonary oedema (35% vs. 93%) and permanent neurological damage (Table 17.4). However, coagulopathy is widespread, and is frequently the major persistent clinical problem, occurring more frequently than previously recognized (see below).

Table 17.4 Comparative review data

	Morgan (1979)[2]	Clark et al (1995)[10]	Howell (Personal data)
n	272	46	135
Mortality (%)	86	61	0
Survival (%)	14	39	100
'Intact' maternal survival (%)	?	15	85
Mean age (years)	32	27	28
Mean gestation (weeks)		39	36
Primiparous (%)	12	39	32
Multiparous (%)	88	61	68
Neonatal survival[a] (%)		79	88[b]
Intact neonatal survival[b] (%)		39	75[b]
Oxytocic uterine stimulation[c] (%)	22	33	31
Initial presentation (%)			
Respiratory	51	30	44[d]
Cardiovascular	27	13	65[d]
Convulsions	10	30	8[d]
Haemorrhage	12	0	15[d]
Fetal distress		17	9[d]
Onset (%)			
Peripartum (vaginal or Caesarean delivery)	>90[e]	93	83
Other (spontaneous +1st and 2nd trimester)		7	17
Timing relative to delivery[f]			
n	<272[e]	43	109
Associated with vaginal delivery (%)	90	83	69
Associated with Caesarean delivery (%)	<10[e]	19	31
In labour before delivery (%)		70	42
In labour after delivery (%)		12[e]	27
During LSCS (%)		19	16
During LSCS after delivery (%)		19	>11
After LSCS (%)		0	16
At or shortly after delivery (%)		53	39
Clinical manifestations (%)			
'Classic' collapse	100	100	50
Hypotension	100	100	87
Cardiac arrest	High	87	25
Pulmonary oedema	24	93	35
Convulsions	>10	48	12
Haemorrhage/coagulopathy	49	83	78
Minimal CVS instability	0	0	11

[a] AFE occurred with viable fetus *in utero*.
[b] Reporting of neonatal outcome not considered reliable.
[c] For induction of labour and augmentation.
[d] Multiple presenting signs and symptoms reported.
[e] Not specified in text.
[f] Excluding spontaneous, and 1st and 2nd trimester cases of AFE.

HAEMODYNAMIC EFFECTS

Severe cardiovascular collapse is one of the characteristic, frequently lethal, features of AFE. Unfortunately, the unexpected nature of the collapse, and the frequent rapidity of ensuing death, has prevented much *in vivo* analysis of the precise haemodynamic sequalae. In the relatively few patients where invasive monitoring has been used, this has almost always been several hours after collapse, and interpretation of data is difficult due to the extent of cardiopulmonary support required. Early concepts of AFE were based on animal studies where the predominant effects reported were of right ventricular failure, although as long ago as 1963 Attwood and Rome reported a case where the right ventricle was flaccid and collapsed, inconsistent with acute pulmonary vascular obstruction.[112] However, in humans, *left ventricular failure* is the consistent finding, with only relatively modest elevations in pulmonary artery pressure (PAP) which could themselves be secondary to reduced left ventricular function.[3,6,12,32,39,60,64,82,94,106,113,114] To quote Clark:

> 'Indeed, to date (left heart failure) seems to be the only significant haemodynamic abnormality consistently documented in human patients; data supporting intrinsic pulmonary artery spasm and secondary cor pulmonale are entirely lacking'.[10]

Biphasic model

In an attempt to reconcile the experimental and clinical haemodynamic findings in AFE, Clark has proposed a biphasic model of AFE (Box 17.4), although notes that there is no evidence in humans of an initial phase of transient pulmonary vasospasm.[4,6,7] However, Shah et al have reported a case of histologically confirmed AFE occurring during elective Caesarean section in a severely hypertensive woman in whom a pulmonary artery catheter had been sited before insertion of the epidural.[85] Immediately prior to delivery, the patient complained of chest pain which was associated with a moderate rise in PAP, and followed by a series of episodes of ventricular tachycardia. Early treatment with glyceryl trinitrate (GTN) infusion and lidocaine boluses were effective and the patient survived.

In the initial phase, amniotic fluid (or a component of amniotic fluid) triggers pulmonary vasospasm which produces acute pulmonary hypertension and profound hypoxia (due to increased ventilation/perfusion mismatch, shunt and a dramatic fall in cardiac output). Animal work suggests that this phase is very transient, lasting less than 30 min,[110,115,116] but the initial period of significant hypoxia may explain the very high early mortality from AFE, and the associated severe neurological deficit reported in survivors.[10]

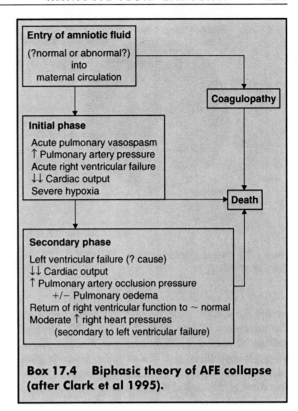

Box 17.4 Biphasic theory of AFE collapse (after Clark et al 1995).

In the secondary phase, right ventricular function returns to normal and the predominant feature is of left ventricular failure, with or without evidence of pulmonary oedema. Whether this is due to hypoxic damage, reduced coronary artery blood flow or direct myocardial depression by factors in amniotic fluid is unknown. Pulmonary vascular pressures may be elevated secondary to impaired left ventricular function.

Pulmonary oedema

Steiner and Lushbaugh considered pulmonary oedema to be one of the cardinal features of AFE, and it has been reported in many cases since.[1] The reported incidence appears very variable, from 93% of patients who did not die in the initial phase,[10] to 24%[2] and 25% in survivors (see Table 17.3). The distinction between pulmonary oedema and acute respiratory distress syndrome (ARDS) is indistinct in these reports, and cases are probably due to either/or a combination of left ventricular dysfunction and pulmonary capillary membrane leak.[39,60]

Cardiac arrest

Cardiac arrest is not uncommon in AFE and was reported in 87% of patients in the US Registry

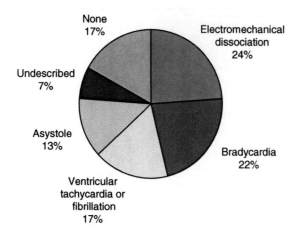

Chart 17.2   Initial dysrhythmias in AFE (after Clark et al 1995).

review, in whom early cardiac dysrhythmias were also common (Chart 17.2).[10] Of the 40 arrested patients, 12 were successfully resuscitated and survived, although only three (i.e. 8% of those who suffered cardiac arrest) survived neurologically intact.[10] Over one-third of the cardiac arrests occurred within 5 min of symptom onset. Compared to these disastrous figures, however, survivors of AFE appear to suffer cardiac arrest less frequently (only 25%) and have a much better intact neurological success rate (53% of those who suffered cardiac arrest).

COAGULOPATHY

Significant coagulopathy, usually labelled as disseminated intravascular coagulation (DIC), is a common occurrence in AFE of all grades of severity, and low levels of plasma fibrinogen have been reported by many authors. Coagulopathy is widely reported to occur in 40% of patients who do not die of the initial haemodynamic insult of AFE, and Morgan reported 49% of patients developed pathological bleeding.[2] However, this may underestimate the problem, since 78% of survivors reviewed here were reported to have developed coagulopathy (Table 17.4). Furthermore, Clark et al reported that out of 46 patients with 'classic' AFE, 38 had laboratory ($n = 34$) or clinical ($n = 4$) evidence of coagulopathy (the other eight died too quickly for assessment), and eight patients had very severe coagulopathy, with undetectable levels of fibrinogen. Some authors consider that AFE is always associated with some form of intravascular coagulopathy and bleeding tendency, even if not clinically apparent.[117,118] Unexpected haemorrhage due to coagulopathy may also be the presenting sign, or

even the only clinical sign, of AFE (as in the 'forme fruste' variant).[71]

The clinical coagulopathy appears to be due to a variable degree of *excessive coagulation, excessive fibrinolysis and/or excessive fibrinogenolysis*.[117,119,120] Excessive fibrinolysis has been demonstrated in AFE[75,120–122] and may result from the direct release of activating factors in amniotic fluid or be secondary to the deposition of fibrin in the circulation caused by the activated clotting process (DIC).[117,119] The relative lack of post-mortem evidence of intravascular thrombi may be due to their breakdown by the exaggerated fibrinolytic process.

Life-threatening haemorrhage is a likely consequence of DIC in AFE and the assistance of a senior haematologist should be sought urgently. Uterine atony is a common finding in AFE and will aggravate haemorrhage due to coagulopathy. Management dilemmas are discussed below.

TIMING

In the great majority of cases, AFE strikes during labour before delivery (70%[10] to 90%[2]), or in the immediate postpartum period. Most cases occur at, or around, term, but AFE has been reported in association with both preterm labour,[50,57,123] termination of pregnancy (including saline abortion)[16,28,55,57,70] and non-labouring 2nd trimester pregnancies.[48,62,91,99]

Data from the US Registry shows that 30% of AFE occurred after delivery (either vaginal or Caesarean), and that in two-thirds of these women it developed very rapidly, within 5 min of delivery.[10] Several cases have been reported during Caesarean section performed for standard obstetric indications, again usually (but not always) occurring immediately after delivery of the neonate.[10,80,85,100] Isolated reports suggest that the post-delivery onset of AFE may be delayed by 1,[59] 2,[53,124] 8,[80] 16[60] or even 24 h.[30]

One striking feature arising from the US Registry was the temporal relationship between the onset of AFE collapse and artificial rupture of the membranes or intra-uterine pressure catheter placement.[10] In five women, collapse occurred within 3 min of the procedure, suggesting iatrogenic trauma was involved. Further information is required. Another interesting point noted by Burrows and Khoo was that in four of five women who developed AFE after delivery, onset occurred very shortly after the administration of an intravenous bolus of syntocinon.[20] Whether the use of bolus syntocinon is related causally or simply coincidental is unclear.

Table 17.5 Unusual associations with AFE (References)	
Prostaglandin/ Saline-induced abortion	16,33,205–209, 210*,214
Curettage abortion	211
Insertion of intra-uterine pressure catheter	10,82
Osmotic cervical dilation prior to abortion	212
Saline amnio-infusion for meconium	33,129,213
Intra-uterine fetal death/missed abortion	1,12,41,50,55,57, 72,90,125,127
Intra-uterine contraceptive device	104,215,216
Blunt abdominal trauma	68
Amniocentesis	31,43,118,217
Castor oil ingestion	89

*Glucose-induced abortion.

PREDISPOSING (OR ASSOCIATED) FACTORS

Many early reports suggested that elderly, multiparous women having short, tumultuous labours, especially when augmented with oxytocic agents, were particularly at risk of AFE.[41,125–127] In fact, there appears to be very little evidence to support any of these long-standing beliefs about predisposing factors for AFE, and, of course, the majority of deliveries occur in multiparous women, and augmentation or induction of labour is extremely common. However, UK data does support the fact that the mortality risk of AFE increases with maternal age.[105]

In his review of 272 cases, Morgan states '*In view of the very wide use of accelerated labour and the rarity of amniotic fluid embolism, it must be concluded that there is no direct association between the two*'.[2] Similarly, data from the US Registry suggests no causative link between hypertonic contractions and the occurrence of AFE, and '*any relation between oxytocin and this syndrome has been refuted on theoretical, statistical and clinical grounds*'.[10] Uterine hypertonus, as occasionally described, is likely to be a secondary phenomenon due to acute uterine hypoxia and massive catecholamine release consequent on the acute haemodynamic collapse (although uterine atony is probably more common).

Other reported associations with AFE are shown in Table 17.5. Without denominator values it is difficult to reliably link AFE with any of these conditions, and causal links are even harder to find. However, there are apparent connections which provoke interesting questions:

- The number of cases reported following saline/ urea abortions in the USA.
- Recent reports that women carrying a male fetus are more likely to develop AFE suggesting an immunological aetiology.[10,128]
- The role of high intra-uterine pressures when infusion devices are used for saline amnio-infusion for meconium – Maher advocates the use of gravity in preference to mechanical pumps.[129]

ANIMAL STUDIES

In view of the difficulties involved in studying human patients, animal models have been used to investigate the potential haemodynamic effects of AFE. However, as Clark[4,5,7,8] and Hankins et al[110] eloquently remonstrate, most of these experimental studies in lower animals have been flawed in design, produced inconsistent results, and have been extrapolated inappropriately to humans. Whole animal studies are summarized in Table 17.6.

Most of these studies involved the use of heterologous, usually human, amniotic fluid injected into animals, many of which were male or non-pregnant females. The amniotic fluid was often not freshly collected, and given in unphysiologically large volumes with very thick (i.e. similarly inappropriate) meconium or particulate contamination. Several of these studies suggested that intravenous injection of (particulate and/or clear) amniotic fluid into the maternal circulation caused rapid death (rabbits and dogs), haematological derangement, or adverse haemodynamic effects. These ranged from transient alterations in systemic and pulmonary artery pressures (PAP) in dogs, sheep, cats and calves to sudden death in rabbits.[7]

In two early animal studies where haemodynamic measurements were taken, PAP, central venous pressure (CVP) and pulmonary vascular resistance (PVR) rose dramatically after intravenous injection of amniotic fluid.[115,116] In both studies there was rapid resolution of pulmonary vascular effects, and no rise in pulmonary artery occlusion pressure (PAOP) and no pulmonary oedema was observed. Evidence from these studies has been used, rather selectively and exclusively, to support the theory that the principal haemodynamic result of AFE in humans is acute cor pulmonale due to severe pulmonary hypertension resulting from occlusive or vasospastic changes in the pulmonary vasculature.[7] However, observation of human cases suggests this is not the whole story (see below).

Table 17.6

Investigator	Ref. no.	Year	Animal	AF species	n	Anaesthetized	Pregnant	AF
Steiner	1	1941	Rabbit	Human	9	No	No	Fresh
Steiner	1	1941	Dog	Human	11	No	No	Fresh
Cron et al	219	1952	Rabbit	Human	14	Variable	No	Stored
Schneider	220	1955	Dog	Human	10	No	No	Stored
Stefanini and Turpini	179	1959	Dog	Dog (homologous)	1	?	No	Stored
Jaques et al	221	1960	Dog	Human/dog	9	Yes	No	Either
Halmagyi et al	222	1962	Sheep	Human	7	Yes	No	Stored
Attwood and Downing	115	1965	Dog	Human	44	Yes	No	Fresh
Stolte et al	131	1967	Monkey	Human/monkey	12	Yes	Yes	Fresh
MacMillan	223	1968	Rabbit	Human	12	No	No	
Reis et al	116	1969	Sheep	Sheep	10	Yes	Yes	Fresh
Dutta et al	177	1970	Rabbit	Human	34	Yes	No	Fresh
Adamsons et al	130	1971	Monkey	Monkey	9	Yes	Yes	Fresh
Kitzmiller and Lucas	154	1972	Cat	Human	?	Yes	No	
Spence and Mason	132	1974	Rabbit	Rabbit (homologous)	26	No	Yes	Fresh
Reeves	224	1974	Calf	Calf (homologous)	14	No	No	Stored
Azegami and Mori	155	1986	Rabbit	Human	36	No	No	Stored
Hankins et al	110	1993	Goat	Goat (autologous)	29	Yes	Yes	Fresh
El-Maradny et al	157	1995	Rabbit	Human	24	No	50%	Stored

Notes: n/e = Not examined, *ml (not ml/kg).
Abbreviations:
$\uparrow$ = increased, $\downarrow$ = reduced, $\rightarrow$ = normal, BP = blood pressure, PAP = pulmonary artery pressure, CO = cardiac
PAOP = pulmonary artery occlusion pressure, RR = respiratory rate, P_aO_2 = arterial oxygen tension, S_aO_2 = arterial

Animal studies

Effects seen with			Volume (ml/kg)	Arterial injection	Pathologic venous	Coagulopathy	Haemodynamic effects
Filtered AF	Raw AF	Meconium					
No	Yes	Yes	1–30*	n/e	Yes	No	n/e
n/e	n/e	Yes	7–4	n/e	Yes	No	n/e
n/e	Yes	Yes	1–8.8	No	Yes	No	n/e
n/e	n/e	Yes		n/e	Yes	5/8	n/e
n/e	mild then severe	n/e	<1	n/e	No then Yes	Yes	Minimal effects 1st dose – ↓ BP, ↓ fibrinogen, ↓ platelets after 2nd dose (1/12 later)
n/e	Yes	n/e	9–50*	n/e	Yes	↓ Fibrinogen 12/13	↑ PAP, → BP
No	Yes	n/e	1–2	n/e	Yes	No	↑ PAP, ↑ PVR, → BP, → CO, → SVR
mild	Yes	Yes	1.7–5.0	Yes	Yes	4/12	↑ PAP, ↑ PVR, → ↑ LAP, ↓ BP, ↓ CO, ↓ SVR
n/e	mild	Yes	2.9–9.2	No	No	No	↓ → BP, → Pulse
n/e	Yes	n/e	1–10*	Yes	Yes	2/12	n/e
Yes	Yes	n/e	<2.5	Yes	Yes	No	↑ PAP, ↑ PVR, → LAP, ↓ BP, ↓ CO, ↓ SVR, → PAOP, ↑ CVP
n/e	Yes	n/e	2.5	n/e	Yes	No	n/e
n/e	No	n/e	<5	n/e	No	No	↑ BP, → Pulse, → RR
No	Yes	No	3	n/e	Yes	No	↓ BP, ↓ Pulse, ↑ CVP
No	No	n/e	2.5	n/e	No	No	→ BP, → Pulse, → RR
n/e	Yes	n/e	0.04–0.07	n/e	Yes		↑ BP, ↑ PAP, → CO, → PAOP
No	Yes	n/e	6.4–9.9	n/e	Yes	No	n/e
Yes	Yes	Yes (severe)	2.5	n/e	Yes		↑ BP, ↑ PAP, ↑ PVR, (meconium ↑↑ SVR, ↓↓ CO, ↑↑ PAOP, ↑ lung water, ↓ P$_a$O$_2$, ↓ SVO$_2$, ↓ S$_a$O$_2$)
Yes	Yes	Yes (maximal)	3	n/e	Yes		↑ Endothelin levels: meconium AF > raw AF > supernatant AF

output, CVP = central venous pressure, PVR = pulmonary vascular resistance, SVR = systemic vascular resistance, oxygen saturation, SVO$_2$ = mixed venous oxygen saturation, LAP = left atrial pressure.

In an important more recent study using invasive monitoring in a pregnant goat model, intravenous injection of autologous amniotic fluid (filtered, filtered and boiled or raw amniotic fluid) produced similar transient rises in both pulmonary and systemic vascular pressures.[110] Maximal effects occurred virtually simultaneously on systemic and pulmonary circulations within 10 min and had generally resolved within 30 min. That these three forms of amniotic fluid produced significantly greater effects than volume infusion in controls suggests that the pressor effects are largely due to a soluble heat-stable compound.

When meconium-stained amniotic fluid was used, however, the pressor effects were significantly greater, and associated with a marked fall in cardiac output and rise in PAOP. Whether this acute left ventricular failure was due to the marked rise in SVR, or due to direct effects from exposure to (meconium-containing) amniotic fluid (e.g. reduced coronary artery flow, acute hypoxaemia or direct myocardial depression) is unclear. Other significant effects observed when meconium-stained amniotic fluid was used to include a transient increase in extravascular lung water and a marked, persistent reduction in oxygen delivery and uptake which outlasted all measured haemodynamic effects.[110]

However, two remarkable studies that undermine all conventional concepts of AFE need highlighting, particularly since they have been largely ignored. Both were performed in monkeys (higher primates, presumably better models for humans), and showed that intravenous injection of *autologous* amniotic fluid did not produce any adverse physiological effects, or signs of AFE syndrome.[130,131] In another study, freshly collected autologous amniotic fluid injected into rabbits produced no changes in heart rate, blood pressure or respiratory rate compared to controls.[132] These studies, in conjunction with growing human evidence that sub-clinical entry of amniotic fluid into the maternal circulation may not be uncommon (see below), suggest that amniotic fluid need not be as dangerous as previously presumed. The concept that the AFE syndrome may result either from the entry of *abnormal* amniotic fluid into the maternal circulation, or from an *abnormal maternal response* to normal amniotic fluid appears more feasible.

DIAGNOSIS

CLINICAL DIAGNOSIS

The initial diagnosis is usually made on clinical grounds following the sudden onset of characteristic signs and symptoms. Clinical diagnosis alone, however, may be unreliable, since there is a significant risk of labelling all unexplained collapses as AFE without valid evidence. In addition, a growing awareness that patients may not show the 'classic' features of AFE has lowered the threshold of suspicion in any woman who develops unexplained cyanosis, hypotension or coagulopathy in pregnancy or after delivery.

HISTOLOGICAL DIAGNOSIS

Since the early descriptions of AFE, the presence of amniotic fluid debris (fetal squamous epithelial cells, mucin, lanugo hair, fat globules, etc.) in maternal lung tissues seen at post-mortem has been considered pathognomonic of AFE.[1,133,134] Squamous cells have been seen in the deep cervical veins in women requiring Caesarean-hysterectomy for AFE.[24,52] Amniotic fluid debris has also been seen in a number of other tissues at post-mortem, including myometrium and broad ligament, kidneys, heart and central nervous system.[125] Standard haematoxylin and eosin staining is unreliable in the detection of amniotic fluid debris,[135] and phloxin tartrazine, Alcian phloxin[136] or Papanicolaou[137] are more reliable general stains (Box 17.5).

Several workers have reported finding amniotic fluid debris in *pulmonary arterial blood* of women suspected of having AFE, suggesting that this may provide confirmed ante-mortem diagnosis.[3,32,60,80,113] Squamous

Squamous cells	Haematoxylin and eosin *Papanicolaou* Phloxin tartrazine Alcian phloxin *also* Rhodamine B Fluorescence[218] Monoclonal antibody TKH-2[150]
NB: difficult to distinguish fetal from maternal squamous cells	
Lanugo hairs from fetal skin	Polarized light
Mucin from fetal gut	Periodic acid–Schiff (PAS) Alcian blue (pH 2.5) Alcian green
Bile from meconium	Haematoxylin and eosin
Fat globules from vernix caseosa	Oil red O stain Sudan black

Box 17.5   Histological diagnosis of AFE.

cells have also been reported in the sputum of patients with AFE.[80,90,93]

An early (1958) study using radio-labelled red blood cells injected into the amniotic sacs of women in early labour suggested that amniotic fluid does not normally enter the maternal circulation.[138] However, autopsies of mothers dying in the perinatal period of other causes, frequently find histological evidence of embolism,[139] and several studies have demonstrated the presence of amniotic fluid debris in pulmonary artery blood of peripartum women *not* considered to have AFE.[4,137,140,141] Squamous cells have also been seen in uterine veins and myometrial tissue in the absence of a clinical diagnosis of AFE.[133]

There is now a growing suspicion that small sub-clinical amounts of amniotic fluid debris, particularly squamous cells, commonly enter the maternal circulation without producing symptoms or being clinically significant.

Minor AFE can be a relatively benign event.[4,139,142,143] It may all be a question of magnitude, where a small amount of amniotic fluid debris represents a common sub-clinical coincident finding, but where '*very considerable contamination of the maternal pulmonary vessels with fetal debris ...*' represents pathological AFE.[136,141]

One compounding difficulty in the histological diagnosis is that there is no easy or reliable way of differentiating fetal from maternal squamous epithelial cells. In addition, contamination of maternal pulmonary blood samples with squamous cells appears to be common.[54,144] However, the absence of Barr bodies or presence of the Y-chromosome (i.e. from a male baby) in squamous cells seen in maternal blood or tissues would strongly suggest that these cells were of fetal origin.

An alternative interpretation of the presence of amniotic fluid debris in pulmonary aspirates of parturients without a diagnosis of AFE (but who are usually unwell enough for other reasons to require invasive monitoring) is that AFE may, in fact, contribute to other pathological conditions (e.g. placental abruption, pulmonary embolism).

In an attempt to ascertain the prevalence and relevance of amniotic fluid debris in maternal pulmonary tissues in the absence of clinical AFE, the authors of the UK 1991–93 triennial mortality report urged pathologists to specifically look for evidence of AFE at post-mortem in all maternal deaths.[105]

It would appear that there may be '*a quantitative continuum of (amniotic fluid material) transported to the central circulation in peripartum patients which may, in part, explain the varied clinical presentations and severity of*

AFE'.[141] In view of the current controversies, therefore, *cytological evidence of AFE should not be considered pathognomonic in the absence of appropriate clinical evidence.* However, at a time when the clinical criteria of suspicion for AFE is being broadened to encompass more varied, less dramatic, non-lethal presentations, this makes the diagnosis of AFE even more uncertain!

OTHER DIAGNOSTIC TESTS

Several *immunohistochemical techniques* have been described which purport to demonstrate evidence of AFE debris (keratin,[145] mucin,[146,149] syncytiotrophoblast cells[147]) more reliably than regular histological staining. Several interesting reports come from Japan. In one, AFE was confirmed post-mortem by the use of a *fetal red blood cell isoantigen marker.*[148]

Kobayashi and colleagues developed a *monoclonal antibody* (TKH-2) to detect the presence of meconium and amniotic fluid derived mucin (sialyl Tn antigen) in maternal serum.[149,150]

Another group showed that *zinc coproporphyrin-I* (ZnCP-I, a component of meconium) is present in the plasma of parturients with or without AFE, but in much higher concentration in those women with AFE (four cases confirmed, three suspected).[46]

Unfortunately, whilst interesting, most of these new tests appear to be little more than research tools.

AETIOLOGY

AMNIOTIC FLUID

In the first trimester, amniotic fluid comprises approximately 50 ml of isotonic solution and represents an extension of fetal and maternal extravascular compartments, without any particulate matter. As pregnancy progresses, amniotic fluid increases in volume and contains increasing amounts of fetal debris, (e.g. squamous epithelial cells, mucin from fetal gastrointestinal and respiratory tracts, lanugo and scalp hair, and lipid material from sebaceous glands), including fetal blood group substances.[31,151] The particulate content of amniotic fluid only becomes significant in the last month of pregnancy.[152] Normal amniotic fluid volume at term is 750–1000 ml.

Vaso-active effects

Amniotic fluid also contains prostaglandins (particularly PGE_2 and $PGF_{2\alpha}$) and other arachidonic acid metabolites in concentrations which vary with the stage of gestation, increasing towards term, with high peak levels occurring in labour.[151] Other related compounds found in amniotic fluid include prostacyclin, thromboxanes and leucotrienes, many of which also increase significantly during labour which is the commonest time for AFE to occur.[153]

Clark has postulated that leucotrienes C4 and D4 may be the agents involved in many of the physiological changes seen in AFE.[3] Labour seems to be an important factor in the vaso-active potential of amniotic fluid.[154] Azegami and Mori showed that suppression of leucotriene production (with a lipoxygenase inhibitor) prevented the experimental development of AFE in rabbits, again suggesting the involvement of a humoral factor in the pathogenesis of AFE.[155] Human amniotic fluid surfactant has been shown to stimulate the production of leucotrienes by both human white blood cells and rabbit lung tissue, and may therefore have a role in stimulating leucotriene production in AFE.[156]

It is interesting that although particulate or meconium-stained amniotic fluid has been shown experimentally to be a more potent cause of haemodynamic disturbance, published cases do not reflect this. Whilst there are many published case reports of severe AFE associated with meconium, Clark reported that most patients in the US Registry who died of 'classic' AFE had clear amniotic fluid (i.e. no meconium).[10] However, the increased morbidity and mortality associated with AFE in the presence of meconium or dead baby suggest that amniotic fluid in these conditions contains substances, which produce a more severe reaction than when clear amniotic fluid is present.

A study by El-Maradny et al showed that injection of human amniotic fluid into rabbits produced a rise in serum *endothelin*, particularly when meconium-stained or supernatant amniotic fluid was used.[157] Endothelin is a highly potent vasoconstrictor, and hence its production as a consequence to the entry of amniotic fluid into the maternal circulation (particularly with meconium) may explain the transient pulmonary hypertension which is thought to characterize the initial phase of AFE.

Coagulation effects

Amniotic fluid contains several pro-coagulant substances, which may trigger excessive coagulation and lead to a consumptive coagulopathy in the event of entry into the maternal circulation. The pro-coagulant effects of amniotic fluid will shorten whole blood clotting time, induce platelet aggregation, activate factor X and behave like thromboplastin, initiating the conversion of prothrombin to thrombin.[158,159] These effects

increase towards term[160–162] and during labour.[163] Lockwood et al demonstrated that amniotic fluid contains tissue factor, which accounted for virtually all the coagulant potential, and that levels of amniotic tissue factor increase with gestational age.[162] Amniotic fluid may also contain maternal trophoblastic tissue, which has strong thromboplastic effects,[75,117,127] and arachidonic acid and metabolites which may induce platelet aggregation.[3] Fibrinolytic mechanisms may also be triggered.[122] Amniotic fluid will activate complement, particularly when taken from mothers with distressed pregnancies.[164] In addition, plasma complement of pregnant women appears to be more easily activated than in non-pregnant controls.

A case report of AFE precipitated by amniocentesis suggests that entry into the maternal circulation of fetal blood group substances contained in amniotic fluid may provoke a severe ABO incompatibility reaction necessitating exchange transfusion.[31] Considering the potential role that ABO incompatibility may play in AFE, it is perhaps surprising that there have been so few reports of its occurrence.

ENTRY OF AMNIOTIC FLUID INTO MATERNAL CIRCULATION

During pregnancy, standard teaching suggests that there is normally no route of access for amniotic fluid to enter the maternal circulation (although recent histological evidence suggests that small amounts of amniotic fluid may commonly enter the maternal circulation during pregnancy with little pathological consequence). However, at delivery, trauma may disrupt the protective barriers. Almost all reports of AFE have occurred after membrane rupture, and several routes of entry may be postulated:

1. *Endocervical and lower uterine veins* – which may be lacerated in normal labour.
2. *Placental separation site* – following normal or premature separation (as in placental abruption).
3. *Uterine wall* – integrity breached at Caesarean section, in uterine rupture and iatrogenic trauma (e.g. amniocentesis or intra-uterine pressure catheter placement). Potential sites of entry of amniotic fluid are sometimes seen on post-mortem inspection of the uterus.[112,165]

   Absence of uterine involution (i.e. uterine atony) would prevent normal postpartum obliteration of uterine veins.

Histological evidence of amniotic fluid debris is most commonly (looked for and) found in the lungs, but occasional reports show that distant organs (i.e. kidney, central nervous system) may also contain amniotic fluid debris.[115,125,133,148] The mechanism by which this occurs is unknown, but an increase in right atrial pressure, (secondary to acute pulmonary vasoconstriction), may allow amniotic fluid to pass through a patent foramen ovale, (which possibly exists in 25% of the population).[166,167]

In the editorial accompanying an Australian review of maternal mortality associated with Caesarean section,[168] in which the only two deaths were due to AFE, it is suggested that the technique of Caesarean section may itself be important. It is postulated that 'undue force by an assistant on the fundus to help deliver the infant's head can cause amniotic fluid embolism'. However, whilst possible, there is no evidence to support this claim, and not all cases of AFE appear to be related to increased intra-uterine pressure or uterine contraction.

Several workers have reported Doppler evidence of micro-air embolism (with or without symptoms) frequently occurring during uterine incision and manipulation at Caesarean section.[169–172] It is therefore recommended that *a small degree of head-up tilt should be employed during* all *Caesarean sections to minimize the risks of embolization occurring during surgery*.

PULMONARY VASCULAR OBSTRUCTION

Early reports of 'classic' AFE presented histological evidence of extensive amniotic fluid debris (mostly squamous cells and mucin) in the pulmonary vasculature.[1,136,143] Physical plugging of the pulmonary vasculature with embolized amniotic fluid was thought to produce acute right heart failure and the 'shock' of AFE. The finding that amniotic fluid can provoke similar responses when given either intravenously, or intra-arterially, suggests that the obliterative effects of particulate matter on the lungs are inconsequential to the development of the syndrome.[7] Hence, it appears more likely that the acute right heart failure produced in AFE is due to triggering of a vasospastic process rather than physical obstruction with amniotic fluid debris in the vast majority of cases. The finding that human endothelial cells produce endothelin on exposure to amniotic fluid material supports this hypothesis.[157]

However, cases of massive pulmonary embolism have been reported in AFE,[35,173] and in other reports of apparently isolated obliterative venous or pulmonary embolism the thrombus has been found to contain extensive evidence of amniotic fluid debris.[174,175] It would appear, therefore, that the distinction between venous thrombo-embolism and AFE may not be entirely discrete, and AFE may be associated with the development of small and large size thrombi. It has been suggested that aortocaval compression causes venous stasis in large vessels such as the inferior vena cava, which, in combination with AFE may produce clots and consequent pulmonary embolism.[176]

IS AFE AN ANAPHYLACTOID REACTION?

Since its first description in 1941, the clinical similarity between AFE and a severe allergic reaction has been apparent to many authors.[7] Clark has also drawn attention to the common features with septic shock.[8] Whilst neither anaphylactic nor anaphylactoid reactions have been proven, there is growing evidence to suggest an immunological or allergic component to the AFE syndrome:

- AFE does not usually appear to be due to physical obstruction of the pulmonary vasculature with amniotic fluid debris.[7]
- Forty-one per cent of patients with AFE in the US Registry had a previous history of drug allergy or atopy, and difficulty in ventilation or bronchospasm was seen in several patients.[10]
- Many of the mediators associated with anaphylactoid reactions are thought to be released in AFE: including histamine, bradykinin, cytokines, leucotrienes, prostaglandins, thromboxanes, and others.[151]
- Arachidonic acid metabolites have been shown experimentally to produce similar physiological and haemodynamic changes to those observed in human AFE.[151]
- Pre-treatment with a leucotriene inhibitor has been shown to prevent experimental (heterologous) AFE collapse and death in rabbits.[155]
- Treatment with an antihistamine reduced the degree of 'shock' and prolonged life in experimental (heterologous) AFE in rabbits.[177]
- Steroids have been used successfully in the management of a number of patients who have survived AFE.

Clark and his colleagues have suggested that the name '*amniotic fluid embolism*' is both inaccurate and unhelpful, and should be discarded in preference for '*the anaphylactoid syndrome of pregnancy*'. This suggests a 'non-immune'-mediated degranulation of mast cells, although other workers consider an antigen–antibody-mediated anaphylactic reaction to be more feasible.[18,178] If, as is suspected, sub-clinical AFE occurs relatively commonly during pregnancy, this would provide obvious opportunity for sensitization to occur. Stefanini and Turpini supports this hypothesis, since they showed that injection of a single bolus of homologous amniotic fluid in a dog produced minimal effects. However, marked hypotension and coagulation defects followed the administration of a second identical dose 1 month later.[179]

Benson and Lindberg have suggested serum should be taken from women with suspected AFE and tryptase levels checked.[180] Elevated levels would be strongly supportive of an anaphylactoid or anaphylactic causation.

RECOGNITION OF AFE

Current understanding of AFE suggests that the clinical presentation of the condition may vary enormously, from the full-blown 'classic' AFE collapse with death occurring within minutes to much more insidious and subtle variants (Boxes 17.1 and 17.2).

It is important to maintain a low threshold of suspicion so that some of the non-classic cases of AFE are picked up in time to make appropriate therapeutic intervention. Although many severe cases appear unsalvageable, the sooner the diagnosis is considered, the sooner optimal care and intensive care support may be offered.

MANAGEMENT OF AFE

The pathophysiological processes in AFE are still poorly understood, and hence the management of suspected AFE is almost entirely supportive, being derived from basic principles. Advice from the most experienced members of the medical teams and the intensive care unit should be sought at an early stage. Successful management may depend on the rapid provision of aggressive therapy (Boxes 17.6 and 17.7).

There are three main therapeutic goals:

- restoration of oxygen delivery to tissues
  - oxygenation of blood
  - restoration of cardiac output;
- treatment of coagulopathy;
- prevention of further complications.

RESTORATION OF OXYGEN DELIVERY

Airway

Following simple ABC guidelines, initial assessment of the patient's level of consciousness and protective airway reflexes will reveal whether immediate protection of the airway with intubation is required.

Breathing

Profound cyanosis is usual, and delivery of a high concentration of oxygen will have several beneficial effects:

- improvement of hypoxaemia,
- improvement in oxygen delivery to tissues,
- minimize hypoxic injury to brain,
- minimize myocardial ischaemia,
- minimize metabolic acidosis,
- minimize hypoxic pulmonary vasoconstriction.

In the mild, or diagnostically equivocal case, where the airway is competent and the patient breathing effectively, 60% oxygen should be administered via a facemask. However, there should be a low threshold for the use of intubation and controlled ventilation since this will allow higher inspired oxygen concentrations and control of P_aCO_2.

The development of pulmonary oedema (cardiogenic, capillary membrane leak or iatrogenic fluid overload) will require early expert management and aggressive monitoring and intervention. Steroids are

---

Venous blood
- Hb
- Platelet count
- Prothrombin time (PT)
- Partial thromboplastin time (PTTK)
- Fibrinogen
- FDP/D-dimer levels
- Tryptase (? anaphylaxis)
    also *U & E, liver function tests*

CVP/PA blood
- Save for histology (? AF debris)

Arterial blood
- Gases (S_aO_2, pH)

Chest X-ray (? Pulmonary oedema)

Box 17.6   Investigations.

ECG
Non-invasive blood pressure
Invasive blood pressure
S_aO_2
End-tidal CO_2
CVP (? right ventricular failure)
Urinary catheter
Cardiotocograph
Pulmonary artery catheter
Cardiac output

Box 17.7   Monitoring.

controversial in the management of acute respiratory failure, but have been used in a number of patients who have survived AFE, with or without pulmonary oedema.

Circulation

A dramatic fall in cardiac output is common, and if Clark's biphasic model is correct, this is associated with early *transient* acute right heart failure followed by more persistent left ventricular failure. In the presence of, (presumed), pulmonary vasospasm the use of pulmonary vasodilators would theoretically have a role. The evanescent nature of the pulmonary vasoconstriction, (lasting less than 30 min), makes it likely that, following an AFE collapse, the pulmonary vasospasm will have passed before the use of such drugs have been thought of and effected. Pulmonary vasodilators except oxygen are also likely to cause significant systemic vasodilation and aggravate hypotension.

Intravenous pulmonary vasodilators that could, in theory, be useful include isoprenaline, GTN, sodium nitroprusside, aminophylline, prostacylin and magnesium sulphate. It must be stressed, however, that despite a theoretical potential there is no clinical evidence to support the use of these drugs to treat (presumed) short-lived pulmonary vasospasm in AFE.

Attention has turned to inhaled therapy, and nitric oxide would seem the potentially ideal agent to use, although it is unlikely to be available for use in the acute collapse situation. *Inhaled aerosolized prostacyclin* has been used successfully in a woman who suffered acute respiratory failure and severe hypoxaemia due to AFE.[95]

Oxygen is an effective pulmonary vasodilator, readily available, safe and easy to use, *and is the clear first therapeutic choice*: it should be administered in the highest concentration possible during the early resuscitative period.

The initial response to hypotension is commonly to infuse fluid, but in the presence of acute right heart failure this is likely to be inappropriate. Early insertion of a CVP line will allow detection of a high CVP, suggestive of pulmonary vasospasm, in which case fluid infusion should not be given.

All human evidence suggests that any right heart failure is very short-lived, and that patients rapidly develop *left heart failure*. Information from a pulmonary artery catheter may be invaluable and guide fluid and inotrope administration, and should be inserted as early as possible once the diagnosis of AFE has been considered.

Loss of intravascular volume due to haemorrhage will reduce cardiac output and requires replacement, preferably under pulmonary artery catheter guidance. Uterine atony will increase the risk of uterine haemorrhage and should be prevented with the use of a syntocinin infusion or ergometrine if necessary. In the event of continuing haemorrhage *due to uterine atony*, the use of carboprost (15-methyl prostaglandin $F_{2\alpha}$ – Hemabate®), or its natural analogue prostaglandin $F_{2\alpha}$) may be considered. However, whilst being well established as effective in the treatment of uterine atony,[181,182] the smooth muscle constriction produced by these drugs may produce a worrying increase in PAP.[183,184] The anticipated beneficial effect of reduced blood loss must be balanced against the potentially detrimental and largely unknown effects that may result from their use in AFE. The risks of haemodynamic catastrophe in AFE are likely to be greatly increased if these drugs are given in overdose.[182,185] In general, however, if continuing haemorrhage due to uterine atony is a major problem, a cautious trial of carboprost seems reasonable in the absence of evidence of raised PAP. Prostaglandin E_2 may theoretically be preferable since it has been shown to have minimal effect on PVR, although it reduces both systemic vascular resistance and blood pressure, and is less commonly available.[184]

Transfer to an *intensive care unit* should be arranged as soon as possible, although an undelivered fetus is likely to need urgent delivery by Caesarean section.

Few specific details are published about the intensive care management of cases or the choice of inotropic support. Where details are given, dobutamine, dopamine and epinephrine are, not surprisingly, the most commonly mentioned. Patients will need to be managed on an individual basis, and the choice of inotropic agents will be guided by local experience, and the response to therapy (including information about oxygen delivery and uptake from pulmonary artery monitoring).

Monitoring

Standard monitoring comprising continuous pulse oximetry and ECG, and intermittent (automatic) non-invasive blood pressure should be rapidly supplemented with early insertion of CVP, pulmonary artery and direct arterial blood pressure catheters (which will facilitate frequent arterial blood gas analysis). Samples of pulmonary microvascular blood should be taken for cytological analysis to help confirm the diagnosis. Intubated, ventilated patients should have full airway monitoring, and, where available, a transoesophageal echo device may offer useful, rapid non-invasive information about cardiac output. If undelivered, fetal heart monitoring is indicated.

Cardiac arrest before delivery

Cardiorespiratory arrest may occur within minutes of the onset of first symptoms in cases of 'classic' AFE collapse. If the mother is undelivered, effective cardiopulmonary resuscitation (CPR) is unlikely due to the inevitable aortocaval compression and the increased oxygen demands of the feto-placental unit. Immediate management will include intubation with cricoid pressure, hyperventilation with 100% oxygen, external cardiac massage, defibrillation and pharmacological support as per standard Advanced Life Support (ALS) guidelines.[186] Aortocaval compression must be minimized by uterine tilt.[187]

Clark et al showed that neonatal outcome following AFE collapse was dependent on a short cardiac arrest-to-delivery interval[10] (Table 17.3). Current ALS Guidelines and a 1997 Advisory Statement from the International Liaison Committee on Resuscitation dicate that *delivery should occur within 5 min of cardiac arrest* if the patient does not respond to initial resuscitation.[67,109,186,188,189–191]

TREATMENT OF COAGULOPATHY

Since both DIC and excessive fibrinolysis may be triggered in AFE, and the treatment of each may be different, early discussion and advice from an experienced haematologist is imperative. Consumptive coagulopathy will cause a fall in levels of platelets, fibrinogen and factors V and VIII, and fibrinolysis will lead to the breakdown of fibrin, fibrinogen and factors V and VIII. Low plasma fibrinogen levels are a common finding, as are elevated fibrin degradation products (FDPs) or D-dimer levels (Box 17.6).

Standard management will include volume resuscitation and replacement of depleted blood products with red blood cells, plasma cryoprecipitate and platelets as considered appropriate. Whilst it is common practice in the face of falling fibrinogen levels to administer fresh frozen plasma or cryoprecipitate, there is a theoretical risk of aggravating intravascular coagulation in the early consumptive phase of DIC.

The early use of *heparin* during the initial, hypercoagulable stage of DIC when intravascular coagulation is occurring has been proposed,[2,119,192] and there are numerous reports of its use in survivors of AFE.[13,17,26,31,32,35,44,49,55,56,58,62,64,68,82,84,90,93] Relatively low doses may be needed during this early

phase, but heparin is less appropriate during the later phase which is characterized by intravascular deposition of fibrin.[119] *The use of heparin in DIC has been controversial for several years, and it has not entered established clinical practice.*

Isolated reports suggest that in the presence of excessive fibrinolysis, as reflected by raised FDPs, *fibrinolytic inhibitors* (e.g. amino-caproic acid, tranexamic acid) may be useful.[17,53,99,119,193] More recently, *aprotinin* has been recommended in two case reports for the acute management of acute massive obstetric haemorrhage[194,195] and has also been used successfully in AFE.[40,48,196] Morgan recommends that the administration of fibrinogen should be accompanied by fibrinolytic inhibitors in the presence of raised FDPs.[2] Aprotinin seems a logical treatment choice if there is evidence that the main haematological problem is of fibrinolysis, and it would be interesting to see further reports of its use in this scenario.

There is little experimental work or current evidence to support the use of heparin, fibrinolytic inhibitors or Dextran 70 in the management of coagulopathy due to suspected AFE, and despite their appeal, their value is currently unclear.

The mainstay of management therefore remains maintenance of circulating intravascular volume with crystalloid, colloid and red cell infusions (to optimize cardiac output and oxygen flux), and transfusion of appropriate blood component coagulation factors (fresh frozen plasma, cryoprecipitate and platelets) to correct the coagulation defect. In view of the complexity and severity of the haematological abnormalities in AFE, the guidance of a senior haematologist should be sought at an early stage. Indeed, it is recommended that a haematologist is contacted at the first indication of the possible diagnosis of AFE, even if coagulopathy is not apparent at that time, since the clinical picture may change with dramatic swiftness.

UNRESOLVED ISSUES

- What is the exact nature of AFE?
- Does sub-clinical AFE occur in normal pregnancy?
- Is it the entry of abnormal amniotic fluid into maternal circulation, or is it an abnormal maternal response to normal amniotic fluid (or both) that causes AFE?
- Does an initial phase of pulmonary vasospasm exist, and if so, is it worth attempting to treat?
- Is AFE an anaphylactoid reaction? Are *steroids* of benefit in treating AFE?

- Does ABO incompatibility, (fetal blood group material entering maternal circulation), play a part in the AFE syndrome?
- Is there a role for the use of *heparin* or *fibrinolytic inhibitors* in the treatment of AFE coagulopathy?
- Is there a relationship between AFE and *placental abruption*? If so, could the coagulopathy of placental abruption be triggered by occult AFE?
- Is there a relationship between AFE and *pulmonary embolism*? If so, could the formation of pulmonary emboli (or peripheral venous thrombosis) be triggered by occult AFE?

SUMMARY

It seems remarkable that AFE, a condition that produces such devastating morbidity and mortality in pregnant women, can still, after 50 years, be such a mystery to us. Perhaps one of the most challenging aspects of this extraordinary condition is the need to change many of the traditional concepts on which AFE was originally established in the light of new information.

Finally, the possibility that minor or sub-clinical AFE is a relatively common occurrence leads one to consider the possible contribution that AFE may make to a whole range of obstetric and peripartum complications and conditions. It is vital, therefore, to maintain a low threshold for considering the diagnosis in a pregnant woman who presents with any of the signs or symptoms of this extraordinary condition.

REFERENCES

1. Steiner PE, Lushbaugh CC. Maternal pulmonary embolism by amniotic fluid. *JAMA* 1941; **117**: 1245–1254, 1340–1345.
2. Morgan M. Amniotic fluid embolism. *Anaesthesia* 1979; **34**: 20–32.
3. Clark SL. Arachidonic acid metabolites and the pathophysiology of amniotic fluid embolism. *Sem Reprod Endocrinol* 1985; **3**: 253–257.
4. Clark SL, Pavlova Z, Greenspoon J et al. Squamous cells in the maternal pulmonary circulation. *Am J Obstet Gynecol* 1986; **154**: 104–106.
5. Clark SL. Amniotic fluid embolism. *Clin Perinatol* 1986; **13**: 801–811.
6. Clark SL, Cotton DB, Gonik B et al. Central hemodynamic alterations in amniotic fluid embolism. *Am J Obstet Gynecol* 1988; **158**: 1124–1126.
7. Clark SL. New concepts of amniotic fluid embolism: a review. *Obstet Gynecol Surv* 1990; **45**: 360–368.
8. Clark SL. Amniotic fluid embolism. *Crit Care Clin* 1991; **7**: 877–881.
9. Clark SL. Successful pregnancy outcomes after amniotic fluid embolism. *Am J Obstet Gynecol* 1992; **167**: 511–512.
10. Clark SL, Hankins GDV, Dudley DA et al. Amniotic fluid embolism: analysis of the national registry. *Am J Obstet Gynecol* 1995; **172**: 1158–1169.
11. Aguillon A, Andjus T, Grayson A et al. Amniotic fluid embolism: a review. *Obstet Gynecol Surv* 1962; **17**: 619–636.
12. Ahmed P, Traube C, Fresko O. Amniotic fluid embolism. *NY State J Med* 1985; **85**: 267–269.
13. Alon E, Atanassoff PG. Successful cardiopulmonary resuscitation of a parturient with amniotic fluid embolism. *Int J Obstet Anesth* 1992; **1**: 205–207.
14. Andrews HJ, Wilson TR. Maternal pulmonary embolism by amniotic fluid. *Ann West Med Surg* 1951; **5**: 127–130.
15. Arnold HR, Gardner JE, Goodman PH. Amniotic pulmonary embolism. *Radiology* 1961; **77**: 629–632.
16. Ballas S, Michowitz M, Lessing JB. Amniotic fluid embolism and disseminated intravascular coagulation complicating hypertonic saline–induced abortion. *Post Grad Med J* 1983; **59**: 127–129.
17. Bates ME, Verma UL, Tejani NA et al. Amniotic fluid embolism. *NY State J Med* 1985; **85**: 265–267.
18. Benson MD. Nonfatal amniotic fluid embolism. *Arch Fam Med* 1993; **2**: 989–994.
19. Botero SD, Holmquist ND. Cytologic diagnosis of amniotic fluid embolism. *Acta Cytological* 1979; **23**(6) 465–466.
20. Burrows A, Khoo SK. The amniotic fluid embolism syndrome: 10 years' experience at a major teaching hospital. *Aust NZ J Obstet Gynaecol* 1995; **35**: 245–250.
21. Cawley LP, Douglass RC, Schneider CL. Nonfatal pulmonary amniotic embolism. *Obstet Gynecol* 1959; **14**: 615–620.
22. Chang M, Herbert WNP. Retinal arteriolar occlusions following amniotic fluid embolism. *Ophthalmology* 1984; **91**: 1634–1637.
23. Chessin H, Greenwald JC. Afibrinogenemia in pregnancy: diagnosis and treatment. *J Mount Sinai Hosp NY* 1953; **20**: 263–266.
24. Cheung ANY, Luk SC. The importance of extensive sampling and examination of cervix in suspected cases of amniotic fluid embolism. *Arch Gynecol Obstet* 1994; **255**: 101–105.
25. Choi DMA, Duffy BL. Amniotic fluid embolism. *Anaesth Intens Care* 1995; **23**: 741–743.
26. Chung AF, Merkatz IR. Survival following amniotic fluid embolism with early heparinization. *Obstet Gynecol* 1973; **42**: 809–814.
27. Cornell SH. Amniotic pulmonary embolism. *Am J Roentgen Rad Ther Nuc Med* 1963; **89**: 1084–1086.

28. Cromey MG, Taylor PJ, Cumming DC. Probable amniotic fluid embolism after first-trimester pregnancy termination. *J Reprod Med* 1983; **28**: 209–211.

29. Dashow EE, Cotterill R, Benedetti TJ et al. Amniotic fluid embolus. A report of two cases resulting in maternal survival. *J Reprod Med* 1989; **34**: 660–666.

30. Devriendt J, Machayekhi S, Staroukine M. Amniotic fluid embolism: another case with non-cardiogenic pulmonary edema. *Intens Care Med* 1995; **21**: 698–700.

31. Dodgson J, Martin J, Boswell J et al. Probable amniotic fluid embolism precipitated by amniocentesis and treated with exchange transfusion. *Br Med J* 1987; **294**: 1322–1323.

32. Dolyniuk M, Orfei E, Vania H et al. Rapid diagnosis of amniotic fluid embolism. *Obstet Gynecol* 1983; **61**: 28S–30S.

33. Dragich DA, Ross AF, Chestnut DH et al. Respiratory failure associated with amnioinfusion during labor. *Anesth Analg* 1991; **72**: 549–551.

34. Ellis GJ, Nunam SP. Amniotic fluid embolism with recovery following laparotrachelotomy. Report of a case. *Med Ann Dist Columbia* 1956; **25**: 375–379.

35. Esposito RA, Grossi EA, Coppa G et al. Successful treatment of postpartum shock caused by amniotic fluid embolism with cardiopulmonary bypass and pulmonary artery thromboembolectomy. *Am J Obstet Gynecol* 1990; **163**: 572–574.

36. Fava S, Galizia AC. Amniotic fluid embolism. *Br J Obstet Gynaecol* 1993; **100**: 1049–1050.

37. Fischbein FI. Ischemic retinopathy following amniotic fluid embolization. *Am J Ophthalmol* 1969; **67**: 351–357.

38. Gad N. Amniotic fluid embolism. *Clin Exp Obst Gyn* 1996; **23**: 248–251.

39. Girard P, Mal H, Laine J-F et al. Left heart failure in amniotic fluid embolism. *Anesthesiology* 1986; **64**: 262–265.

40. Graeff H, Hafter R, Von Hugo R. Molecular aspects of defibrination in a case of amniotic fluid embolism. *Thrombos Haemostas* 1977; **38**: 724–727.

41. Gregory MG, Clayton EM. Amniotic fluid embolism. *Obstet Gynecol* 1973; **42**: 236–244.

42. Hager HF, Davies SD. Nonfatal maternal pulmonary embolism by amniotic fluid. *Am J Obstet Gynecol* 1952; **63**: 901–904.

43. Hasaart THM, Essed GGM. Amniotic fluid embolism after transabdominal amniocentesis. *Eur J Obstet Gynecol Reprod Biol* 1983; **16**: 25–30.

44. Hogberg U, Joelsson I. Amniotic fluid embolism in Sweden, 1951–1980. *Gynecol Obstet Invest* 1985; **20**: 130–137.

45. Howes LJ. Anaphylactoid reaction possibly caused by amniotic fluid embolism. *Int J Obstet Anesth* 1995; **4**: 51–54.

46. Kanayama N, Yamazaki T, Naruse H et al. Determining zinc coproporphyrin in maternal plasma – a new method for diagnosing amniotic fluid embolism. *Clin Chem* 1992; **38**: 526–529.

47. Kates RJ, Schifrin BS. Self-limited acute defibrination in pregnancy: case report. *Am J Obstet Gynecol* 1976; **124**: 432–434.

48. Kelly MC, Bailie K, McCourt KC. A case of amniotic fluid embolism in a twin pregnancy in the second trimester. *Int J Obstet Anesth* 1995; **4**: 175–177.

49. Kircher KF, Roberts WD, Tye JG. Nonfatal amniotic pulmonary embolism. *Am J Roentgen Rad Ther Nucl Med* 1966; **98**: 434–435.

50. Koegler A, Sauder P, Marolf A et al. Amniotic fluid embolism: a case with non-cardiogenic pulmonary edema. *Intens Care Med* 1994; **20**: 45–46.

51. Kumar B, Christmas D. Plasma fibronectin levels in amniotic fluid embolism. *Intens Care Med* 1985; **11**: 273–274.

52. Laforga JBM. Amniotic fluid embolism. Report of two cases with coagulation disorder. *Acta Obstet Gynecol Scand* 1997; **76**: 805–806.

53. Lalos O, Von Schoultz B. Amniotic fluid embolism: a review of the literature with two case reports. *Int J Gynaecol Obstet* 1977; **15**: 48–53.

54. Lee KR, Catalano PM, Ortiz-Giroux S. Cytologic diagnosis of amniotic fluid embolism. *Acta Cytol* 1986; **30**: 177–182.

55. Lees DE, Shin Y, MacNamara TE. Probable amniotic fluid embolism during curettage for a missed abortion. *Anesth Analg* 1977; **56**: 739–742.

56. Lumley J, Owen R, Morgan M. Amniotic fluid embolism. Report of three cases. *Anaesthesia* 1978; **34**: 33–36.

57. Mainprize TC, Maltby JR. Amniotic fluid embolism: a report of four probable cases. *Can Anaesth Soc J* 1986; **33**: 382–387.

58. Maki M, Tachita K, Kawasaki Y et al. Heparin treatment of amniotic fluid embolism. *Tohoku J Exp Med* 1969; **97**: 155–160.

59. Margarson MP. Delayed amniotic fluid embolism following Caesarean section under spinal anaesthesia. *Anaesthesia* 1995; **50**: 804–806.

60. Masson RG, Ruggieri J, Siddiqui MM. Amniotic fluid embolism: definitive diagnosis in a survivor. *Am Rev Resp Dis* 1979; **120**: 187–192.

61. Masson RG. Amniotic fluid embolism. *Clin Chest Med* 1992; **13**: 657–665.

62. Meier PR, Bowes WA. Amniotic fluid embolus-like syndrome presenting in the second trimester of pregnancy. *Obstet Gynecol* 1983; **61**(suppl 3): 315–345.

63. Miles LM. Amniotic fluid pulmonary embolism. Report of a presumptive case with recovery. *West J Surg Obstet Gynecol* 1951; **59**: 403–404.

64. Moore PG, James OF, Saltos N. Severe amniotic fluid embolism: case report with haemodynamic findings. *Anaesth Intens Care* 1982; **10**: 40–44.

65. Newton M. Amniotic fluid embolism: the nonfatal case. *J Mississippi State Med Assoc* 1966; **7**: 607–609.

66. Noble WH, St-Amand J. Amniotic fluid embolus. A report of two cases resulting in maternal survival. *Can J Anaesth* 1993; **40**: 971–980.

67. Oates S, Williams GL, Rees GAD. Cardiopulmonary resuscitation in late pregnancy. *Br Med J* 1988; **297**: 404–405.

68. Olcott C, Robinson AJ, Maxwell TM et al. Amniotic fluid embolism and disseminated intravascular coagulation after blunt abdominal trauma. *J Traum* 1973; **13**: 737–740.

69. Phuapradit W, Nilprapussorn P, Srivannaboon S. Amniotic fluid embolism: a case report with definite diagnosis in a survivor. *J Med Ass Thailan* 1985; **68**: 609–611.

70. Pollak L, Schiffer J, Leonov Y et al. Acute subdural haematoma following disseminated intravascular coagulation associated with an obstetric catastrophe. *Israel J Med Sci* 1995; **31**: 489–491.

71. Porter TF, Clark SL, Dildy GA et al. Isolated disseminated intravascular coagulation and amniotic fluid embolism. *Am J Obstet Gynecol* 1996; **172**: 486.

72. Price TM, Baker VV, Cefalo RC. Amniotic fluid embolism. Three case reports with review of the literature. *Obstet Gynecol Surv* 1985; **40**: 462–475.

73. Pritchard JA, Dugan RJ. Presumed amniotic fluid embolism with recovery. *Ohio State Med J* 1956; **52**: 379–381.

74. Quinn A, Barrett T. Delayed onset of coagulopathy following amniotic fluid embolism: two case reports. *Int J Obstet Anesth* 1993, **2**: 177–180.

75. Ratnoff OD, Vosburgh GJ. Observations of the clotting defect in amniotic fluid embolism. *New Engl J Med* 1952; **247**: 970–973.

76. Ratten GJ. Amniotic fluid embolism – 2 case reports and a review of maternal deaths from this cause in Australia. *Aust NZ Obstet Gynaecol* 1988; **28**: 33–35.

77. Reid DE, Weiner AE, Roby CC. Intravascular clotting and afibrinogenaemia. The presumptive lethal factors in the syndrome of amniotic embolism. *Am J Obstet Gynecol* 1953; **66**: 465–474.

78. Reid DE, Weiner AE, Roby CC. Presumptive amniotic fluid infusion with resultant post-partum hemorrhage due to afibrinogenemia. *JAMA* 1953; **152**: 227–230.

79. Resnik R, Swartz WH, Plumer MH et al. Amniotic fluid embolism with survival. *Obstet Gynecol* 1976; **47**: 295–298.

80. Ricou B, Reper P, Suter PM. Rapid diagnosis of amniotic fluid embolism causing severe pulmonary failure. *Intens Care Med* 1989; **15**: 129–131.

81. Rodgers GP, Heymach GJ. Cryoprecipitate therapy in amniotic fluid embolization. *Am J Med* 1984; **76**: 916–920.

82. Schaerf RHM, de Campo T, Civetta JM. Hemodynamic alterations and rapid diagnosis in a case of amniotic fluid embolism. *Anesthesiology* 1977; **46**: 155–157.

83. Scott MM. Cardiopulmonary considerations in nonfatal amniotic fluid embolism. *JAMA* 1963; **183**: 989–993.

84. Seltzer LM, Schuman W. Nonfatal pulmonary embolism by amniotic fluid contents with report of a possible case. *Am J Obstet Gynec* 1947; **54**: 1038–1046.

85. Shah K, Karlman R, Heller J. Ventricular tachycardia and hypotension with amniotic fluid embolism during cesarean section. *Anesth Analg* 1986; **65**: 533–535.

86. Skjodt P. Amniotic fluid embolism. A case investigated by coagulation and fibrinolysis studies. *Acta Obstet Gynecol Scand* 1965; **44**: 437–457.

87. Spapen HD, Umbrain V, Braekmans P et al. Use of Swan-Ganz catheter in amniotic fluid embolism. *Intens Care Med* 1988; **14**: 678.

88. Sprung J, Rakic M, Patel S. Amniotic fluid embolism during epidural anaesthesia for cesarean section. *Acta Anaesth Belg* 1991; **42**: 225–231.

89. Steingrub JS, Lopez T, Teres D et al. Amniotic fluid embolism associated with castor oil ingestion. *Crit Care Med* 1988; **16**: 642–643.

90. Stromme WB, Fromke VL. Amniotic fluid embolism and disseminated intravascular coagulation after evacuation of missed abortion. *Obstet Gynecol* 1978; **52**(suppl): 76S–80S.

91. Syed SA, Dearden CH. Amniotic fluid embolism: emergency management. *J Accid Emerg Med* 1996; **13**: 285–286.

92. Taenaka N, Shimada Y, Kawai M et al. Survival from DIC following amniotic fluid embolism. Successful treatment with a serine proteinase inhibitor, FOY. *Anaesthesia* 1981; **36**: 389–393.

93. Tuck CS. Amniotic fluid embolus. *Proc Roy Soc Med* 1972; **65**: 94–95.

94. Van Haeften TW, Van Schijndel RJM, Thijs LG. Severe lung damage after amniotic fluid embolism: a case with haemodynamic measurements. *Nether J Med* 1989; **35**: 317–320.

95. Van Heerden PV, Webb SAR, Hee G et al. Inhaled aerosolized prostacyclin as a selective pulmonary vasodilator for the treatment of severe hypoxaemia. *Anaesth Intens Care* 1996; **24**: 87–90.

96. Wasser WG, Tessler S, Kamath CP et al. Nonfatal amniotic fluid embolism: a case report of post-partum respiratory distress with histopathologic studies. *Mount Sinai J Med* 1979; **46**: 388–391.

97. Weksler N, Ovadia L, Stav A et al. Continuous arteriovenous hemofiltration in the treatment of amniotic fluid embolism. *Int J Obstet Anesth* 1994; **3**: 92–96.

98. Willocks J, Mone JG, Thomson WJ. Amniotic fluid embolism: case with biochemical findings. *Brit Med J* 1966; **2**: 1181–1182.

99. Woodfield DG, Galloway RK, Smart GE. Coagulation defect associated with presumed amniotic fluid embolism in the mid-trimester of pregnancy. *J Obstet Gynaec Br Commw* 1971; **78**: 423–429.

100. Zipser G. Amniotic fluid embolism. *Med J Aust* 1971; **2**: 953–956.

101. Department of Health, and others. *Why mothers die. Report on confidential enquiries into maternal deaths in the United Kingdom 1994–1996.* The Stationary Office, 1998.

102. Gabel HD. Maternal mortality in South Carolina from 1970 to 1984: an analysis. *Obstet Gynecol* 1987; **69**: 307–311.

103. Thompson WB, Budd JW. Erroneous diagnoses of amniotic fluid embolism. *Am J Obstet Gynecol* 1965; **91**: 606–620.

104. McLeod AGW. Fatal amniotic fluid embolism in Dade County: an unusual incidence. *Am J Obstet Gynecol* 1972; **113**: 1103–1107.

105. Department of Health, and others. *Report on confidential enquiries into maternal deaths in the United Kingdom 1991–1993.* The Stationary Office, 1996.

106. Vanmaele L, Noppen M, Vincken W et al. Transient left heart failure in amniotic fluid embolism. *Intens Care Med* 1990; **16**: 262–271.

107. Duffy BL. Does amniotic fluid embolism recur? *Anaesth Intens Care* 1998; **26**: 333.

108. Barrows JJ. A documented case of amniotic fluid embolism presenting as acute fetal distress. *Am J Obstet Gynecol* 1982; **143**: 599–600.

109. Katz VL, Dotters DJ, Droegemueller W. Perimortem cesarean section. *Obstet Gynecol* 1986; **68**: 571–576.

110. Hankins GDV, Snyder RR, Clark SL et al. Acute hemodynamic and respiratory effects of amniotic fluid embolism in the pregnant goat model. *Am J Obstet Gynecol* 1993; **168**: 1113–1130.

111. Quance D. Amniotic fluid embolism: detection by pulse oximetry. *Anesthesiology* 1988; **68**: 951–952.

112. Attwood HD, Rome RM. Amniotic embolism and uterine rupture. *Aust NZ J Obstet Gynaecol* 1963; **3**: 73–77.

113. Duff P, Engelsjerd B, Zingery LW et al. Hemodynamic observations in a patient with intrapartum amniotic fluid embolism. *Am J Obstet Gynecol* 1983; **146**: 112–115.

114. Dib N, Bajwa T. Amniotic fluid embolism causing severe left ventricular dysfunction and death. *Cath Cardiovasc Diag* 1996; **39**: 177–180.

115. Attwood HD, Downing SE. Experimental amniotic fluid and meconium embolism. *Surg Gynecol Obstet* 1965; **120**: 255–262.

116. Reis RL, Pierce WS, Behrendt DM. Hemodynamic effects of amniotic fluid embolism. *Surg Gynecol Obstet* 1969; **129**(1): 45–48.

117. Beller BK. Disseminated intravascular coagulation and consumptive coagulopathy in obstetrics. *Obstet Gynecol Ann* 1974; **3**: 267–281.

118. Geoghegan FJ, O'Driscoll MK, Comerford JB. Amniotic fluid infusion. *J Obstet Gynaecol Br Commonw* 1964; **71**: 673–680.

119. Rodriguez-Erdmann F. Bleeding due to increased intravascular blood coagulation. *New Engl J Med* 1965; **273**(2S): 1370–1378.

120. Willoughby MLN. Obstetric hypofibrinogenaemia. A report of 17 cases. *J Obstet Fynaec Brit Cwlth* 1966; **73**: 940–953.

121. Albrechtsen OK, Storm O, Trolle D. Fibrinolytic activity in the circulating blood following amniotic fluid infusion. *Acta Haemat* 1955; **14**: 309–313.

122. Albrechtsen OK. Hemorrhagic disorders following amniotic fluid embolism. *Clin Obstet Gynec* 1964; **7**: 361–371.

123. Pevey WJ. An unusual occurrence of amniotic fluid embolism. *J Louisiana State Med Soc* 1990; **142**: 31–32.

124. Boyd EF, Mulder JI. Amniotic fluid embolism: an overview and case report. *Am J Obstet Gynecol* 1985; **152**: 430–435.

125. Peterson EP, Taylor HB. Amniotic fluid embolism. An analysis of 40 cases. *Obstet Gynecol* 1970; **35**: 787–793.

126. Russell WS, Jones WN. Amniotic fluid embolism. A review of the syndrome with a report of 4 cases. *Obstet Gynecol* 1965; **26**: 476–485.

127. Courtney LD. Amniotic fluid embolism. *Obstet Gynecol Surv* 1974; **29**: 169–177.

128. Martin RW. Amniotic fluid embolism. *Clin Obstet Gynecol* 1996; **39**: 101–106.

129. Maher JE, Wenstrom KD, Hauth JC et al. Amniotic fluid embolism after saline amnioinfusion: two cases and review of the literature. *Obstet Gynecol* 1994; **83**: 851–854.

130. Adamsons K, Mueller-Heubach E, Myers RE. The innocuousness of amniotic fluid infusion in the pregnant rhesus monkey. *Am J Obstet Gynec* 1971; **109**: 977–984.

131. Stolte L, Van Kessel H, Seelen J et al. Failure to produce the syndrome of amniotic fluid embolism by infusion of amniotic fluid and meconium into monkeys. *Am J Obstet Gynecol* 1967; **98**: 694–697.

132. Spence MR, Mason KG. Experimental amniotic fluid embolism in rabbits. *Am J Obstet Gynecol* 1974; **119**: 1073–1078.

133. Liban E, Raz S. Clinicopathologic study of fourteen cases of amniotic fluid embolism. *Am J Obstet Gynecol* 1969; **51**: 477–486.

134. Roche WD, Norris HJ. Detection and significance of maternal pulmonary amniotic fluid embolism. *Obstet Gynecol* 1974; **43**: 729–731.

135. Attwood HD. Fatal pulmonary embolism by amniotic fluid. *J Clin Path* 1956; **9**: 38–46.

136. Attwood HD. The histological diagnosis of amniotic fluid embolism. *J Path Bact* 1958; **LXXVI**: 211–215.

137. Lee W, Ginsburg KA, Cotton DB et al. Squamous and trophoblastic cells in the maternal pulmonary circulation identified by invasive hemodynamic

monitoring during the peripartum period. *Am J Obstet Gynecol* 1986; **155**: 999–1001.

138. Sparr RA, Pritchard JA. Studies to detect the escape of amniotic fluid into the maternal circulation during parturition. *Surg Gynecol Obstet* 1958; 560–564.

139. Thurlbeck WM, Miller RR. The respiratory system. In: Rubin E, Farber JL (eds) *Pathology*. Philadelphia: JB Lippincott Co., 1988, 620 pp.

140. Plauche WC. Amniotic fluid embolism. *Am J Obstet Gynecol* 1983; **147**: 982–983.

141. Kuhlman K, Hidvegi D, Ralph KT et al. Is amniotic fluid material in the central circulation of peripartum patients pathologic? *Am J Perinatol* 1985; **4**: 295–299.

142. Lau G, Chui PPS. Amniotic fluid embolism. A review of 10 fatal cases. *Singapore Med J* 1994; **35**: 180–183.

143. Anderson DG. Amniotic fluid embolism. A re-evaluation. *Am J Obstet Gynecol* 1967; **98**: 336–348.

144. Giampaolo C, Schneider V, Kowalski BH et al. The cytological diagnosis of amniotic fluid embolism: a critical reappraisal. *Diagnos Cytopathol* 1987; **3**: 126–128.

145. Garland IWC, Thompson WD. Diagnosis of amniotic fluid embolism using an antiserum to human keratin. *J Clin Pathol* 1983; **36**: 625–627.

146. Ohi H, Kobayashi H, Terao T. A new histological diagnosis for amniotic fluid embolism by monoclonal antibody TKH-2 that recognizes mucin-type glycoprotein. Nippon Sanka Fujinka Gakkai Zasshi – *Acta Obstet Gynaecol Japon* 1993; **45**: 464–470.

147. Lunetta P, Penttila A. Immunohistochemical identification of syncytiotrophoblastic cells and megakaryocytes in pulmonary vessels in a case of fatal amniotic fluid embolism. *Int J Legal Med* 1996; **108**: 210–214.

148. Ishiyama I, Mukaida M, Komuro E et al. Analysis of a case of generalized amniotic fluid embolism by demonstrating the fetal isoantigen (A blood type) in maternal tissues of B blood type, using immunoperoxidase staining. *Am J Clin Path* 1986; **85**: 239–241.

149. Kobayashi H, Ohi H, Terao T. A simple, non-invasive, sensitive method for diagnosis of amniotic fluid embolism by monoclonal antibody TKH-2 that recognizes NeuAcalpha2-6GalNAc. *Am J Obstet Gynecol* 1993; **168**: 848–853.

150. Kobayashi H, Ooi H, Hayakawa H et al. Histological diagnosis of amniotic fluid embolism by monoclonal antibody TKH-2 that recognizes NeuAcalpha2-6 GalNAc epitope. *Hum Pathol* 1997; **28**: 428–433.

151. Dudney TM, Elliott CG. Pulmonary embolism from amniotic fluid, fat, and air. *Prog Cardiovasc Dis* 1994; **36**: 447–474.

152. Westbrook OC, Thomas JR. Amniotic fluid embolism complicating late abortion. *Am J Obstet Gynecol* 1956; **71**: 447–448.

153. Pulkkinen MO, Eskola J, Kleimola V et al. Pancreatic and catalytic phospholipase A2 in relation to pregnancy, labor and fetal outcome. *Gynecol Obstet Invest* 1990; **29**: 104–107.

154. Kitzmiller JL, Lucas WE. Studies on a model of amniotic fluid embolism. *Obstet Gynecol* 1972; **39**: 626–627.

155. Azegami M, Mori N. Amniotic fluid embolism and leukotrienes. *Am J Obstet Gynecol* 1986; **155**: 1119–1124.

156. Lee H-C, Yamaguchi M, Ikenoue T et al. Amniotic fluid embolism and leukotrienes – the role of surfactant in leukotriene production. *Prostaglan Leukotr Essen Fat Acid* 1992; **47**: 117–121.

157. El Maradny E, Kanayama N, Halim A et al. Endothelin has a role in early pathogenesis of amniotic fluid embolism. *Gynecol Obstet Invest* 1995; **40**: 14–18.

158. Phillips LL, Davidson EC. Procoagulant properties of amniotic fluid. *Am J Obstet Gynecol* 1972; **113**: 911–919.

159. Weiner AE, Reid DE, Roby CC. The hemostatic activity of amniotic fluid. *Science* 1949; **110**: 190–191.

160. Heyes H, Leucht W, Musch K. Evaluation of fetal lung maturity by measurement of the procoagulant activity in amniotic fluid. *Arch Gynecol* 1982; **233**: 7–14.

161. Hastwell GB. Accelerated clotting time: an amniotic fluid thromboplastic activity index of fetal maturity. *Am J Obstet Gynecol* 1978; **131**: 650–654.

162. Lockwood CJ, Bach R, Guha A et al. Amniotic fluid contains tissue factor, a potent initiator of coagulation. *Am J Obstet Gynecol* 1991; **165**: 1335–1341.

163. Strickland MA, Bates GW, Whitworth NS et al. Amniotic fluid embolism: prophylaxis with heparin and aspirin. *South Med J* 1985; **78**: 377–379.

164. Hammerschmidt DE, Ogburn PL, Williams JE. *Amniotic fluid* activates complement. A role in amniotic fluid embolism syndrome? *J Lab Clin Med* 1984; **104**: 901–907.

165. Attwood HD. Matthew Baillie – a possible early description of amniotic fluid embolism. *Aust NZ J Obstet Gynaec* 1979; **19**: 176–177.

166. Konstadt SN, Louie EK, Black S et al. Intraoperative detection of patent foramen ovale by transesophageal echocardiography. *Anesthesiology* 1991; **74**: 212–216.

167. Hagen PT, Scholz DG, Edwards WD. Incidence and size of patent foramen ovale during first 10 decades of life: an autopsy study of 965 normal hearts. *Mayo Clin Proc* 1984; **59**: 17–20.

168. Broe S, Khoo SK. How safe is Caesarean section in current practice? A survey of mortality and serious morbidity. *Aust NZ J Obstet Gynaecol* 1989; **29**: 93–98.

169. Fong J, Gadalla F, Gimbel AA. Precordial Doppler diagnosis of haemodynamically compromising air embolism during Caesarean section. *Can J Anaesth* 1990; **37**: 262–264.

170. Fong J, Gadalla F, Druzin M. Venous emboli occurring during Caesarean section: the effect of patient position. *Can J Anaesth* 1991; **38**: 191–195.

171. Younker D, Rodriguez V, Kavanaugh J. Massive air embolism during cesarean section. *Anesthesiology* 1986; **65**: 77–79.

172. Malinow AM, Naulty JS, Hunt CO et al. Precordial ultrasonic monitoring during cesarean section. *Anesthesiology* 1987; **66**: 816–819.

173. Bauer P, Lelarge P, Hennequin L et al. Thrombo-embolism during amniotic fluid embolism. *Intens Care Med* 1995; **21**: 384–388.

174. Turner R, Gusack M. Massive amniotic fluid embolism. *Ann Emerg Med* 1984; **13**: 359–361.

175. Kern SB, Duff P. Localized amniotic fluid embolism presenting as ovarian vein thrombosis and refractory post-operative fever. *Am J Clin Path* 1981; **76**: 476–480.

176. Kool MJ. Successful treatment of postpartum shock caused by amniotic fluid embolism with cardiopulmonary bypass and pulmonary artery thrombo-embolectomy (comment). *Am J Obstet Gynecol* 1991; **164**: 701–702.

177. Dutta D, Bhargava KC, Chakravarti RN et al. Therapeutic studies in experimental amniotic fluid embolism in rabbits. *Am J Obstet Gynecol* 1970; **106**: 1201–1208.

178. Benson MD. Anaphylactoid syndrome of pregnancy. *Am J Obstet Gynecol* 1996; **175**: 749.

179. Stefanini M, Turpini RA. Fibrinogenopenic accident of pregnancy and delivery: a syndrome with multiple etiological mechanisms. *Ann NY Acad Sci* 1959; **75**: 601–625.

180. Benson MD, Lindberg RE. Amniotic fluid embolism, anaphylaxis, and tryptase. *Am J Obstet Gynecol* 1996; **175**: 737.

181. Hayashi RH, Castillo MS, Noah ML. Management of severe post partum hemorrhage with a prostaglandin F2alpha analogue. *Obstet Gynecol* 1984; **63**: 806–808.

182. O'Leary AM. Severe bronchospasm and hypotension after 15-methyl prostaglandin F2alpha in atonic post partum haemorrhage. *Int J Obstet Anesth* 1994; **3**: 42–44.

183. Weir EK, Greer B, Smith S et al. Bronchoconstriction and pulmonary hypertension during abortion induced by 15-methyl prostaglandin F2alpha. *Am J Med* 1976; **60**: 556–561.

184. Secher NJ, Thayassen P, Arnsbo P et al. Effect of prostaglandin E2 and F2alpha on the systemic and pulmonary circulation in pregnant and anesthetised women. *Acta Obstet Gynecol Scand* 1981; **61**: 213–218.

185. Douglas MJ, Farquharson DF, Ross PLE et al. Cardiovascular collapse following an overdose of prostaglandin F2alpha: a case report. *Can J Anaesth* 1989; **36**: 466–469.

186. Resuscitation Council UK. Cardiac arrest in special circumstances. In: Handley AJ, Swain A (eds) *Advanced life support* 1994, pp 53–57.

187. Rees GAD, Willis BA. Resuscitation in late pregnancy. *Anaesthesia* 1988; **43**: 347–349.

188. International Liaison Committee on Resuscitation. Special resuscitation situations. *Resuscitation* 1997; **34**: 129–149.

189. Lindsay SL, Hanson GC. Cardiac arrest in near-term pregnancy. *Anaesthesia* 1987; **42**: 1074–1077.

190. Davies MG, Harrison JC. Amniotic fluid embolism: maternal mortality revisited. *Br J Hosp Med* 1992; **47**: 775–776.

191. Anonymous. Amniotic fluid embolism and emergency cardiac care. *Ann Emerg Med* 1984; **13**(12): 1172–1173.

192. Brandjes DPM, Schenk BE, Buller HR et al. Management of disseminated intravascular coagulation in obstetrics. *Eur J Obstet Gynecol Reprod Biol* 1991; **42**: S87–S89.

193. Hoedt HT. Case of amniotic fluid embolism treated with epsilon-amino-caproic acid. *Nederl Tijdschr Verlosk Gynaec* 1962; **62**: 331–337.

194. Sher G, Statland BE. Abruptio placentae with coagulopathy: a rational basis for management. *Clin Obstet Gynecol* 1985; **28**: 15–23.

195. Valentine S, Williamson P, Sutton D. Reduction of acute haemorrhage with aprotinin. *Anaesthesia* 1993; **48**: 405–406.

196. Oney T, Schander K, Muller N et al. Amniotic fluid embolism with coagulation disorder – a case report (in German). *Geburtsh Frauenheilk* 1982; **42**: 25–28.

197. National Health and Medical Research Council. *Report on maternal deaths in Australia 1988–1990*. Australian Government Publishing Service.

198. Jenkins DM, Carr C, Stanley J et al. Maternal mortality in the Irish Republic, 1989–1991. *Irish Med J* 1996; **89**: 140–141.

199. Shinagawa S, Katagiri S, Noro S et al. An autopsy study of 306 cases of maternal death in Japan. *Acta Obstet Gynaec Jpn* 1983; **35**: 194–200.

200. Ravindran J. Sudden maternal deaths probably due to obstetrical pulmonary embolism in Malaysia for 1991. *Med J Malaysia* 1994; **49**: 53–61.

201. Moldin P, Hokegard K, Nielsen TF. Cesarean section and maternal mortality in Sweden 1973–1979. *Acta Obstet Gynecol Scand* 1984; **63**: 7–11.

202. Kaunitz AM, Hughes JM, Grimes DA et al. Causes of maternal mortality in the United States. *Obstet Gynecol* 1985; **65**: 605–612.

203. Dorfman SF. Maternal mortality in New York City, 1981–1983. *Obstet Gynecol* 1990; **76**: 317–323.

204. Guha-Ray DK. Maternal mortality in an urban hospital. *Obstet Gynecol* 1976; **47**: 430–433.

205. Schiffer MA, Pakter J, Clahr J. Mortality associated with hypertonic saline abortion. *Obstet Gynecol* 1973; **42**: 759–764.

206. Mirchandani HG, Mirchandani IH, Parikh SR. Hypernatremia due to amniotic fluid embolism during a saline-induced abortion. *Am J Foren Med Path* 1988; **9**: 48–50.

207. Lawson HW, Atrash HK, Franks AL. Fatal pulmonary embolism during legal induced abortion in the United States from 1972 to 1985. *Am J Obstet Gynecol* 1990; **162**: 986–990.

208. Guidotti RJ, Grimes DA, Cates W. Fatal amniotic fluid embolism during legally induced abortion, United States, 1972 to 1978. *Am J Obstet Gynecol* 1981; **141**: 257–261.

209. Goldstein PJ. Amniotic fluid embolism complicating intrauterine saline abortion. *Am J Obstet Gynecol* 1968; **101**: 858–859.

210. Lee HA, Frampton J. Case of intramniotic glucose induction followed by non-fatal amniotic fluid embolism and acute renal failure. *Am J Obstet Gynecol* 1964; **90**: 554–555.

211. Cates W, Boyd C, Halvorson-Boyd G et al. Death from amniotic fluid embolism and disseminated intravascular coagulation after a curettage abortion. *Am J Obstet Gynecol* 1981; **141**: 346–347.

212. Hern WM. Laminaria versus Dilapan osmotic cervical dilators for outpatient dilation and evacuation abortion: randomized cohort comparison of 1001 patients. *Am J Obstet Gynecol* 1994; **171**: 1324–1328.

213. Dibble LA, Elliott JP. Possible amniotic fluid embolism associated with amnioinfusion. *J Mater Fetal Med* 1992; **1**: 263–266.

214. Less A. Vaginal prostaglandin E2 and fatal amniotic fluid embolism. *JAMA* 1990; **263**: 3259–3260.

215. Thomsen RJ. Pregnancy in the presence of an intrauterine contraceptive device and amniotic fluid embolism: a possible association. *Am J Obstet Gynecol* 1975; **121**: 279–280.

216. Scott RB. Critical illnesses and deaths associated with intrauterine devices. *Obstet Gynecol* 1968; **31**: 322–327.

217. Paterson WG, Grant KA, Grant JM et al. The pathogenesis of amniotic fluid embolism with particular reference to transabdominal amniocentesis. *Eur J Obstet Gynecol Reprod Biol* 1977; **7**: 319–324.

218. Shapiro SH, Wessely Z. Rhodamine B fluorescence as a stain for amniotic fluid embolism and fetal lungs. *Ann Clin Lab Sci* 1988; **18**: 451–454.

219. Cron RS, Kilkenny GS, Wirthwein C et al. Amniotic fluid embolism. *Am J Obstet Gynecol* 1952; **64**: 1360–1363.

220. Schneider CL. Coagulation defects in obstetric shock: meconium embolism and heparin, fibrin embolism and defibrination. *Am J Obstet Gynecol* 1955; **69**: 758–775.

221. Jaques WE, Hampton JW, Bird RM et al. Pulmonary hypertension and plasma thromboplastin antecedent deficiency in dogs. *Arch Pathol* 1960; **69**: 248–256.

222. Halmagyi DFJ, Starzecki B, Shearman RP. Experimental amniotic fluid embolism: mechanism and treatment. *Am J Obstet Gynecol* 1962; **84**: 251–256.

223. MacMillan D. Experimental amniotic fluid infusion. *J Obstet Gynaecol Br Commonw* 1968; **75**: 849–852.

224. Reeves JT, Daoud FS, Estridge M et al. Pulmonary pressor effects of small amounts of bovine amniotic fluid. *Respir Physiol* 1974; **20**: 231–237.

ANAESTHESIA DURING PREGNANCY

Michael Hudspith

INTRODUCTION

Anaesthesia during pregnancy presents the anaesthetist with a number of complicating issues. Perhaps the most fundamental questions are:

- How does anaesthesia affect the fetus and mother?
- How does the pregnant state influence the maternal response to drugs used in anaesthesia?

The reported incidence of non-obstetric surgery during pregnancy varies widely. A US study[1] found that as many as 2% of pregnant women underwent non-obstetric surgery between 1968 and 1978. A more recent study,[2] reported 5405 operations performed on 720 000 Swedish women between 1973 and 1981, an overall surgery rate of 0.75%. Between 1980 and 1989, in a further US study,[3] the reported incidence was 0.15% suggesting that overall incidence may be declining. These figures suggest that in the UK with a crude birth rate of 12.9/1000[4] and approximately 750 000 births per annum, between 1000 and 6000 women, with a pregnancy continuing to term, may undergo anaesthesia each year. A recent study reported an unrecognized pregnancy rate in menstruating women presenting for ambulatory non-obstetric surgery of 0.3%[5] and pregnancy testing is strongly recommended when admitting women of a child bearing age, to an intensive care unit.

The most common indications for non-obstetric surgery with an ongoing pregnancy are appendicectomy, cholecystectomy and pelvic laparoscopy[2,3,6] although a broad spectrum of procedures including cardiac surgery, neurosurgery and orthotopic liver transplantation have been performed with successful outcome to the pregnancy.

Examination of product licence information from the ABPI Data Sheet Compendium[7] reveals that few (if any) drugs used in anaesthesia are specifically licensed for use in pregnancy, although only a small number are relatively or absolutely contraindicated as a consequence of definitive adverse effects upon fetal outcome. The anaesthetist must weigh up the relative risks and benefits of any individual anaesthetic technique, depending upon the circumstances.

The safety of the mother and maintenance of maternal pregnant physiology are of primary importance. The most acute risk to the fetus under anaesthesia is maternal hypoxaemia and/or a reduction in placental perfusion. Optimal anaesthesia during pregnancy necessitates a consideration of the potential direct and indirect toxic effects of anaesthetic drugs upon the feto-placental unit.

ANAESTHETIC EFFECTS ON THE FETO-PLACENTAL UNIT

Anaesthetic effects upon the fetus can be broadly subdivided into:

- Direct toxic effects of drugs upon the fetus (including teratogenicity).
- Indirect effects; essentially a reduction in placental perfusion and/or oxygenation resulting from adverse anaesthetic effects upon maternal physiology. It should be recognized that alterations in maternal physiology, for example chronic hypercarbia or hyperthermia[8] may in themselves be teratogenic.
- Anaesthesia, surgery and the disease that requires intervention may threaten the ongoing pregnancy by increasing the chance of premature labour.

DIRECT FETOTOXICITY AND TERATOGENICITY

Drugs should only be prescribed in pregnancy if the benefits to the mother and unborn child outweigh the risks.[9] Many drugs used in anaesthesia interfere with fundamental intercellular and intracellular signalling mechanisms: these involve neurotransmitters, receptor mechanisms, Ca^{2+}-signalling and second messenger function.[10-13] Such systems are involved in organogenesis and cellular differentiation. Furthermore, anaesthetic drugs are known to affect cellular mitosis and DNA synthesis.[14-16] We need therefore to consider whether drugs commonly used in anaesthesia are fetotoxic or teratogenic in a clinical scenario.

Shepard[17] has defined teratogenicity as any significant change in post-natal *form* or *function* in an offspring after pre-natal treatment. This definition does not limit the term to structural defects but encompasses behavioural teratology. Teratological effects are dose dependent, and the precise nature of any change in form or function will be determined by the duration and gestational stage of exposure:

- Exposure to teratogenic agents during the early pluripotential stage of development may result in all or nothing effects, i.e. embryonic death and resorption or survival of an unaffected embryo.
- Later exposure during the period of organogenesis (which corresponds in the human to days 31–71 after the last menstrual period) may result in structural malformation.
- After this period, interference with ongoing maturation of the central nervous system has the potential for altered post-natal behaviour and development (Fig. 18.1).

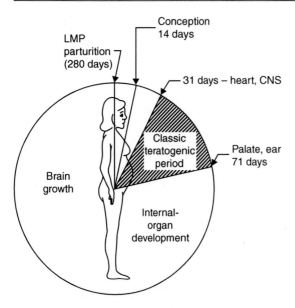

Figure 18.1 The gestational clock showing the classic teratogenic period (from Niebyl JR. *Drug use in pregnancy,* 2nd edn. Philadelphia: Lea & Febiger, 1988: 2).

There is tenuous retrospective data associating increased incidence of hydrocephalus and neural tube defects with first trimester anaesthesia in human pregnancy.[19,20] A causal link has not been established and it is unclear which, if any, anaesthetic drug or combination may be responsible. Prospective clinical studies in this field are impractical as any increase over the background rate of malformations is likely to be small[19,20] and enormous numbers would be required.[21] Much emphasis has therefore been placed upon prospective animal studies, but the finding of teratogenesis in animals following either the administration of a single extremely high dose of a drug or protracted exposure to low doses, does not unequivocally indicate that a single brief anaesthetic exposure, in the clinical scenario, would carry a similar risk. Marked inter-species differences exist in teratogenic sensitivity and animal data cannot be directly applied to human pregnancy.

The precise evaluation of the fetal safety of drugs used in anaesthesia thus requires the cautious interpretation of animal data, retrospective human studies and epidemiological surveys of occupational exposure.

VOLATILE ANAESTHETICS

Volatile anaesthetics have been reported to have teratogenic and embryotoxic effects in experimental animals. Such studies have included a variety of techniques encompassing both prolonged gestational exposure to trace concentrations of anaesthetics and single or repeated high dose exposure. It is essential to note that many studies have not controlled for teratogenicity arising from maternal hypoxia, hypercarbia, hypothermia and nutritional deficiency that complicates prolonged anaesthesia in experimental animals.[8,22] Most studies demonstrating teratologic effects of volatile agents have reported high maternal mortality associated with derangement of maternal physiology and metabolism rather than specific embryo-toxicity.[22] Extrapolation of such data to clinical anaesthesia in human pregnancy is therefore of questionable relevance. For example, Basford and Fink[23] demonstrated an increase in skeletal abnormalities in rats exposed to 0.8% halothane for 12 h on days 8 and 9 of gestation. Exposure of mice to 4 MAC h per day of halothane during days 6–15 resulted in major developmental malformations in surviving embryos, although this was attributed to hypothermia and metabolic derangement.[24] Repeated but less protracted exposure to anaesthetic concentrations may be less embryotoxic: Kennedy et al[25] found no adverse effects of five consecutive 1 h exposures to 1.5% halothane at various stages of rodent pregnancy. A similar lack of developmental abnormalities was reported following three consecutive 6 h exposures to halothane in rats.[26] Although it is difficult to exclude confounding metabolic effects in a number of the above studies, there is limited evidence to suggest that enflurane[27] and isoflurane[26] may have lower embryotoxic and teratogenic potential than halothane.

There are no published studies documenting the teratogenic potential of the newer agents sevoflurane and desflurane. Manufacturer's data on file indicate that fetotoxic effects in rodents (increased post-implantation loss, decreased weight gain and skeletal abnormalities) with either agent, occurred only at concentrations or cumulative doses associated with maternal toxicity. These data would appear to support the conclusion made in 1986 by Mazze and colleagues that volatile anaesthetics *per se* are not teratogenic.[26]

A number of studies[24,27–31] have examined the teratogenic and fetotoxic potential of chronic low dose administration of volatile anaesthetics in rodents. Epidemiological data suggest increases in spontaneous abortion and congenital anomalies amongst female personnel experiencing occupational exposure to trace concentrations of both volatiles and nitrous oxide.[32,33] Animal studies however demonstrated that when the influence of derangements to maternal physiological status were excluded, subanaesthetic concentrations of volatile agents did not increase the rates of macroscopic congenital anomalies. Some studies,[34–37]

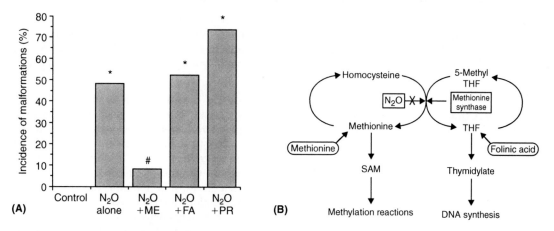

Figure 18.2 (A) Incidence of malformations induced by N_2O alone and N_2O plus methionine (ME), folinic acid (FA), or prazosin (PR). *Value significantly higher than control: $P < 0.05$. #Value significantly less than N_2O alone: $P < 0.05$. (B) Pathway of inhibition of methionine synthase by N_2O and its potential metabolic consequences. SAM = S-adenosyl-methionine; THF = tetrahydrofolate (from Fujinaga M, Baden JM. Methionine prevents nitrous oxide-induced teratogenicity in rat embryos grown in culture. *Anesthesiology* 1994; **81**: 184–189).

however, have reported ultrastructural degenerative changes in cerebral cortical neurones in rats exposed *in utero* to trace concentrations of halothane throughout gestation. The human significance of these findings is unclear, but persisting changes in rat behaviour had been previously reported following *in utero* exposure to halothane[38] and its potential behavioural teratogenicity have been considered.[39] Certain authors have strongly recommended that halothane should not be inhaled in pregnancy[34] and it may be prudent to use isoflurane, enflurane or the newer volatile agents where practicable for anaesthesia in pregnancy.

NITROUS OXIDE

Since the study of Fink et al in 1967,[40] adverse reproductive and teratogenic effects have been associated with prolonged exposure to nitrous oxide.[41–44] With the exception of a study by Viera, who reported skeletal abnormalities in rats exposed continuously to 0.1% N_2O throughout gestation,[45] exposures to in excess of 50% N_2O for greater than 24 h have generally been required to demonstrate teratogenic effects *in vivo*.

Definitive studies have demonstrated that the specific pattern of skeletal anomalies associated with N_2O exposure is dependent upon the time of gestational exposure.[46–48] The use of rat whole-embryo cultures has enabled detailed investigation of the mechanisms of N_2O teratogenicity and it is now clear that it is not a simple consequence of inhibition of methionine synthase–tetrahydrofolate reductase and reduced DNA synthesis. Folinic acid supplementation (which reverses

the haematological toxicity of N_2O) does not prevent its teratogenic potential.[49] Rather a decrease in methionine availability may be causal as methionine supplementation was protective against N_2O teratogenicity in embryo cultures (Fig. 18.2).[50] The interesting observation that volatile anaesthetics such as halothane[49] and isoflurane[51] prevent N_2O teratogenicity, but do not prevent the decrease in methionine synthase activity, suggests that other mechanisms are involved.

Nitrous oxide is a sympathomimetic agent[52] known to activate central noradrenergic pathways[53] via opioid receptors. Alpha-adrenergic receptor-mediated mechanisms have been implicated in the production of situs inversus in the rat[54] and N_2O potentiates the production of this anomaly by the α_1-agonist phenylephrine. This potentiation is reversed by the α_1-antagonist prazosin.[50] That volatile agents and N_2O may have opposing actions on central opioid and noradrenergic mechanisms, is supported by the intriguing demonstration that pre-emptive analgesia with N_2O can be reversed by co-administration of isoflurane or halothane.[55]

INTRAVENOUS ANAESTHETICS

In contrast to the plethora of studies on inhalational anaesthetics, the fetotoxicity of intravenous agents appears to have received only limited attention. Shepard[8] stated that anaesthetic doses of thiopentone administered to rats or mice were devoid of teratogenic effects; low doses of other barbiturates are not teratogenic and methohexitone may be similarly safe. Nevertheless, anticonvulsant barbiturates have been shown to be teratogenic in high doses in animals. The fetal dysmorphism associated with barbiturate anticonvulsant use may at least in part be attributable to drug effects, rather than maternal epilepsy.[56] Etomidate appears to be devoid of teratogenic effect,[57] as does ketamine.[8]

Propofol has been shown not to affect fertilization and early embryonic development,[58] and there is neither clinical nor animal data to suggest that it is teratogenic (ICI/Zeneca data on file). However, reproductive studies suggest adverse effects upon perinatal survival and its manufacturers state that it should not be used in pregnancy.

BENZODIAZEPINES

There are concerns regarding the safety of benzodiazepine (BDZ) usage in pregnancy.[59] Animal studies indicate that, (at least at high doses), direct effects mediated by both central and peripheral type BDZ receptors may mediate both structural and behavioural teratogenicity,[60] resulting in orofacial clefts and abnormal behaviour.

Retrospective data from the 1970s suggested a causal link between first trimester BDZ administration and cleft lip and palate[61,62] however a subsequent prospective study[63] failed to confirm this. Bergman et al[64] commented on the confounding effects of drugs of abuse and alcohol in the 'fetal BDZ syndrome' and Shepard in the *Catalog of teratogenic agents*[8] states that Diazepam is not teratogenic.

Long-term maternal administration may be associated with fetal BDZ dependence and withdrawal[65] and peripartum administration is well known to cause fetal hypotonia, hypothermia, respiratory depression and feeding difficulties.[56]

It is extremely unlikely that a single dose of a short acting BDZ, given as premedication or for perioperative sedation, has the potential for embryo- or fetotoxicity. Their safety with prolonged high dose administration, for example sedation in intensive care is less well defined and consideration should be given to the use of other agents.[66]

OPIOIDS

Many early studies using rodents, suggested that opioid administration in pregnancy was teratogenic, causing craniofacial and neural tube defects. Such studies did not adequately control for prolonged hypoxia, hypercarbia, hypothermia, and nutritional derangements, resulting from repeated administration of opioids. Definitive studies, mainly by Fujinaga and colleagues,

which avoided these confounding factors by using implanted osmotic minipumps have failed to show structural teratogenicity with fentanyl,[67] alfentanil and sufentanil,[68] morphine,[69] pethidine and phenoperidine.[70]

Long-lasting behavioural effects in the neonate may follow chronic maternal opioid administration: for example altered analgesic responses and preference for sweet solutions in the rat persist to adulthood.[71] This may be associated with abnormalities in central noradrenergic mechanisms.[72] Such behavioural teratogenic effects are likely to be receptor mediated,[73] but their clinical significance remains obscure. There is no evidence that the intraoperative administration of opioids, or their use for acute pain carries fetal risk (besides respiratory depression at delivery). The safety of longerterm high dose administration in intensive care or in the management of chronic pain is less clear. It must be appreciated that long-term administration may be associated with fetal dependence and withdrawal, which has been well documented with maternal methadone and diamorphine abuse.[74-76] One case report describes the long-term use of intrathecal morphine to avoid these complications in a pregnancy complicated by neuropathic pain of malignant origin.[77]

NON-STEROIDAL ANTI-INFLAMMATORY AGENTS

Aspirin has been shown to be teratogenic in high doses in rodent studies, but with the exception of a single study reporting a possible reduction in IQ following high consumption in pregnancy,[78] it is not considered a human teratogen.[8] The follow-up of 'CLASP' (collaborative low dose aspirin study in pregnancy) confirms this earlier conclusion.[79] Non-steroidal anti-inflammatory agents, (NSAID), commonly used in the peri-operative period, have not been associated with problems, except the possibility of vascular malformations associated with ketorolac in animal studies, (product literature).

This suggests that NSAIDs, other than ketorolac, may be safe in the first and second trimester. NSAIDs when given in the third trimester of pregnancy, may however cause premature closure of the fetal ductus arteriosus, tricuspid incompetence and pulmonary hypertension or non-closure of the ductus arteriosus post-natally which may be resistant to medical management.[80-82] Manufacturer's product literature also describe myocardial degenerative changes; platelet dysfunction with resultant bleeding; intracranial bleeding; renal dysfunction or failure; renal injury; dysgenesis; oligohydramnios; gastrointestinal bleeding or perforation; increased risk of necrotising enterocolitis; and delayed labour or birth following third trimester administration. It is recommended that NSAIDs are not used after 32 weeks gestation.[82]

NEUROMUSCULAR BLOCKING AGENTS

It has been stated that 'muscle relaxants are difficult to test for reproductive toxicity ... because of the respiratory depression that they cause in the mother'.[83] This has necessitated the use of either sub-paralysing doses[84] or prolonged intubation and ventilation[85] with potential confounding factors such as hypoxia and/or hypercarbia – themselves teratogenic.

Despite these problems, non-depolarizing muscle relaxants appear not to be teratogenic at clinically relevant doses. The use of cultured embryo techniques demonstrated that concentrations 30-fold greater than clinically used were required to produce developmental toxicity with pancuronium, atracurium or vecuronium.[83] Given that serum concentrations in the fetus are only ~10% of maternal, there is a large margin of safety.

Whilst brief exposure to muscle relaxants are likely to be benign, there is some evidence that prolonged disruption of cholinergic neuromuscular function may produce limb malformations in the chick.[86,87] Although this has not been reproduced in mammals, it should be noted that arthrogryposis was reported in an infant born to a mother treated with d-tubocurarine (for tetanus) during the first trimester.[88] Whether this association was causal remains open to conjecture, given maternal hypoxia, hyperthermia and polypharmacy in this case.

LOCAL ANAESTHETICS

Procaine, lidocaine and bupivacaine are cytotoxic in vitro[15] and cocaine is a teratogen[89] with maternal cocaine abuse linked to adverse fetal outcome.[8] Reproductive and teratogenic studies in rats indicate that lidocaine is devoid of both structural[90] and behavioural teratogenicity.[91] These studies did not extend to bupivacaine, but exhaustive reproductive and teratological tests undertaken with ropivacaine (Astra product data), show no evidence of adverse effects upon organogenesis, early or late fetal development.

If the confounding effect of alcohol and other drugs of abuse associated with maternal cocaine abuse are disaccounted, fetotoxic effects of cocaine may reflect altered maternal cardiovascular status and sympathomimetic actions in the fetus, as opposed to sodium-channel-mediated mechanisms, common to other local anaesthetics.

ANTIEMETICS

Hyperemesis gravidarum and pregnancy-associated nausea of lesser severity has meant that many of the antiemetics commonly used in the peri-operative period have been tried in human pregnancy.[92]

Metoclopramide has been widely used throughout pregnancy and has not been demonstrated to have teratogenic effects in animals or humans. Although its efficacy in the treatment of post-operative nausea and vomiting is questionable, it is perhaps the safest and least controversial agent in pregnancy.

Prochlorperazine appears to have little fetotoxic potential and Milkovich[93] considered that prochlorperazine was not teratogenic in a large prospective human study. However, its manufacturers caution that jaundice and prolonged extra-pyramidal disturbance have been reported following high doses in late pregnancy. Similar caution has been recommended regarding other phenothiazines and the butyrophenone antiemetics.[94]

Cyclizine has not been shown to be a human teratogen,[8,93] but a closely related antihistamine meclizine is, at high doses, a teratogen in the rat.[8]

Ondansetron and other $5HT_3$ antagonists are not teratogenic in animal studies. There is no available human safety data and manufacturers caution against their use, especially during the first trimester of pregnancy.

TRANSPLACENTAL CARCINOGENICITY

Volatile anaesthetic agents such as halothane, enflurane and isoflurane are known to affect DNA synthesis and mitosis in a variety of mammalian cell types[14,16,95] and nitrous oxide may have similar actions.[95] Related halogenated alkanes and ethers (e.g. chloroform, trichloroethylene) are well-known carcinogens,[96] and the administration of certain chemicals during pregnancy can result in transplacental carcinogenesis. Despite the effects upon DNA synthesis and mitosis of inhalational anaesthetics, there is no evidence that any anaesthetic agent available for clinical use is mutagenic, nor does their use entail a risk of transplacental carcinogenicity.

CONCLUSION

Reassuringly, there is very limited evidence for teratogenicity of the commonly used drugs in anaesthesia at dosage and duration encountered in most surgical scenarios. Although, the evidence for teratogenicity of nitrous oxide is stronger, the duration of exposure required for teratogenicity is such that concern regarding its bone marrow suppressant and neurological toxicity may only be significant during long

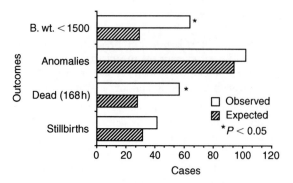

Figure 18.3 Total number of observed and expected adverse outcomes among women having non-obstetric operations during pregnancy. Incidences of infants with birth weights <1500 g and of infants born alive and dying within 168 h of birth were significantly increased (P < 0.05) (from Mazze RI, Kallen B. Reproductive outcome after anesthesia and operation during pregnancy: a registry study of 5405 cases. *Am J Obstet Gynecol* 1989; **161**: 1178–1185).

procedures. Prolonged sedation and analgesia in intensive care does require consideration of the potential direct fetotoxic effect, but under such circumstances acute disturbances to maternal physiology represent an enormously greater risk to the fetus than does potential teratogenicity.

Nevertheless, outcome data from human studies[2] (Fig. 18.3) indicate a clear risk of adverse outcome after anaesthesia and surgery in pregnancy, not manifest by teratogenicity but as increases in abortions, stillbirth, intrauterine growth retardation and prematurity.

INDIRECT TOXICITY: EFFECTS UPON UTERO-PLACENTAL PERFUSION

The aim of anaesthesia during pregnancy is to provide maternal amnesia, analgesia and muscle relaxation appropriate to the procedure undertaken. This is frequently accompanied by a reduction in fetal heart rate (FHR) variability, particularly following the use of intravenous anaesthetic agents and opioids.[97] Although this effect is attributable to fetal anaesthesia,[98] fetal distress may also manifest as changes in FHR variability[99] and it is necessary to consider the effects of maternal anaesthesia upon utero-placental perfusion.

Fetal survival is critically dependent upon placental perfusion with oxygenated maternal blood. Significant maternal hypoxia represents the most acute risk to the fetus: anaesthetic causes for maternal hypoxia are

well recognized and include airway obstruction, intubation problems, aspiration, laryngospasm, equipment problems together with hypoventilation arising from opioid overdose or excessively high spinal/epidural anaesthesia.

Utero-placental hypoperfusion from *any cause* will result in fetal hypoxaemia and acidosis. The commonest and under-recognized cause of uterine hypoperfusion is aortocaval compression (which may *not* manifest as overt systemic hypotension) and occurs as early as 18–20 weeks of gestation.[100] Other physical causes of reduced uterine blood-flow include haemorrhage and uncompensated sympathetic blockade from regional anaesthesia.

OXYGENATION AND ACID–BASE BALANCE

Hypoxaemia

Although the calibre of uterine vessels alters in response to oxygen tension *in vitro*,[101,102] moderate hypoxaemia does not result in a compensatory increase in uteroplacental perfusion *in vivo*.[103,104] The fetus may compensate for temporary reductions in maternal oxygen delivery by increased oxygen extraction.[105] The high concentration in the fetal circulation of HbF and its high affinity for maternal oxygen provide a significant 'oxygen margin of safety'[106] and experimental data suggests that a mild to moderate reduction in oxygen delivery of several minutes duration[107] is well tolerated by the fetus. Severe or prolonged maternal hypoxaemia causes utero-placental vasoconstriction and a redistribution of blood flow away from the utero-placental bed (despite increasing maternal cardiac output)[108] resulting in fetal hypoxaemia, hypotension and acidosis and ultimately leading to fetal death.

Hyperoxia

Hyperoxia causes uterine vasoconstriction *in vitro*,[101,102,109] but this potentially detrimental effect does not appear relevant in human pregnancy, where elevation of maternal P_aO_2 has been reported to result in increased fetal scalp PO_2.[110] A large materno-fetal oxygen gradient, high placental oxygen consumption and poor matching of fetal and maternal blood-flow limit the maximal elevation of fetal P_aO_2, with increased maternal FiO_2. Fetal P_aO_2 rarely exceeds 45 mmHg and never exceeds 60 mmHg. Premature closure of the ductus arteriosus or retrolental fibroplasia does not therefore occur with maternal exposures to FiO_2 approaching 1.0.

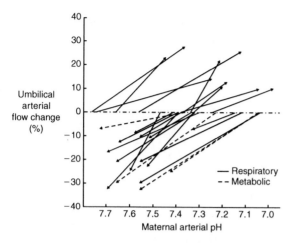

Figure 18.4 Effect on blood flow in one umbilical artery of changes in maternal arterial pH expressed as per cent change of initial flow. Closed circles and triangles represent values before and during changes in maternal pH, respectively. Solid lines indicate pH changes produced by respiratory alkalaemia, and acidaemia, and broken lines, by metabolic alkalaemia (from Motoyama EK, Rivard G, Acheson F, Cook CD. The effect of changes in maternal pH and PCO_2 on the PO_2 of fetal lambs. *Anesthesiology* 1962; **28**: 891–903).

Hypercarbia

Carbon dioxide diffuses freely across the placenta and maternal respiratory and/or metabolic acid–base imbalance may adversely affect fetal well-being. Maternal hypercarbia directly causes fetal respiratory acidosis, mild degrees of which are of little significance provided that the fetus remains normoxaemic. In the acidotic fetus, the reduction in fetal cardiac output in response to hypoxia is more profound[111] and combined hypercarbia and hypoxia is poorly tolerated. Severe respiratory acidosis is associated with myocardial depression even in the normoxaemic fetus. Although chronic hypercapnia has been shown in animals to be teratogenic,[8] it is extremely unlikely that durations of hypercapnia encountered in the anaesthetic scenario carry such a risk. Uterine blood-flow is modulated by maternal P_aCO_2 and pH. Moderate hypercapnia may initially increase uterine blood-flow, although above a P_aCO_2 of 8 kPa, uterine vasoconstriction resulted in reduced uterine blood-flow in sheep.[112]

Hypocarbia

Maternal alkalaemia, whether of respiratory or metabolic origin is equally sinister, with an almost linear

reduction in uterine blood-flow in response to a reduction in maternal P_aCO_2 or H^+ concentration (Fig. 18.4).[113,114] This reduction in uterine blood-flow in conjunction with a leftward shift in maternal oxygen-dissociation curve, results in fetal acidosis. Maternal hyperventilation and hypocapnia must therefore be avoided, which necessitates careful control of minute ventilation during anaesthesia together with optimal peri-operative analgesia to prevent hyperventilation due to inadequate pain relief.[115]

Drugs used in anaesthesia have the potential to directly and indirectly influence uterine blood-flow. This can be a consequence of both a reduction in maternal cardiac output and redistribution of maternal blood-flow.

GENERAL ANAESTHESIA

Thiopentone

Induction of anaesthesia with barbiturates has been reported to be associated with transient reductions in uterine blood-flow of 20–35% (Fig. 18.5)[116,117] Studies performed in sheep[118] evaluated the combined effect of intravenous induction together with laryngoscopy and tracheal intubation. Airway manipulation is a potent cause of sympathetic stimulation causing a 90% increase in arterial norepinephrine concentrations in pregnant sheep.[116,119] The resultant maternal hypertension and vasoconstriction could in part account for a reduction in uterine blood-flow.

Propofol

A similar study with propofol[117] suggests that sympathetic stimulation alone may not account for the reduction of uterine blood-flow seen at barbiturate induction. Propofol induction and endotracheal intubation resulted in no change in uterine blood-flow despite a significant maternal hypertensive response. Maintenance of anaesthesia using propofol and 50% nitrous oxide for up to 2 h uterine showed that blood-flow remained unchanged (Fig. 18.5).

Ketamine

In sheep, induction doses of ketamine result in increases in blood pressure and cardiac output.[120,121] Ketamine has consistently been shown to increase uterine blood-flow in the third trimester. Ketamine may be less benign during the second trimester, as it has been reported to cause uterine hypertonus of a similar magnitude to ergometrine,[122] which might be expected to significantly impair uterine blood-flow.

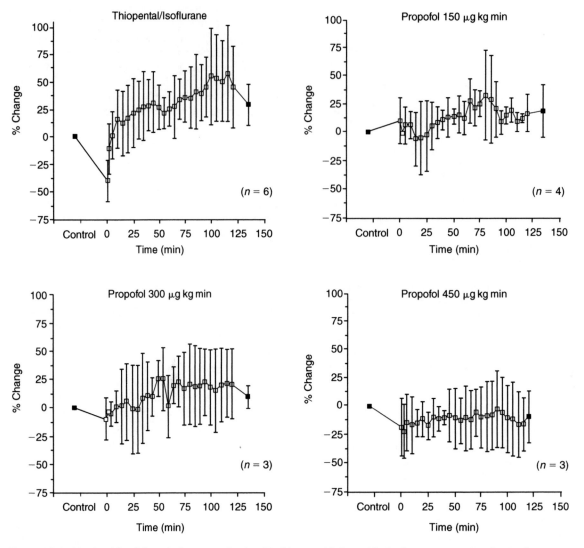

Figure 18.5 Uterine blood-flow during anaesthesia with thiopental followed by isoflurane or varying doses of propofol. Percentage change from baseline values obtained during pre-anaesthesia control period was calculated. All data are expressed as mean ± SD (from Alon E, Ball RH, Gillie MH, Parer JT, Rosen MA, Shnider SM. Effects of propofol and thiopental on maternal and fetal cardiovascular and acid-base variables in the pregnant ewe. *Anesthesiology* 1993; **78**: 562–576).

Etomidate

Although etomidate has been recommended as an induction agent for Caesarean section,[123] its effects upon the fetus early in gestation have not been reported. Its use at Caesarean section may cause suppression of neonatal cortisol levels and increase the incidence of hypoglycaemia.[124] Whilst maternal plasma glucose will ensure normoglycaemia in an unstressed fetus, endogenous glucose synthesis may be inadequate in the stressed fetus,[125] and it remains possible that etomidate might cause or accentuate fetal hypoglycaemia under conditions of stress.

Volatile agents

The volatile anaesthetics are uterine relaxants (with halothane probably the most potent) and this in conjunction with direct effects upon maternal regional blood-flow will affect uterine perfusion.

Below 1.5 MAC halothane, uterine relaxation and vasodilatation maintain uterine blood-flow, despite reductions in maternal cardiac output.[126] With low concentrations of halothane (0.5% in 50% nitrous oxide), increases in uterine blood-flow of 20% have been reported.[119] Above 2 MAC, falling maternal cardiac output predominates and this is associated with progressive fetal hypoxaemia and acidosis.[126] Data with isoflurane is essentially similar, with 1% isoflurane/50% N_2O producing a 25% increase in uterine blood-flow.[117,126] While enflurane appears not to increase uterine blood-flow, fetal acid–base status remained stable with concentrations below 1%.[119]

There is a little data regarding the influence of the newer inhalational agents desflurane and sevoflurane[127,128] upon uterine perfusion. Both have been used at Caesarean section and are not associated with adverse fetal outcome.[129,130] Preliminary data in sheep suggest that sevoflurane may better maintain maternal haemodynamics and increase uterine blood-flow to a greater extent than isoflurane.[131] Rapid increases in inspired concentrations of desflurane are associated with transient cardiovascular stimulation and hypertension,[128] which might influence uterine perfusion. The effects of this sympathetic-mediated phenomena on fetal well-being have not been documented.

REGIONAL ANAESTHESIA

If systemic hypotension is avoided, regional anaesthesia is well tolerated by the fetus.

Using a pregnant sheep model, uterine blood-flow remained stable during epidural anaesthesia near term.[132] Many studies of women undergoing Caesarean section under epidural[133–136] or spinal[137] blockade have confirmed these findings. One study,[138] suggested that the drop in peripheral vascular resistance with epidural blockade, was associated with a possible reduction in utero-placental perfusion. This is not supported by data from women receiving epidural analgesia in labour where either no change[139] or improvement in placental blood-flow[140,141] is reported.

Maintenance of utero-placental perfusion requires that hypotension is avoided, as reduction in mean arterial pressure proportionately reduces uterine blood-flow.[133,142] Adverse effects of hypotension on uterine blood-flow and the development of fetal hypoxaemia and acidosis may be more marked during maternal haemorrhage,[143] thus maternal circulating volume must be maintained at all times during epidural and spinal anaesthesia during pregnancy.

Epidural administration of opioids including morphine,[144] fentanyl[145] and sufentanil[146] has been found not to affect utero-placental perfusion or fetal acid–base balance. Provided that fetal oxygenation is not compromised by maternal respiratory depression, there is no evidence to suggest that they are contraindicated in ongoing pregnancy. Placental transfer of opioids occurs rapidly after maternal epidural administration and this should be considered where delivery is to be imminent. Epidural and intrathecal fentanyl appears not to cause a clinically significant respiratory or behavioural effects in the neonate, when bolus doses are less than 100 μg.[147,148] However higher doses have been associated with fetal respiratory depression.[149]

CATECHOLAMINES AND VASOACTIVE DRUGS

Maternal hypertension may adversely affect uterine perfusion: for example, stress sufficient to induce hypertension causes significant increases in circulating norepinephrine and marked reductions in uterine blood-flow in sheep.[150] The observation that anxiety in labouring women is associated with elevated levels of plasma catecholamines and abnormal fetal heart rate recordings,[151] suggests that pre-operative anxiety, (frequently associated with hypertension), may be detrimental to fetal well-being.

Exogenous administration of vasoactive agents will affect uterine perfusion. α-adrenergic agonists are believed to accentuate uterine hypoperfusion, despite restoring maternal systemic blood pressure to normal or supra-normal levels.[152–154] In contrast, the indirect sympathomimetic ephedrine may be used to treat maternal hypotension, whilst restoring uterine perfusion to normal or near normal levels.[152,154,155] This reflects both positive chonotropic and inotropic actions mediated via β-stimulation. α-receptor-mediated maternal venoconstriction, (and therefore restoration of cardiac pre-load), with phenylephrine may occur before adverse uterine vasoconstriction.[156] The careful use of α-agonists can therefore be considered, particularly in conjunction with invasive monitoring of maternal cardiovascular parameters.

ANTIHYPERTENSIVE AGENTS

Surgical requirements – notably during neurosurgical emergencies – may necessitate the use of systemic vasodilators and antihypertensive agents.

Labetolol

The combined α- and β-antagonist labetalol is widely used to induce hypotension or treat hypertension in the peri-operative period. Its intravenous administration has been shown to maintain uterine blood-flow in pregnant hypertensive rats[157] and a similar effect on uterine perfusion is seen during the use of labetalol in pre-eclamptic women.[158,159] It may therefore be the agent of choice during anaesthesia in pregnancy.[160]

Hydralazine

When labetalol is contraindicated (e.g. asthma) or is ineffective, a direct acting vasodilator may be required. Hydralazine has been shown in pregnant sheep to both reduce maternal hypertension, and attenuate reductions in uterine blood-flow following infusion of phenylephrine.[161]

Glyceryl trinitrate

Glyceryl trinitrate has similar properties and there were no adverse effect upon fetal circulation or acid–base balance during infusions of up to 2 h.[162]

Sodium nitroprusside

Sodium nitroprusside has been used clinically to induce hypotension during neurosurgical anaesthesia in pregnancy.[163,164] It does not improve low uterine blood-flow caused by maternal hypertension[161] and the potential for fetal cyanide toxicity[165] makes its use unappealing in the pregnant patient.

Esmolol

Maternal β-blockade may be associated with fetal β-blockade and bradycardia[166] but there may also be a significant reduction in uterine blood-flow and fetal hypoxaemia.[167] This may reflect significant reductions in maternal cardiac output associated with β-blockade and suggests that potent short acting agents such as esmolol should be used cautiously during pregnancy.

Calcium-channel blockers

L-type calcium-channel blockers such as nifedipine and nimodipine may be used to treat hypertension in the peri-operative period and have beneficial effect upon both cerebral and coronary perfusion. Although both have been used effectively to treat hypertension in pregnancy,[168–170] an infusion of nifedipine and similar calcium-channel blockers has recently been associated with the development of fetal hypoxaemia and acidosis, which may persist even after cessation of the drug.[171] This suggests that calcium-channel blockers should not be routinely used in the management of peri-operative hypertension in the pregnant patient unless their effects upon coronary and more importantly, cerebral perfusion are specifically required.[160,172] Nimodipine should be used to attenuate cerebral vasospasm as part of the standard management of this neurosurgical emergency.[173]

Magnesium sulphate

The administration of magnesium sulphate causes systemic vasodilatation and the recent reappraisal of its efficacy in eclampsia,[174,175] together with its potential neuroprotective actions[10] suggests that its use as a hypotensive agent in pregnancy may be appropriate. In both normotensive and hypertensive animals, $MgSO_4$ administration attenuated maternal hypertension and increased uterine blood-flow by approximately 10%,[176] and it has been effectively used to maintain haemodynamic control in a pregnant woman undergoing resection of phaeochromocytoma.[177]

CHANGES IN ANAESTHETIC TECHNIQUE

PHYSIOLOGICAL CONSIDERATIONS

Respiratory

Pregnancy represents a state of controlled hyperventilation which results in a chronic, partially compensated respiratory alkalosis, with a P_aCO_2 of 3.7–4.3 kPa, pH 7.44 and a reduction in bicarbonate and buffer base. P_aO_2 remains within the normal range or may be mildly elevated. The associated 25% fall in FRC creates the potential for airway closure and markedly reduces pulmonary oxygen reserve. This in conjunction with increased oxygen consumption and a reduction in plasma buffering capacity means that there is a rapid onset of maternal hypoxaemia and acidosis during apnoea or airway obstruction.

Weight gain, breast development and pharyngeal capillary engorgement throughout the third trimester increase the potential for airway management problems as pregnancy progresses.[178,179]

An increased respiratory rate and a reduced FRC in pregnancy, (together with a reduction in MAC for volatile anaesthetics), will permit a more rapid inhalational induction of anaesthesia and/or change in depth of anaesthesia.

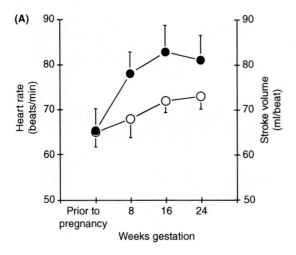

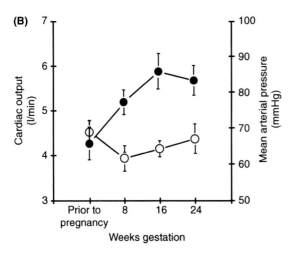

Figure 18.6 (A) Stroke volume (filled circles) and heart rate (open circles) components of cardiac output are presented for four study periods. (B) Cardiac output (filled circles) and mean arterial pressure (open circles) components of systemic vascular resistance are presented for four study periods (from Capeless EL, Clapp JF. Cardiovascular changes in early phase of pregnancy. Am J Obstet Gynecol 1989; **161**: 1449–1453).

Cardiovascular

Pregnancy is associated with an increase in stroke volume and blood volume such that cardiac output increases by 30–50% throughout pregnancy. These changes are essentially complete by 16 weeks of gestation (Fig. 18.6).[180]

Of greater concern to the anaesthetist is aortocaval compression.[100] Almost complete compression of the inferior vena cava by the gravid uterus[181] results in a

marked reduction in cardiac output of 25–30%, with venous return being maintained in part by the dilated plexus of epidural veins (Fig. 18.7). Although aorto-caval compression and the supine-hypotensive syndrome are most clearly recognized in the late third trimester, significant reductions in cardiac output can occur from 18 to 20 weeks of gestation.[100]

The supine position should therefore be avoided from the mid-trimester onward. MRI images demonstrate that the lateral position restores the inferior vena cava to its pre-pregnant calibre.[181] Where the lateral positioning is inappropriate for surgical access, lateral uterine displacement should be used.

Gastrointestinal changes

The precise stage of gestation at which prophylactic antacid and H_2-antagonist administration together with rapid sequence induction becomes mandatory remains uncertain. Gastric volumes and pH at less than 20 weeks gestation have been reported not to differ from the non-pregnant state.[182] However, reduced lower oesophageal sphincter tone may be evident as early as 15 weeks gestation, particularly in patients with symptomatic heartburn.[183] It seems prudent to recommend that antacid prophylaxis and rapid-sequence induction be used in all patients beyond 20 weeks gestation, and in any patient with symptomatic reflux.

PHARMACOLOGICAL CHANGES

Volatile anaesthetics

Pregnancy is associated with an increased sensitivity to volatile anaesthetic agents, which occurs early in gestation. In a study comparing women undergoing termination of pregnancy at 8–12 weeks gestation with equivalent non-pregnant patients, the MAC for isoflurane was reduced from 1.1% to 0.78% (Fig. 18.8).[184] There have been similar results from animal studies in which reductions in MAC for volatile agents between 16% and 40% have been reported, dependent upon the species and stage of gestation.[185,186]

The mechanism of this reduction in MAC is uncertain, but the possibility that it reflects a neuro-steroid anaesthetic effect of progesterone has been proposed.[187] Subtle changes in $GABA_A$ and BDZ receptors have been described in pregnancy,[188] and $GABA_A$ receptors play a key role in the mechanism of anaesthesia.[189] Clinically, the reduction in MAC may reduce the potential for intra-operative awareness in patients

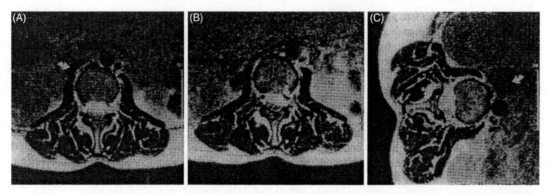

Figure 18.7   T2-weighted MR image showing an axial section at the level of the lamina of L2 in the same subject. A = Non-pregnant, B = pregnancy-supine, C = pregnancy-lateral. The inferior vena cava (curved arrow) was identified in the non-pregnant state (A) and in the pregnant-lateral position (C). The lateral components of the anterior internal vertebral veins (vertical arrow) are noted to engorge in the supine position (B), whereas there is no engorgement of the extradural veins in the lateral position (C). The cauda equina was positioned at the posteromedial region of the dural sac in the supine position, while it migrated to the dependent side within the dural sac in the left lateral position (from Hirabayashi et al. Effects of the pregnant uterus on the extradural venous plexus in the supine and lateral positions, as determined by magnetic resonance imaging. *Br J Anaesth* 1997; **78**: 317–319). © The Board of Management and Trustees of the British Journal of Anaesthesia. Reproduced by permission of Oxford University Press/British Journal of Anaesthesia.

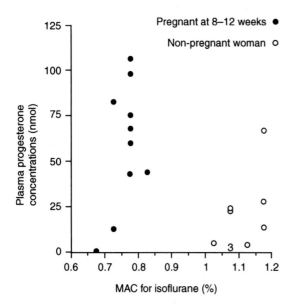

Figure 18.8   Minimum alveolar concentrations (MAC) for isoflurance (percentage) and plasma progesterone concentrations (nanomolar) in ten non-pregnant women (open circles) and ten pregnant women at 8–12 weeks' gestation (filled circles). Number 3 5 three overlapping data points in the non-pregnant group (from Gin T, Chan MT. Decreased minimum alveolar concentration of isoflurane in pregnant humans. *Anesthesiology* 1994; **81**: 829–832).

in whom we might wish to minimize exposure to anaesthetic agents.

Intravenous anaesthetics

A similar increase in sensitivity to thiopentone during pregnancy has been reported.[190] The dose requirement for anaesthesia during the first trimester is reduced by 18%, when compared to non-pregnant women (Fig. 18.9). Other induction agents have not been studied. Whilst this effect of pregnancy upon thiopentone requirements may be a similar pharmacodynamic effect to that seen with isoflurane[184] and might extend to other intravenous induction agents, the possibility that pregnancy results in altered pharmacokinetics of thiopentone has not been excluded.

Neuromuscular blockade

The haemodynamic and hormonal changes of pregnancy have the potential to alter the duration of action of neuromuscular blocking drugs.

The duration of action of the steroid vecuronium is prolonged by approximately 40% in the early postpartum period and a similar effect is seen with rocuronium.[191,192] This may reflect pregnancy-induced changes in hepatic blood-flow or competition for liver uptake by the sex hormones. The duration of action

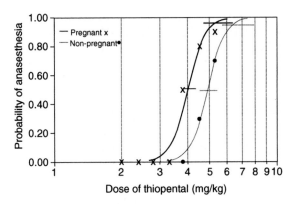

Figure 18.9 Calculated dose–response curves (log dose scale) for anaesthesia in pregnant and non-pregnant women. The 95% confidence intervals for the $Ed_{50}s$ and $ED_{95}s$ are also displayed, slightly offset for clarity. Raw data shown by x (pregnant group) and • (non-pregnant group) (from Gin T, Mainland P, Chan MT, Short TG. Decreased thiopental requirements in early pregnancy. *Anesthesiology* 1997; **86**: 73–78).

of atracurium is unaffected by pregnancy, reflecting its breakdown by Hoffman degradation.[191]

Plasma cholinesterase levels decrease by approximately 25% from the first trimester, until the early post-partum period. Prolonged neuromuscular blockade with suxamethonium is uncommon due to an increased volume of distribution in pregnancy.[193] Nevertheless, monitoring of the return of neuromuscular function with a peripheral nerve stimulator is strongly recommended.

Local anaesthesia

Pregnancy is associated with both pharmacodynamic and pharmacokinetic changes in the response to local anaesthetics. The onset of local anaesthetic block with bupivacaine is accelerated in nerve fibres from pregnant animals[194] and lidocaine content in peripheral nerves is lower in pregnant animals at any given stage of block.[195] Total dosage of local anaesthetics may therefore need to be reduced by 25–30% in pregnancy. This pharmacodynamic alteration in sensitivity to amide local anaesthetics may in part account for the increased spread of epidural anaesthesia, which has been reported as early as 8–12 weeks gestation.[196] Later in pregnancy, engorgement of epidural veins[181] may further contribute to increased spread of epidural local anaesthetics.

Pharmacokinetic changes may enhance the toxicity of amide local anaesthetics during pregnancy. Convulsions and cardiovascular collapse occur at lower total bupivacaine concentrations in pregnant than in non-pregnant sheep.[197] This may reflect a reduction in protein binding and increased free drug availability. A reduction in volumes of distribution of both bupivacaine and ropivacaine during pregnancy[198] may increase peak plasma concentrations after inadvertent intravascular injection. The reduced cardiotoxicity of ropivacaine when compared with bupivacaine persists in pregnancy,[199] suggesting that it may be a safer drug for surgical anaesthesia during pregnancy, although because of reduced potency this effect may not be as marked as first thought.

Opioids

Pain threshold increases in human pregnancy,[200,201] an opioid-mediated effect.[202,203] This may reflect a functional upregulation of both δ-opioid[204] and κ-opioid[205] receptor mechanisms. Levels of substance P, a neuropeptide associated with nociception are reduced in human pregnancy,[206] which may also contribute to changes in pain perception in pregnancy.

The clinical significance of changes in opioid pharmacodynamics is uncertain. A reduction in opioid requirement together with the increased respiratory drive of pregnancy would suggest an increased margin of safety in opioid use. Nevertheless, it should be noted that one case report[207] described opioid-rigidity after ~1 μg/kg fentanyl in pregnancy. The pharmacodynamic changes outlined above, may therefore reduce the threshold for this adverse effect normally seen only with high doses of opioids.

SPECIFIC ANAESTHETIC CONSIDERATIONS

The largest study to date of anaesthesia and surgery during pregnancy indicates an increased risk of delivery of low birth weight infants and early perinatal death[2] (Fig. 18.3). The combination of surgery, disease and anaesthesia may all promote premature onset of labour in the third trimester, but evidence is lacking to support the prophylactic use of tocolytic agents.[3] It is impossible to determine the relative contributions of the pathology necessitating surgery, operation and anaesthesia to adverse outcome, but it should be clear that elective surgery is contraindicated during pregnancy.

When maternal pathology is serious or life threatening, optimal maternal treatment is paramount and the management of such surgical conditions is essentially unchanged by pregnancy. Procedures such as cardiopulmonary bypass,[208,209] including circulatory

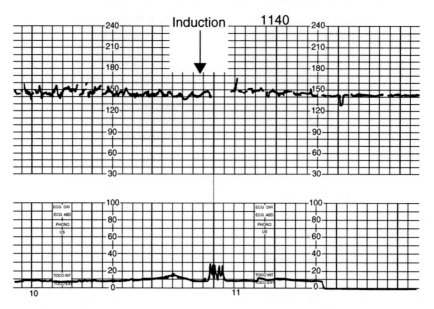

Figure 18.10   Peri-operative fetal heart rate and uterine tocodynamic recording. Normal beat-to-beat FHR variation (left upper tracing) diminished within 1 min after induction of anaesthesia (from Liu PL, Warren TM, Ostheimer GW, Weiss JB, Liu LMP. Foetal monitoring in partrurients undergoing surgery unrelated to pregnancy. *Canad Anaesth Soc J* 1985; **32**: 525–532).

arrest;[210] neurosurgical resection of aneurysm and arteriovenous malformation,[160,172] orthotopic liver transplantation,[211] and resection of phaeochromocytoma[177] have all been performed with continuation of pregnancy and birth of normal infants. Providing maternal oxygenation and utero-placental blood-flow are maintained, the fetus is remarkably tolerant of anaesthesia and surgical insult.

Fetal monitoring

The fetal heart is audible by transabdominal doppler by 12 weeks and continuous intraoperative monitoring is feasible after 18–20 weeks gestation.[212] Where patient position and surgical approach permit, intra-operative FHR monitoring should be performed. There should be an appropriate plan of action should fetal distress become evident. For procedures performed after 24 weeks gestation, the feasibility of proceeding to Caesarean delivery (and appropriate neonatal intensive care facilities) should be considered before surgery is undertaken.

Fetal anaesthesia as a consequence of maternal opioid and volatile administration may directly affect FHR variability.[98] A reduction in baseline variability (normally considered an index of fetal well-being)[99] alone may not reflect fetal compromise (Fig. 18.10). Persistent fetal tachycardia or bradycardia is a more specific indicator of fetal distress and may reflect maternal hypoxaemia (Fig. 18.11). In the absence of maternal hypoxaemia, fetal distress may indicate aortocaval compression or surgical interference with uterine blood-flow.

Intra-operative monitoring of uterine contractions (external tocography) has been recommended,[212,214] although technical considerations may limit its feasibility. External tocography should be undertaken for at least 48 h post-operatively, and is mandatory if post-operative regional analgesia is used, as the mother may be unable to report the onset of contractions.

ANAESTHETIC TECHNIQUE

No study has demonstrated the advantage of any individual anaesthetic technique with regard to fetal outcome, but from a teratogenic viewpoint, exposure to drugs *per se* should be minimized, particularly during the first trimester of pregnancy.

Although there is no firm evidence for human teratogenicity of inhalational and intravenous anaesthetics, animal studies suggest that exposure to anaesthetic drugs should be minimized during the period of organogenesis. Given the absence of evidence of teratogenicity of amide local anaesthetics, regional anaesthesia should be considered in all cases where maternal and surgical demands permit.

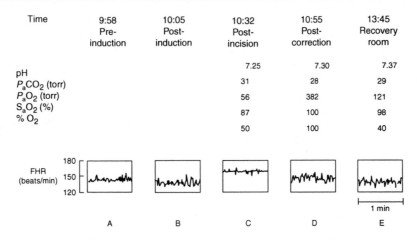

Time	9:58 Pre-induction	10:05 Post-induction	10:32 Post-incision	10:55 Post-correction	13:45 Recovery room
pH			7.25	7.30	7.37
P_aCO_2 (torr)			31	28	29
P_aO_2 (torr)			56	382	121
S_aO_2 (%)			87	100	98
% O_2			50	100	40

Figure 18.11   Serial samples of fetal heart rate: A and B, Baseline fetal heart at 140 beats/min, with normal beat-to-beat variability. C, Fetal tachycardia and stabilization of the beat-to-beat interval at maternal P_aO_2 = 56 torr. D, Following correction of maternal ventilation there is a return to baseline fetal heart rate and variability. E, Normal baseline post-operatively (from Katz JD, Hook R, Barash PG. Fetal heart rate monitoring in pregnant patients undergoing surgery. *Am J Obstet Gynecol* 1976; **125**: 267–269).

Abdominal surgery extending above the umbilicus usually requires general anaesthesia, with muscle relaxation and endotracheal intubation. Precautions against regurgitation and aspiration are necessary after 20 weeks gestation or earlier if the mother is symptomatic of reflux.

The intravenous induction agent of choice is thiopentone. Where thiopentone is contraindicated (for example: hypersensitivity or porphyria), etomidate should be considered as the product licence does not preclude its use in pregnancy. The use of propofol is not recommended except in neurosurgery where maternal benefits outweigh fetal risk.[66,160]

Where possible, the use of halothane should be avoided in pregnancy: isoflurane or enflurane are the volatile agents of choice for maintenance and sevoflurane is recommended for inhalational induction of anaesthesia. While from a theoretical perspective nitrous oxide should be avoided, (at least in the first trimester), and air/oxygen/volatile techniques used, there is no human data to support or refute this viewpoint.[215]

Laparoscopy

There is increasing emphasis on the use of laparoscopic techniques in pregnancy,[216–219] which are considered safe.[220] Animal studies have demonstrated the development of fetal acidosis during CO_2 pneumoperitoneum,[221] and adverse fetal outcome has been attributed to this in a clinical setting.[217] Recent data[222] indicates that an increasing maternal P_aCO_2 to $P_{Ei}CO_2$ gradient occurs during laparoscopy in pregnancy, but when P_aCO_2 is maintained within normal limits, fetal acidosis does not occur. Standard minimal monitoring[223] for such procedures such as non-invasive blood pressure, electro-cardiogram, pulse oximetry, temperature and capnography may be inadequate in pregnancy. Invasive arterial monitoring permits accurate assessment of P_aCO_2 and is recommended during all but the briefest laparoscopic and other abdominal surgery.

Post-operative analgesia

Post-operative analgesia must be of the highest standard to minimize the risk of maternal and fetal hypoxaemia and consideration should be given to the use of epidural local anaesthetic and opioid techniques. Excellent analgesia will attenuate elevated circulating catecholamine levels arising from pain and stress, which adversely affect utero-placental perfusion in this critical early post-operative period.

REFERENCES

1. Brodsky JB, Cohen EN, Brown BW. Surgery during pregnancy and fetal outcome. *Am J Obstet Gynec* 1980; **138**: 1165–1167.

2. Mazze RI, Kallen B. Reproductive outcome after anesthesia and operation during pregnancy: a registry study of 5405 cases. *Am J Obstet Gynecol* 1989; **161**: 1178–1185.

3. Kort B, Katz VL, Watson WJ. The effect of nonobstetric operation during pregnancy. *Surg Gynecol Obstet* 1993; **177**: 371–376.

4. World Health Organisation. *World Health Statistics Annual 1995*. Geneva, World Health Organisation 1996.

5. Manley S, De Kelaita G, Joseph NJ, Salem R, Heyman HJ. Preoperative pregnancy testing in ambulatory surgery. *Anesthesiology* 1995; **83**: 690–693.

6. Mazze RI, Kallen B. Appendectomy during pregnancy: a Swedish registry study of 778 cases. *Obstet Gynecol* 1991; **77**: 835–840.

7. Association of British Pharmaceutical Industries. *Compendium of data sheets*. London: Datapharmn Publications Ltd, 1998.

8. Shepard TH. *Catalog of teratogenic agents*. Baltimore: The Johns Hopkins University Press, 1989.

9. Committee on safety of medicines. Drug-induced birth defects. *Curr Prob Pharmacovigil* 1997; **23**: 11.

10. Hudspith MJ. Glutamate: a role in normal brain function, anaesthesia, analgesia and CNS injury. *Br J Anaesth* 1997; **78**: 731–747.

11. Kress HG. Effects of general anaesthetics on second messenger systems. *Eur J Anaesth* 1995; **12**: 83–97.

12. Langmoen IA, Larsen M, Berg-Johnsen J. Volatile anaesthetics: cellular mechanisms of action. *Eur J Anaesth* 1995; **12**: 51–58.

13. Richards CD. The synaptic basis of general anaesthesia. *Eur J Anaesth* 1995; **12**: 5–19.

14. Sturrock JE, Nunn JF. Mitosis in mammalian cells during exposure to anesthetics. *Anesthesiology* 1975; **43**: 21–33.

15. Sturrock JE, Nunn JF. Cytotoxic effects of procaine, lignocaine and bupivacaine. *Br J Anaesth* 1979; **51**: 273–281.

16. Sturrock JE, Nunn JF. Effects of halothane on DNA synthesis and the pre-synthetic phase (G1) in dividing fibroblasts. *Anesthesiology* 1976; **45**: 413–420.

17. Shepard TH. Human teratogens: how can we sort them out? *Ann N Y Acad Sci* 1986; **477**: 105–115.

18. Niebyl JR. *Drug use in pregnancy*. Philadelphia: Lea & Febiger, 1988.

19. Sylvester GC, Khoury MJ, Lu X, Erickson JD. First-trimester anesthesia exposure and the risk of central nervous system defects: a population-based case-control study. *Am J Public Health* 1994; **84**: 1757–1760.

20. Kallen B, Mazze RI. Neural tube defects and first trimester operations. *Teratology* 1990; **41**: 717–720.

21. Miller RW. How environmental effects on child health are recognized. *Pediatrics* 1974; **53**: 792–799.

22. Friedman JM, Polifka JE. *Teratogenic effects of drugs*. Baltimore: The Johns Hopkins University Press, 1994.

23. Basford AB, Fink BR. The teratogenicity of halothane in the rat. *Anesthesiology* 1968; **29**: 1167–1173.

24. Wharton RS, Wilson AI, Mazze RI, Baden JM, Rice SA. Fetal morphology in mice exposed to halothane. *Anesthesiology* 1979; **51**: 532–537.

25. Kennedy GL, Jr, Smith SH, Keplinger ML, Calandra JC. Reproductive and teratologic studies with halothane. *Toxicol Appl Pharmacol* 1976; **35**: 467–474.

26. Mazze RI, Fujinaga M, Rice SA, Harris SB, Baden JM. Reproductive and teratogenic effects of nitrous oxide, halothane, isoflurane, and enflurane in Sprague-Dawley rats. *Anesthesiology* 1986; **64**: 339–344.

27. Wharton RS, Mazze RI, Wilson AI. Reproduction and fetal development in mice chronically exposed to enflurane. *Anesthesiology* 1981; **54**: 505–510.

28. Pope WD, Halsey MJ, Lansdown AB, Bateman PE. Lack of teratogenic dangers with halothane. *Acta Anaesthesiol Belg* 1975; **23**(suppl): 169–173.

29. Wharton RS, Mazze RI, Baden JM et al. Fertility, reproduction and postnatal survival in mice chronically exposed to halothane. *Anesthesiology* 1978; **48**: 167–174.

30. Green CJ, Monk SJ, Knight JF, Dore C, Luff NP, Halsey MJ. Chronic exposure of rats to enflurane 200 p.p.m.: no evidence of toxicity or teratogenicity *Br J Anaesth* 1982; **54**: 1097–1104.

31. Mazze RI, Wilson AI, Rice SA, Baden JM. Fetal development in mice exposed to isoflurane. *Teratology* 1985; **32**: 339–345.

32. Cohen EN, Brown BW, Wu ML et al. Occupational disease in dentistry and chronic exposure to trace anesthetic gases. *J Amer Dental Assoc* 1980; **101**: 21–31.

33. Knill-Jones RP, Rodrigues LV, Moir DD. Anaesthetic practice and pregnancy: controlled survey of women anaesthetists in the UK. *Lancet* 1972; **i**: 1326–1328.

34. Baeder C, Albrecht M. Embryotoxic/teratogenic potential of halothane. *Int Arch Occup Environ Health* 1990; **62**: 263–271.

35. Chang LW, Dudley AW, Jr, Katz J. Pathological changes in the nervous system following *in utero* exposure to halothane. *Environ Res* 1976; **11**: 40–51.

36. Chang LW, Dudley AW, Jr, Lee YK, Katz J. Ultrastructural changes in the nervous system after chronic exposure to halothane. *Exp Neurol* 1974; **45**: 209–219.

37. Uemura E, Ireland WP, Levin ED, Bowman RE. Effects of halothane on the development of rat brain: a golgi study of dendritic growth. *Exp Neurol* 1985; **89**: 503–519.

38. Smith RF, Kurkjian MF, Mattran KM, Kurtz SL. Behavioral effects of prenatal exposure to lidocaine in the rat: effects of dosage and of gestational age at administration. *Neurotoxicol Teratol* 1989; **11**: 395–403.

39. Butcher RE. Halothane – a behavioral teratogen? *Anesthesiology* 1978; **49**: 308–309.

40. Fink BR, Shepard TH, Blandau RJ. Teratogenic activity of nitrous oxide. *Nature* 1967; **214**: 146–148.

41. Shepard TH, Fink BR. Teratogenic activity of nitrous oxide in rats. In: Fink BR (ed) *Toxicity of anesthetics*. Baltimore: Williams & Wilkins, 1968, pp 308–323.

42. Fujinaga M, Baden JM, Mazze RI. Susceptible period of nitrous oxide toxicity in Sprague-Dawley rats. *Teratology* 1989; **40**: 439–444.

43. Lane GA, Nahrwold ML, Tait AR, Taylor Busch M, Cohen PJ, Beaudoin AR. Anesthetics as teratogens: nitrous oxide is fetotoxic, xenon is not. *Science* 1980; **210**: 899–901.

44. Mazze RI, Wilson AI, Rice SA, Baden JM. Reproduction and fetal development in rats exposed to nitrous oxide. *Teratology* 1984; **30**: 259–265.

45. Vieira E, Cleaton Jones P, Austin JC, Moyes DG, Shaw R. Effects of low concentrations of nitrous oxide on rat fetuses. *Anesth Analg* 1980; **59**: 175–177.

46. Fujinaga M, Baden JM, Mazze RI. Susceptible period of nitrous oxide teratogenicity in Sprague-Dawley rats. *Teratology* 1989; **40**: 439–444.

47. Fujinaga M, Mazze RI, Baden JM, Fantel AG, Shepard TH. Rat whole embryo culture: an *in vitro* model for testing nitrous oxide teratogenicity. *Anesthesiology* 1988; **69**: 401–404.

48. Baden JM, Fujinaga M. Effects of nitrous oxide on day 9 rat embryos grown in culture. *Br J Anaesth* 1991; **66**: 500–503.

49. Mazze RI, Fujinaga M, Baden JM. Halothane prevents nitrous oxide teratogenicity in Sprague-Dawley rats; folinic acid does not. *Teratology* 1988; **38**: 121–127.

50. Fujinaga M, Baden JM. Methionine prevents nitrous oxide-induced teratogenicity in rat embryos grown in culture. *Anesthesiology* 1994; **81**: 184–189.

51. Fujinaga M, Baden JM, Yhap EO, Mazze RI. Reproductive and teratogenic effects of nitrous oxide, isoflurane, and their combination in Sprague-Dawley rats. *Anesthesiology* 1987; **67**: 960–964.

52. Ma D, Wang C, Pac-Soo CK, Chakrabarti MK, Whitwam JG. Dissociation between the effect of nitrous oxide on spontaneous and reflexly evoked sympathetic activity in dogs. *Br J Anaesth* 1997; **79**: 525–529.

53. Guo T-Z, Poree L, Golden W, Stein J, Fujinaga M, Maze M. Antinociceptive response to nitrous oxide is mediated by supraspinal opiate and spinal α_2 adrenergic receptors in the rat. *Anesthesiology* 1996; **85**: 846–852.

54. Fujinaga M, Maze M, Hoffman BB, Baden JM. Activation of α-1 adrenergic receptors modulates the control of left/right sidedness in rat embryos. *Develop Biol* 1992; **150**: 419–421.

55. Goto T, Marota JJA, Crosby G. Nitrous oxide induced preemptive analgesia in the rat that is antagonized by halothane. *Anesthesiology* 1994; **80**: 409–416.

56. Palmer PG. Sedatives and anticonvulsants in pregnancy. In: Hawkins DF (ed) *Drugs and pregnancy: human teratogenesis and related problems*, 2nd edn. Edinburgh: Churchill Livingstone, 1987, pp 128–147.

57. Janssen PA, Niemegeers CJ, Marsboom RP. Etomidate, a potent non-barbiturate hypnotic. Intravenous etomidate in mice, rats, guinea-pigs, rabbits and dogs. *Arch Int Pharmacodyn Ther* 1975; **214**: 92–132.

58. Alsalili M, Thornton S, Fleming S. The effect of the anaesthetic, propofol, on *in-vitro* oocyte maturation, fertilization and cleavage in mice. *Human Reproduction* 1997; **12**: 1271–1274.

59. Committee on safety of medicines. Reminder: avoid benzodiazepines in pregnancy and lactation. *Curr Prob Pharmacovigil* 1997; **23**: 10.

60. Jurand A, Martin LV. Cleft palate and open eyelids inducing activity of lorazepam and the effect of flumazenil, the benzodiazepine antagonist. *Pharmacol Toxicol* 1994; **74**: 228–235.

61. Saxen I. Associations between oral clefts and drugs taken during pregnancy. *Int J Epidemiol* 1975; **4**: 37–44.

62. Saxen I, Saxen L. Association between maternal intake of diazepam and oral clefts. *Lancet* 1975; **2**: 498.

63. Shiono PH, Mills JL. Oral clefts and diazepam use during pregnancy. *N Engl J Med* 1984; **311**: 919–920.

64. Bergman U, Rosa FW, Baum C, Wiholm BE, Faich GA. Effects of exposure to benzodiazepine during fetal life. *Lancet* 1992; **340**: 694–696.

65. Athinarayanan P, Pierog SH, Nigam SK, Glass L. Chloriazepoxide withdrawal in the neonate. *Am J Obstet Gynecol* 1976; **124**: 212–213.

66. Bacon RC, Razis PA. The effect of propofol sedation in pregnancy on neonatal condition. *Anaesthesia* 1994; **49**: 1058–1060.

67. Fujinaga M, Stevenson JB, Mazze RI. Reproductive and teratogenic effects of fentanyl in Sprague-Dawley rats. *Teratology* 1986; **34**: 51–57.

68. Fujinaga M, Mazze RI, Jackson EC, Baden JM. Reproductive and teratogenic effects of sufentanil and alfentanil in Sprague-Dawley rats. *Anesth Analg* 1988; **67**: 166–169.

69. Fujinaga M, Mazze RI. Teratogenic and postnatal developmental studies of morphine in Sprague-Dawley rats. *Teratology* 1988; **38**: 401–410.

70. Martin LV, Jurand A. The absence of teratogenic effects of some analgesics used in anaesthesia. Additional evidence from a mouse model. *Anaesthesia* 1992; **47**: 473–476.

71. Gagin R, Cohen E, Shavit Y. Prenatal exposure to morphine alters analgesic responses and preference for sweet solutions in adult rats. *Pharmacol Biochem Behav* 1996; **55**: 629–634.

72. Siddiqui A, Haq S, Shah BH. Perinatal exposure to morphine disrupts brain norepinephrine, ovarian cyclicity, and sexual receptivity in rats. *Pharmacol Biochem Behav* 1997; **58**: 243–248.

73. Jurand A. The interference of naloxone hydrochloride in the teratogenic activity of opiates. *Teratology* 1985; **31**: 235–240.

74. Rajegowda BK, Glass L, Evans HE, Maso G, Swartz DP, Leblanc W. Methadone withdrawal in newborn infants. *J Pediatr* 1972; **81**: 532–534.

75. Glass L, Rajegowda BK, Kahn EJ, Floyd MV. Effect of heroin withdrawal on respiratory rate and acid–base

status in the newborn. *N Engl J Med* 1972; **286**: 746–748.

76. Zelson C, Kahn EJ, Neumann L, Polk G. Heroin withdrawal syndrome. *J Pediatr* 1970; **76**: 483–484.

77. Wen YR, Hou WY, Chen YA, Hsieh CY, Sun WZ. Intrathecal morphine for neuropathic pain in a pregnant cancer patient. *J Formos Med Assoc* 1996; **95**: 252–254.

78. Streissguth AP, Treder RP, Barr HM, Shepard TH, Blew WA, Sampson PD, Martin DC. Aspirin and acet-aminophen use by pregnant women and subsequent child IQ and attention decrements. *Teratology* 1987; **35**: 211–219.

79. CLASP Collaborative Group. Low dose aspirin in pregnancy and early childhood development: follow up of the collaborative low dose aspirin study in pregnancy. *Br J Obstet Gynaecol* 1995; **102**: 861–868.

80. Heymann MA. Non steroidal anti-inflammatory agents. In: Eskes TKA, Finister M. *Drug therapy during pregnancy*. London: Butterworths, 1985, p 85.

81. Wright RG, Shnider SM, Fong CJ. Fetal and neonatal effects of maternally administered drugs. In: Shnider SM, Levinson G (eds) *Anesthesia for obstetrics*, 3rd edn. Baltimore: Williams & Wilkins, 1996, pp 709–722.

82. Ostesen M. Optimisation of antirheumatic drug treatment in pregnancy. *Clinical Pharmacokinetics* 1994; **27**: 486–503.

83. Fujinaga M, Baden JM, Mazze RI. Developmental toxicity of nondepolarizing muscle relaxants in cultured rat embryos. *Anesthesiology* 1992; **76**: 999–1003.

84. Skarpa M, Dayan AD, Follenfant M, James DA, Moore WB, Thomson PM, Lucke JN, Morgan M, Lovell R, Medd R. Toxicity testing of atracurium. *Br J Anaesth* 1983; **55**(suppl 1): 27S–29S.

85. Jacobs RM. Failure of muscle relaxants to produce cleft palate in mice. *Teratology* 1971; **4**: 25–30.

86. Meiniel R. Neuromuscular blocking agents and axial teratogenesis in the avian embryo: can axial morphogenetic disorders be explained by pharmacological action upon muscle tissue. *Teratology* 1981; **23**: 259–271.

87. Drachman DB, Coulombre AJ. Experimental club foot and artrogryphosis multiplex congenita. *Lancet* 1962; **ii**: 523–526.

88. Jago RH. Arthrogryposis following treatment of maternal tetanus with muscle relaxants. *Arch Disease in Childhood* 1970; **45**: 227–229.

89. Koren G, Gladstone D, Robeson C, Robieux I. The perception of teratogenic risk of cocaine. *Teratology* 1992; **46**: 567–571.

90. Fujinaga M, Mazze RI. Reproductive and teratogenic effects of lidocaine in Sprague-Dawley rats. *Anesthesiology* 1986; **65**: 626–632.

91. Teiling AKY, Mohammed AK, Monior BG, Jarbe TUC, Hiltunen AJ, Archer T. Lack of effect of prenatal exposure to lidocaine on development of behaviour in rats. *Anesth Anal* 1987; **66**: 533–541.

92. Sidle NR. Anti-emetics in pregnancy. In: Hawkins DF (ed) *Drugs and pregnancy: human teratogenesis and related problems*. Edinburgh: Churchill Livingstone, 1987, pp 115–127.

93. Miklovich L, van den Berg BJ. An evaluation of the teratogenicity of certain antinauseant drugs. *Am J Obstet Gynecol* 1976; **125**: 244–248.

94. Sitland-Marken PA, Rickman LA, Welss BG, Mabie WC. Pharmacologic management of acute mania in pregnancy. *J Clin Psychopharmacol* 1989; **9**: 78–87.

95. Rodier PM, Aschner M, Lewis LS, Koeter HB. Cell proliferation in developing brain after brief exposure to nitrous oxide or halothane. *Anesthesiology* 1986; **64**: 680–687.

96. Sittig M. *Handbook of toxic and hazardous chemicals and carcinogens*. New Jersey: Noyes Publications, 1985.

97. Johnson ES, Colley PS. Effects of nitrous oxide and fentanyl anesthesia on fetal heart rate variability intra- and postoperatively. *Anesthesiology* 1980; **52**: 429–430.

98. Liu PL, Warren TM, Ostheimer GW, Weiss JB, Liu LMP. Foetal monitoring in partrurients under-going surgery unrelated to pregnancy. *Canad Anaesth Soc J* 1985; **32**: 525–532.

99. Reiss RE, Gabbe SG, Pelic RH. Intrapartum fetal evaluation. In: Gabbe SG, Niebyl JR, Simpson JL. *Obstetrics: normal and problem pregnancies*, 3rd edn. Churchill Livingstone 1997, pp 397–424.

100. Kinsella SM, Lohmann G. Supine hypotensive syndrome. *Obstet Gynecol* 1994; **83**: 774–788.

101. Nyberg R, Westin B. The influence of oxygen tension and some drugs on human placental vessels. *Acta Physiol Scand* 1957; **39**: 216–227.

102. Tominaga T, Page EW. Accomodation of the human placenta to hypoxia. *Am J Obstet Gynecol* 1966; **94**: 679–691.

103. Greiss FCJ, Anderson JG, King LC. Uterine vascular bed: effects of acute hypoxia. *Am J Obstet Gynecol* 1972; **113**: 1057–1064.

104. Makowski EL, Hertz RH, Meschia G. Effect of acute maternal hypoxia and hyperoxia on the bloodflow to the pregnant uterus. *Am J Obstet Gynecol* 1973; **115**: 624–629.

105. Edelstone DI. Fetal compensatory responses to reduced oxygen delivery. *Seminars in Perinatology* 1984; **8**: 184–191.

106. Richardson B. Fetal adaptive responses to asphyxia. *Clin Perinatol* 1989; **16**: 595–611.

107. Itskovitz J, LaGamma EF, Rudolph AM. The effect of reducing umbilical bloodflow on fetal oxygenation. *Am J Obstet Gynecol* 1983; **145**: 813–818.

108. Dilts PVJ, Brinkman CRI, Kirschbaum TH, Assali NS. Uterine and systemic interrelationships and the response to hypoxia. *Am J Obstet Gynecol* 1966; **103**: 138–157.

109. Panigel M. Placental perfusion experiments. *Am J Obstet Gynecol* 1962; **84**: 1664–1683.

110. Khazin AF, Hon EH, Hehre FW. Effects of maternal hyperoxia on the fetus. I. Oxygen tension. *Am J Obstet Gynecol* 1971; **109**: 628–637.

111. Iwamoto HS. Cardiovascular effects of acute fetal hypoxia and asphyxia. In: Hanson MA, Spencer JAD, Rodeck CH *Fetus and neonate: physiology and clinical applications*. Cambridge: Cambridge University Press, 1993, pp 197–214.

112. Walker AM, Oakes GK, Ehrenkranz R, McLaughlin M, Chez RA. Effects of hypercapnia on uterine and umbilical circulation in conscious pregnant sheep. *J Appl Physiol* 1976; **41**: 727–733.

113. Motoyama EK, Rivard G, Acheson F, Cook CD. The effect of changes in maternal pH and PCO_2 on the PO_2 of fetal lambs. *Anesthesiology* 1967; **28**: 891–903.

114. Levinson G, Shnider SM, deLorimier AA, Steffenson JL. Effects of maternal hyperventilation on uterine blood-flow and fetal oxygenation and acid-base status. *Anesthesiology* 1974; **40**: 340–347.

115. Bonica JJ. Pain of partruition. *Clinics in Anesthesiology* 1986; **4**: 1–32.

116. Palahniuk RJ, Cumming M. Foetal deterioration following thiopentone-nitrous oxide anaesthesia in the pregnant ewe. *Canad Anaesth Soc J* 1977; **24**: 361–370.

117. Alon E, Ball RH, Gillie MH, Parer JT, Rosen MA, Shnider SM. Effects of propofol and thiopental on maternal and fetal cardiovascular and acid-base variables in the pregnant ewe. *Anesthesiology* 1993; **78**: 562–576.

118. Jouppila P, Kuikka J, Jouppila R, Hollmen A. Effect of induction of general anesthesia for cesarean section on inter-villous bloodflow. *Acta Anaesth Scand* 1979; **58**: 249–253.

119. Warren TM, Datta S, Ostheimer GW, Naulty SJ, Weiss JB, Morrison JA. Comparison of the maternal and neonatal effects of halothane, enflurane and iso-flurane for cesarean delivery. *Anesth Anal* 1983; **62**: 516–520.

120. Levinson G, Shnider SM, Gildea JE, deLorimier AA. Maternal and foetal cardiovascular and acid-base changes during ketamine anaesthesia in pregnant ewes. *Br J Anaesth* 1973; **45**: 1111–1113.

121. Craft JBJ, Coaldrake LA, Yonekura JL, Dao SD, Co EF, Roizen MF, Mazel P, Gilman R, Shokes L, Trevor AJ. Ketamine, catecholamines and uterine tone in pregnant ewes. *Am J Obstet Gynecol* 1983; **146**: 429–434.

122. Oats JN, Vasey DP, Waldron BA. Effects of ketamine on the pregnant uterus. *Br J Anaesth* 1979; **51**: 1163.

123. Downing JW, Buley RJ, Brock-Utne JG, Houlton PC. Etomidate for induction of anaesthesia at caesarean section: comparison with thiopentone. *Br J Anaesth* 1979; **51**: 135–140.

124. Crozier TA, Flamm C, Speer CP, Rath W, Wuttke W, Kuhn W, Kettler D. Effects of etomidate on the adreno-cortical and metabolic adaptation of the neonate. *Br J Anaesth* 1993; **70**: 47–53.

125. Philips AF. Carbohydrate metabolism in the fetus. In: Polin RA, Fox WW (eds) *Fetal and neonatal physiology*. Philadelphia: W.B. Saunders, 1992, pp 373–383.

126. Palahniuk RJ, Shnider SM. Maternal and fetal cardiovascular and acid-base changes during halothane and isoflurane anesthesia in the pregnant ewe. *Anesthesiology* 1974; **41**: 462–472.

127. Patel SS, Goa KL. Sevoflurane. A review of its pharmacodynamic and pharmacokinetic properties and its clinical use in general anaesthesia. *Drugs* 1996; **51**: 658–700.

128. Patel SS, Goa KL. Desflurane. A review of its pharmacodynamic and pharmacokinetic properties and its efficacy in general anaesthesia. *Drugs* 1995; **50**: 742–767.

129. Abboud TK, Zhu J, Richardson M, Peres da Silva E, Donovan M. Desflurane: a new volatile anesthetic for cesarean section. Maternal and neonatal effects. *Acta Anaesthesiol Scand* 1995; **39**: 723–726.

130. Gambling DR, Sharma SK, White PF et al. Use of sevoflurane during elective caesarean birth: a comparison with isoflurane and spinal anaesthesia. *Anesth Anal* 1995; **81**: 90–95.

131. Stein D, Masaoka T, Wlody D, Santos A, Pedersen H, Morishima HO, Finster M. The effects of sevoflurane and isoflurane in pregnant sheep: uterine bloodflow and fetal well-being. *Anesthesiology* 1995; **75**: A851.

132. Wallis KL, Shnider SM, Hicks JS, Spivey HT. Epidural anesthesia in the normotensive pregnant ewe. *Anesthesiology* 1976; **44**: 481–487.

133. Jouppila R, Jouppila P, Kiukka J, Holmen A. Placental bloodflow during caesarean section under lumar extradural analgesia. *Br J Anaesth* 1978; **50**: 275–278.

134. Giles WB, Lah FX, Trudinger BJ. The effect of epidural anaesthesia for caesarean section on maternal uterine and fetal umbilical artery bloodflow velocity waveforms. *Br J Obstet Gynaecol* 1987; **94**: 55–59.

135. Turner GA, Newnham JP, Johnson C, Wwestmore M. Effects of extradural anaesthesia on umbilical and uteroplacental arterial flow velocity waveforms. *Br J Anaesth* 1991; **67**: 306–309.

136. Alahunta S, Rasanen J, Jouppila P, Jouppila R, Westerling P, Hollmen A. The effects of epidural ropivacaine and bupivacaine for cesarean section on uteroplacental and fetal circulation. *Anesthesiology* 1995; **83**: 23–32.

137. Jouppila P, Jouppila R, Barinoff T, Koivula A. Placental bloodflow during caesarean section under subarachnoid blockade. *Br J Anaesth* 1984; **56**: 1379–1382.

138. Baumann H, Alon E, Atanassof P, Pash T, Huch A, Huch R. Effect of epidural anesthesia for cesarean section on maternal femoral arterial and venous, uteroplacental and umbilical bloodflow velocities and waveforms. *Obstet Gynecol* 1990; **75**: 194–198.

139. Jouppila R, Jouppila P, Hollmen A, Kiukka J. Effect of segmental extradural analgesia on placental bloodflow during normal labour. *Br J Anaesth* 1978; **50**: 563–567.

140. Hollmen AI, Jouppila R, Jouppila P, Koivula A, Vierola H. Effect of extradural analgesia using bupivacaine and 2-chlorprocaine on intervillous bloodflow during normal labour. *Br J Anaesth* 1982; **54**: 837–842.

141. Jouppila P, Jouppila R, Hollmen A, Koivula A. Lumbar epidural analgesia to improve intervillous bloodflow during labor in severe preeclampsia. *Obstet Gynecol* 1982; **59**: 158–162.

142. Greiss FCJ. Pressure-flow relationship in the gravid uterine vascular bed. *Am J Obstet Gynecol* 1966; **96**: 41–47.

143. Vincent RDJ, Chestnut DH, Sipes SL, DeBruyn CS, Chatterjee P, Thompson CS. Epidural anesthesia worsens uterine bloodflow and fetal oxygenation during hemorrhage in gravid ewes. *Anesthesiology* 1992; **76**: 799–806.

144. Craft JB, Bolan JC, Coaldrake LA, Mondino M, Mazel P, Gilman RM, Shokes LK, Woolf WA. The maternal and fetal cardiovascular effects of epidural morphine in the sheep model. *Am J Obstet Gynecol* 1982; **142**: 835–839.

145. Craft JBJ, Robichaud AG, Kim H-S, Thorpe DH, Mazel P, Woolf WA, Stolte A. The maternal and fetal cardiovascular effects of epidural fentanyl in the sheep model. *Am J Obstet Gynecol* 1984; **148**: 1098–1104.

146. Vetommen JD, Marcus MA, Van-Aken H. The effects of intravenous and epidural sufentanil in the chronic maternal-fetal sheep preparation. *Anesth Anal* 1995; **80**: 71–75.

147. Fernando R, Bonello E, Gill P, Urquhart J, Reynolds F, Morgan B. Neonatal welfare and placental transfer of fentanyl and bupivacaine during ambulatory combined spinal epidural analgesia for labour. *Anaesthesia* 1997; **52**: 517–524.

148. Loftus JR, Hill H, Cohen SE. Placental transfer and neonatal effects of epidural sufentanil and fentanyl administered with bupivacaine during labor. *Anesthesiology* 1995; **83**: 300–308.

149. Carrie JES, O'Sullivan GM, Seegobin R. Epidural fentanyl in labour. *Anaesthesia* 1981; **36**: 965–969.

150. Shnider SM, Wright RG, Levinson G, Roizen MF, Wallis KL, Rolbin SH, Craft JBJ. Uterine bloodflow and plasma norepinephrine changes during maternal stress in the pregnant ewe. *Anesthesiology* 1979; **50**: 524–527.

151. Lederman RP, Lederman E, Work BA, McCann DS. Anxiety and epinephrine in multiparous labour: relationship to duration of labour and fetal heart rate pattern. *Am J Obstet Gynecol* 1985; **153**: 870–877.

152. Ralston DH, Shnider SM, deLorimier AA. Effects of equipotent ephedrine, metaraminol, mephentermine and methoxamine on uterine bloodflow in the pregnant ewe. *Anesthesiology* 1974; **40**: 354–370.

153. Greiss FCJ, Gobble FLJ. Effect of sympathetic nerve stimulation on the uterine vascular bed. *Am J Obstet Gynecol* 1967; **97**: 962–967.

154. Eng M, Berges PU, Ueland K, Bonica JJ, Parer JT. The effects of methoxamine and ephedrine in normotensive pregnant primates. *Anesthesiology* 1971; **35**: 354–360.

155. James FMI, Greiss FCJ, Kemp RA. An evaluation of vasopressor therapy for maternal hypotension during spinal anesthesia. *Anesthesiology* 1970; **33**: 25–34.

156. Ramanathan S, Grant GJ. Vasopressor therapy for hypotension due to epidural anesthesia for cesarean section. *Acta Anaesthesiol Scand* 1988; **32**: 559–565.

157. Ahokas RA, Mabie WC, Sibai BM, Anderson GB. Labetalol does not decrease placental perfusion in the hypertensive term-pregnant rat. *Am J Obstet Gynecol* 1988; **160**: 480–484.

158. Nylund L, Lunell N-O, Lewander R, Sarby B, Thornstrom S. Labetalol for the treatment of hypertension in pregnancy. *Acta Obstet Gynaecol Scand* 1984; **118**: S71–S73.

159. Joupilla P, Kirkinen P, Koivula A, Ylikorkala O. Labetalol does not alter the placental and fetal bloodflow or maternal prostanoids in pre-eclampsia. *Br J Obstet Gynaecol* 1986; **93**: 543–547.

160. Hudspith MJ, Popham PA. The anaesthetic management of intracranial haemorrhage from arteriovenous malformations in pregnancy: three cases. *Int J Obstet Anesth* 1996; **5**: 189–193.

161. Ring G, Krames E, Shnider SM, Wallis KL, Levinson G. Comparison of hydralazine and nitroprusside in hypertensive pregnant ewes. *Obstet Gynecol* 1977; **50**: 598–602.

162. Bootstaylor BS, Roman C, Parer JT, Heymann MA. Fetal and maternal hemodynamic and metabolic effects of maternal nitroglycerin infusions in sheep. *Am J Obstet Gynecol* 1997; **176**: 644–650.

163. Willoughby JS. Sodium nitroprusside, pregnancy and multiple intracranial aneurysms. *Anaesth Intensive Care* 1984; **12**: 351–357.

164. Donkin Y, Amirav B, Sahar A, Yarkoni S. Sodium nitroprusside for aneurysm surgery in pregnancy. *Br J Anaesth* 1978; **50**: 849–851.

165. Curry SC, Carlton MW, Raschke RA. Prevention of fetal and maternal cyanide toxicity from nitroprusside with coinfusion of sodium thiosulfate in gravid ewes. *Anesth Anal* 1997; **84**: 1121–1126.

166. Larson CP, Jr, Shuer LM, Cohen SE. Maternally administered esmolol decreases fetal as well as maternal heart rate. *J Clin Anesth* 1990; **2**: 427–429.

167. Eisenach JC, Castro MI. Maternally administered esmolol produces fetal beta-adrenergic blockade and hypoxemia in sheep. *Anesthesiology* 1989; **71**: 718–722.

168. Childress CH, Katz VL. Nifedipine and its indications in obstetrics and gynecology. *Obstet Gynecol* 1994; **83**: 616–624.

169. Belfort MA, Saade GR, Moise KJJ, Cruz A, Adam K, Kramer W, Kirshon B. Nimodipine in the management of preeclampsia: maternal and fetal effects. *Am J Obstet Gynecol* 1994; **171**: 417–424.

170. Anthony J, Mantel G, Johanson R, Dommisse J. The haemodynamic and respiratory effects of intravenous

nimodipine used in the treatment of eclampsia. *Br J Obstet Gynaecol* 1996; **103**: 518–522.

171. Blea CW, Barnard JM, Magness RR, Phernetton TM, Hendricks SK. Effect of nifedipine on fetal and maternal hemodynamics and blood gases in the pregnant ewe. *Am J Obstet Gynecol* 1997; **176**: 922–930.

172. Dias MS, Sekhar LN. Intracranial hemorrhage from aneurysms and arteriovenous malformations during pregnancy and the puerperium. *Neurosurgery* 1990; **27**: 855–865.

173. Law JA, Gelb AW. Anaesthetic management of aneurysms and arteriovenous malformations. In: Van Aken H (ed) *Neuroanaesthetic practice*. London: BMJ Publishing group, 1995, pp 193–213.

174. Saunders N, Hammersley B. Magnesium for eclampsia. *Lancet* 1995; **346**: 788–789.

175. Duley L, Carroli G, Belizan J, Gonzalez L, Campodonico L, Bergel E, Taillades P, Ayers S, Wincott L, Gallagher K, Fredrick K, Reynolds J, Adadevoh S, Atallah A, George K, Grant A, Mahomed K, Mehta S, Mmiro F, Moodley J, Neilson J, Sheth S, Walker G, Chalmers I, Collins R et al. Which anticonvulsant for women with eclampsia – evidence from the collaborative eclampsia trial. *Lancet* 1995; **345**: 1455–1463.

176. Dandavino A, Woods JRJ, Murayam L, Brinkman CRI, Assali NS. Circulatory effects of magnesium sulfate in normotensive and renal hypertensive pregnant sheep. *Am J Obstet Gynecol* 1977; **127**: 769–774.

177. Hamilton A, Sirrs S, Schmidt N, Onrot J. Anaesthesia for phaeochromocytoma in pregnancy. *Can J Anaesth* 1997; **44**: 654–657.

178. Pilkington S, Carli F, Dakin MJ, Romney M, De Witt KA, Dore CJ, Cormack RS. Increase in Mallampati score during pregnancy. *Br J Anaesth* 1995; **74**: 638–642.

179. Farcon EL, Kim MH, Marx GF. Changing Mallampati score during labour. *Can J Anaesth* 1994; **41**: 50–51.

180. Capeless EL, Clapp JF. Cardiovascular changes in early phase of pregnancy. *Am J Obstet Gynecol* 1989; **161**: 1449–1453.

181. Hirabayashi Y, Shimizu R, Fukuda H, Saitoh K, Igarashi T. Effects of the pregnant uterus on the extradural venous plexus in the supine and lateral positions, as determined by magnetic resonance imaging. *Br J Anaesth* 1997; **78**: 317–319.

182. Wyner J, Cohen SE. Gastric volume in early pregnancy. *Anesthesiology* 1982; **57**: 209–212.

183. Brock-Utne JG, Dow TGB, Dimopoulos GE, Welman S, Downing JW, Moshal MG. Gastric and lower oesophageal sphincter (LOS) pressures in early pregnancy. *Br J Anaesth* 1981; **53**: 381–384.

184. Gin T, Chan MT. Decreased minimum alveolar concentration of isoflurane in pregnant humans. *Anesthesiology* 1994; **81**: 829–832.

185. Palahniuk RJ, Shnider SM, Eger EII. Pregnancy decreases the requirement for inhaled anesthetic agents. *Anesthesiology* 1974; **41**: 82–83.

186. Strout CD, Nahrwold ML. Halothane requirement during pregnancy and lactation in rats. *Anesthesiology* 1981; **55**: 322–323.

187. Datta S, Migliozzi RP, Flanagan HL, Krieger NR. Chronically administered progesterone decreases halothane requirements in rabbits. *Anesth Analg* 1989; **68**: 46–50.

188. Weizman R, Dagan E, Snyder SH, Gavish M. Impact of pregnancy and lactation on $GABA_A$ receptor and central-type and peripheral-type benzodiazepine receptors. *Brain Research* 1997; **752**: 307–314.

189. Franks NP, Lieb WR. Molecular and cellular mechanisms of general anaesthesia. *Nature (London)* 1994; **367**: 607–614.

190. Gin T, Mainland P, Chan MT, Short TG. Decreased thiopental requirements in early pregnancy. *Anesthesiology* 1997; **86**: 73–78.

191. Khuenl-Brady KS, Koller J, Mair P, Puhringer F, Mitterschiffthaler G. Comparison of vecuronium- and atracurium-induced neuromuscular blockade in postpartum and non-pregnant patients. *Anesth Analg* 1991; **72**: 110–113.

192. Puhringer FK, Sparr HJ, Mitterschiffthaler G, Agoston S, Benzer A. Extended duration of action of rocuronium in postpartum patients. *Anesth Analg* 1997; **84**: 352–354.

193. Leighton BL, Cheek TG, Gross JB et al. Succinylcholine pharmacodynamics in peripartum patients. *Anesthesiology* 1986; **64**: 202–205.

194. Datta S, Lambert DH, Gregus J, Gissen AJ, Covino BG. Differential sensitivities of mammalian nerve fibres during pregnancy. *Anesth Analg* 1983; **62**: 1070–1072.

195. Popitzbergez FA, Leeson S, Thalhammer JG, Strichartz GR. Intraneural lidocaine uptake compared with analgesic differences between pregnant and non-pregnant rats. *Regional Anaesthesia* 1997; **22**: 363–371.

196. Fagraeus L, Urban BJ, Bromage PR. Spread of epidural analgesia in early pregnancy. *Anesthesiology* 1983; **58**: 184–187.

197. Santos AC, Pedersen H, Harmon TW, Morishima HO, Finster M, Arthur GR, Covino BG. Does pregnancy alter the systemic toxicity of local anesthetics. *Anesthesiology* 1989; **70**: 991–995.

198. Santos AC, Arthur GR, Lehning EJ, Finster M. Comparative pharmacokinetics of ropivacaine and bupivacaine in nonpregnant and pregnant ewes. *Anesth Analg* 1997; **85**: 87–93.

199. Santos AC, Arthur GR, Wlody D, De Armas P, Morishima HO, Finster M. Comparative systemic toxicity of ropivacaine and bupivacaine in nonpregnant and pregnant ewes. *Anesthesiology* 1995; **82**: 734–740.

200. Cogan R, Spinnato JA. Pain and discomfort thresholds in late pregnancy. *Pain* 1986; **27**: 63–68.

201. Whipple B, Josimovich JB, Komisaruk BR. Sensory thresholds during the antepartum, intrapartum and post-partum periods. *Int J Nursing Studies* 1990; **27**: 213–221.

202. Iwasaki H, Collins JG, Saito Y, Kerman-Hinds A. Naloxone-sensitive, pregnancy-induced changes in behavioural responses to colorectal distension: pregnancy-induced analgesia to visceral stimulation. *Anesthesiology* 1991; **74**: 927–933.

203. Jarvis S, Mclean KA, Chirnside J, Deans LA, Calvert SK, Molony V, Lawrence AB. Opioid-mediated changes in nociceptive threshold during pregnancy and parturition in the sow. *Pain* 1997; **72**: 153–159.

204. Dawsonbasoa M, Gintzler AR. Involvement of spinal cord delta opiate receptors in the antinociception of gestation and its hormonal simulation. *Brain Research* 1997; **757**: 37–42.

205. Sander HW, Portoghese PS, Gintzler AR. Spinal K-opiate receptor involvment in the analgesia of pregnancy: effects of intrathecal nor-binaltorphimine, a K-selective antagonist. *Brain Research* 1988; **474**: 343–347.

206. Dalby PL, Ramanathan S, Rudy TE, Roy L, Amenta JS, Aber A. Plasma and saliva substance p levels – the effects of acute pain in pregnant and non-pregnant women. *Pain* 1997; **69**: 263–267.

207. Viscomi CM, Bailey PL. Opioid-induced rigidity after intravenous fentanyl. *Obstet Gynecol* 1997; **89**: 822–824.

208. Pomini F, Mercogliano D, Cavalletti C, Caruso A, Pomini P. Cardiopulmonary bypass in pregnancy. *Ann Thorac Surg* 1996; **61**: 259–268.

209. Strickland RA, Oliver WC, Jr, Chantigian RC, Ney JA, Danielson GK. Anesthesia, cardiopulmonary bypass, and the pregnant patient. *Mayo Clin Proc* 1991; **66**: 411–429.

210. Buffolo E, Palma JH, Gomes WJ, Vega H, Born D, Moron AF, Carvalho AC. Successful use of deep hypothermic circulatory arrest in pregnancy. *Ann Thorac Surg* 1994; **58**: 1532–1534.

211. Fair J, Klein AS, Feng T, Merritt WT, Burdick JF. Intrapartum orthotopic liver transplantation with successful outcome of pregnancy. *Transplantation* 1990; **5**: 534–535.

212. Steinberg ES, Santos AC. Surgical Anesthesia during pregnancy. *Int Anesth Clin* 1990; **28**: 58–66.

213. Katz JD, Hook R, Barash PG. Fetal heart rate monitoring in pregnant patients undergoing surgery. *Am J Obstet Gynecol* 1976; **125**: 267–269.

214. Biehl DR. Foetal monitoring during surgery unrelated to pregnancy. *Canad Anaesth Soc J* 1985; **32**: 455–459.

215. Fujinaga M. Anesthetics. In: Kavlock RJ, Daston GP (eds) *Advances in understanding mechanisms of birth defects: mechanistic understanding of human developmental toxicants. Handbook of experimental pharmacology*, Vol 124. Springer Verlag, 1997, pp 295–331.

216. Lanzafame RJ. Laparoscopic cholecystectomy during pregnancy. *Surgery* 1995; **118**: 627–631.

217. Amos JD, Schorr SJ, Norman PF, Poole GV, Thomae KR, Mancino AT, Hall TJ, Scott Conner CE. Laparoscopic surgery during pregnancy. *Am J Surg* 1996; **171**: 435–437.

218. Steinbrook RA, Brooks DC, Datta S. Laparoscopic cholecystectomy during pregnancy. Review of anesthetic management, surgical considerations. *Surg Endosc* 1996; **10**: 511–515.

219. Lemaire BMD, Vanerp WFM. Laparoscopic surgery during pregnancy. *Surgical Endoscopy – Ultrasound & Interventional Techniques* 1997; **11**: 15–18.

220. Reedy MB, Galan HL, Richards WE, Preece CK, Wetter PA, Kuehl TJ. Laparoscopy during pregnancy – a survey of laparoendoscopic surgeons. *J Reprod Med* 1997; **42**: 33–38.

221. Hunter JG, Swanstrom L, Thornburg K. Carbon dioxide pneumoperitoneum induces fetal acidosis in a pregnant ewe model. *Surg Endosc* 1995; **9**: 272–277.

222. Cruz AM, Southerland LC, Duke T, Townsend HG, Ferguson JG, Crone LA. Intraabdominal carbon dioxide insufflation in the pregnant ewe. Uterine blood flow, intraamniotic pressure, and cardiopulmonary effects. *Anesthesiology* 1996; **85**: 1395–1402.

223. Association of Anaesthetists of Great Britain and Ireland. *Recommendations for standards of monitoring during anaesthesia and recovery, revised 1994*. London: Association of Anaesthetist's, 1994.

MIDWIFERY EDUCATION AND THE ANAESTHETIST

John Urquhart

INTRODUCTION

Midwives in training need to be instructed about anaesthesia and analgesia. Information on this subject should, ideally, be given by an obstetric anaesthetist. The qualified midwife has different educational requirements. Although an annual 'epidural lecture' is perceived as an update, it has more significance than this. Firstly, in most centres midwives run the antenatal classes and need to be able to provide up-to-date information about pain relief and even anaesthesia (ideally women should also receive this information from an obstetric anaesthetist). Secondly, with access to the media and Internet, women are increasingly aware of what is new and all midwives should be informed of new techniques, even if they are not available locally. Finally, in most centres it is the midwife who assists the insertion of regional analgesia, and to whom maintenance of that analgesia is delegated.

MIDWIFERY TRAINING

CERTIFICATE, DIPLOMA AND DEGREE

Midwifery education has changed markedly over the past 20 years. Most maternity units are likely to employ midwives with a variety of training, (and/or those who have been trained overseas). In the UK, senior staff are likely to have qualified at certificate level, as State Certified Midwifes (SCM). This training was of 1 year or, latterly, 18 months duration, and entry was from State Registered Nurse (SRN) or Registered General Nurse (RGN). A few midwives were trained as 'direct entrants' with no previous nursing qualification and undertook a 3-year training period.

In 1990, a number of changes occurred within nursing and allied professions. The United Kingdom Central Council for Nursing, Midwifery and Health Visiting (UKCC) superseded the various bodies previously responsible for the registration of each type of professional and the term Registered Midwife (RM) replaced SCM. Seven hospitals in England and Wales were selected to develop training of midwives to Diploma level. Significantly, entry to training no longer requires previous nursing qualifications; applicants must be at least 17 years and 6 months of age, (exceptionally, 17 years), and have a minimum of five subjects to grade A, B or C at General Certificate of School Education (GCSE) level, including English and a science subject. The course lasts 3 years leading to the award of Diploma of Health Education (Dip HE) in midwifery.

Midwives with this diploma can now study for a Degree (BSc) in midwifery. It is envisaged that in the future, all training in midwifery will be to Degree level. Training is organized on a module system. One module involves one half-day session of study per week over a 12-week period, and results in the award of 20 credits. For midwives at RM level, progression to the award of Dip HE would require the accumulation of 240 credits, with some recognition (typically 120 credits) for existing training and experience. Progression to BSc entails the accumulation of 360 credits.

ANAESTHETIC TRAINING

At the University College Suffolk, the amount of time devoted to training in anaesthesia and analgesia within the syllabus amounts to several sessions throughout the 3-year period. These are organized by midwifery tutors with the involvement of anaesthetic staff. Practical experience is limited to observation on labour ward and in theatre, although there are opportunities for assisting the anaesthetist on labour ward under certain supervised circumstances.

Continuing education for post-registration midwives

Since 1995 the UKCC has required midwives and nurses to complete 5 days of study during each 3-year registration period. The individual practitioner decides the subject and content. It is recommended that subjects should be taken from five broad categories:

- patient, client and colleague support;
- care enhancement;
- practice development;
- reducing risk;
- education development.

The midwife's Professional Portfolio is a record of continuing education and is subject to scrutiny by the UKCC at 3-yearly intervals, analogous to the anaesthetist's record of continuing medical education in the UK.

In addition, it is a statutory requirement that midwives 'refresh their midwifery knowledge' every 5 years. This can be done by attending an English Nursing Board (ENB) approved 5-day refresher course, other modules or courses approved by the ENB or by attending 7 assorted study days. The institutions providing these study days must either be approved by the ENB or given approval by a Supervisor of Midwives. This statutory requirement was superceded in 2001.

A midwife, who had not practised as a midwife for at least the equivalent of 12 working weeks during the preceding 5 years, was required to complete an approved course of a minimum period of 4 weeks before she could notify her intention to practice. From 1 April 2000 this was extended to nurses, and the period of time increased to 750 h or 100 working days.

WHAT PAIN RELIEF ARE MIDWIVES ALLOWED TO ADMINISTER?

The guidance for administration of medicines and other forms of pain relief[1] state *'A practising midwife shall not on her own responsibility administer any medicine, including analgesics unless in the course of her training, whether before or after her registration as a midwife, she has been thoroughly instructed in its use and is familiar with its dosage and methods of administration and application'*. An anaesthetist envisaging the setting up of an epidural service where none previously existed, or adapting an existing service by, for example, the introduction of a 'walking epidural' service, will therefore have to incorporate a training program for midwifery staff in the plans. Once instruction has been provided, the midwife is empowered to administer analgesia after prescription by a medical practitioner, or to follow the protocols laid down within an institution. Indeed, Section 16 of The Midwife's Code of Practice refers to Rule 40[2] and states that *'... mutual respect should enhance care and practice must be based upon agreed standards to ensure effective communication and co-operation in care'*.

Midwives may administer epidural top-ups and replace infusions for epidural analgesia as long as such instruction has been provided; and also, that in observing the spirit of Rule 40, midwives should attend to epidurals in accordance with instructions provided by anaesthetists, whether written as individual prescriptions or institutional protocols.

It is also worth noting that nowhere does it state that midwives may not, for example, administer infusions or top-ups containing opioids. Rule 41 continues to emphasize the importance of adherence to The Misuse of Drugs Regulations 1985 and the Medicines Act 1968, and states that *'The administration of controlled drugs by a midwife working in a hospital should be in accordance with locally agreed policies and procedures'*.

THE IMPORTANCE OF INFORMED MATERNAL CHOICE ON PAIN RELIEF IN LABOUR

Within the past decade government publications have stressed the importance of giving women clear, unambiguous information about different methods of pain relief available in labour. It was notable that there was no anaesthetic representation on the authorship of either 'Changing Childbirth'[3,4] or the Audit Commission report, *First Class Delivery*.[5] Both documents were received with much interest by both decision-makers and consumers. What is the appropriate source of information for women to enable to make them informed choices about pain relief in labour? It has been argued that the appropriate individual to discuss analgesia in parentcraft classes is the obstetric anaesthetist.[6] Experience has shown that it is helpful to have an anaesthetic run antenatal class on pain relief. Questions can be answered well in advance of the onset of pain, and misconceptions about regional analgesia, and its complications such as paralysis and nerve damage, can be resolved. Involvement of obstetric anaesthetists has however been associated with an increase in the uptake of anaesthetic services, which has associated resource implications.

In most centres, however, this information comes from a midwife. In rural communities parentcraft is often locally provided, in the main by community midwives. The importance of these midwives being informed of current practice in anaesthesia is clear and consistency of information is important.

PRACTICAL CONDUCT OF MIDWIFERY EDUCATION

A regular time should be allocated for teaching, when a consultant anaesthetist is available. Interest will soon diminish if lectures are cancelled at short notice. It is important to include all midwifery staff and where a permanent night shift is in operation evening teaching sessions should be arranged. The support of the Head of Midwifery in setting up such a teaching programme, in advertising the teaching and in making staff available to attend, is invaluable. A record of attendance is useful, and can form the basis of a record of those midwives accredited in managing epidural analgesia in labour.

An informal setting is appropriate, and a comprehensive 'handout' is appreciated and discourages frantic note taking during the talk. Props such as regional analgesia packs of the type used locally and a plastic model of the lumbar spine are useful.

CONTENT OF PAIN-RELIEF LECTURE

Anne May in Leicester has written concisely[7] on the syllabus for post-registration midwives. It is the author's practice to stress the concept of partnership between anaesthetist and midwife in the management of pain in labour. It is important to make clear that it must be the *mother* who decides the type of analgesia, a decision made in conjunction with her attendants. This provides an opportunity to emphasize the point that this decision must be made in the context of *all* the information available, which must be presented in as impartial and fair way as possible.

PAIN PATHWAYS AND NON-REGIONAL METHODS OF PAIN RELIEF

The segmental nature of the pathways in the first stage and second stages of labour is a good starting point. A contrast needs to be drawn between the type of nerve fibres involved. A description of the differing vulnerability of nerve fibres to local anaesthetics (LAs) can be used as part of the explanation of how analgesia can be produced without the numbness and paralysis still expected by not only a proportion of parturients, but their midwives as well. At this juncture, it is possible to describe other forms of pain relief and the point in the pain pathway where they have their effect.

ANATOMY

The anatomy of the epidural space and its boundaries, and the difference between epidural, and spinal compartments should be discussed (Fig. 19.1).

MECHANISM OF ACTION OF EPIDURAL ANALGESIA

An explanation of the mechanism of action of epidural analgesia can be enhanced using epidurograms to explain phenomena such as unilateral blockade and failed block. The distinction between epidural and spinal anaesthesia should emphasize the different doses of LA required in each case, which in turn may be used to explain inadvertent spinal block and total spinal. The relative safety of low-dose top-ups (10–12.5 mg bupivacaine with fentanyl) is illustrated by the study by Cox et al.[8] These authors deliberately injected 10 ml of 0.1% bupivacaine with fentanyl into the intrathecal spaces of a group of women having elective Caesarean section. None developed a dangerously high block.

VENOUS CANNULATION

This is a skill which midwifery staff need to acquire for independent, community-based practice. Practical training should start with practice on one of the many suitable training mannequins available.

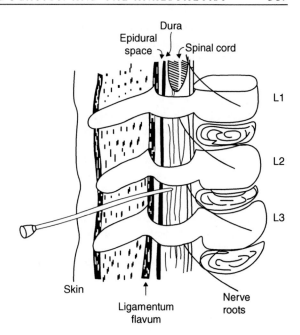

Figure 19.1   Anatomy for epidural and spinal placement.

Midwives need instruction on the use of local infiltration prior to cannula insertion. Choice of cannulation site should be discussed, with emphasis on choosing a convenient, comfortable and reliable site.

ASSISTANCE AT EPIDURAL INSERTION

Initial instruction should have been possible at the pre-registration stage. The key points to emphasize can be grouped under 'preparation for epidural insertion', and 'assistance during the procedure'.

Midwives must be aware of any investigations required prior to regional blockade, especially the mother with pre-eclampsia or one who has been on an anticoagulant.

What should be stocked on the 'epidural' trolley should be listed. The purpose of each piece of equipment should be explained. It must be emphasized that the process of epidural insertion must be under strictly sterile conditions.

COMPLICATIONS

Each complication should be discussed in relation to incidence, recognition and management:

- The high-dense block that will follow inadvertent intrathecal injection of 'low-dose' top-up (10–12 mg bupivacaine) should be described. A clear distinction needs to be made between this situation and the misplacement of an epidural bolus intended to create anaesthesia for operative delivery. The latter is clearly the responsibility of the attending anaesthetist.

- Inadvertent intravenous administration of a labour epidural top-up may elicit symptoms of dizziness and circumoral paraesthesia but cardiovascular sequelae should not occur with low-dose top-ups.
- The subject of hypotension following epidural administration needs to be discussed along with the relative safety of the use of ephedrine to prevent or control the situation. It must be explained that placental hypoperfusion resulting in fetal bradycardia can occur despite normal maternal blood pressure. The need for careful positioning to avoid any aorto-caval compression should be reiterated.

Although the fact that deranged coagulation is a recognized contraindication to regional analgesia, the rarity of neurological sequelae attributable to anaesthesia (at 1:13 000 maternities)[9] should be a reassurance. Nevertheless, the concept of the spinal haematoma, its cause, recognition and management need explanation. Peripheral neuropathy associated with difficult child-birth is relatively common (1 in 1–2000) and it is useful to discuss this. The characteristics of post-dural puncture headache (PDPH) and the management must be explained.

Recovery of post-operative mothers

Little time in the syllabus is devoted to instruction on post-operative recovery.

This is of particular concern in complicated cases and when general anaesthesia is used. The guidelines for recovery of non-obstetric cases should be described and adhered to.

Resuscitation

Resuscitation of the pregnant woman is an important issue and can be taught by the obstetric anaesthetist.

CONCLUSION

Provision of high-quality epidural analgesia for women in labour is dependent on co-operation between anaesthetists, midwives and obstetricians. Regular but informal instruction by senior anaesthetic staff can help to enhance the quality of analgesia as well as improving the efficiency of the service.

APPENDIX: NOTES FOR MIDWIVES

These are the notes used by the author for midwifery education and may be reproduced.

PHYSIOLOGY OF PAIN IN LABOUR

In the first stage of labour, pain comes from uterine contractions and from cervical dilatation. The uterus is innervated by nerves that enter the spinal cord at thoracic (T)10, T11, T12 and lumbar (L)1. Nerves from the abdominal wall immediately above and below the umbilicus enter at the same levels, which allows for testing of the spread of block by testing loss of sensation over the skin there. In the second stage, in addition to this, the pain is transmitted from the perineum, to nerves entering the spinal cord at sacral (S)2, S3 and S4.

The pain message can be interrupted at a number of sites:

- locally, in the wall of the uterus, or on the perineum, by infiltration;
- at the level of the spinal nerve peripherally, for example, by pudendal block;
- at the nerve root, where the nerve emerges from the spinal cord, by an epidural block;
- at the spinal nerve within the cerebro-spinal fluid (CSF), by a spinal block;
- within the spinal cord, and within the brain, with opiates; or
- on the cerebral cortex, by a general anaesthetic.

The mixed spinal nerve

This consists of motor and autonomic (sympathetic) as well as sensory fibres. The latter include fibres that relay other types of sensation in addition to pain, but it is necessary to know about the different types and their sizes to understand how LAs, for example, work.

LAs block small fibres before large ones. Thus in order to block both types of pain fibres – both the C and the Aδ, the pre-ganglionic fibres will also be blocked, hence the inevitability of some sympathetic block. The action of sympathetic nerves is to provide tone to peripheral blood vessels. In the presence of a sympathetic block, the blood vessels will dilate, and the blood pressure may drop as a result.

Motor block can be minimized by keeping the dose as low as possible. If, however, the pain fibres are embedded in the core of a large nerve root, the dose of LA may have to be increased for an effective concentration to reach those fibres leading to unwanted motor block.

Class	Function	Size (μm diameter)	Velocity (m/s)
Aα	Somatic motor	12–20	70–120
Aβ	Touch, pressure, proprioception	5–12	30–70
Aγ	Spindle afferents	3–6	15–30
Aδ	Sharp pain	2–5	12–30
B	Pre-ganglionic autonomic	<3	3–15
C	Dull pain, temperature	0.4–1.2	0.5–2.0

Central pathways

The pain signals become messages at the cerebral cortex.

Once the C pain fibres enter the spinal cord, they synapse in the area of the spinal cord known as the dorsal horn. Within the dorsal horn there is an area called the substantia gelatinosa. From here fibres ascend in the spinothalamic tract to the thalamus and then to the cerebral cortex, which is where the pain is imposed on the consciousness.

Within the spinal cord there are large molecules on the surface of nerve cells that, if stimulated appropriately, affect the performance of the cell. This may be with the effect of enhancing the electrical activity of the cell, so that more messages are passed, or the opposite. These large molecules are receptors, and those of one type, found on cells especially in the substantia gelatinosa and in the thalamus, are called opiate receptors. They cause a reduction in the messages being sent to the cortex. There are a number of sub-types of opiate receptor, the most relevant for this discussion being the μ-receptor.

The natural ligand (stimulant) for the μ-type of opiate receptor is β-endorphin, which is both a neurotransmitter, acting locally, and a neurohormone, being blood-borne and affecting sites all over the body. It is a natural painkiller, and drugs such as morphine, pethidine and fentanyl have similar chemical structures to β-endorphin and so act in the same way, by binding to μ-receptors on cells in the substantia gelatinosa and thalamus, and reducing the ability of those cells to transmit pain messages.

By giving an opioid intrathecally or epidurally the drug is delivered very close to the site of action. The advantages of doing so are twofold. Firstly, the effective dose required is greatly reduced compared with that if given systemically (intravenously or intramuscularly). Secondly, because only a small proportion of this small dose will reach the blood stream, side effects in the mother and fetal exposure are reduced. Side effects include reduced gastrointestinal motility with nausea and vomiting, and respiratory depression.

Descending pathways

There are nerves that descend to the substantia gelatinosa and other parts of the dorsal horn from higher up the central nervous system (CNS) that modify the way the cells operate, rather as opiates do. Such pathways are activated by cerebral activity. This means the individual is distracted from the pain, or, paradoxically, by pain itself. The 'Gate' theory describes this; in the normal situation, pain is transmitted in C fibres in the way described above. Other fibres can reduce the C-fibre transmission as if closing a 'gate' although, obviously, there is no mechanical closure involved.

A combination approach: LAs and opiates

The use of LAs alone will certainly provide analgesia by affecting pain transmission but to get complete relief the amount of LA used will affect motor fibres as well, which is undesirable. If opiates are used alone, again, to get complete analgesia the amount of pethidine or morphine used will cause maternal respiratory depression, nausea, and neonatal depression. If, however, a low dose of LA is used, a partial block will be achieved, which can be completed by a low dose of opiate; so that neither will the LA cause a motor block, nor the opiate any significant side effect. The LA and the opiate acting at different sites, the LA to reduce nerve conduction, and the opiate at the dorsal horn to reduce onward transmission of any pain messages that get past the LA.

METHODS OF PROVIDING PAIN RELIEF IN LABOUR

Transcutaneous electrical nerve stimulation

This works by means of the gate theory described above and is often perfectly adequate for mothers in early and sometimes advanced labour. Electrodes are placed on dermatomes corresponding to the source of pain, (the uterus); T10–L1. Low-frequency high-amplitude stimulation of the Aβ fibres 'closes the gate', thus reducing transmission of pain.

Inhalation methods

These operate at a cortical and thalamic level, and affect conscious level. The effect is, however, very transient but inhaled agents will reach the fetus. At present, the only widely used inhalation agent is Entonox, which is 50% nitrous oxide in oxygen. The cylinders are blue with blue and white shoulders and are available in sizes D (500 l) F (2000 l) and G (5000 l). Delivery is from a demand valve operated by maternal inspiration. Only about 50% of mothers who use Entonox derive adequate analgesia. There are two problems. Firstly, the use of the valve requires some teaching, and must be co-ordinated with the beginning of the contraction since the analgesic effect takes 45 s to be maximal. Secondly, there is a tendency to hyperventilate, which can reduce oxygen delivery to the fetus.

Intramuscular opiates

When administering controlled drugs in the National Health Service, midwives should comply with locally agreed policies and procedures. This will usually permit the administration of intramuscular pethidine up to 150 mg. The major objections to the use of pethidine are that it is sedative rather than analgesic, it accumulates in the fetus and causes neonatal respiratory depression. Metabolites of pethidine may be detected in the neonate for a prolonged period post-delivery.

Regional analgesia

This is the most effective means of providing analgesia and is safe for the fetus. In pre-eclampsia it can help control of blood pressure. Also in multiple births regional block enables the second twin to be delivered in better condition. Its use in complicated cases can reduce the need for general anaesthesia.

There are only three situations when a regional technique must never be used. These are maternal refusal, bleeding disorder and known allergy to one the drugs. Sepsis, hypovolaemia and urgency of delivery are all relative contraindications. Neither aspirin nor back surgery are contraindications.

Onset of regional blockade

The sacral segments are the last to be blocked. This is significant and is often the explanation for the so-called 'missed segment' and for second stage pain when the epidural has been allowed to wear off. The use of an opiate such as fentanyl will often retrieve this situation.

When testing a block it is the reduction or absence of ice sensation which is the blockade of C fibres that is the most useful to note for labour analgesia. Confirmation of a well spread block from T10 to the

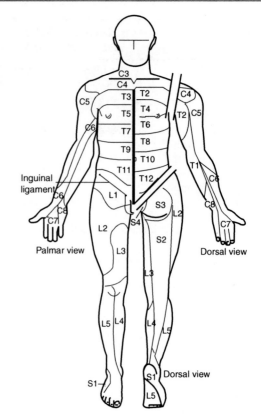

Figure 19.2   Dermatomes for assessment of a region block.

sacral roots should be recorded with reference to a dermatome map (Fig. 19.2).

Complications of regional blockade

Early
- Failure, including one-sided blocks. Incidence approximately 5%. Low threshold for resisting.
- Dural tap. Incidence approximately 0.5–1%. Blood patch is the definitive treatment for PDPH. Rest and epidural infusion just delay onset. Avoidance of pushing makes no difference.
- Total spinal, respiratory failure, aspiration. Recognition and rapid management with intubation, assisted ventilation and vasopressors.
- Inadvertent intravenous injection with cardiovascular toxicity. The cardiac collapse (CC) to CNS toxicity (CC/CNS) ratio dictates the relative safety of different agents; it is 7:1 for lidocaine but only 3:1 for bupivacaine. The treatment of LA-induced arrhythmia is bretylium, 7 mg/kg.
- Anaphylaxis: very rare.
- Sympathetic block, shivering, and pruritis.

Late

- *Neurological: cord compression or ischaemia.* Epidural haematoma is very rare and can occur in the absence of a regional block. Inappropriate motor block, which is dense or prolonged, is an ominous sign. It is a neurosurgical emergency. Cord ischaemia is more usually a complication of epidurals in the elderly, rather than the young.
- *Neurological: single nerve palsies.* These are often indistinguishable from those caused by obstetric trauma.
- *Bladder dysfunction:* retention of urine and bladder dystonia. Great care must be taken to ensure that over distension does not occur.
- *Backache:* this is a frequent complication of pregnancy and the puerpurium whether or not regional analgesia is used. Local discomfort from the puncture site needs to be explained beforehand to the mother and is self-limiting.

Fetal

- *Instrumental delivery:* In the first series of epidurals for labour, in the 1960s, there was a 90% instrumental delivery. The technique used large volumes of high-concentration LA and inevitably produced a dense motor block. Modern techniques minimize motor block. The nature of the association between this mode of delivery and regional analgesia is not known for certain: 'impact studies' which look prospectively at the effect of introducing regional analgesia services *de novo* suggest that regional analgesia is not necessarily associated with a greater incidence of instrumental deliveries.
- *Prolongation of the second stage:* Most centres do allow a longer second stage in women with regional analgesia to give time for the head to descend. There remains controversy over the risk benefit ratio how long this period should be.

- *Maternal core temperature and/or intra-uterine temperature:* may be increased in women receiving traditional, high-dose regional analgesia in labour. This may result in fetal tachycardia. Whether this is indicative of any adverse effect to the fetus is not known but there are concerns that it might result in needless investigations. There is a reduced risk of hyperthermia with low-dose epidurals.

REFERENCES

1. Midwives Rules, 1993.

2. The Midwife's Code of Practice, 1994.

3. Anderson MM, Court S, Farmer P et al. In: Cumberledge J (ed) *Changing Childbirth: Part 1: Report of the Expert Maternity Group.* London: HMSO, Department of Health, 1993, 1. Changing Childbirth. 0-11-321623-8.

4. Rolf L, MacFarlane L, Farrall M, Lee N. In: Cumberledge J (ed) *Changing Childbirth: Part 2: Survey of Good Communications Practice in Maternity Services.* London: HMSO, Department of Health, 1993, 2. Changing Childbirth. 0-11-321623-8.

5. Audit Commission. *First Class Delivery: Improving Maternity Services in England and Wales.* London: Audit Commission, 1997.

6. Urquhart JC. Ethics in obstetric anaesthesia. *Anaesthesia* 1996; **51**: 1183.

7. May AE. *Epidurals for Childbirth*, vol. 1. Oxford: Oxford University Press, 1994, p 1, 0-19-262438-5.

8. Cox M, Lawton G, Morgan BM. Let us re-examine the safety of midwife top-ups. *Anaesthesia* 1995; **50**: 570.

9. Holdcroft A, Gibberd FB, Hargrove RL, Hawkins DF, Dellaportas CI. Neurological complications associated with pregnancy. *Br J Anaesth* 1995; **75**: 522–526.

Index

Lightning Source UK Ltd.
Milton Keynes UK
24 March 2011

169798UK00001B/58/P